To C

enjoy

his halo.

Homoeopathic
Psychiatry

Understanding the use and meaning of the *Delusion* rubrics in Case Analysis

Liz Lalor

BJAIN archibel

B. Jain Archibel s.p.r.l.

Rue Fontaine St. Pierre 1E, Zoning Industriel de la Fagne,
5330 Assesse, Belgium, Europe

HOMOEOPATHIC PSYCHIATRY

First Edition: 2011
1st Impression: 2011

Published by Kuldeep Jain for
B. JAIN ARCHIBEL S.P.R.L.
Rue Fontaine St. Pierre 1E, Zoning Industriel de la Fagne,
5330 Assesse, Belgium Europe
Tel.: +32 8266 55 00 • *Fax:* +32 83 65 62 82
Email: info@bjain.com • *Website:* **www.bjain.com**

B. JAIN PUBLISHERS (P) LTD.
An ISO 9001 : 2000 Certified Company
1921/10, Chuna Mandi, Paharganj, New Delhi 110 055 (INDIA)
Tel.: +91-11-4567 1000 • *Fax:* +91-11-4567 1010
Email: info@bjain.com • *Website:* **www.bjain.com**

Printed in India by
J.J. Offset Printers

ISBN: 978-2-87491-016-6

Foreword

Most recently, a young Belgian homeopath asked me how to get more out of the Repertory. I suggested she slowly read through the *Delusion* rubrics; making sure to understand each one. It is this insight which makes me very happy to endorse this enormous work of Liz Lalor.

The *Delusion* rubrics are treasures which need to be unlocked. Some homeopaths dismiss them altogether as delusions which are too difficult to understand, or too difficult to rely upon. Liz Lalor has come up with a most interesting concept to not only understand these critical rubrics but to effectively use them in practice.

I am proud that she prefers using our team's work to do so. When editing the repertory, we have spent much time to remain faithful to the source texts. These efforts are complementary to the wisdom and work, generously explained in Liz's book. I trust that the reader of "Homeopathic Psychiatry" will find the repertory to be an even more accurate tool.

Dr Frederik Schroyens
Gent, October 26, 2010

Foreword

Most recently a young Belgian homeopath asked me how to get more out of the Repertory. I suggested she slowly read through the Delusion rubrics, making sure to understand each one. It is this insight which makes me very happy to endorse this enormous work of Liz Lalor.

The Delusion rubrics are treasures which need to be unlocked. Some homeopaths dismiss them altogether as delusions which are too difficult to understand or too difficult to rely upon. Liz Lalor has come up with a most interesting concept to not only understand these crucial rubrics but to effectively use them in practice.

I am proud that she prefers using our team's work to do so. When editing the repertory, we have spent much time to remain faithful to the source texts. These efforts are complementary to the wisdom and work, generously explained in Liz's book. I trust that the reader of "Homeopathic Psychiatry" will find the repertory to be an even more accurate tool.

Dr Frederik Schroyens
Gent October 26, 2010

Contents

What is Homoeopathic Psychiatry?

Homoeopathic psychiatry is the psychoanalytical study of the meaning and application of the *Delusion* rubric in homoeopathic case-taking and case analysis.

A delusion is an illusion which misrepresents the truth. Psychology is the science that deals with emotional and mental processes and behaviors. A psychological delusion[1] is a perception or opinion which is exaggerated or disproportionate to reality. In psychiatry, a 'delusion of grandeur' is viewed as a symptom of mental illness and is applied to the patient who is displaying hallucinatory exaggeration of their personality or status. For example: *he suffers from the delusion he is a great singer*. In psychiatry, the patient's psychological delusion is treated because it indicates an abnormality or illness in the affected person's thought processes. In both modalities – psychiatry and homoeopathy – the psychological delusion exists, and is diagnosed (in the case analysis) because the patient needs to avoid reality.

In homoeopathy, the psychological delusion is viewed as an exaggeration of personality status which indicates an abnormality or an illness. The *Mind* section of the repertory contains the *Delusion* rubrics. These are the rubrics which are applicable in the case analysis if the patient displays psychological delusions. The rubrics in the repertory[2] which resonate with a conflict matching the psychological delusions can only be *Delusion* rubrics because these rubrics indicate an abnormality or illness in the affected person's thought processes. A *Delusion* rubric applies to the case analysis when a patient misrepresents and misinterprets reality in a disproportionate way consistent with the psychiatric definition of a psychological delusion.

In the application of a *Delusion* rubric (in case-taking) the homoeopath seeks to understand why the patient has set up the delusional state and why they need to maintain the misrepresentation of reality. This understanding in homoeopathic case analysis is an integral part of case-taking which will indicate the simillimum in the case. In a psychiatric consultation, the psychoanalyst also seeks to understand the need behind why the patient has created the psychological delusion to avoid reality. In both modalities – psychiatry and homoeopathy – the psychological delusion is recognized as being injurious to health and recognized as the first indicator of potential illness across all levels – the emotional, mental and physical. That is where the similarity between the two modalities end.

The treatment of the patient in homoeopathy is based on the cure from the simillimum. The psychotherapeutic understanding of the patient's need for the psychological delusion is the indicator of, and explanation for, the simillimum.

For example, to continue the delusion of being a great singer: the patient will say, *I am a great singer. I have the most spectacularly beautiful baritone voice of all time, but it has not been recognized by the world. I have not been able to sing for the last ten years that is why I need you to treat me with homoeopathic remedies. The reason I am not able to sing so well at the moment is that I am suffering from an allergy to the tree outside my flat. In fact this tree is causing me such weakness that it has made me feel incredibly vulnerable. I have suffered terribly from these allergies. This tree has caused me to be rejected by all the music academies, they have deliberately not recognized the beauty in my voice.* In homoeopathic case analysis this case would be analysed using the following *Delusion* rubrics.

- *Delusion* rubric: *beautiful*: *Sulph*.
- *Delusion* rubric: *persecuted; he is persecuted*: *Sulph*.
- *Delusion* rubric: *poisoned; he; has been*: sulph.

In both modalities – psychiatry and homoeopathy – this patient would be seen to be suffering 'delusions of grandeur'. The psychological delusion has been maintained and created to avoid the reality that his voice is not as incredible as he thinks it is. The psychological delusion is also the cause behind his need to create or manifest his allergy to the tree outside his flat. This case analysis is a typical rubric-repertorisation which would be applicable to the remedy picture of *Sulphur*. His 'delusions of grandeur' have led to him exaggerating his allergy reaction or potentially manifesting his allergy in the first place. His physical weakness is needed to explain why he has been unable to move out of his flat. If he becomes physically well he will have to face the reality that his voice is not good enough to be recognized by the opera houses of the world. It is to his advantage to maintain the psychological delusion that the tree is the cause of his failure to be recognized. His psychological 'delusions of persecution' are to his advantage because they help maintain and protect his 'delusions of grandeur'.

Homoeopathic psychiatry is the study of the psychotherapeutic application of the *need* for the psychological delusions within each of the constitutional remedy profiles.

Sulphur[3] has a psychotherapeutic need to avoid personal responsibility for failure which manifests as an intense psychological need to delude themselves into believing they are great. This *Sulphur* patient has developed, and stayed in, the mental and physical disability of the allergy to avoid the emotional reality that his voice is not as beautiful as he thinks.

My purpose in writing *Homeopathic Psychiatry* is to use my thirty years of experience in counselling patients to offer insights into the psychological meaning of the *Delusion* rubrics and into the psychodynamic illusions of the mind that each patient reveals within their disease state and their psyche. *Homeopathic Psychiatry* explores the application and meaning of the *Delusion* rubrics in case-repertorisation. The ability to find the simillimum is based on *exacting* listening, and understanding the true psychiatric meaning of the *Delusion* rubrics. For too long in homoeopathy we have held on to a literal and limited psychological understanding of the *Delusion* rubrics.

In the first section: **What is Homoeopathic Psychiatry?** I define the psychotherapeutic role that the *Delusion* rubrics have in case-taking, and outline four necessary requirements for the *use* of the *Delusion* rubrics in a patient's case analysis.

In the **Rubric-categories** I outline the psychodynamic application of the *Delusion* rubrics in case-development. I have identified five stages that a patient will progress through in case-taking. I have formulated these stages into a psychotherapeutic model which follows the psychological steps that the patient will move through in a homoeopathic consultation as they struggle to acknowledge, or resign themselves to, their loss of good health. I use these stages to group the rubrics accordingly. The rubric-categories match the psychological delusions and the psychological stages which all patients manifest in an illness.

Recognizing the psychological stages will assist in finding the simillimum because it allows you to narrow down the remedies being considered in case-taking to the remedies listed in those particular rubric-categories.

In the **Rubric-categories** I take the most commonly used *Delusion* rubrics that I have found in my practice, group them according to the five rubric headings and explain their delusional use.

In analyzing and explaining the meaning of each individual *Delusion* rubric, I offer previously unexplored explanations of the psychological delusional state inherent in each *Delusion* rubric.

Furthermore, I explain their psychotherapeutic meaning and application by analyzing how each remedy listed under the rubric heading has utilized the delusional stance to its advantage. The reasons why each constitutional remedy is listed under a rubric will often be vastly different. Understanding the need for the psychological delusions within each of the constitutional remedy profiles will aid in remedy recognition.

In the **Case Companion to Homoeopathic Psychiatry** I present several cases from my practice. In the case analysis I explain why the patient has set up the delusional state and why they need to maintain the misrepresentation of reality. In the cases presented I identify the *Delusion* rubrics and explain how the patient has used the psychological delusion to construct and to maintain their disease state. In each case analysis, I unravel the significant events in the patient's life and repertorise each poignant emotional event to give an explanation of the causation within the case and an explanation of the rubric-repertorisation which justifies the use of the *Delusion* rubrics. As in the above example of the *Sulphur* case, this analysis of the *Delusion* rubrics aims to give insight into the psychological modeling of why a patient has chosen to concoct a complicated system of excuses to justify their psychological delusions which help formulate their existing pathology.

The Four Requirements of a *Delusion* Rubric

In this section I define the psychotherapeutic role that the *Delusion* rubrics have in case-taking and outline four necessary prerequisites for the *use* of the *Delusion* rubrics in a patient's case analysis and not just the *Mind* rubrics.

You can only use a *Delusion* rubric in the case analysis if the following four prerequisites have been noted in the patient's case-development.

1. Evidence that the patient has notable inner conflict and evidence of self-destruction and pathology which is proof of the need for a *Delusion* rubric to be used in the rubric-repertorisation.

2. Evidence that the patient has used the psychological delusion in a disproportionate way to misinterpret reality.

3. Evidence that the delusional stance is maintained by the patient because it is to their advantage to delude themselves of reality.

4. The 'never-well-since-event' confirming the primary psychodynamic trauma.

1. Evidence that the Patient has Notable Inner Conflict and Self-destruction

The patient must display destructive evidence of dispropor-tionate disturbance which will often be the primary source of present or future pathologies. The first prerequisite emphasizes that all pathology has its foundation in delusional disturbance.

This is acknowledged in the modalities of psychiatry and homoeopathy.

The homoeopath must be able to identify destructive pathology in either the emotional, mental, or physical. The rubrics that point to the correct remedy to cure all the destructive pathologies that I have treated in my homoeopathic practice are found within the *Delusion* rubrics because these are the rubrics which resonate with conflict, self-destruction and disorder; they match the very nature of the disordered disease state.

For a *Delusion* rubric to be relevant in a case analysis the reasons behind the patient developing the psychological delusion have to be confirmed by the homoeopath to be the primary and continual source of pain and confusion across all levels of the patient's life – emotionally, mentally, and physically.

2. Evidence of a Disproportionate Misinterpretation of Reality

The second necessary prerequisite is to find the inner disturbance which is the core of our case-taking, and it is always reflective of what is unusual or disturbing to *your* (the homoeopath's) inner sensibilities. The homoeopath must identify what is disproportionate to reality in their patient's story. Hahnemann said in aphorism 153 of *The Organon*, that in the search for a homoeopathic specific remedy we should concentrate on "the *more striking, singular, uncommon and peculiar* signs and symptoms of the case". The disturbance which reverberates with a *striking* symptom, will be when the patient reveals how they have constructed their mental and emotional outlook around the first *disproportionate* analysis of their lives. In unraveling the significant events in the lives of your patients, and repertorising each poignant emotional event, the simillimum will be evident in every case once you identify the disproportionate interpretation of the patient's life. The key to unraveling your patient's story in case-taking is listening, asking the right questions, and finding the disproportionate disturbance or the *peculiar* interpretation each patient has developed around their trauma.

I have been able to repertorise the *peculiar* signs and symptoms of the patient's case using the *Delusion* rubrics because these are the rubrics which resonate with disruption. I have found it invaluable in case-taking to be able to understand the significant psychological meaning and application of the *Delusion* rubrics. In Radar,™ Dr Luc De Schepper's concepts of the *Delusion* rubrics give a modern-day translation which you can use to interpret your patient's language. Dr Luc De Schepper's list of delusions and concepts is an invaluable thesaurus. I do not aim to repeat or expand that list. In my work I make *an important distinction in the use* of *Delusion* rubrics in case analysis. If a patient says in the consultation, *I feel all alone in the world*, or *I am not as important as my colleagues at work*, or *my parents favored my brother,* that should be repertorised as the *Mind* rubric: *forsaken*. If a patient says *no one understands me*, this is the *Mind* rubric: *forsaken* and should be repertorised as such until you can uncover the misrepresentation and the disturbance in the case. It is not correct to assume that because a patient says, *I have no family in the world and no one to help me*, that it should be repertorised as the *Delusion* rubric: *forsaken*. In psychiatry, the definition of a psychological delusion is that *it is a falsified belief* which is *used* by the patient as self-deception. The false perception of the delusional person is held regardless of reality or proof to the contrary, and the homoeopath must see evidence of this in the case-taking. If a patient says in the consultation, *I feel all alone in the world*, or *I am not as important as my colleagues at work*, or *my parents favored my brother* – those statements could all be true or realistic perceptions. It is not repertorised as a *Delusion* rubric (in the case-taking) until the patient uses their stance as a psychological delusion or misrepresentation and it is this understanding and distinction which I wish to impart. If a patient says *I can't stop spending my money because when I deny myself of what I want, I feel deprived*, it should be repertorised as the *Mind* rubric: *forsaken*. It should be repertorised as a *Mind* rubric and not a *Delusion* rubric because the patient is not self-delusional. The patient is clearly stating they have feelings of deprivation. If the patient is self-deluding of their behavior then it should be repertorised as the *Delusion* rubric: *forsaken*. It is not a *Delusion* rubric until the patient uses the stance as an avoidance, which forms the basis of an excuse, which then forms the basis of a misrepresentation of reality. If the patient cannot correctly assess how much money they have spent or if the patient is disproportionately sensitive to feeling deprived if they are not *continually* spending money on themselves, then there is evidence of deception. It only becomes a *Delusion* rubric (in case-taking) when the patient uses it as a self-deception or their perception is disproportionate to reality. The patient's deception or exaggerated mental and emotional needs are evidence of "the *more striking, singular, uncommon and peculiar* signs and symptoms of the case".

If within the patient's interpretation of their life there is a disturbance which is reflective of inner conflict then a *Delusion* rubric should be used in the case analysis. In homoeopathy we do not prescribe on a disease state or the miasmic presentation of the disease state, we prescribe on how the patient has interpreted those events or that disease state in a *peculiar* and individualistic way. Disturbance within a patient can cause conflict and pain which can eventuate in a physical illness or mental and emotional illness which is reflective of the intensity of the conflict. The reason why it is important to know the disturbance in a case is because any severe disease state can often be a reflection of our deep subconscious struggles. This disturbance can form the foundation of our inner angst and form the basis of future pathology.

The key point within case-taking is confirming that the patient has a *peculiar* avoidance of reality which is a psychological delusion. This is the core basis of the use of a *Delusion* rubric in the case analysis.

3. Evidence that the Delusional Stance is Maintained because it is Advantageous

The third key point within the case is confirming that the patient *needs to maintain their avoidance of reality*. Regardless of whether the psychological delusion has positive or negative consequences, the patient *must* be seen to maintain the delusional stance because they believe it is *advantageous* to delude themselves. For example, the *Sulphur* singer who believed his voice was spectacular suffered from a 'delusion of grandeur'. His need to protect his psychological 'delusion of grandeur' resulted in him exaggerating his allergy reaction or potentially manifesting his allergy in the first place. This patient will not become physically well until the simillimum in the case can make him strong enough to face the reality that his voice is not good enough to be recognized by the best opera houses of the world. An indication of cure is when it will no longer be to his advantage to maintain the psychological 'delusion of persecution' that the tree is the cause of his failure to be recognized as a great singer. The homoeopath in this case should not point out to this *Sulphur* patient that he could just move out of his flat and away from the tree which is causing him the allergies. Nor should the homoeopath point out the obvious fact that he has chosen to continue to live next to a tree which has caused him to become unwell. Both of those observations are valid and may at some point become important to discuss. The cure in this case is for the *Sulphur* patient to be able to find his mental and emotional strength again. The simillimum will enable the patient to move to a place of strength within himself so that he can make those observations for himself.

The character of Lars, in the film *Lars and the Real Girl*, is another example of psychological modeling being adopted because it is advantageous. Lars sets up a delusional relationship with a life-like plastic doll which he names Bianca. His underlying need for the delusion is based on his fears of the future loss of a real girlfriend because his own mother died giving birth to him. To avoid the loss of a real wife he has a relationship with a life-like plastic doll. With the help of a psychologist he is able to slowly unravel his need for the psychological delusion. He then allows the plastic doll to die so he can be released from the relationship and fall in love with a real girl.

In the analysis of a *Delusion* rubric (in case-taking) you have to see and understand, within the case and within the nature of the constitutional remedy profile, why the patient needs the delusional state.

Lars's psychological delusion is needed to avoid grief. The *Delusion* rubrics for Lars would be the following, to confirm the remedy *Arnica*.

*   *Delusion* rubric: *fancy, illusions of.*
*   *Delusion* rubric: *visions, has; fantastic.*
*   *Mind* rubric: *fear: touched; of being.*
*   *Skin* rubric: *coldness.*
*   *Skin* rubric: *coldness; sensation, of.*
*   *Delusion* rubric: *dead: persons, sees.*
*   *Delusion* rubric: *die: about to die; one was.*

In taking Lars's case the above list of rubrics appear in the order in which they are revealed in the film. The first rubric, the *Delusion* rubric: *illusions of fancy*, is a psychological 'delusion of grandeur'. The *Delusion* rubric: *illusions of fancy,* is used (in the rubric-repertorisation) for a patient who is suffering with grand visions of persona: their expectations of what they can achieve, or what they *have* achieved, or who they are in the world are exaggerated. Lars's fanciful illusions allows him to imagine that the life-like plastic doll called Bianca is a real girlfriend. The next piece of information we find out about him is his fear of being touched. The patient needing *Arnica* is fearful of being approached, fearful of being touched, and their whole body is over-sensitive. Lars wears several layers of clothing to protect him from being touched. Lars experiences being touched as cold and physically painful, as well as being emotionally painful. *Arnica* have the *Mind* rubric: *fear of being touched* and the *Skin* rubric: *coldness on skin*. *Arnica* is a homoeopathic remedy commonly used to treat shock. The Lars character is a beautiful portrayal of the remedy *Arnica* and if Lars was my patient in a homoeopathic consultation I could surmise that he has been in emotional shock since his mother died giving birth to him. Although I would prescribe *Arnica* for shock, I would only prescribe it on the basis of the above five rubrics in the rubric-repertorisation. I would not assume anything about Lars being in shock about his mother's death until Lars tapped into his unconscious in the follow-up consultations and revealed that element in the case analysis.

I would also repertorise the case systematically, chronologically compiling the above rubrics in the precise order in which they were revealed in the case-taking. This is case-development.

The psychologist in the film did not uncover his unresolved grief about his mother's death or his overwhelming fear that a future real wife could die in childbirth until several consultations had occurred. *Arnica* also have the *Delusion* rubric: *one was about to die*, and *sees dead persons*, both of these rubrics reinforce his fear of having a real relationship with a real girl. If Lars gets close to someone, the psychological delusion is they could die; this is the meaning of the *Delusion* rubric: *he sees dead persons*. In a homoeopathic consultation the same process unfolds. It is not until the follow-up consultations that I compile all the rubrics or understand all of the patient's delusional needs for the *Delusion* rubrics attached to a particular remedy profile. Although I might surmise that Lars could have been in shock since his birth I would not use the *Delusion* rubrics: *one was about to die*, and *sees dead persons*, in the rubric-repertorisation until Lars revealed his fear of a real future wife dying in the case-taking.

Lars's *illusions of fancy*, enabled him to believe that the life-like plastic doll Bianca, was a real girlfriend, and although this was obviously a self-delusion it was also advantageous to him to be able to imagine his girlfriend Bianca was real. The profoundly touching aspect of the film is that everyone in his small town went along with his psychological delusion and did not confront or try to dispel his illusions.

If the patient has a psychological delusion, then the patient also has a *need* for the delusional stance.

A patient's need will reside in their conscious and subconscious mind, and it is more than likely that the patient is aware and able to verbalize their need for the avoidance. The avoidance is advantageous because it covers up, and helps distract the patient from, underlying and potentially overwhelming emotions like fear, hurt, rage, or jealousy. If the patient is not aware of the feeling they are trying to avoid the answer will often reside in their subconscious or unconscious mind. The need is often a complicated system of psychological avoidances and the patient has chosen to concoct a complex system of excuses to cover up their mental and emotional trauma. If the patient needs an avoidance tactic they will have developed a complicated set of excuses and justifications for their psychological need to maintain the avoidance.

In case-taking, the homoeopath needs to understand the excuses and avoidances which maintain the patient's psychological avoidance of reality. Psychological denial is adopted by the patient when they need to maintain their psychological delusion to avoid reality. The deceptive motivations which form the basis of this mental and emotional need will fall into two categories; avoidance or self-deluding denial. I have used the following two models to define avoidance and self-delusion.

Avoidance: You have to see that it is advantageous to the patient to have their mental or emotional belief. The definitive reason behind the avoidance for each constitution will point the homoeopath in the direction of the simillimum. Their need for avoidance will reside in their conscious and subconscious mind, and it is more than likely that the patient is aware and able to verbalize their need for the avoidance. The avoidance is advantageous because it will cover up, and help distract the patient from potentially overwhelming emotions like fear, hurt, rage, or jealousy.

Self-Deluding: In the case analysis there must be evidence that the patient has used their delusional stance to their own advantage. For self-delusion to be applicable you have to see that the patient has hidden the psychological delusion from themselves. Self-delusion will often reside in the patient's subconscious or unconscious mind and the patient is often not aware of their psychological delusion. Lars would fit into this category because his need to avoid the death of his mother and the potential death of a girlfriend resided in his unconscious mind.

The psychological delusions will always be psychologically needed by the patient to avoid the first psychodynamic trauma. However, the homoeopath might not understand until the third or fourth consultation why the patient needed to maintain their avoidance or self-delusion. If the homoeopath does not understand the patient's need for their psychological delusion and proceeds to attack the patient's logic or their need for maintaining their psychological delusions the homoeopath could undermine the integrity of the patient's mental or emotional well-being.

4. The 'Never-well-since-event' confirming the Primary Psychodynamic Trauma

As a student of homoeopathy I was taught not to ask leading or inquiring questions which would cross the boundaries of psychotherapy. The irony is that the *Delusion* section of the *Mind* in our repertory has for centuries contained a psychotherapeutic analysis which is the basis of homoeopathic psychiatry.

Inherent in the very nature of a psychological delusion and the use of the *Delusion* rubrics in case analysis is that the patient's perception is *not correct*, it is a psychological delusion. In a homoeopathic consultation the psychological delusion is recognized as the first indicator of potential illness in the case-taking and is labeled the 'never-well-since-symptom'. The *Delusion* rubrics reflect and mirror psychodynamic trauma and they have always been significant markers in a patient's life which point us in the direction of the simillimum.

If you don't ask leading questions you will struggle in the rubric-repertorisation. If these causation events are interpreted by the patient in a way which is disproportionate to reality, then they are events which become a misrepresentation and they form the platform of disturbance which has to be repertorised as a *Delusion* rubric. The primary *Delusion* rubric is the first rubric which matches the first trauma in the patient's life which is misinterpreted in a disproportionate way by the patient. Another way to identify these markers in a patient's life is to label them as significant 'layers' in the patient's case-taking. The term 'layers' is frequently used by homoeopaths to identify an event which causes a film or layer which comes in and settles over the case. This 'layer' influences the simillimum in the case. The original psychodynamic trauma will always indicate the primary *Delusion* rubric and this is always where we start questioning our patient.

The role of the homoeopath in analyzing the case is to find the causation in the case which forms the primary *Delusion* rubric, and all the subsequent *Delusion* rubrics which support their disproportionate view of reality.

In the cases presented in the *Case Companion* to *Homoeopathic Psychiatry* I emphasize repeatedly the need to understand the causation or the 'never-well-since-event'. Chronological events are crucial in case-development. They are important because they show us the cause and meaning of the 'how, why, and when,' of the significant events in our patients' lives. The homoeopath needs to ask the patient "why do you think you are sick?" or "what event has happened in your life which you think has contributed to your illness?" or simply "tell me about your life and what has happened to you in your life". I prefer to ask the last question because then the patient will tell me about the events in their life which they think are crucial to their case.

The first consultation is often on the conscious level. It is often not until patients have had several consultations that they are able to reveal deep traumatic events in their life which have formulated psychological delusions. Until I discover the primary trauma in a patient's life I am never *totally* sure of a simillimum prescription. The case analysis should initially be formulated using the above three points which confirm mental and emotional disturbance and physical pathology.

In the follow-up consultations if the remedy is the simillimum the patient will often reveal in the consultation the formation of their psychological delusions. The cure of, and from the simillimum will always elicit the 'never-well-since-event'. It is what I refer to as the 'eye of the storm'. The 'eye of the storm', is when your patient reveals to you their primary traumatic event in their lives. The patient might not reveal the 'never-well-since-event' until the third or the fourth consultation.

It occurs during a consultation when everything stops in the case-taking and you know you have arrived at the centre of your patient's internal storm.

The character of Lars in the film *Lars and the Real Girl,* quietly and at the same time dramatically revealed after several consultations with the psychologist his overwhelming fear behind having a real girlfriend was that she could die in childbirth like his mother. A patient facing illness and death whether it is non-fatal or fatal will journey through an emotional typhoon. It is both the moment of great calm and great turmoil because it is the centre of the inner disturbance inside of your patient. In a psychotherapeutic process the subconscious mind is what the patient enters into when they uncover pain. Significantly, the exact same process happens in a homoeopathic consultation, especially if the situation is made urgent by a serious or fatal illness. Joseph Conrad wrote a story about a crew's journey through a typhoon. Conrad[4] wrote in *Typhoon*: "But the quietude of the air was startlingly tense and unsafe, like a slender hair holding a sword suspended over his head. By this awful pause the storm penetrated the defense of the man and unsealed his lips." The transcripts of patient's follow-up consultations which I present in the *Case Companion* to *Homoeopathic Psychiatry* capture this *exact* moment of revelation which Conrad identified when the captain faced the loss of his ship.

When you face your psychological delusional state it is like a sword suspended above your head forcing you to reveal the disruption inside your whole being. It is a moment of self-reflection and inner knowing. It is also proof that the action of the simillimum has been able to penetrate the defenses of the delusional trauma in the subconscious and unconscious. The simillimum must be noted by the homoeopath to be peeling back the layers of the psychological delusions one after the other.

Good case analysis and good case-development will have prepared the homoeopath to know why each psychological delusion has been *needed* by the patient. A patient will see that it is advantageous to maintain the psychological delusion because if they drop their psychological delusions they will have to face the pain of their primary psychodynamic trauma.

It is crucial in case-development and treatment that the homoeopath is prepared and able to be supportive when the patient starts to see they can let go of maintaining their psychological delusion. The simillimum will undo the layers of psychological delusions and undo the need for the delusions in the reverse order of their development. This is evidence of Dr. Hering's Law of Cure[5]: in the reverse order of their coming.

Below is my story. In relaying a snippet of my own case I will outline my case-taking framework. I will outline each poignant emotional event in the first few years of my life to explain the case analysis technique and the relevant rubrics which help to develop the simillimum in the case-development. Over the years, I have listened to my patients telling similar stories. Each case I present in the *Case Companion* will follow a similar pattern which will enable you to construct the primary *Delusion* rubric which developed from the patient's first psychodynamic trauma.

In homoeopathy I have discovered that when you delve into the original crisis or psychodynamic trauma in your patient that created the primary *Delusion* rubric, you highlight the simillimum.

Trauma in a patient's life usually starts when they are a child, and frequently the trauma forms the subconscious and unconscious responses which govern the assimilation and misinterpretation of the first pain in our life. It is also possible that a child is born after having an in-vitro trauma. If the in-vitro trauma or a subsequent birth trauma is the original trauma then the patient will not necessarily be able to relay a conscious or subconscious experience from their life. The primal memory will be buried in the unconscious memory which will still unconsciously influence the patient but it will not be able to be explained consciously by the patient in the case-taking. If the trauma is in-vitro or a birth trauma the patient will have other significant early indicators which will confirm that they are emotionally still in an early psychologically arrested infant state. A primal or birth trauma is not a psychological delusion until the patient uses the trauma to delude themselves. A primal or birth trauma may predispose the patient to future psychological delusions. A primal or birth trauma may also predispose the person to a definitive psychodynamic trauma which becomes the primary *Delusion* rubric.

It is a relevant *Delusion* rubric in a case when you are able to notice that the patient has internalized the trauma and is using the trauma in a disproportionate way to misrepresent reality. The psychological delusion must be able to be traced back by the patient to a specific event in their life. The psychodynamic trauma is the basis of the primary *Delusion* rubric even if there were predisposed circumstances and early in-vitro primal traumas in the patient's life which predisposed them to a psychological delusion or psychological trauma.

Assimilation of the first psychodynamic trauma and the intricacies which develop from that interpretation form our stance in this life. This interpretation then develops our conscious reactions to the world. In the unconscious we lock away secrets and thought processes from ourselves that we can't easily access, even though they can still influence our behavior and thoughts. In the subconscious mind, thoughts which are not fully conscious, but still able to influence and offer explanations of our behavior, sit just under the surface. In case-taking, the patient will dip into their subconscious world, and it is in this world that you will find the meaning of the 'causations' or the '*how, why,* and *when*' in the case. As an adult, I found out my feelings of abandonment were real when I learned I was rejected at birth. In my case the *Mind* rubric: *forsaken* must have formed an unconscious foundation from birth which definitely predisposed me to a psychological 'delusion of abandonment'.

Notably, it is not a *Delusion* rubric in the case-development until a delusional stance is formed by the patient. In both modalities – psychiatry and homoeopathy – it is accepted that a baby is not born with a psychological delusion, rather a psychological delusion is developed by the child or adult as a result of the child or adult misinterpreting the precipitating event.

For example, if the mother, while carrying the child, was in turmoil over whether she wanted to keep the baby, or if she had wanted to miscarriage, or if she had wanted to abort the child and had not been able to for various reasons, it would be possible to assume in case-taking that the baby could be born with primal feelings and this could be reflected in the rubric-repertorisation by using the *Mind* rubrics: *anxiety, forsaken,* or *frightened easily* or *fear of being neglected.* The remedy *Pulsatilla* will appear in all those rubrics. In a *Pulsatilla* case an in-vitro primal trauma or birth trauma could be repertorised by using the *Mind* rubric: *fear of being neglected,* which would confirm the psychological trauma of being neglected in-vitro. Although *Pulsatilla* will also be listed in the *Delusion* rubric: *forsaken* it is not correct for the homoeopath to use the *Delusion* rubric: *forsaken* in the case-taking if the *Pulsatilla* patient does *not* have a psychological delusion.

My role as a homoeopath is to repertorise a patient's story and to find the correct *Mind* rubrics in the case, or the correct *Delusion* rubrics. My role in case-taking is not to assume anything unless the patient shows evidence of a psychological delusion or confirms a psychological delusion in their story.

The first conscious memory I would be able to relay in case-taking is of being left in hospital to have my eyes operated on when I was two years old. I vividly remember seeing my mother leave the hospital ward. I remember her looking back at me in the cot and then leaving through the door. I remember the long row of cots, all the other children and babies and the nurse at the nurse's station. I wanted desperately to have my cot moved closer to the baby next to me so I could hold her hand. The nurse misunderstood me and thought I wanted to get into her cot and she scolded me and told me I had to stay in my own cot. I was left by my mother but the despair of being left *alone* in a cot is what I remember being fixated on. It is important to emphasize that it is not helpful to point out to the patient that they were not alone because other children and the nurse were in the ward with them. Here, the homoeopath shouldn't correct the patient by telling them that they were not permanently abandoned by their mother as she did in fact come back, and that they were being looked after by a nurse. I remember as a two-year-old the nurse scolding me and saying, "What are you upset about, you can see the little girl next to you in the other cot". In taking such a case, the first rubric a homoeopath would look up would be the rubric for abandonment, which is the *Mind* rubric: *forsaken*. The precise and correct sub-section is the *Mind* rubric: *forsaken, sensation of isolation*. We pick that *precise and particular* rubric because it was not just that my mother left; the essence of the case-taking so far is that I wanted to be able to *touch* the baby in the next cot. What distressed me was being *alone* in my cot and not being able to *touch* the baby next to me. The correct rubric to address my particular sensation of abandonment is the *Mind* rubric: *forsaken, sensation of isolation* from others.

- *Mind*: rubric: *forsaken*: *isolation; sensation of.*

The next conscious memory I have is when I was four years of age and I had to walk home alone after kindergarten; the rubric in the case-repertorisation is still the *Mind* rubric: *forsaken, sensation of isolation.* In my next significant memory I was once again in hospital at five years of age. I had my teeth removed by a local dentist who thought the best way for poor children living in the country to avoid tooth decay was to remove perfectly healthy molars (back teeth) before they could develop decay. The premise was that my family would not be able to afford fillings in the future. I woke up in a bed and vomited blood all over the bed. I was terrified. My mother was in the room and she nearly fainted at the sight of the blood. The nurse attended to her distress and not to *mine*. Observing the nurse's actions, I concluded that no one would look after me. My psychological interpretation of my life, and my story, developed into the assumption that I was alone in the world. This is a psychological delusion, and this is how the primary *Delusion* rubric came into play in my case.

The primary *Delusion* rubric is based on the patient's conscious understanding of the first psychodynamic trauma which is of significance to them. In the patient relaying their life story it is more than likely that they do not know the meaning, significance, or importance of that event until they reveal it to you in the consultation. The primary event must contain the event which forms the basis of the patient's *misrepresentation of reality* in their life. Their *misinterpretation* or misrepresentation of the event will then form the basis of their revisionist rewriting of the mental and emotional 'baggage' they carry with them. In homoeopathy we develop a case around this primary event and we call it the 'never-well-since-symptom' of the case.

The homoeopath should never correct a delusional perception that the patient has revealed in the case-taking because that disproportionate perception is the first formation of a potential *Delusion* rubric in the case.

The simillimum in my case must emphasize abandonment. The *Delusion* rubric: *he is separated from the world*, should be the next rubric used, since I assumed an *exaggerated and disproportionate* forsaken and isolated stance. The feeling became a mental and emotional stance whereby I believed that no one would ever understand my distress or my need to be comforted. If I had just interpreted this event as being abandoned by my mother then the rubric would still be the *Mind* rubric: *forsaken,* or the *Mind* rubric: *forsaken, sense of isolation.* The fact that I presumed that no-one would ever help me is the reason the rubric used has to be a *Delusion* rubric which in particular emphasizes abandonment. This is how I psychotherapeutically analyze the use of a *Delusion* rubric in case-taking. I adopted the stance that I was all alone in the world and this is a psychological delusion or misrepresentation of reality. The emotional stance I took then formed my approach to the world and I subsequently used this as the self-deluding excuse to separate myself from the world.

The original psychodynamic trauma is when the perception becomes a misrepresentation of reality; this is the meaning of a psychological delusion.

- *Delusion* rubric: *world*: *separated; from the.*

My constitutional remedy (simillimum) is not listed under the *Mind* rubric: *forsaken* nor, most importantly, is it listed

under the *Delusion* rubric: *forsaken*. The first correct rubric in
the case-repertorisation is the *Mind* rubric: *forsaken, sensation
of isolation* because my distress came from not being able to
touch the little baby in the next cot.

Acknowledgment and listening to how *the patient* interprets their life
experiences is crucial in case-taking in order to be able to understand the
peculiar interpretation each patient has of their story.

The *Mind* rubric: *forsaken, sensation of isolation*, is
used as the first rubric in the case-taking. It then became a
Delusion rubric in my case because psychologically I took
the delusional stance of believing that I was *always* going to
be alone and abandoned. In case-taking, the homoeopath
has to be able to see how the patient used this psychological
delusion as a misinterpretation of reality. This has to be *seen*
for the repertorisation and case-development to include
Delusion rubrics. I did not consciously think that I was literally,
physically separated from the world, but in my psychodynamic
interpretation of the world, which governed my emotional
responses, I felt I was isolated and alone. I then developed
a complicated mesh of excuses and avoidances around that
persecution which were advantageous to maintain. This is how
I interpret the *Delusion* rubrics. If the sense of separation is
not used as a delusion of reality then it remains an emotional
stance which is not a psychological delusion and the rubric
choice in the case-repertorisation would be simply the *Mind*
rubric: *forsaken*. The *Delusion* rubric: *he is separated from the
world* is not meant to be taken literally. A literal interpretation
would mean that the *Delusion* rubrics have not been used
correctly in the case analysis.

If I ask myself as a patient, "Why do you think you felt isolated
from the world?", I would give an answer from my inner-child's
psyche which resides in my subconscious world. My answer
would not be an adult's logical understanding of the situation
because the event is the primary psychodynamic trauma which

is arrested and frozen in the psyche of a five-year-old child. In case-taking it is obviously not appropriate to say to your patient that their perception is not a correct assumption of the situation because the nurse would have eventually attended to their needs.

Knowing why you felt isolated from the world as a five-year-old will not be a logical understanding; it will be an understanding that lives in the subconscious mind of a small child. The majority of children will wrongly assume that they are bad or that they are *The Ugly Duckling* from the fairytale by Hans Christian Anderson and that is why they believe they have been abandoned by their mother. This was certainly true in my own case. The *Delusion* rubric: *he is separated from the world* immediately results in inner conflict and disturbance because the child, as in my own case, formed an incorrect perception of being bad. The *Delusion* rubric for the assumption of being bad is the *Delusion* rubric: *he has committed a crime* or the *Delusion* rubric: *he has done wrong.* I have found that the *Delusion* rubrics of sin, or self-blame, will always be the relevant causations in all cases which involve psychological delusions. An assumption that one is bad or evil forms the subconscious disturbance within the mental and emotional processing of the majority of adults when they are faced with an illness.

The primary source of this psychological disturbance will often be found in childhood, and it is the role of the homoeopath to discover their primary 'never-well-since-event' which compounds their illness.

In my own case analysis, the journey began in the conscious memory with the *Mind* rubric: *forsaken, sensation of isolation*, and continued into the subconscious world with delusional feelings of isolation of a five-year-old, which is the *Delusion* rubric: *separation from the world.* Why this happened in the subconscious mind of a five-year-old is incorrectly explained by the next psychological delusion of being bad or evil. The *Delusion* rubric we use for that is the *Delusion* rubric *he has done wrong.* To conclude, we have now collected several chronological rubrics in the case which is how I analyze all cases in my practice and in the *Case Companion* to *Homoeopathic Psychiatry*.

- *Mind* rubric: *forsaken*: *isolation; sensation of.*
- *Delusion* rubric: *world*: *separated; from the.*
- *Delusion* rubric: *crime*: *committed; he had.*
- *Delusion* rubric: *wrong*: *done wrong; he has.*

My first abandonment at birth helped unconsciously form the *Mind* rubric: *forsaken*. The first hospital visit at two years of age helped consciously form the *Mind* rubric: *forsaken, sensation of isolation*, but it was not until the later event in the hospital at five years of age that my delusional interpretation of the primary trauma indicated a *Delusion* rubric. Although abandonment might cause suffering it will not, in my experience, present years later as the foundation of abnormal emotional, mental, or physical pathology, *unless* it moves into avoidance or self-denial and eventually self-destruction in the subconscious or unconscious. The first prerequisites emphasizes that all pathology has its foundation in delusional disturbance. I have been fortunate to find the simillimum to end my mental and emotional conflict with being separated from the world as well as finding the simillimum to end my physical conflict and pending auto-immune disease. In an auto-immune disease, anti-bodies produced by the body attack the body's own connective tissue and organs. The excess anti-nuclear anti-bodies subsequently become self-destructive. The rubrics that point to the correct remedy to cure the numerous auto-immune cases which I have treated within my practice are found within the *Delusion* rubrics because these are the rubrics which resonate with conflict, self-destruction and disorder; they match the very nature of the disordered disease state.

The primary trauma which caused the primary *Delusion* rubric is the causation in the case. Then *there must be evidence* in the case-taking of self-destruction and pathology which is proof of the need to use a *Delusion* rubric in the rubric-repertorisation.

This is confirmed in the pending development of an auto-immune condition. There are another two notable elements to the case which must be present to justify a *Delusion* rubric being used in the case-repertorisation. You can only use a *Delusion* rubric in the case analysis if you can identify how the patient has used the psychological delusion as a revisionist misinterpretation of reality. A patient might have been abandoned but it is not correct to repertorise this event as a *Delusion* rubric until you have evidence in the case-taking of a psychological delusion. Lastly, you have to see evidence that the patient used the feelings of abandonment as a psychological delusion and perverted it into an often complicated system of psychological avoidances or self-delusions. Psychological modeling is an assumed mental or emotional attitude which is adopted because it is primarily advantageous to the patient. In my own case I felt abandoned and alone but this only became a psychological delusion or misrepresentation of reality because it formed my assumption[6] that I would always be alone. I subsequently used this as the self-deluding excuse to separate myself from the world to avoid further abandonment. This is evidence in the case-development of the psychological delusion being advantageous. The simillimum has to undo the need to maintain the psychological delusion. The simillimum first cured the psychological stance which produced the *Delusion* rubric: *I had done wrong,* then the psychological stance which produced the *Delusion* rubric: *separated from the world.* This was evidence of Hering's Law of Cure.

The constitutional remedy chosen must contain within the make-up of the remedy profile the same psychological delusions as the patient otherwise it is not the simillimum.

The simillimum in my case emphasized abandonment as a key causation. If the homoeopath does not understand the case-development or understand the psychological development of the rubric-repertorisation or the importance of the patient's need to maintain the avoidance or self-delusion, then the case will be lost. The primary trauma constitutes a significant event in your patient's life and this marker will be the significant event which will define the simillimum in the case.

What are the Rubric-categories?

In my **Rubric-categories** I have identified five rubric-categories. The rubric-categories match the psychological delusions and the psychological stages which all patients manifest in an illness.

In all homoeopathic consultations the patient will move through *some or all* of these five states as they struggle to acknowledge that they are suffering an illness. A patient will often start their story from the arrogant assumption, or misapprehension of immortality; we all assume that we are entitled to health and long life. This is denial.

Denial

"I am not sick."

"I will be cured."

"I will cure myself."

"*I* should not have got sick."

"This should not have happened to *me*."

Forsaken

"My body has let me down." (abandonment).

"My illness has been caused by others." (persecution).

"I have been cheated of my life." (abandonment and persecution).

"I have been singled out for punishment." (abandonment and persecution).

Causation

"I have caused my disease."

"This is my fault."

"I must have done something wrong to deserve this."

"I have been bad."

"I have sinned."

Depression

"I will never become well."

"I will never succeed."

"I will always fail."

"This is my fate."

Resignation

"I am dying."

"I am sure I have cancer."

"I am sure I have a terrible disease."

"I am too weak to survive this world."

In the **Rubric-categories** I take the most commonly used *Delusion* rubrics that I have found in my practice, group them according to the five rubric headings and explain their delusional use.

1. Denial: 'hubristic denial' of disease.
2. Forsaken: disproportionate feelings of abandonment, or persecutory delusional beliefs.
3. Causation: disproportionate guilt.
4. Depression: predictions of failure.
5. Resignation: overblown resignation to disease and death, or exaggerated hypochondriacal fears of illness.

They encompass respectively, the psychological 'delusions of grandeur', 'delusions of abandonment', 'delusions of persecution', 'delusions of original sin', 'delusions of impending doom' and the 'delusions of hypochondria'.

The purpose of understanding these five psychological stages is to match the simillimum to the psychological presentation of your patient's delusional state, whether it be 'delusions of persecution' or 'delusions of hypochondria', etc. If you learn how to recognize these five psychological stages in the consultation within your patient, it will help you in the rubric-repertorisation and in finding the simillimum.

1. I have allocated all the *Delusion* rubrics which pertain to 'delusions of grandeur' into Denial. If the patient's trauma starts with denial of, and disbelief in, their illness/sickness, then the simillimum is listed in Denial. If the trauma inside your patient starts with martyrdom and/or delusional belief in divine cure then the simillimum is listed in Denial. If your patient unrealistically believes they are so *great* or *superior* that they will not die then the simillimum is listed in all the *Delusion* rubrics: *immortality, in communication with God, under an all powerful influence*, or *being divine*.

2. I have allocated all the *Delusion* rubrics which pertain to psychological 'delusions of abandonment' or 'delusions of persecution' into Forsaken. If the trauma inside your patient starts with them feeling alone and abandoned, or singled out for punishment by their illness then the simillimum is listed in all the *Delusion* rubrics: *forsaken* or *persecution*.

3. I have allocated all the *Delusion* rubrics which pertain to psychological 'delusions of original sin' or self-blame into Causation. If the trauma inside your patient starts with them feeling guilty and unrealistically responsible for their illness then the simillimum is listed in the all the *Delusion* rubrics: *he is sinful, he has committed a crime* or *he has done wrong*, and is allocated to the section Causation.

4. I have allocated all the *Delusion* rubrics which pertain

to psychological 'delusions of impending doom' into Depression. If the trauma inside your patient starts with them feeling hopeless doom about being sick or them feeling like they will never succeed in becoming well in life, then the simillimum is listed in the *Delusion* rubrics: *failure* and *he will not succeed* and is allocated to the section Depression.

5. I have allocated all the *Delusion* rubrics which pertain to psychological 'delusions of hypochondria' into Resignation. If the patient's trauma starts with hypochondria or delusional doom about being sick, or you feel that your patient is exaggerating their weakness or sickness then the simillimum is listed in the *Delusion* rubrics: *death*, and *disease* and is allocated to the section Resignation.

Each remedy profile will present in one, or all, of the psychological stages.

Each patient will have a tendency to be *predominately* in denial, forsakenness, persecutory paranoia, guilt, depression, or hypochondria.

The simillimum *must* have *Delusion* rubrics which match the delusional state of mind of the patient.

If the constitutional remedy that the homoeopath has chosen has *Delusion* rubrics allocated into Denial, the patient *must* display psychological 'delusions of grandeur'.

If the constitutional remedy that the homoeopath has chosen has *Delusion* rubrics allocated into Forsaken, the patient *must* display psychological 'delusions of abandonment', or 'delusions of persecution'.

If the constitutional remedy that the homoeopath has chosen has *Delusion* rubrics allocated into Causation, the patient *must* display psychological 'delusions of original sin'.

If the constitutional remedy that the homoeopath has chosen has *Delusion* rubrics allocated into Depression, the patient *must* display psychological 'delusions of impending doom'.

If the constitutional remedy that the homoeopath has chosen has *Delusion* rubrics allocated into Resignation, the patient *must* display psychological 'delusions of hypochondria'.

For example, the simillimum will not be *Veratrum album* unless the patient believes that they are God-like or that they are in contact with divine spiritual-like energy. The hardest issue to tackle in *Veratrum album* is their belief in God's punishment. The hardest issue to tackle in *Veratrum album* is also their belief in their God-like status. *Veratrum album* will not trust or work with the homoeopath unless they believe that the homoeopathic practitioner is in contact with a 'divine energy' which is able to guide their prescription. The simillimum will only be *Veratrum album* if the patient has psychological 'delusions of grandeur'.

Aurum muriaticum natronatum have no *Delusion* rubrics allocated into Denial. *Aurum muriaticum natronatum* have numerous *Delusion* rubrics allocated into Forsaken and Causation. *Aurum muriaticum natronatum* exaggerate their delusions of unworthiness. *Aurum muriaticum natronatum* demonstrate exaggerated hyper-vigilant fears, and predictions of being abandoned. They base these 'delusions of persecution' on their 'delusions of original sin'. The simillimum will only be *Aurum muriaticum natronatum* if the patient believes that they can't, or don't deserve to be treated or cured.

Anhalonium do not have any *Delusion* rubrics pertaining to self-blame or 'delusions of original sin'. If your patient blames themselves for their illness then the simillimum is not *Anhalonium*. *Anhalonium* does not necessarily blame anyone else either. If your patient is fearful about their fatal illness, or death, the simillimum is not *Anhalonium*. *Anhalonium* are not interested in, and do not cope with, the earthly plane of existence; they only feel depressed if they are *hindered* from leaving. *Anhalonium* feel like they are suffering by being forced to live on this earthly plane. *Anhalonium* have numerous

Delusion rubrics allocated into Denial. The simillimum will only be *Anhalonium* if the patient has psychological 'delusions of grandeur'.

Elaps corallinus do not fight for their life. The Brazilian coral snake is found in South America. It is a shy and timid reptile that is easily captured in comparison to other snakes. If gently tapped on the head with a stick it will coil itself up and lie still, only raising its tail and rattling. It is then easily captured. *Elaps corallinus* are not able to motivate themselves. *Elaps corallinus* behave as if they are *being beaten* into submissiveness. *Elaps corallinus* in the face of adversity immediately surrender, they lack the 'hubristic denial' of the other snake remedy profiles. *Elaps corallinus* lack *Delusion* rubrics allocated into Denial. The simillimum will not be *Elaps corallinus* if the patient has psychological 'delusions of grandeur'.

Natrum muriaticum do *not* have any *Delusion* rubrics pertaining to disproportionate guilt. They have no *Delusion* rubrics allocated into Causation. If your patient disproportionately over-exaggerates self-blame for their illness, then the simillimum is not *Natrum muriaticum*. *Natrum muriaticum* will exaggerate their failure. But their failure is attributed to others who have neglected and/or insulted them. *Natrum muriaticum* will always attribute blame for their mental and emotional mental pain to everyone else who has caused them hurt. *Natrum muriaticum* have numerous *Delusion* rubrics pertaining to 'delusions of persecution'.

Lac-equinum are *trapped* in their own depression because they believe they will *always* fail. *Lac-equinum* have numerous *Delusion* rubrics allocated into Depression. When *Lac-equinum* are sick they sink into a depressive anxiety which has such a tight grip on their psyche that they believe there is *no* hope of cure. *Lac-equinum* remain in suffocating servitude because they have no *Delusion* rubrics allocated into Denial. *Lac-equinum* have no *Delusion* rubrics allocated into psychological 'delusions of grandeur' which would enable them to have a grandeur vision of themselves.

Xanthoxylum wants to die because they do not have enough mental and emotional energy to desire life. Boericke notes that the remedy is for mental depression. *Xanthoxylum* would rather sink into decline and die, than make the choice to live. *Xanthoxylum* have predominantly *Delusion* rubrics allocated into Depression and Resignation. The simillimum will be only *Xanthoxylum* if the patient displays evidence of extreme depressive weakness across all levels – emotionally, mentally, and physically. The simillimum will only be *Xanthoxylum* if the patient is a depressive hypochondriac.

The advantage in identifying and understanding the psychological processing that your patient is moving through is that it allows you to narrow the remedies being considered to the remedies listed in those particular rubric-categories.

Denial

"I am not sick."

"I will be cured."

"I will cure myself."

"*I* should not have got sick."

"This should not have happened to *me*."

I have allocated all the *Delusion* rubrics which pertain to 'delusions of grandeur' into Denial.

If the patient's trauma starts with denial of, and disbelief in, their illness/ sickness, then the simillimum is listed in Denial.

If the trauma inside your patient starts with martyrdom and/ or delusional belief in divine cure then the simillimum is listed in Denial. If your patient unrealistically believes they are so *great* or *superior* that they will not die then the simillimum is listed in all the *Delusion* rubrics: *immortality, in communication with God, under an all powerful influence,* or *being divine.*

A patient who is struggling to come out of denial or who refuses to believe they are sick is suffering psychological 'delusions of grandeur'. Although we know we are all eventually going get sick and die, it is always something which is going to happen to someone else, never us. Cancer is always something which someone else is going to die from – not us. A heart attack is not going to happen to us because we now have cholesterol-lowering medications. Since the development of modern medicine and the technical revolution we have developed a delusional belief in our own hubristic power over mortality and our bodies. In my practice I run a significant fertility program[7]. The most distressing psychological delusions I see in this program are those in which couples blame themselves or each other for their infertility even when they have clearly passed the realistic, medically accepted, ideal age for conception. The couple who is struggling to acknowledge the time-frame of their fertile years is suffering psychological delusions of immortality. The patient who refuses to accept that they have something as simple as a gluten allergy, for example, is suffering psychological 'delusions of grandeur'.

The patient who refuses to accept ageing or illness is suffering psychological denial. It is invaluable to consider the rubrics in this category for the patient who believes they are invincible and that they will never die.

I have noticed that it is very common amongst health practitioners, especially homoeopaths, to have psychological delusions of immortality. My patients who are also homoeopaths are frequently very shocked if they become ill. 'Hubristic denial' of illness is a denial of our death; this is the *Delusion* rubric: *immortality*.

Acknowledging illness and death is emotionally challenging. It is normal to struggle with the acceptance of illness and disease. When faced with illness and death, patients commonly move into psychological denial. Illness and diagnosis of pending death fuel psychological delusions of believing in God or an equivalent 'higher spirit' who will perform a miraculous cure.

The Denial list is relevant to consider in case-taking when the patient presents with an *unrealistic belief* that they can be cured by divine intervention; this is a psychological delusion of 'hubristic denial'. It is invaluable to consider the rubrics in this category for the patient struggling to *realistically* acknowledge or assess the gravity of the situation concerning their health. Rather than face our human frailty, which we have to acknowledge when we face disease and death, we commonly choose to believe we can be cured of our fatal diseases and delude ourselves that we will live forever. Believing you can cure a fatal disease is a psychological 'delusion of denial' and a psychological 'delusion of grandeur'. Delusional belief in *superiority* is where one aligns oneself with God. These are the *Delusion* rubrics which relate to being *under a powerful influence*, as well as all the *Delusion* rubrics of *greatness, superiority,* and *power over all diseases.*

A patient's delusional belief in a miraculous cure, or arrogant assumption of continuous good health, are psychological 'delusions of grandeur'. God is synonymous with our 'inner spiritual guide' and synonymous with our 'higher self'. God can also be synonymous with a 'divine entity' or a 'spiritual energy' or 'fate', it can be a personage like Buddha, or Mohammad or Jesus. Most commonly, I have found that a patient's ancestors are the guardian angels who come to them in their dreams telling them that they will be cured. Consequently, in this section I have included all the *Delusion* rubrics of *beautiful visions* and *illusions*. A patient facing an incurable dilemma with their health, who believes they will live to a ripe old age, is easily identifiable as suffering a psychological delusion of 'hubristic denial'. A patient who believes they can cure themselves by getting in touch with their 'higher spiritual self' is not so easily identifiable as suffering psychological 'delusions of grandeur' or 'hubristic denial'. I certainly acknowledge that whether or not a patient is in denial when they place their faith in God, or a spiritual force or their own 'spirit' curing them, is a contentious issue which could fuel many discussions and arguments. My aim is to identify *delusional hubristic denial* in relation to 'spiritual saviors'.

'Spiritualistic belief' is the marketing of denial. If a patient aligns his or herself with God, then they use their 'delusions of grandeur' to believe they are either God, so therefore are not sick, or else they will believe God will cure them of their illness.

When a patient alludes to being God they will say in the

consultation: *you know Liz I did not expect this to happen to someone like me. I have always seen myself as having total control over my destiny. I did not perceive this in my future. I really do think that it cannot be something which is going to be really serious because I am very pure in my diet and in my heart. I am a good person and have always been good, I have no bad inside of me. I am not tempted by bad things in life and I have always been in charge of counselling everyone around me to do good. In fact I have great foresight, so I am sure I will be able to resolve this health problem by myself.* This is 'hubristic denial'. These are the 'hubristic denial' *Delusion* rubrics: *of greatness.*

All 'delusions of grandeur' are self-deluding denials of feelings of inadequacy. You *have* to ask why each constitutional remedy needs to believe they are *superior*, or *a great person*, or *distinguished*. You have to know how, and why, each constitutional remedy is using the psychological delusion, and what would happen if they did not put the psychological energy into believing they were so *great*. If a patient needs to identify themselves as a 'spiritual person' then the homoeopathic practitioner needs to know if their need for 'spiritualism' is based on avoidance and/ or denial.

In the seventies, I remember Gurus would warn against hubris. A 'spiritual person' was commonly identified as having a 'spiritual ego'. Nowadays that derogatory label no longer exists within spiritual organizations. The various 'New-Age' philosophies that exist now encourage hubris. 'Hubristic denial' is applicable for the patient who uses their identification with 'spiritualism' to avoid reality and deny inadequacy. These are the 'hubristic denial' *Delusion* rubrics: *illusions of fancy,* and *visions.*

A patient's belief that they will be spared or cured of a fatal disease by their 'spiritual enlightenment' or 'spiritual awakening' is a psychological avoidance of reality and their mortality. The various 'New-Age' philosophies of 'you are what you think', and 'you can cure your disease', have put incredible pressure on patients.

In 1969, when Kübler-Ross identified her five stages of grief, her patients did not have the pressure that various 'New-Age' philosophies have put on modern-day patients. **Since the emergence of 'New-Age' philosophies, the patient has become a victim of the belief that *they should be able to cure themselves.***

The relevant question that the homoeopath needs to ask the patient is, "What happens if you lose this battle?" Asking this question forces the patient to acknowledge the reality of their disease. **Acknowledging one's mortality is the opposite of denial.** I recently read an account of a woman who was told that she had an incurable brain tumor (Gioblastoma-multiforme). The notable dilemma in the story was that even though the woman was a medic, and knew the truth about her medical prognosis, she was extremely angry at being told it was fatal because she believed this took away her hope. She was emphatic that cancer patients need to be given hope rather than medical prognoses. Hope is an emotional need to look forward with expectation to the promise of cure. Hope is also the inspiration behind our desire to embrace life. A *Delusion* rubric is only used in the case analysis if the patient needs to deny reality.

If the desire for hope of cure is extreme in the face of overwhelming evidence to the contrary, it can become self-destructive. It would be self-destructive because it would prevent the patient from finding the mental and emotional peace which comes from being able to accept death.

The consequence of denial is that the patient expends more energy trying to avoid acknowledging their disease than they would expend in acknowledging their mortality. I have always noted that when the patient moves out of psychological denial they have markedly more energy to dedicate to their last few weeks or months of living. This doesn't mean that the patient has no more hope – they

do. In fact they have more hope than before. For example, they tell me they go to sleep every night hoping that they will be able to enjoy one more day.

Delusional hope of cure **i.e. denial, can be an illusion which robs one of the energy to live** *now.* **The irony is that the patient who moves out of denial not only has more energy, they also usually live longer.**

The homoeopath who has a vested interest, emotionally and philosophically, in the patient healing themselves can easily fall into the patient's delusional belief in the power of their spiritual inner world and not recognize that their patient's belief is evidence of psychological denial. The remedies in this category of rubrics are invaluable for the homoeopathic practitioner suffering from 'delusions of grandeur' or delusions of miraculous cure. Homoeopathy cannot cure the incurable. Many homoeopaths suffer with psychological 'delusions of grandeur' when they believe that their dying patient can be cured by homoeopathy. 'Hubristic denial' is found within all the omnipotent *Delusion* rubrics of self-alignment with God or personal greatness.

The homoeopath must learn how to recognize delusional denial to be able to know when and how to use the *Delusion* rubrics which are all aligned to spiritual greatness.

My aim in highlighting the *peculiar* denial process of each constitutional remedy is to identify the *striking* peculiarities of denial *specific* to each constitutional remedy profile. If there is evidence of notable inner conflict, and evidence of self-destruction and pathology, this indicates that the rubric-repertorisation and case analysis must contain a *Delusion* rubric. If there are contradictions and inconsistencies in the rubrics pertaining to a remedy profile then there is *also* inner conflict which is indicative of the psychological pathology of suppression or denial.

'Hubristic denial' is evident in the inconsistencies between the Denial rubrics pertaining to 'delusions of grandeur' or cure, and the Resignation rubrics pertaining to disease, and death or 'delusions of hypochondria'.

In particular, if there are inconsistencies between Stage one and Stage five, then there is evidence of self-denial and suppression which will either accelerate present pathology or precede future pathology.

Example of inconsistencies:

1. Denial: *Delusion* rubric: *well, he is*: puls.

   Versus

5. Resignation: *Delusion* rubric: *sick: being*: **PULS**.

Example of inconsistencies:

1. Denial: *Delusion* rubric: *great person, is a*: Cann-i.

   Versus

5. Resignation: *Delusion rubric*: *maelstrom[8]; carried down a psychical*: cann-i.

Example of inconsistencies:

1. Denial: *Delusion* rubric: *distinguished; he is*: verat.

   Versus

5. Resignation: *Delusion* rubric: *disease*: *deaf, dumb and has cancer; he is*: verat. [1] 1.[9]

The importance of understanding the contradictions and inconsistencies within each constitutional remedy profile is that they provide psychological insight into how each constitutional remedy profile will behave when sick. For example, *Pulsatilla* in Denial will present believing they are *well*, and *Pulsatilla* in Resignation will present with over-exaggerated predications of illness and fragility and over-blown predictions that they are *sick*. *Cannabis indica* will alternate between invincible denial, *Delusion* rubric: *great person*, and delusional destruction,

Delusion rubric: *carried down a maelstrom. Veratrum album* will alternate between delusional superiority that they are too important to accept your help, and delusional self-denigration that they are too *dumb* to be worthy of your help.

Inconsistencies between *Delusion* rubrics pertaining to grandeur and *Delusion* rubrics pertaining to destruction in the rubric-repertorisation indicate that the constitutional remedy has a vested psychological, delusional interest in suppression and denial. If the patient displays evidence of disproportionate disturbance and contradictions this will often be an indication of future pathologies which the homoeopath must be able to identify and predict in the treatment.

The constitutional remedy profiles which contain inconsistencies indicate that the patient will have a vested interest in maintaining their illness. Pathology has its foundation in delusional disturbance. This is acknowledged in the modalities of psychiatry and homoeopathy.

The homoeopath must be aware of the patient's destructive need to maintain their illness. Under every self-delusion is a specific need to maintain the denial. Homoeopaths need psychological foresight to unravel the various processes of psychological denial. If we develop this foresight, it not only helps us to understand the development or causation within the constitutional remedy, it also helps in the management of the patient. For example, *Thuja* will alternate between denial of their helplessness, *Delusion* rubric: *I am powerful*, and delusional existential doom, *Delusion* rubric: *she can no longer exist. Thuja* will stop taking the homoeopathic remedy and stop consultations because they believe they are so *powerful* that they do not believe they need the homoeopathic treatment.

Example of inconsistencies:

1. Denial: *Delusion* rubric: *power: all-powerful; she is*: thuj.
   Versus

5. Resignation: *Delusion* rubric: *existence: longer; she cannot
    exist any:* thuj. [1] 1.

If a patient has 'delusions of grandeur' their belief and reliance on
homoeopathic treatment will be compromised if the homoeopath does
not recognize the pretensions and pitfalls of the inconsistencies in
the remedy profile. Self-delusion is maintained because the patient
cannot psychologically acknowledge reality. It is important in the case-
management and case analysis to fully understand the exact nature of
the psychodynamic crisis your patient needs to protect. The homoeopath
has to protect the denial process of their patient until the simillimum has
lifted the need to maintain the self-delusion. This is the responsibility that
all homoeopaths need to acknowledge; this responsibility can only come
about through understanding the meaning of homoeopathic psychiatry.

Delusion Rubrics in Denial

In this section I analyze and explain the meaning of each individual *Delusion* rubric. I offer previously unexplored explanations of the psychological delusional state inherent in each *Delusion* rubric. Furthermore, I explain their psychotherapeutic meaning and application by analyzing how each remedy listed under the rubric heading has utilized the delusional stance to its advantage. The reasons why each constitutional remedy is listed under a rubric will often be vastly different. Understanding the need for the psychological delusions within each of the constitutional remedy profiles will aid in remedy recognition.

Each selection of *Delusion* rubrics discussed are shaded. Analyses of the remedy profiles follow each sub-section. The psychological development of *Delusion* rubrics for each constitutional remedy profile is analyzed according to either **avoidance** or **self-deluding** need.

- *Delusions: Christ, himself to be*: cann-i. **VERAT.**
- *Delusions: God: communication with God; he is in*: chord-umb. olib-sac. psil. stram. thres-a. verat.
- *Delusions: God: messenger from God; he is a*: verat. [1] 1.
- *Delusions: heaven: is in; talking with God*: verat. [1] 1.
- *Delusions: heaven, is in*: calc-ar. cann-i. hydrog. op. *Verat.*
- *Delusions: eternity: he was in*: cann-i. [1] 1.
- *Delusions: God: presence of God; he is in the*: hydrog. [1] 1.

- *Delusions*: *God*: *sees God*: aether. ol-eur.
- *Delusions*: *divine, being*: cann-i. glon. ignis-alc. stram.
- *Delusions*: *Iris*: *being the goddess*: irid-met. [1] 1.
- *Delusions*: *Mary*: *Virgin*: *she is*: cann-i. stram. verat.
- *Delusions*: *prince, he is a*: verat. [1] 1.
- *Delusions*: *queen, she is a*: cann-i. olib-sac. oncor-t.
- *Delusions*: *emperor*: *is an*: cann-i. [1] 1.
- *Delusions*: *spirit, he is a*: cann-i. ignis-alc.
- *Delusions*: *lifted; she was being*: ozone. plut-n.
- *Delusions*: *transparent*: *he is*: anh. bell. cann-i. falco-pe. urol-h.
- *Delusions*: *superhuman; is*: cann-i. ignis-alc. psil.
- *Delusions*: *power*: *all-powerful; she is*: adam. cann-i. thuj. verat.
- *Delusions*: *born into the world*; *he was newly*: cori-r. lac-h. olib-sac. plut-n.
- *Delusions*: *beautiful*: anh. bell. *Cann-i*. coca *Lach*. op. petr-ra. positr. *Sulph*. taosc.
- *Delusions*: *delightful*: *she is or wants to be delightful*: stram. [1] 1.
- *Delusions*: *beautiful*: *she is beautiful and wants to be*: stram.[1] 1.
- *Delusions*: *angels, seeing*: aether cann-i. irid-met. olib-sac. stram.
- *Delusions*: *choir; he is in a cathedral on hearing music of a*: cann-i. [1] 1.
- *Delusions*: *bewitched, he is*: cann-i. loxo-recl. rhus-t.
- *Delusions*: *cathedral; he is in a*: *choirs; on hearing*: cann-i. [1] 1.
- *Delusions*: *creative power; has*: agath-a. cann-i. ignis-alc. psil.
- *Delusions*: *cathedral; he is in a*: olib-sac. [1] 1.
- *Delusions*: *nun; she is a*: olib-sac. [1] 1.
- *Delusions*: *consciousness*: *higher consciousness; unification with*: hydrog. podo.
- *Delusions*: *religious*: alum-sil. *Anac*. *Ars*. aur. bell. croc. *Hyos*. *Kali-br*. lach. lyc. med. merc. nux-v. olib-sac. plat. *Puls*. *Stram*. *Sulph*. tarent. *Verat*.

Self-Deluding: Megalomaniacal righteousness and the belief that 'God is on your side', or psychological delusions that one is God, help allay underlying fears and doubts about one's safety in the world. Each constitutional remedy will need God in order to avoid a different psychological delusion, and each remedy in their own *peculiar* way will believe they are divinely blessed. If the delusion is self-deluding it is hidden from oneself and protected and maintained because the patient *needs* to hide from reality. I discuss *Cannabis indica, Hydrogenium, Olibanum sacrum, Stramonium* and *Veratrum album. Cannabis indica* need to believe they are a heavenly queen in a beautiful cathedral listening to choirs of angels because they suffer from 'delusions of annihilation'. Conversely, *Hydrogenium* desire death so they can be merged with God in a higher consciousness. *Olibanum sacrum* need to believe they are in communication with God because when they are ill and dying they are fearful that they will not find peace and beauty in death. *Stramonium* need the intervention of a higher power because they suffer from psychosomatic illusions and delusions that their own body is dismembered. *Veratrum album* use their belief that 'God is on their side', to protect themselves. Underlying their righteousness is fear of God's vengeance. Of all the *Delusion* rubrics listed above, the one *Delusion* rubric: *religious,* is the most important rubric to understand. It is one of the most important rubrics to understand because the need for religion becomes paramount when one is facing disease and death. I am yet to experience a dying patient who has not needed to either find God or find peace within a spiritual practice. (My intention is to relay my experience only. I acknowledge that atheists believe that when faced with death they will not need to believe in any other heavenly realm. I have not treated any dying atheists.) Religiosity can take the form of conventional religious practices or 'New-Age positive thinking', or Eastern meditative practices. The reference to God is synonymous and applicable to all religions and all personifications of God. God can refer to Buddha, Jesus or Mohammed, to name just a few. It is important to note here that I am not attacking the need, or the validity of the need, for religion or any meditative practice. The *Delusion* rubric: *religious* is specifically and only, used in case analysis if there is a notable *disproportionate* need to use religious faith to deny disease and death. If there is *not* a notable *disproportionate* need to use religious faith then the homoeopath should use the *Mind* rubric: *religious affections* in the rubric-repertorisation. Psychological delusions of religiosity are a form of 'delusion of hubristic denial' because they allow the patient to believe that God will save them from their disease or death. Religiosity or spirituality allows the patient to believe that God or their 'spiritual practice' will annul their sins, or in the case of Eastern religions, 'clear their karma'. I have placed denial of illness amongst the rubrics of communication with God because the first stage of denial for a sick patient will be righteous religiosity which vindicates, and annuls them of, their sins. Conversely, each remedy profile listed in the *Delusion* rubric: *religious*, can become obsessed with the sins they have committed. If your patient believes that they truly deserve their illness and this is why they are sick, then they are delusional and representative of the *Delusion* rubrics of having sinned and committed a crime. The remedies listed in the *Delusion* rubric: *religious* each have a tendency to self-persecution. Self-persecution is commonly referred to as psychological 'delusions of original sin'. 'Delusions of original sin' will always be the reason for avoidance which fuels the need for all delusional religious 'inspirational ideologies'. If your patient *obsessively* needs to find God before they die (whether it be within Eastern meditation practices, or within the confessional) then the simillimum will be one of the remedies listed in this *Delusion* rubric. Underlying the need for religion will be a need for absolution[10]. This is why it is so important to allow your patient to tell you why they have become sick. I have dedicated the Causation chapter to psychological 'delusions of original sin' because disproportionate guilt and self-blame is often the causation of psychological disturbance.

Cannabis indica is a homoeopathic remedy derived from the drug Cannabis sativa *var. indica*. The constitutional remedy profile of *Cannabis indica* is synonymous with the hallucinations of hubristic grandeur commonly associated with the consumption of the drug hashish.

Cannabis indica delight in their belief in their omnipotence.

They believe they are a heavenly queen in a beautiful cathedral listening to choirs of angels. Consumers of Cannabis often tell me that the reason they smoke Cannabis is to feel elevated above their worldly troubles. *Cannabis indica* have the *Delusion* rubric: *transferred to another world.* [1] 1. *Cannabis indica need* to believe they are in another world listening to angels singing in a cathedral whilst they are surrounded by friends. *Cannabis indica* need to create an omnipotent belief in their own greatness because they have stark inconsistencies between their hubristic grandeur and their psychological delusions of disease and death. Underneath denial are the over-exaggerated, hyper-vigilant fears and predictions of being forsaken and abandoned. If there are stark inconsistencies between Stage one ('delusions of grandeur') and the other Stages (two to five) then the psychological 'delusions of grandeur' or 'hubristic denial' are maintained to protect themselves from annihilation from external or internal sources. *Cannabis indica* have 'delusions of persecution'. They believe they will be *murdered.* In the repertory there are numerous *Delusion* rubrics pertaining to fears: *murdered, surrounded by enemies, strangers, watched, pursued by the devil, criminals,* and *enemies, haunted by specters, ghosts and spirits, insulted, persecuted, criticized, betrayed, threatened, deceived, poisoned,* and *choked.* These *Delusion* rubrics should not be interpreted literally. The homoeopath should not expect that a patient will literally say that someone is going to murder them. These rubrics are applicable to any case analysis in which the patient displays psychological 'delusions of persecution'. 'Delusions of persecution', or a 'persecution complex', are a delusional belief that others are pursuing you in order to harm you. 'Delusions of persecution' can be applicable in case analysis for all incorrect perceptions and imaginings that someone is going to embarrass you or cause you embarrassment in society. 'Delusions of persecution' are imaginary rejections and over-exaggerated imaginings of abandonment. A patient who pre-empts real or perceived rejection or abandonment and responds to this incorrect perception by either aggressive behavior or self-imposed exile is suffering a 'persecution complex'. 'Delusions of abandonment' can be a precursor to, or the cause of, paranoiac 'delusions of persecution'. *Cannabis indica* need to allay their fear of being *annihilated* and *psychically carried down a maelstrom*. *Cannabis indica* have the *Delusion* rubric: *existence without form in space*. [1] 1.

Cannabis indica maintain their delusional grandeur to avoid feeling abandoned and alone in this world without a form and without the right to an existence.

Cannabis indica also suffer from 'delusions of deprivation'. They fear they will be left penniless in *rags*, abandoned on a *bier*, left without any existence of great importance. The rubric-repertorisation for *Cannabis indica* is good to do because it will indicate the underlying motivations behind their need to believe that they are a great person of notoriety. Underneath the acknowledgment of being forsaken is disproportionate guilt for sins committed.

Cannabis indica also delude themselves they are God to cover up their fears of being internally undermined by their own fears that they are aligned to the devil. *Cannabis indica* have the *Delusion* rubric: *he is the devil*.

Following acknowledgment of disproportionate guilt are psychological delusions of self-destructive depression and predictions of failure.

Cannabis indica fear they will not be important and successful [*diminished*].

Their belief in their own omnipotence will become extremely important if they have to face the reality that they are sick. *Cannabis indica* will have contradictory responses if they have to face illness. On the one hand they can believe they are so great that they cannot possibly die: – *Delusion* rubric: *body covers the whole earth.* On the other hand they can sink into over-exaggerated fears of being *annihilated* and *diminished* by their disease. *Cannabis indica* have 'delusions of impending doom' and 'delusions of hypochondria'. *Cannabis indica* have the *Delusion* rubric: *he is dying.* I have noticed in patients who smoke Cannabis regularly that they are more likely to become depressed and anxious about their health. I have also noticed in patients who smoke Cannabis regularly that they are more likely to be in denial about how bad their health is.

1. Denial: *Delusion* rubric: *body: covers: earth; covers the whole*: cann-i. [1] 1.

   Versus

5. Resignation: *Delusion rubric: existence: own existence; he doubted his*: cann-i. [1] 1.

1. Denial: *Delusion* rubric: *divine, being*: cann-i. *Delusion* rubric: *great person, is a: Cann-i. Delusion* rubric: *heaven, is in*: cann-i. *Delusion* rubric: *knowledge; he possesses infinite*: cann-i. *Delusion* rubric: *transferred: world, to another* :cann-i. [1] 1. *Delusion* rubric: *argument, making an eloquent*: cann-i. [1] 1. *Delusion* rubric: *body: covers: earth; covers the whole*: cann-i. [1] 1. *Delusion* rubric: *body: greatness of, as to: Cann-i. Delusion* rubric: *commander; being a*: cann-i. *Delusion* rubric: *friend: surrounded by friends; being*: cann-i. *Delusion* rubric: *journey; he is on a*: cann-i. *Delusion* rubric: *opiate: influence of an opiate; he were under the*: cann-i.

2. Forsaken: *Delusion* rubric: *want: they had come to*: cann-i.
    Delusion rubric: *clothes: rags; is clad in: Cann-i.* [2] 1.
    Delusion rubric: *bier, is lying on a*: cann-i. *Delusion* rubric:
    forsaken; is: cann-i. *Delusion* rubric: *existence: without
    form in vast space*: cann-i. [1] 1. *Delusion* rubric: *murdered:
    will be murdered; he: bribed to murder him; persons are*:
    cann-i. [1] 1. *Delusion* rubric: *injury: about to receive injury;
    is*: cann-i.
3. Causation: *Delusion* rubric: *devil: he is a devil*: cann-i.
    Delusion rubric: *hell: in; is*: cann-i.
4. Depression: *Delusion* rubric: *annihilation; about to sink into*:
    cann-i. *Delusion* rubric: *diminished: all is*: cann-i. *Delusion*
    rubric: *bier, is lying on a*: cann-i. [This rubric can pertain
    to suffering or can allude to feelings of deprivation and
    abandonment.] *Delusion* rubric: *existence: own existence;
    he doubted his*: cann-i. [1] 1. [This rubric can pertain to
    depression of fear of death.]
5. Resignation: *Delusion* rubric: *dead; he himself was*: cann-i.
    Delusion rubric: *maelstrom; carried down a psychical*:
    cann-i. [1] 1. *Delusion* rubric: *dying: he is*: cann-i. *Delusion*
    rubric: *dissected, he will be*: cann-i. [1] 1. *Delusion* rubric:
    existence: own existence; he doubted his: cann-i. [1] 1.

Hydrogenium find it difficult to live on the worldly plane.

Hydrogenium have the *Delusion* rubric: *separated from the world* because they choose to live in the presence of God, united with a higher consciousness.

Hydrogenium experience a psychological delusional conflict between their higher consciousness of God and their existence in the world. *Hydrogenium* have the *Mind* rubrics: *conflict between higher consciousness and worldly existence* and *confusion of mind as to his personal boundaries and identity*. *Hydrogenium* have the *Delusion* rubric: *body is separated from soul*. *Hydrogenium* have separated themselves from their own psyche. They have 'nihilistic delusions'. A 'nihilistic delusion' is the delusion that everything, including the self, does not exist, and that everything outside of the self is also unreal. *Hydrogenium* have the *Mind* rubric: *depersonalization*, and the *Delusion* rubrics: *everything seems unreal, out of body* and *all is diminished*. *Hydrogenium* have the *Delusion* rubric: *everything seems unreal*, because they believe that the world does not exist and that they do not exist in the world. *Hydrogenium* have the *Delusion* rubric: *energy moving around in the air*. [1] 1.

Hydrogenium will not come down to earth and acknowledge they are sick. If your patient is *not* in denial about being sick then the simillimum can't be Hydrogenium.

Hydrogenium have the *Mind* rubric: *vacancy of thoughts*, and the *Mind* rubric: *sensation of death*, because they nihilistically abandon their own somatic body. *Hydrogenium* desire death so they can be merged with God in a higher consciousness.

1. Denial: *Delusion* rubric: *God: presence of God; he is in the*: hydrog: [1] 1. *Delusion* rubric: *consciousness: higher consciousness; unification with*: hydrog. [1] 2. *Delusion* rubric: *beautiful: thinks look*: hydrog. *Delusion* rubric: *heaven, is in*: hydrog. *Delusion* rubric: *enlarged*: hydrog. *Delusion* rubric: *energy: air, moving around in the*: hydrog. [1] 1. *Delusion* rubric: *separated: body: soul; body is separated from*: Hydrog.

2. Forsaken: *Delusion* rubric: *separated: world; from the*: *he is separated*: **HYDROG**. *Delusion* rubric: *repudiated; he is*: *society; by*: hydrog. [1] 1. *Delusion* rubric: *despised; is*: hydrog. *Delusion* rubric: *insane: people think him being insane*: hydrog.

3. Causation: *Delusion* rubric: *frightening others; that she is*: hydrog. [1] 1.

4. Depression: *Delusion* rubric: *hell: in; is*: hydrog. *Delusion* rubric: *insane: become insane; one will*: hydrog. *Delusion* rubric: *unreal: everything seems unreal*: hydrog.

5. Resignation: *Delusion* rubric: *diminished*: *all is*: hydrog.
    [I have allocated this rubric to this section because
    Hydrogenium have the 'nihilistic delusion' that their somatic
    body does not exist.] *Delusion* rubric: *body*: *out of the body*:
    Hydrog.

Olibanum sacrum is a homoeopathic remedy derived
from frankincense[11]. *Olibanum sacrum* have exchanged their
soul for beauty – *Delusion* rubric: *soul was exchanged*. *Olibanum
sacrum* are the only remedy listed in the *Mind* rubric: *sensation
of beauty of the soul, beautiful things*. *Olibanum sacrum* need
to communicate with God to allay their guilt for needing position
and power and beauty. *Olibanum sacrum* are the only remedy
listed in the *Mind* rubrics: *desire for seduction*, and *imaginary
love for a person*. *Olibanum sacrum* are in love with God.

Olibanum sacrum have the theme that they are a gift *from* God and a gift
to God.

Olibanum sacrum have the *Delusion* rubric: *he was newly
born into the world*. *Olibanum sacrum* perceive that they are
pure [*she is a nun*] and as yet untouched by the world. They
feel responsible for any lack of harmony and they believe
they are dutifully bound to bring harmony and peace to man.
Olibanum sacrum are the only remedy listed in the *Delusion*
rubric: *restlessness with anxiety*. *Olibanum sacrum* are also
the only remedy listed in the *Mind* rubric: *anger about disorder*.
Communication with God brings peace, order and a heightened
awareness of meditative beauty which they crave. *Olibanum
sacrum* have psychological 'delusions of original sin' in relation
to only one sin: that their soul was exchanged for the ability to
be in communication with God. God is synonymous with power
and beauty – *Delusion* rubric: *she is a queen*. God is also
synonymous with religious power and religious responsibility –
Delusion rubric: *she is a nun*.

When *Olibanum sacrum* are ill and dying they are fearful that they will not
find peace and beauty in death. They fear being trapped [*she is a prisoner*]
and divided between heaven and earth.

1. Denial: *Delusion* rubric: *God: communication with God; he is in*: olib-sac. *Delusion* rubric: *queen, she is a*: olib-sac. *Delusion* rubric: *religious*: olib-sac. *Delusion* rubric: *nun; she is a*: olib-sac. [1] 1. *Delusion* rubric: *cathedral; he is in a*: olib-sac. [1] 1. *Delusion* rubric: *apparition; he would see an*: olib-sac. *Delusion* rubric: *flying: church; in the*: olib-sac. [1] 1. *Delusion* rubric: *convent, she will have to go to a*: olib-sac. *Delusion* rubric: *born into the world; he was newly*: olib-sac. *Delusion* rubric: *clothes*: beautiful; clothes are: olib-sac. *Delusion* rubric: *apparition; he would see an*: olib-sac. [1] 2. [brom] *Delusion* rubric: *visions, has: grandeur, of magnificent*: olib-sac.

2. Forsaken: *Delusion* rubric: *misunderstood; she is*: olib-sac. *Delusion* rubric: *watched, she is being*: olib-sac. [This rubric (in relation to *Olibanum sacrum*) can pertain to persecutory fears or the desire to be admired and be allocated into 'delusions of grandeur'.]

3. Causation: *Delusion* rubric: *soul: exchanged; was:* olib-sac. [1] 1.

4. Depression: *Delusion* rubric: *danger, impression of*: olib-sac. *Delusion* rubric: *prisoner; she is*: olib-sac. *Delusion* rubric: *restlessness with anxiety*: olib-sac. [1] 1. *Delusion* rubric: *drugged; as if*: olib-sac. *Delusion* rubric: *dirty: he is*: olib-sac. [*Olibanum sacrum* get depressed if they are not dressed magnificently.]

5. Resignation: *Delusion* rubric: *dissolving, she is*: olib-sac. *Delusion* rubric: *body: divided, is*: olib-sac. *Delusion* rubric: *body: lighter than air, body is*: olib-sac. *Delusion* rubric: *old: feels old*: olib-sac.

Stramonium need to align themselves with God to allay their overwhelming fears of being attacked. *Stramonium* have numerous 'delusions of persecution'. *Stramonium* believe they are going to be attacked by people or by a multitude of animals. They also believe they are going to be attacked from within, by the devil and the darkness of their own unstable mind.

Stramonium believe they will be saved from their illness and death by the intervention of a higher power. *Stramonium* need to believe they have power over all disease to allay their often irrational and disproportionate fear that they are about to die. If your patient is not fearful about their disease attacking them and consuming their whole psyche then the simillimum is not *Stramonium.*

Stramonium have a conflict between themselves and the world. Neurotic psychoses or mental derangements stem from a conflict between the 'ego' and the external world. The *Delusion* rubrics which cover psychoses are the *Delusion* rubrics: forsaken, depression and resignation. These *Delusion* rubrics emphasize the threat that the world poses to the self or 'ego'. They encompass respectively, the 'delusions of abandonment', 'delusions of persecution', 'delusions of impending doom' and the 'delusions of hypochondria'. *Stramonium* are consumed with internal neurotic psychoses and mental derangement. *Stramonium* have the *Delusion* rubric: *he is God, then he is the devil.* [3] 1. 'Transference neurosis' is a conflict between the rational and realistic 'ego' and the unconscious somatically driven 'id'. A neurosis is an inability to have a rational or realistic, objective view of one's life. Transference is characterized by unconscious self-deluding denial which allows for the redirection of feelings on to another person. 'Transference neuroses' are found in the *Delusion* rubrics of 'hubristic denial' in which the patient transfers 'cause and effect' on to God or their own 'delusions of grandeur'. These are the *Delusion* rubrics: *in communication with God.* 'Transference neuroses' are also found in the *Delusion* rubrics of sin in which the patient transfers 'cause and effect' on to the devil. These are the *Delusion* rubrics: *in communication with the devil. Stramonium* transfer their neuroses on to God and the devil. This is why *Stramonium* have the *Delusion* rubric: *he is God, then he is the devil.* [3] 1.

Stramonium have internal conflict and fear of themselves as well as conflict with the outer world.

This is why they have so many 'delusions of abandonment', 'delusions of persecution', 'delusions of impending doom', and 'delusions of hypochondria'. When *Stramonium* are sick they are terrified. *Stramonium* need their *communication with God* to allay their all consuming deranged fears. *Stramonium* have the *Mind* rubric: *religious affections, wants to read the bible all day*. When a patient first finds out that they have a life threatening disease, it is common for them to be consumed with overwhelming fears about the loss of their own life. It is also common for them to turn to God or religious practices to save them. Sankaran, in *The Soul of Remedies,* writes that *Stramonium* "is a remedy that tends to be over-prescribed because it deals with one of the most basic fears of man, the feeling of being left alone in the wilderness." Feeling alone and abandoned and thinking that no one else can understand how you feel is a normal response to loss of health. Given that *Stramonium* have numerous 'delusions of abandonment', 'delusions of persecution', 'delusions of impending doom' and 'delusions of hypochondria', it would seem appropriate to discuss the remedy profile of *Stramonium* in the *Delusion* rubrics: forsaken, depression and resignation. The distinguishing *peculiarity* specific to *Stramonium* is that when *Stramonium* are sick they are also neurotic about their disease robbing them of their beauty. *Stramonium* have the *Delusion* rubrics: *she is beautiful and wants to be beautiful* [1] 1., and *poses as a statue to be admired.* [2] 1. *Stramonium* also have the *Delusion* rubric: *imaginary appearance at catches.* [3] 2.

The reason why *Stramonium* have so many *Delusion* rubrics pertaining to psychological delusions of dismemberment is that they are terrified of the destructive consequences that any disease will have on their body. *Stramonium* have the *Delusion* rubric: *body is cut through.* [2] 1. The most common presentations of anxiety and depressive disorders are somatic. *Stramonium* disproportionately exaggerate the physical effects of all illnesses. When sick they suffer from psychosomatic illusions and delusions that their own body is dismembered.

Stramonium are consumed with internal neurotic psychoses which they transfer on to God and the devil. The *Delusion* rubric: *he is God then he is the devil*, can be interpreted as a psychosomatic representation of the divide between the divine and the devil in the split *Stramonium*.

The simillimum will not be *Stramonium* unless the patient is terrified of themselves. *Stramonium* need to align themselves with God (or any spiritual practice) to feel safe.

If there is a contradiction between Stage one ('delusions of grandeur') and Stage five ('delusions of hypochondria') then there will always be evidence of neuroses.

1. Denial: *Delusion* rubric: *power. diseases; he had power of all*: *Stram*.

    Versus

5. Resignation: *Delusion rubric: disease: every disease; he has*: stram.

1. Denial: *Delusion* rubric: *God: communication with God; he is in*: stram. *Delusion* rubric: *religious*: *Stram*. *Delusion* rubric: *delightful: she is or wants to be delightful*: stram. [1] 1. *Delusion* rubric: *beautiful: she is beautiful and wants to be*: stram.[1] 1. *Delusion* rubric: *great person, is a*: stram. *Delusion* rubric: *pleasing delusions*: stram. *Delusion* rubric: *divine, being*: stram. *Delusion* rubric: *power. diseases; he had power of all*: *Stram*. [2] 1. *Delusion* rubric: *pure; she is*: stram. *Delusion* rubric: *influence; one is under a powerful*: *Stram*. [This rubric can pertain to God or the devil.]

2. Forsaken: *Delusion* rubric: *alone, being: wilderness; alone in a*: stram.[1] 1. *Delusion* rubric: *dogs: attack him*: **STRAM**. [3] 1. *Delusion* rubric: *specters, ghosts, spirits: pursued by, is*: stram. *Delusion* rubric: *animals: devoured by: being*: *Stram*. *Delusion* rubric: *animals: persons are animals*: stram. *Delusion* rubric: *bitten, will be*: stram. *Delusion* rubric: *creeping things; full of*: stram. [1] 1. *Delusion* rubric: *cockroaches swarmed about the room*: stram. *Delusion*

rubric: *cats*: *sees*: *Stram*. *Delusion* rubric: *devil*: *sees*: stram. *Delusion* rubric: *forsaken; is*: *Stram*. *Delusion* rubric: *suffocated; she will be*: *Stram*. *Delusion* rubric: *murdered*: *will be murdered; he*: *Stram*. *Delusion* rubric: *murdered*: *being murdered; he is*: *roasted and eaten; he was murdered*: stram. [1] 1. *Delusion* rubric: *persecuted*: *he is persecuted*: stram. *Delusion* rubric: *poisoned*: *he*: *has been*: stram. *Delusion* rubric: *wilderness; being in*: stram. [1] 1. *Delusion* rubric: *injury*: *being injured; is*: **STRAM**. *Delusion* rubric: *snakes*: *in and around her*: stram.

3. Causation: *Delusion* rubric: *devil*: *possessed of a devil; he is*: stram.

4. Depression: *Delusion* rubric: *inconsolable; being*: stram. [1] 1. *Delusion* rubric: *dark*: **STRAM**. *Delusion* rubric: *doomed, being*: stram. *Delusion* rubric: *fright*: *as if in a fright*: stram. *Delusion* rubric: *flight from objects*: *Stram*. [2] 1. *Delusion* rubric: *joy*: *nothing could give her any joy*: stram. [1] 1.

5. Resignation: *Delusion* rubric: *dead*: *he himself was*: stram. *Delusion* rubric: *disease*: *every disease; he has*: stram. *Delusion* rubric: *dying*: *he is*: stram. *Delusion* rubric: *sick*: *being*: stram. *Delusion* rubric: *body*: *cut through; he is*: *Stram*. [2] 1. *Delusion* rubric: *body*: *cut through; he is*: *two; in*: stram. *Delusion* rubric: *body*: *divided, is*: *Stram*. *Delusion* rubric: *body*: *parts*: *absent; parts of body are*: stram. *Delusion* rubric: *body*: *scattered about; body was*: stram.

Veratrum album use their belief that 'God is on their side' to protect themselves. Underlying their righteousness is fear of God's vengeance. *Veratrum album* have the opposing *Delusion* rubrics: *he is a messenger of God* versus *he has done wrong*. *Veratrum album* have the *Delusion* rubric: *hears the ringing of bells*. *Veratrum album* feel they are doomed to die. The *Veratrum album* (case) in the *Case Companion* to *Homoeopathic Psychiatry* would not seek treatment for her cancer because she saw the cancer as God's punishment and she did not dare go against God's retribution.

The simillimum will not be *Veratrum album* unless the patient believes that they are God-like or that they are in contact with divine God-like energy. The hardest issue to tackle in *Veratrum album* is their belief in God's punishment. The hardest issue to tackle in *Veratrum album* is also their belief in their God-like status. *Veratrum album* will not trust or work with the homoeopath unless they believe that the homoeopathic practitioner is in contact with 'divine energy' which is able to guide their prescription.

1. Denial: *Delusion* rubric: *God: communication with God; he is in*: verat. *Delusion* rubric: *God: messenger from God; he is a*: verat. [1] 1. *Delusion* rubric: *religious*: Verat. *Delusion* rubric: *Christ, himself to be*: **VERAT**. *Delusion* rubric: *Mary; Virgin: she is*: verat. *Delusion* rubric: *heaven: is in; talking with God*: verat. [1] 1. *Delusion* rubric: *distinguished; he is*: verat. *Delusion* rubric: *vow: keep it, must*: verat. [1] 1.

2. Forsaken: *Delusion* rubric: *home: away from home; he is*: verat. *Delusion* rubric: *enemy: surrounded by enemies*: verat. *Delusion* rubric: *murdered: will be murdered; he*: verat. *Delusion* rubric: *persecuted: he is persecuted*: verat. *Delusion* rubric: *pursued; he was*: verat.

3. Causation: *Delusion* rubric: *criminal, he is a*: verat. *Delusion* rubric: *wrong: done wrong; he has*: verat.

4. Depression: *Delusion* rubric: *doomed, being*: Verat. *Delusion* rubric: *misfortune: approaching; as if some misfortune were*: Verat. *Delusion* rubric: *misfortune: inconsolable over imagined misfortune*: Verat. [2] 2. [calc-s.] *Delusion* rubric: *unfortunate, he is*: verat. *Delusion* rubric: *ruined: is ruined; he*: verat.

5. Resignation: *Delusion* rubric: *disease: deaf, dumb and has cancer; he is*: verat. [1] 1. *Delusion* rubric: *die: about to die; one was*: verat. *Delusion* rubric: *cancer, has a*: verat. *Delusion* rubric: *sick: being*: verat. *Delusion* rubric: *bells; hears ringing of*: verat. [This rubric is reminiscent of saying 'the bell tolls for thee'.]

- *Delusions*: *visions, has*: absin. agar. alum-sil. alum. ambr. anac. anh. antip. arg-n. arn. *Ars.* atro-s. *Atro.* aur. **BELL.** borx. calc-ar. *Calc-s. Calc.* camph. **CANN-I.** cann-s. cann-xyz. canth. carb-an. carb-v. carbn-o. *Carbn-s.* carc. caust. cench. cham. chlol. chlorpr. cic. cimic. *Cina.* cocain. coff. con. convo-s. cortico. *Crot-c.* dig. dros. dulc. graph. hell. *Hep.* hippoc-k. *Hyos.* kali-br. kali-c. *Lach.* lact. lyc. mag-m. mag-s. merc. methys. *Morph.* naja. nat-c. *Nat-m.* nat-sal. nit-ac. nux-m. *Nux-v.* olib-sac. olnd. *Op.* orot-ac. past. *Ph-ac.* phos. plat. psil. *Puls.* rhod. rhus-t. sanguis-s. santin. sec. sep. *Sil.* spong. *Stram. Sulph.* tarent. ther. valer. verat.

- *Delusions*: *fancy, illusions of*: Acon. Aeth. agar. alum-sil. alum. am-c. *Ambr.* anac. ang. anh. ant-c. ant-t. apis. arn. ars-i. *Ars.* aur-ar. aur-s. *Aur.* bar-c. bar-i. *Bell.* berb. bism. bit-ar. bry. bufo bufo-s. calc-ar. calc-p. calc-sil. calc. camph. **CANN-I.** cann-s. *Cann-xyz.* canth. carb-an. carb-v. carbn-s. caust. cham. chin. chinin-ar. chinin-s. cic. *Cina Cocc.* coff. colch. coloc. con. croc. *Crot-c.* cupr. cycl. dig. dros. dulc. euphr. *Fl-ac.* graph. hell. hep. **HYOS. IGN.** indg. iod. kali-ar. *Kali-br.* kali-c. *Kali-p.* kali-sil. lac-c. **LACH.** lact. *Laur.* led. lyc. *Lyss.* mag-c. *Mag-m.* mag-s. *Merc.* nat-c. nat-m. *Nit-ac. Nux-m.* nux-v. olib-sac. olnd. *Op.* par. petr. *Ph-ac.* phos. *Plat.* plb. positr. psil. puls. rheum rhod. *Rhus-t. Sabad.* samb. sec. sep. sil. spong. stann. *Staph.* **STRAM.** sul-ac. sul-i. **SULPH.** *Tarent.* thuj. valer. verat. verb. viol-o. visc. zinc-p. zinc.

- *Delusions*: *pleasing delusions*: aeth. atro. cann-i. nitro-o. op. phos. psil. stram.

- *Delusions*: *visions, has*: *beautiful*: bell. *Cann-i.* coca. lac-c. lach. olib-sac. olnd. **OP.** psil.

- *Delusions*: *visions, has*: *grandeur, of magnificent*: cann-i. carbn-s. coff-t. coff. olib-sac.

- *Delusions*: *visions, has*: *power, of imaginary*: cann-i. psil.

- *Delusions*: *visions, has*: *wonderful*: anh. calc. camph. cann-i. lach. oxal-a. psil.

- *Delusions*: *visions, has*: *fantastic*: ambr. arn. ars.. bell. *Chlol.* hyos. lach. nit-ac. op. psil. stram. verat.

Self-deluding: If a patient suffering from an incurable disease tells you in a consultation that their grandmother visited them in a dream and told them, "everything will work out for the best and not to worry because they will become well", this should be repertorised as the *Delusion* rubric: *has visions*. The *Delusion* rubric: *illusions of fancy*, alludes to a patient's belief that if they create positive visions of being well in their meditation practices then their visions will manifest in real life. The patient's symptom should be acknowledged in the case analysis as evidence of a psychological need for denial. Each remedy will have and need the visions, and create the visions, for vastly different reasons.

The *Delusion* rubric: *illusions of fancy*, alludes to the ability to be able to side-step tragedies. In modern-day 'New-Age language' this *Delusion* rubric is code for having a 'positive take on things'.

It is a *Delusion* rubric which I commonly use for patients who side-step or refuse to acknowledge the gravity of their illness by continually needing to look at the 'lesson' they will learn from their 'experience' of being sick and dying. **The obsessive need to always feel positive and have a 'positive take' on every situation is a denial of grief as well as a 'hubristic denial' which helps the patient feel like they are in total control of the situation.** The *Delusion* rubric: *illusions of fancy* alludes to the need to create in one's fantasy a grander vision of the world which one aspires to, i.e. one's ideal world. (Their need for inspirational hope can be emotionally driven, intellectually driven, or politically driven.) A patient who is suffering from *illusions of fancy* is someone who has grand visions of persona; their expectations of what they can achieve are idealistic and often unrealistic. The *Delusion* rubric: *illusions of fancy* should be used in case-repertorisation for the patient who believes that they should be able to cure themselves.

Arnica suffer from persecutory illusions as well as fanciful illusions. The *Delusion* rubric: *illusions of fancy* alludes to the need to create in one's fantasy a grander vision of the world which one aspires to, i.e. one's ideal world. In the Introduction I outlined a simple rubric-repertorisation of the character of Lars, from the film *Lars and the Real Girl*. The character of Lars is a good example of psychological modeling being adopted because it is advantageous. Lars sets up a delusional relationship with a life-like plastic doll which he names Bianca. His underlying need for the delusion is based on his fears of the future loss of a real girlfriend because his own mother died giving birth to him. To avoid the loss of a real wife he has a relationship with a life-like plastic doll. With the help of a psychologist he is able to slowly unravel his need for the psychological delusion. He then allows the plastic doll to die so he can be released from the relationship and fall in love with a real girl. In the analysis of a *Delusion* rubric (in case-taking) you have to see and understand, within the case and within the nature of the constitutional remedy profile, why the patient needs the delusional state. Lars's psychological delusion is needed to avoid grief. The *Delusion* rubrics for Lars would be the following, to confirm the remedy *Arnica*.

- *Delusion* rubric: *fancy, illusions of.*
- *Delusion* rubric: *visions, has; fantastic.*
- *Mind* rubric: *fear: touched; of being.*
- *Skin* rubric: *coldness.*
- *Skin* rubric: *coldness; sensation, of.*
- *Delusion* rubric: *dead: persons, sees.*
- *Delusion* rubric: *die: about to die; one was.*

In taking Lars's case the above list of rubrics appear in the order in which they are revealed in the film. The first rubric, the *Delusion* rubric: *illusions of fancy*, is a psychological 'delusion of grandeur' which allow the patient who is suffering with grand visions of persona to create a vision of their expectation of their world. Lars's fanciful illusions allows him to imagine that the life-like plastic doll called Bianca is a real girlfriend. The next piece of information we find out about him is his fear of being touched. The patient needing *Arnica* is fearful of being approached, fearful of being touched, and their whole body is over-sensitive. Lars wears several layers of clothing to protect him from being touched. Lars experiences being touched as cold and physically painful, as well as being emotionally painful. *Arnica* have the *Mind* rubric: *fear of being touched* and the *Skin* rubric: *coldness on skin*. *Arnica* is a homoeopathic remedy commonly used to treat shock. The Lars character is a beautiful portrayal of the remedy *Arnica* and if Lars was my patient in a homoeopathic consultation I could surmise that he has been in emotional shock since his mother died giving birth to him. Although I would prescribe *Arnica* for shock, I would only prescribe it on the basis of the above five rubrics in the rubric-repertorisation. I would not assume anything about Lars being in shock about his mother's death until Lars tapped into his unconscious in the follow-up consultations and revealed that element in the case analysis. I would also repertorise the case systematically, chronologically compiling the above rubrics in the precise order in which they were revealed in the case-taking. This is case-development. The psychologist in the film did not uncover his unresolved grief about his mother's death or his overwhelming fear that a future real wife could die in childbirth until several consultations had occurred. *Arnica* also have the *Delusion* rubric: *one was about to die*, and *sees dead persons*, both of these rubrics reinforce his fear of having a real relationship with a real girl. If Lars gets close to someone, the psychological delusion is they could die; this is the meaning of the *Delusion* rubric: *he sees dead persons*. In a homoeopathic consultation the same process unfolds. It is not until the follow-up consultations that I compile all the rubrics or understand all of the patient's delusional needs for the *Delusion* rubrics attached to a particular remedy profile. Although I might surmise that Lars could have been in shock since his birth I would not use the *Delusion* rubrics: *one was about to die*, and *sees dead persons*, in the rubric-repertorisation until Lars revealed his fear of a real future wife dying in the case-taking.

Lars's *illusions of fancy*, enabled him to believe that the life-like plastic doll Bianca, was a real girlfriend, and although this was obviously a self-delusion it was also advantageous to him to be able to imagine his girlfriend Bianca was real. The profoundly touching aspect of the film is that everyone in his small town went along with his psychological delusion and did not confront or try to dispel his illusions. Psychological denial is adopted by the patient when they need to maintain their psychological delusion and illusion to avoid reality.

The simillimum will only be *Arnica* if the patient needs to create an illusionary fantasy to help them escape reality. *Arnica* need to rely upon their fanciful illusions because they are undermined by persecutory illusions of ill health and death.

If there are contradictions and inconsistencies between Stage one ('delusions of grandeur') and Stage five ('delusions of hypochondria') then the remedy profile will contain undermining illusionary and delusionary psychoses and neuroses. The simillimum will only be *Arnica* if the patient is undermined by their own persecutory illusions and delusions. *Arnica* suffer exaggerated persecutory fears and delusional beliefs that others are pursuing them in order to harm. *Arnica* also suffer exaggerated fear about diseases and obsessive fear that they are going to die. A psychosis is a severe mental derangement. The *Delusion* rubrics which cover psychoses are the *Delusion* rubrics: forsaken, depression and resignation. All these *Delusion* rubrics emphasize the threat that the world poses to the 'ego'. All these *Delusion* rubrics contain the 'delusions of abandonment', 'delusions of persecution', 'delusions of impending doom', and the 'delusions of hypochondria', in that order.

Arnica is a homoeopathic remedy which is commonly used for shock because inherent within the psychological profile is the need to dissociate from reality. *Arnica* have the *Delusion* rubric: *floating in air.*

The *Delusion* rubric: *lumps in bed* confirm the depth of their sensitivity. *Arnica* is a remedy which should be used for the patient who is suffering from dissociative trauma as a result of having experienced post traumatic stress disorder. The simillimum will only be *Arnica* if the patient presents with dissociative psychoses. The simillimum will only be *Arnica* if the patient presents with physical neuroses. Lars was terrified of being touched. This particular presentation will not be the specific for every *Arnica* case but the patient must show evidence of psychosomatic physical trauma. Freud analyzed a neurosis as a conflict between the 'ego' and the 'id'. Neuroses, relate to psychosomatic conditions, and psychosis, relate to mental conflict between the 'ego' and the external world.

The simillimum will only be *Arnica* if the patient presents with psychosomatic trauma. *Arnica* shroud themselves in psychosomatic neuroses as a way of protecting their psyche from coming in touch with the shock and trauma that they have experienced in the past. *Arnica* also envelop themselves in psychoses to protect themselves from the shock and trauma that they expect to experience in the future. The patient needing *Arnica* is fearful of being approached, fearful of being touched, and their whole body is over-sensitive, and over-reactive to all outside influences.

The 'never-well-since-event' in an *Arnica* case must contain evidence of emotional, mental, or physical, abuse or trauma. *Arnica* enshroud themselves in fanciful illusions in order to create a fantasy of a grander [*fantastic*] vision of an ideal world. The homoeopath working with an *Arnica* patient must have patience because the trauma is enshrouded in their unconscious traumatized past, and is not assessable to their subconscious or conscious mind. The action of the simillimum will slowly unravel the psychodynamic need to create and maintain their illusions and delusions. The action of the simillimum will slowly heal their traumatized psyche. The action of the simillimum will also slowly unravel their need to create and maintain their numerous psychosomatic neuroses.

As a consequence of having no 'delusions of original sin' or no concept of personal guilt or self-blame *Arnica* experience trauma more intensely than a lot of other remedy profiles. *Arnica* are often left feeling confused as to why they have been singled out for persecution.

1. Denial: *Delusion* rubric: *well, he is*: **ARN**.

   Versus

5. Resignation: *Delusion* rubric: *disease: incurable disease; he has an*: arn.

1. Denial: *Delusion* rubric: *visions, has*: arn. *Delusion* rubric: *visions, has: fantastic*: arn. *Delusion* rubric: *fancy, illusions of*: arn. *Delusion* rubric: *floating: air, in*: arn. *Delusion* rubric: *well, he is*: **ARN**.

2. Forsaken: *Delusion* rubric: *dead: persons, sees*: arn. *Delusion* rubric: *dead: corpse: mutilated corpse*: arn. *Delusion* rubric: *arrested, is about to be*: arn. *Delusion* rubric: *bed: lumps in bed*: arn. *Delusion* rubric: *images, phantoms; sees: frightful*: arn. *Delusion* rubric: *mutilated bodies; sees*: arn. *Delusion* rubric: *thieves: seeing*: arn. *Delusion* rubric: *churchyard: visits a*: arn. *Delusion* rubric: *objects; about: lean forward and about to fall; high places*: arn. [1] 1.

3. Causation: NONE.

4. Depression: *Delusion* rubric: *council; holding a*: arn. [1] 2. *Delusion* rubric: *succeed, he does everything wrong; he cannot*: arn. *Delusion* rubric: *objects; about: lean forward and about to fall; high places*: arn. [1] 1. [This rubric can pertain to predictions of failure or persecutory paranoia.]

5. Resignation: *Delusion* rubric: *disease: incurable disease; he has an*: arn. *Delusion* rubric: *die: about to die; one was*: arn. *Delusion* rubric: *heart: disease: going to have a heart disease and die; is*: arn.

   Arsenicum album suffer from 'delusions of hypochondria', and numerous 'delusions of persecution', and 'delusions of deprivation'. The illusions of *seeing accidents*, seeing *rats*, seeing *insects*, and *worms in the bed*, *teeth gnashing wild beasts around the bed* and *policeman coming into the house* are just a few of conspiracies against *Arsenicum album*. *Arsenicum album* suffer from a multitude of real and imagined hypochondriacally orientated fears which torment them especially if they feel financially insecure. They believe everything they touch is contaminated and their body will putrefy. *Arsenicum album* feel overwhelmed with fear of the day of atonement. *Arsenicum album* have the *Delusion* rubrics: *she is lost for salvation*, and *time has come to die*. Underlying their intense need to create another vision of reality is the fear that they have sinned away their day of grace. *Arsenicum album* have the *Delusion* rubric: *sees devil*.

When faced with disease and death *Arsenicum album* believe in and create *visions of fantastic* grandeur to overcome their crippling 'delusions of hypochondria'. *Arsenicum album* delude themselves with *fantastic visions* of wellness to help them cover up their exaggerated fears of persecution.

Within their *illusions of fancy Arsenicum album* create an obsessively perfected grand vision of their persona. *Arsenicum album* have the *Mind* rubrics: *anger about his mistakes, increased ambition to make money*, and *wanting elegance*. When they are sick *Arsenicum album* are crippled by the reality of disease because it threatens their need to create a perfected persona and perfect world. Psychoses are a conflict between the 'ego' and the external world. A psychosis is a severe mental derangement in which the patient believes that their psyche is under threat. The *Delusion* rubrics which cover psychoses are the *Delusion* rubrics: Forsaken, Depression and Resignation. These *Delusion* rubrics emphasize the threat that the world poses to the self or 'ego'. *Arsenicum album* need their grand visions of persona to cover up numerous 'delusions of hypochondria', 'delusions of persecution' and 'delusions of deprivation'. *Arsenicum album* suffer psychotic delusions of their own decaying body abandoning them, and of the world being full of creatures attacking them.

If a particular remedy profile is weighted heavily in persecution rubrics, as is the case with *Arsenicum album*, then they will need *religion* to protect them. *Arsenicum album* have the *Mind* rubric: *too occupied with religion*. It is important to note that 'religion' does not necessarily pertain to institutionalized religious practices. The most common religious practices that I have noted in *Arsenicum album* patients is the 'religion of alternative health practices'.

1. Denial: *Delusion* rubric: *visions, has: Ars*. *Delusion* rubric: *religious*: *Ars*. *Delusion* rubric: *well, he is*: ars. *Delusion* rubric: *visions, has: fantastic*: ars.

2. Forsaken: *Delusion* rubric: *conspiracies: against him; there are conspiracies*: ars. *Delusion* rubric: *starve: family will*: ars. *Delusion* rubric: *bed: drawn from under her, alighted on the floor, and she had*: ars. [1] 1. *Delusion* rubric: *faces, sees*: ars. *Delusion* rubric: *beetles, worms etc.*: ars. *Delusion* rubric: *faces, sees*: ars. *Delusion* rubric: *fire: visions of*: ars. *Delusion* rubric: *beetles, worms etc.*: ars. *Delusion* rubric: *worms: bed; are in*: ars. [1] 1. *Delusion* rubric: *insects, sees*: **ARS**. *Delusion* rubric: *bugs; sees: bed; crawling over*: ars. [1] 1. *Delusion* rubric: *noise: gnashing their teeth around his bed; hears wild beasts*: ars. [1] 1. *Delusion* rubric: *policeman: coming into house; he sees a policeman*: ars. *Delusion* rubric: *arrested, is about to be*: ars. *Delusion* rubric: *pursued; he was: enemies, by*: ars. *Delusion* rubric: *vermin: bed is covered with; his*: ars. [1] 1. *Delusion* rubric: *thieves: house, in: bed is full of thieves; and space under. Ars*. [2] 1.

3. Causation: *Delusion* rubric: *friend: offended; has*: ars. [1] 1. *Delusion* rubric: *wrong: done wrong; he has: Ars*. *Delusion* rubric: *sinned; one has: day of grace; sinned away his*: ars. *Delusion* rubric: *crime: committed a crime; he had*: ars.

4. Depression: *Delusion* rubric: *hang himself, wants to: Ars*. [2] 1. *Delusion* rubric: *suicide; impelled to commit*: ars. *Delusion* rubric: *doomed, being*: ars. *Delusion* rubric: *lost;*

she is: ars. *Delusion* rubric: *happy in his own house, he will never be*: ars. [1] 1.

5. Resignation: *Delusion* rubric: *dead*: *he himself was*: ars. *Delusion* rubric: *contaminated*: *everything one is touching is contaminated*: ars. *Delusion* rubric: *body*: *putrefy, will*: *Ars*. *Delusion* rubric: *sick*: *being*: *Ars*.

Calcarea silicata are only listed in one of the rubrics pertaining to 'delusions of grandeur' – *Delusion* rubric: *illusions of fancy*. A patient who is suffering with *illusions of fancy* is someone who has grand visions of persona: their expectations of what they can achieve, or what they *have* achieved, or who they are in the world, are over-exaggerated because they have a disproportionate idealistic need to exaggerate them. The psychodynamic consequence of *illusions of fancy* is that the patient will always be left wanting in their *own eyes*. They will always feel anxious. They will feel anxious about themselves and this in turn predisposes them to being easily undermined by others' opinions of them. The reason *Calcarea silicata* have so many rubrics pertaining to being haunted by ghosts and phantoms is that they feel unable to support themselves or defend themselves. *Calcarea silicata* have the *Delusion* rubrics: *sees horrible visions, images and phantoms,* and *sees dead people*. A homoeopathic practitioner will not have a *Calcarea silicata* patient come into a consultation and say that they are hearing or seeing dead people. *Calcarea silicata* will relay the following: *I am extremely anxious about what my friends say about me. I do not think I have any friends, I only have 250 friends on Facebook, how many do you have? I am sure they think I am stupid. What do you think about how I look? I don't think what I have done is any good. I am sure everyone is saying that they do not think I am as popular as others. I am often not sure that what I am doing is okay. I am scared about failing. Everyone else says that they are much smarter than me. I often talk to myself. Sometimes out loud, but most of the time in my head. I go over all the conversations that I have had,* *and that I am going to have beforehand to work out what to say.* A *Delusion* rubric is used in the case-repertorisation if, and when, you identify an over-exaggerated or disproportionate troubling issue for the patient.

Calcarea silicata need to look outside of themselves to be reassured.

Calcarea silicata have the *Mind* rubric: *desire to be magnetized.* The *Mind* rubric: *desire to be magnetized* means that the patient has a desire to surrender themselves to someone else's opinion. *Calcarea silicata* need and want to be influenced by the opinions of others. This need becomes predictably undermining for *Calcarea silicata* because it then means they are easily influenced by all around them. The negative consequences of surrendering your will to another is that it reinforces that you are unable to know your own truth. *Calcarea silicata* have the *Mind* rubrics: *loss of will power, yielding disposition,* and *mental insecurity.* If you identify a disproportionate element in the case it will be this psychodynamic trauma which will cause the patient to create a psychological delusion. *Calcarea silicata* need their *illusions of fancy* to deny how influenced they are by others' opinions.

If the *illusions of fancy* or grand visions of persona are in place then *Calcarea silicata* will believe in, and aspire to achieve, grandeur. If they do *not* achieve grandeur, they will feel easily undermined. *Calcarea silicata* fear that they will be abandoned by their family dying. *Calcarea silicata* have the *Delusion* rubric: *dead corpse of husband, brother,* or *child.* *Calcarea silicata* fear being forsaken by family because their psyche struggles to exist without the support of friends or family. *Calcarea silicata* undermine themselves by not supporting their opinions, therefore they need support from *talking to the dead. Calcarea silicata* have the *Mind* rubric: *reproaching oneself from trifles.* [1] 2. *Calcarea silicata* have a disproportionately high expectation of what they should achieve. If an expectation is *very* grand, it can become a self-fulfilling prophecy of doom or expected failure. Grand visions and *illusions of fancy* predispose the patient to suffering from anticipatory anxiety and insecurity. *Calcarea silicata* always desire things which they haven't got because they need to reinforce their *illusions of fancy*. *Calcarea silicata* also have the *Mind* rubric: *full of desires, things not present*. [1] 1. As soon as *Calcarea silicata* feel deprived or insecure they need to acquire more possessions of *fancy*.

Calcarea silicata have a unique defense mechanism: when anxious they refuse to listen to anyone. If you stubbornly refuse to listen to anyone, it immediately reinforces your belief in your own *illusions of fancy*. *Calcarea silicata* are the only remedy listed in the *Mind* rubric: *inclination to sit on the same place, looks into space and does not answer*. [1] 1. *Calcarea silicata* are also boldly listed in the *Delusion* rubric: *talking with dead people*. They only listen to dead people because they refuse to listen to the living. The theme of *Calcarea silicata* is: if I listen to your opinion or advice, it could prove that my *illusions of fancy* about what I have achieved are not correct. The theme of *Calcarea silicata* is insecurity and the need to find security inside themselves. *Calcarea silicata* need to only trust their own opinion. Their refusal to listen to advice is particularly notable when they are sick, or dying from an incurable disease. *Calcarea silicata* need to believe that if they listen to your opinion or advice then it could prove that they are not fully confident in their own *illusions of fancy*. For a *Delusion* rubric to be used you have to see within the remedy profile that the patient needs to maintain their avoidance of reality. Regardless of whether the psychological delusion has positive or negative consequences, it must be maintained because the patient believes the delusional stance is advantageous. A *Delusion* rubric should be used when you detect self-deceit and/or excuses which misrepresent reality. This is regardless of whether the misinterpretation of reality is positive or negative. If the homoeopathic practitioner understands why *Calcarea silicata* need to deny their need for help, the practitioner will be able to sensitively devise methods to make the patient feel more in control and empowered by being able to look after their health.

In the rubric-repertorisation, *Calcarea silicata* have no psychological 'delusions of original sin', no *Delusion* rubrics of aligning themselves to the devil, and no *Delusion* rubrics of having committed crimes or wrongs. Each remedy profile will be different but for *Calcarea silicata* the fact that they have no psychological delusions of being evil is indicative of their need to maintain their grand *illusions of fancy*. *Calcarea silicata* are extremely idealistic.

1. Denial: *Delusion* rubric: *fancy, illusions*: calc-sil. *Delusion* rubric: *voices: hearing*[12]: *answers; and*: calc-sil. *Delusion* rubric: *voices: hearing*: calc-sil. *Delusion* rubric: *faces, sees*: calc-sil.

2. Forsaken: *Delusion* rubric: *dead: corpse: husband, corpse of*: calc-sil. [1] 2. *Delusion* rubric: *dead: corpse: brother and child, corpse of*: calc-sil. [1] 3. *Delusion* rubric: *images, phantoms; sees*: calc-sil. *Delusion* rubric: *visions, has: horrible*: calc-sil. *Delusion* rubric: *dead: persons, sees*: calc-sil.

3. Causation: NONE.

4. Depression: *Delusion* rubric: *talking: dead people; with*: **CALC-SIL**.

5. Resignation: *Delusion* rubric: *disease: incurable disease; he has an*: calc-sil.

The above rubric-repertorisation highlights all the aspects of the need for security and protection within *Calcarea silicata* which Sankaran has emphasized in the quote below.

Sankaran, in *The Soul of Remedies* says, "Calcarea silicata is a salt and represents a combination of feelings of both Calcarea and Silicea. Like Calcarea the person feels insecure, with the need for protection and like Silicea he feels the need to maintain a particular standard. Hence the feeling of Calcarea silicata is: 'I need to keep up to a particular standard to get the security and protection I need'. The Calcarea silicata patient has a fear of poverty and so he has to be careful about spending money. Being poor puts him at a disadvantage. The need to maintain a certain standard gives Calcarea silicata its sensitivity to reprimands. This sensitivity to reprimands keeps him from confrontation and getting fired and hence maintains the standard that his superior sets for him. He also becomes timid, bashful, yielding, irresolute, hesitant, since this will help him. Also, he has a lot of anticipatory anxiety before exams, interviews, meeting people or before beginning a new job. When he comes to the doctor the patient has the fear of a serious disease, but subconsciously he uses this fear to do nothing. If he is told he has no problem he can get irritated ("Consolation aggravates"). He wants support but doesn't want to be told he has no problem. This sounds contradictory."

Cina: Underlying any contradictory behavior is an inner conflict with the self which is the basis or source of a psychological delusion. In understanding a remedy profile it is crucial to look at the psychological need and the psychological avoidances which fuel conflicting behavior. Cina have the Mind rubrics: *aversion to being carried,* and *desire to be carried.* On the one hand Cina have a desire to be carried, and on the other hand they have an aversion to being carried. The understanding which is crucial in a Cina case is the perversity of this contradiction. Cina have convulsions from being reprimanded or punished and this is the 'never-well-since-event', or the underlying psychological trigger to Cina needing to avoid intimacy. Cina have a fear of being approached. Cina have the Mind rubrics: *ailments from reproaches,* and *anxiety from being touched.* Cina also have physical convulsions from being scolded. Cina need to emphasize physical abandonment and exaggerate physical abuse because they suffer from self-disgust.

Underlying their capricious need for attention, and their immediate rejection of that attention, is a psychological need to avoid their self-disgust. *Cina* have the *Delusion* rubric: *body looks ugly*. For the remedy profile to be *Cina*, the patient must display body disgust.

Cina have the *Delusion* rubric: *has visions*. The belief that one is aligned with God is a hubristic vision of oneself. The next phase they sink into are psychological 'delusions of abandonment'. They believe that since they are sick no one will love them because they are *ugly*. Their ill health is subsequently turned in on themselves in the form of self-blame for being so bad. They then move into persecutory imaginings. *Cina* have the *Mind* rubric: *cannot bear to be looked at*, and the *Delusion* rubric: *seeing figures*. Finally, they capriciously reject help because they believe they will be harmed. *Cina* have the *Delusion* rubric: *about criminals*. *Cina* have the *Mind* rubric: *capriciousness, rejecting things he has been longing for*. It is advantageous for *Cina* to maintain their capriciousness because this is how they protect themselves from physical harm. These are the psychological avoidance techniques of *Cina*. Their hubristic vision of themselves indicates a need to separate themselves from others and align themselves with God. The *Delusion* rubric: *has visions*, can be interpreted as evidence of hubristic illusions or evidence of persecutory illusions. This understanding highlights the perversity of their need to maintain their capriciousness.

On the one hand they suffer from fears of persecutory attack from being helped or touched, and on the other hand they have illusions of hubristic visions of grandeur which fuel the need to capriciously reject all help because they are superior.

1. Denial: *Delusion* rubric: *visions, has*: *Cina*. *Delusion* rubric: *figures*: *seeing figures*: cina.

2. Forsaken: *Delusion* rubrics: *criminals, about:* cina. *Delusion* rubrics: *images, phantoms; sees, frightful:* cina. *Delusion* rubric: *figures*: *seeing figures*: cina. *Delusion*

rubric: *visions, has*: *Cina*. [The last two rubrics can indicate hubristic visions or persecutory visions.]

3. Causation: *Delusion* rubric: *crime*: *committed a crime; he had*: cina. *Delusion* rubric: *criminal, he is a*: cina. *Delusion* rubric: *wrong: done wrong; he has*: cina.

4. Depression: *Delusion* rubric: *body: ugly; body looks:* cina. [*Cina* are very depressed about body image.]

5. Resignation: *Delusion* rubric: *body: ugly; body looks:* cina.

All homoeopaths treating *Cina* need to understand that *Cina* have intense reactions to being reprimanded or punished; this is the 'never-well-since-event'.

Cina, because of their conflict over wanting to be carried and then feeling averse to being carried, will be capricious in their approach to treatment. *Cina* will deliberately stop taking the homoeopathic remedy. If you scold them for this they will have succeeded in setting you up and it will be the self-fulfilling prophecy of reprimand they were looking for. *Cina* have the *Mind* rubric: *easily offended*, because they need to protect themselves. They are emotionally fearful. It is crucial to predict these stages to protect *Cina*. If you use the five psychological steps in your case analysis as soon as you identify a remedy, you will immediately be able to predict and understand your patient's psychological denial and avoidance techniques. This is why homoeopathic psychiatry and understanding the *Delusion* rubrics will help you in understanding and protecting your patient.

Crotalus cascavella have visions and dreams of hearing voices.

Clairvoyance and clairaudience are needed by most snake remedies because it alerts them to potential attackers.

The venom of this Brazilian rattlesnake in potentised form produces a euphoric state wherein the patient feels that his clairaudient sensibilities and his personal power have increased. In a proving of *Crotalus cascavella* by Sankaran, in Similia Similibus Curentur, Radar™, he quotes the prover as saying: "I felt God would help me so that one day they will realize my importance." *Crotalus cascavella* have 'delusions of superiority'. *Crotalus cascavella* believe their clairaudience and clairvoyance will help them realize personal *greatness* and importance. If God is personally speaking to one it immediately protects one and warns one of a possible attack so one can counter-attack. This is why *Crotalus cascavella* have such strong clairaudience and why they are listed in the *Mind* rubric: *clairvoyance,* and the *Delusion* rubric: *hearing voices.* The persecutory *Delusion* rubric: *hearing footsteps behind him,* highlights their fear of attack. *Crotalus cascavella* need to maintain *superiority* in all situations. Underpinning their 'delusions of grandeur' are numerous *Delusion* rubrics pertaining to 'delusions of abandonment' and 'delusions of persecution'. *Crotalus cascavella* have a contradiction between Stage one ('delusions of grandeur') and Stage five ('delusions of hypochondria').

They have psychological delusions of being *tall* and above everything and in control of everything, as well as fears that they are *small* and able to be attacked.

Crotalus cascavella have the *Mind* rubric: *anxiety about health. Crotalus cascavella* view illness with fear. Illness will make them feel vulnerable and too weak to retaliate or protect themselves. If the homoeopath confronts them with the need to acknowledge their illness, it will be viewed as a criticism. *Crotalus cascavella* will retaliate because they cannot afford to feel small and weak, which is how they feel when they have to acknowledge disease and death. *Crotalus cascavella* have the *Mind* rubric: *ailments from embarrassment.* They are the only remedy listed in the *Mind* rubric: *destructiveness alternating with fear of being harmed.* [1] 1.

Crotalus cascavella feel like they are *insulted* and *being looked down upon* when they are sick. *Crotalus cascavella* will continually need to maintain their 'hubristic visions' and their 'hubristic denial' so they can feel secure.

1. Denial: *Delusion* rubric: *visions, has*: Crot-c. *Delusion* rubric: *voices: hearing*: Crot-c. *Delusion* rubric: *voices: hearing*: *follow, that he must*: crot-c. *Delusion* rubric: *superiority, of*: crot-c. *Delusion* rubric: *great person, is a*: crot-c. *Delusion* rubric: *tall*: *he or she is tall*: crot-c. *Delusion* rubric: *people*: *conversing with absent people*: crot-c.

2. Forsaken: *Delusion* rubric: *forced; that she is*: crot-c. [1] 1. *Delusion* rubric: *outcast; she were an*: crot-c. *Delusion* rubric: *persecuted*: *he is persecuted*: crot-c. *Delusion* rubric: *forsaken; is*: crot-c. *Delusion* rubric: *neglected*: *he or she is neglected*: crot-c. *Delusion* rubric: *deceived; being*: crot-c. *Delusion* rubric: *snakes*: *in and around her*: crot-c.

3. Causation: *Delusion* rubric: *criminal, he is a*: crot-c. *Delusion* rubric: *neglected*: *duty; he has neglected his*: crot-c. *Delusion* rubric: *wrong*: *done wrong; he has*: crot-c.

4. Depression: *Delusion* rubric: *forced; that she is*: crot-c. [1] 1. *Delusion* rubric: *insulted, he is*: *looked down upon*: crot-c. [1] 1. [Both of these rubrics can pertain to 'delusions of persecution'.]

5. Resignation: *small*: *body is smaller*: crot-c.

Natrum muriaticum need to protect their inner emotional sensitivity and vulnerability to being hurt. It is well recognized that *Natrum muriaticum* is a good homoeopathic remedy to use for grief and loss. When a patient is faced with loss of health, the first stage which they move into is denial. When *Natrum muriaticum* is faced with loss, the first stage which they move into is denial. *Natrum muriaticum* patients, more than any other remedy group, tell me that they have developed a deep inner connection to their spiritual self and that their lost relatives have visited them in their dreams to reassure them that they are in total control and are on the right path to becoming well. *Natrum muriaticum* are listed in the *Delusion* rubrics: *visions*, and *illusions of fancy*. 'Hubristic visions' indicates a need to create an illusion of oneself which is grander than reality. *Natrum muriaticum* have the *Delusion* rubric: *visions during sleep*. [2] 1.

Natrum muriaticum have visions of themselves being well in the future to reassure themselves they have complete control.

Another *Delusion* rubric to consider for *Natrum muriaticum* is the *Delusion* rubric: *pitied on account of his misfortune and he wept*. [2] 1. *Natrum muriaticum* cannot stand losing control. *Natrum muriaticum* have the *Delusion* rubrics: *talking with spirits*, and *talking with dead people. Illusions of fancy*, alludes to the ability that *Natrum muriaticum* have of defensively deflecting negativity by always having 'a positive take on the situation'.

The obsessive need to always feel positive and have a 'positive take' on every situation is a denial of reality. This well developed defensiveness can protect them from having to acknowledge that they are ill. This is hubristic visionary revisionism.

Natrum muriaticum have the *Delusion* rubric: *as if in a net*. They are one of only two remedies listed under this rubric. Illness will be perceived as a lack of personal control or freedom for *Natrum muriaticum*.

Natrum muriaticum do not have any *Delusion* rubrics pertaining to disproportionate guilt. The importance of acknowledging this is that if your patient disproportionately over-exaggerates self-blame for their illness, then the simillimum is not *Natrum muriaticum*. *Natrum muriaticum* will exaggerate their failure. But their failure is attributed to others who have neglected and/or insulted them. Most commonly, *Natrum muriaticum* feel a sense of injustice when others don't believe that they are able to cure themselves.

Natrum muriaticum will always attribute blame for their mental and emotional mental pain to everyone else who has caused them hurt. The obsessive need to have a 'positive take' on every situation is also a denial of personal responsibility.

Natrum muriaticum have numerous *Delusion* rubrics pertaining to 'delusions of persecution'. Following the rubric-repertorisation according to the model of the five psychological processing steps makes this immediately obvious. The *Delusion* rubric: *illusions of fancy*, can allude to the ability that *Natrum muriaticum* have of never acknowledging self-blame.

1. Denial: *Delusion* rubric: *fancy, illusions, of*: nat-m.
2. Forsaken: *Delusion* rubric: *neglected: he or she is neglected*: nat-m. *Delusion* rubric: *criticized, she is*: nat-m. *Delusion* rubric: *insulted, he is*: nat-m. *Delusion* rubric: *persecuted: he is persecuted*: nat-m. *Delusion* rubric: *thieves: house, in*: *Nat-m.*
3. Causation: NONE.
4. Depression: *Delusion* rubric: *succeed, he does everything wrong; he cannot*: nat-m. *Delusion* rubric: *doomed, being*: nat-m. *Delusion* rubric: *pitied on account of his misfortune and he wept; he is*: *Nat-m.* [2] 1. *Delusion* rubric: *head: belongs to another*: nat-m. [This rubric should be interpreted literally. It indicates that *Natrum muriaticum* attribute blame for their action on to others.]
5. Resignation: *Delusion* rubric: *wretched; she looks*: **NAT-M**. *Delusion* rubric: *wretched; she looks*: *looking in a mirror; when*: **NAT-M**.

Nux vomica have the *Delusion* rubrics: *has visions, illusions of fancy*, and *religious*.

Nux vomica have hubristic visions fueled by a zealous belief in their need to succeed – as if they have *taken a stimulant*.

Nux vomica have the *Delusion* rubric: *he can live without a heart*. [2] 1. It is incorrect to interpret this rubric literally; rather it should be analyzed in the context of the hubristic profile of *Nux vomica*. *Nux vomica* need to remain unattached to their emotions. *Nux vomica* need to remain unattached so they can avoid personal failure and succeed. *Nux vomica* need to maintain their zealous belief in being successful because underpinning their 'delusions of grandeur' are intense fears of 'loss of face'. Preceding illness in *all Nux vomica* patients I have treated has been an event in their lives which has caused them to 'lose face' and feel socially *disgraced*. Commonly I ask *Nux vomica* if they feel like they have ever failed. Invariably they will recall that it has been *once only* and it was recent. The 'never-well-since-event' or causation in *Nux vomica* will be exaggerated guilt over being *disgraced*. *Nux vomica* will feel physically undermined and threatened – *as if their body is made of threads – as if someone has sold their bed*. I cannot emphasize enough how crucial it is to know and understand the *Delusion* rubrics attached to a constitutional remedy. *Nux vomica* are a mass of contradictions – *strong will power* – versus – *weakness of will*. *Nux vomica* are listed in numerous *Mind* rubrics pertaining to ailments from loss of position – *being neglected by mother and father – deceived ambition – anger when contradicted.*

Underpinning all the *Mind* rubrics pertaining to anxiety of illness, fear of illness, and anger with illness, is the *Delusion* rubric: *he is dying*. When *Nux vomica* are sick they literally lose all their inner fiber – *inside of body is made of threads*.

If homoeopaths are looking for a remedy profile of the strong willed *Nux vomica*[13], then the simillimum will be missed because that is not what will present in the first consultation *if* they are sick. *Nux vomica* are also listed in the *Delusion* rubrics: *horrible visions,* and *sees mutilated bodies*. *Nux vomica* suffer from 'delusions of hypochondria'.

Nux vomica have the *Delusion* rubric: *he is revolving around his axis.* [1] 1. *Nux vomica* constantly check and recheck their own safety and position, they never feel secure. When *Nux vomica* are sick they shrink inside themselves –

body is smaller. When *Nux vomica* are physically well they elevate themselves above the mundane emotions in the world and are fueled by grandiose visions of what they are going to create next – *walking on air* – *illusions of fancy.*

1. Denial: *Delusion* rubric: *fancy, illusions of:* nux-v. *Delusion* rubric: *visions, has:* Nux-v. *Delusion* rubric: *religious:* nux-v. *Delusion* rubric: *stimulant; had taken a:* nux-v. [1] 2. *Delusion* rubric: *enlarged:* nux-v. *Delusion* rubric: *walking: air: on air; walks:* nux-v. *Delusion* rubric: *heart: live without; he can:* Nux-v. [2] 1.

2. Forsaken: *Delusion* rubric: *home: away from home; he* is: *Nux-v. Delusion* rubric: *bed: sold his bed; someone has:* nux-v. [1] 1. *Delusion* rubric: *laughed at and mocked at; being:* nux-v. *Delusion* rubric: *poisoned: he: has been:* nux-v. *Delusion* rubric: *persecuted: he is persecuted:* nux-v. *Delusion* rubric: *disgraced: she is:* nux-v.

3. Causation: *Delusion* rubric: *disgraced: she is:* nux-v. [In relation to *Nux vomica* being disgraced is synonymous with an admission of guilt.] *Delusion* rubric: *crime: committed a crime; he had:* nux-v.

4. Depression: *Delusion* rubric: *depressive:* nux-v. *Delusion* rubric: *wealth, of: purchases; and make useless:* Nux-v. [2] 1. [This rubric reemphasizes wrong decisions.] *Delusion* rubric: *interest in anything; felt no:* nux-v. [1] 1. *Delusion* rubric: *wrong: everything goes wrong:* nux-v. *Delusion* rubric: *fail, everything will:* nux-v.

5. Resignation: Delusion rubric: *die: must; she:* nux-v. [1] 1. *Delusion* rubric: *body: threads; body inside is made of:* nux-v. [1] 1. *Delusion* rubric: *body: ugly; body looks:* Nux-v. *Delusion* rubric: *dying: he is:* nux-v. *Delusion* rubric: *small: body is smaller:* nux-v.

   • *Delusions: beautiful: landscape; of:* coff-t. coff. irid-met. Lach. olib-sac. petr-ra.

- *Delusions*: *visions*: *has*: *grandeur, of magnificent*: cann-i. carbn-s. coff-t. coff. olib-sac.
- *Delusions*: *paradise, seeing*: coff-t. coff.

Self-Deluding: If one has overwhelming fears of death then the psychological delusion of believing in, and seeing paradise is a psychological 'delusion of grandeur' which will be needed to deny death.

Coffea cruda have numerous and wonderful fantasies of omnipotence. *Coffea cruda* is a homoeopathic remedy derived from coffee. Coffee is a psychotropic stimulant which elevates mood. Most people have a drink of coffee first thing in the morning to help them 'face the day'.

Coffea cruda have the *Delusion* rubrics: *has visions*, and *illusions of fancy*. *Coffea cruda* dissociate themselves from mundane reality. *Coffea cruda* have the *Delusion* rubric: *walking on air*. *Coffea cruda* need their hubristic visions because underlying their 'hubristic denial' are disproportionate reactions to fear.

In the case-development of *Coffea cruda,* the *Mind* rubrics: *fear of death,* and *fear of pain* indicate the somatic need that *Coffea cruda* have to delude themselves about the reality of disease and death. When *Coffea cruda* have to face the reality of illness they literally cannot think about it. *Coffea cruda* have the *Mind* rubric: *when very sick, says he is well. Coffea cruda* have the *Delusion* rubric: *whirling in head when thinking*. Coffee addicts use coffee to stimulate creative thought processes. Often those creative processes are exaggerated illusions. Excessive coffee consumption also causes an agitated nervous system resulting in the person over-exaggerating or reacting inappropriately to stressors. Coffee (the substance) stimulates the production of cortisone and adrenaline, two stimulating hormones. Cortisol is a corticosteroid hormone or glucocorticoid produced by the adrenal cortex. It is usually referred to as the 'stress hormone' as it is involved in response to stress and anxiety. It increases blood pressure and blood sugar, and reduces immune responses. Cortisol production inhibits the secretion of corticotropin-releasing hormone (CRH), resulting in feedback inhibition of ACTH (Adrenocorticotropic hormone) secretion. This normal feedback system is crucial to being able to appropriately respond to 'flight or fight' stressors. *Coffea cruda* are locked in to an inappropriate flight response. Cortisol production resulting from chronic stress inhibits or blocks the body's ability to be able to deal with chronic inflammation. *Coffea cruda* have the *Mind* rubrics: *fear of death from pain*, and *fear of others approaching lest he be touched*. *Coffea cruda* have the following *Mind* rubrics (listed below) which pertain to over-exaggerated somatic responses to sudden frights, even if the fright is a pleasant surprise. *Coffea cruda* overreact to persecutory illusions. *Coffea cruda* have the *Delusion* rubrics: *he is away from home,* and *about criminals.*

Underlying their visions of grandeur are fears of isolation and abandonment which need to be hidden with *grand visions of magnificent grandeur.*

The causation or 'never-well-since-event' in *Coffea cruda* will have its foundation in abandonment during childhood. *Coffea cruda* have the somatic responses of a frightened child. They are so frightened that they create a fantasy world which is a beautiful vision of paradise. As adults, the psychosomatic response to stressors is to dissociate. As a child the psychosomatic response to stressors is to create a fantasy world.

- *Mind: ailments from: surprises: pleasant:* **COFF**.
- *Mind: ailments from: joy: sudden:* **COFF**.
- *Mind: ailments from: fear:* coff.
- *Mind: ailments from: excitement: sudden:* coff. [1] 1.
- *Mind: alert: Coff.*
- *Mind: fear: death, of: pain, from:* **COFF**.
- *Mind: fear: approaching; of: others; of: touched, lest he be:* coff.

- *Mind: starting: fright; from and as from:* coff.

1. Denial: *Delusion* rubric: *beautiful: landscape; of.* coff. *Delusion* rubric: *visions, has: grandeur, of magnificent:* coff. *Delusion* rubric: *paradise: seeing:* coff. *Delusion* rubric: *strong; he is:* coff. *Delusion* rubric: *walking: air. on air; walks:* coff. *Delusion* rubric: *excited; as if.* coff. [1] 1. *Delusion* rubric: *fancy, illusions:* coff.

2. Forsaken: *Delusion* rubric: *home: away from home; he* is: *Coff. Delusion* rubric: *criminals, about:* coff.

3. Causation: *Delusion* rubric: *criminal, he is a:* coff.

4. Depression: *Delusion* rubric: *head: whirling in head: thinking; when:* coff. [1] 1.

5. Resignation: Delusion rubric: *light: is light; he:* coff.

   - *Delusions: immortality, of.* anh.[1] 1.
   - *Delusions: body: immaterial, is:* anh. thuj.

Self-Deluding: Believing one can cure one's disease or live forever is a psychological 'delusion of grandeur' which helps to deny having to live on an 'earthly plane'.

Anhalonium choose to connect to their *immortal* soul. *Anhalonium* have a psychic connection to a spiritual world and actively disconnect themselves from an earthly external world. Other *Delusion* rubrics to consider in *Anhalonium* would be, *out of the body* and the following *Delusion* rubrics: *separated from the world*, and *decomposition of space and shape. Anhalonium* feel *separated from the world* and believe they have been rejected by the world because they are so different. They also choose to *separate themselves from the world* to connect to the ethereal.

Anhalonium have *wonderful visions* of the spirit world which are much more attractive to *Anhalonium* than this earthly world.

Anhalonium will embrace death because they believe they are going to live forever in 'spirit'. If your patient is fearful about their fatal illness and death the simillimum is not *Anhalonium*.

Anhalonium are not interested in, and do not cope with, the earthly plane of existence; they only feel depressed if they are *hindered* from leaving. *Anhalonium* feel like they are suffering by being forced to live on this earthly plane. They feel like they are waiting to die so they can be an *immortal* soul *merged in eternity*. *Anhalonium* have the *Delusion* rubric: *he had to wait*. [1] 1. *Anhalonium* do not have any *Delusion* rubrics pertaining to self-blame or 'delusions of original sin'.

If your patient blames themselves for their illness then the simillimum is not *Anhalonium*. *Anhalonium* does not necessarily blame anyone else either.

1. Denial: *Delusion* rubric: *immortality, of*: anh. [1] 1. *Delusion* rubric: *body: immaterial, is*: anh. *Delusion* rubric: *eternity, merged with present*: anh. [1] 1. *Delusion* rubric: *floating, air, in*: anh. *Delusion* rubric: *visions, has: wonderful*: anh. *Delusion* rubric: *transparent, everything is*: Anh. *Delusion* rubric: *beautiful*: anh. *Delusion* rubric: *hearing: illusions of*: anh. *Delusion* rubric: *visions, has: beautiful: kaleidoscope changes; varied*: anh. *Delusion* rubric: *space: decomposition of space and shape*: anh. *Delusion* rubric: *transparent: he is*: anh. *Delusion* rubric: *body: immaterial, is*: anh.

2. Forsaken: *Delusion* rubric: *separated: world; from the*: *he is separated*: Anh.

3. Causation: NONE.

4. Depression: *Delusion* rubric: *hindered; he is*: anh. *Delusion* rubric: *waiting: had to wait; he*: anh. [1] 1.

5. Resignation: *Delusion* rubric: *dead: he himself was*: anh. *Delusion* rubric: *body: immaterial, is*: anh. *Delusion* rubric: *body: out of the body*: Anh.

- *Delusions: superhuman: is: control; is under superhuman*: agar. anac. carc. cypra-eg. des-ac. falco-pe. kali-br. *Lach. Naja*. op. petr-ra. plat. psil. sal-fr. *Thuj.*

- *Delusions: influence; one is under a powerful*: ambr. brass-n-o. carc. cere-b. dream-p. foll. *Hyos*. irid-met. kali-br. *Lach*. ozone positr. psil. *Sal-fr. Stram*. thuj. verat.

- *Delusions: someone else: she was someone else: power; and in the hands of a strong*: lach. [1]1.
- *Delusions: charmed and cannot break the spell: Lach* [2]1.
- *Delusions: voices: hearing: follow, that he must*: anac. crot-c. lach. thuj.
- *Delusions: sight and hearing, of*: anac. bell. eup-pur. kali-br.
- *Delusions: divided: two parts; into: which part he has possession on waking; and could not tell*: thuj. [1] 1.

Self-deluding: Believing one is controlled by someone else can be avoidance of personal responsibility or a pretentious psychological 'delusion of grandeur'. Transference is characterized by unconscious self-deluding denial which allows for the redirection of feelings on to another person.

A 'transference neurosis' is found in the *Delusion* rubrics of 'hubristic denial' in which the patient transfers 'cause and effect' on to God. A 'transference neurosis' is also found in the *Delusion* rubrics of sin in which the patient transfers 'cause and effect' on to the devil. This *Delusion* rubric: *is under superhuman control*, and the *Delusion* rubric: *one is under a powerful influence*, can be transferred on to God, or the devil. In everyday language, transference is referred to as 'dumping your shit on to someone else'. In everyday language a 'transference neurosis' refers to 'not owning your shit'.

Kali bromatum are undermined by their feelings of helplessness so they need to believe they have 'God on their side' to make themselves feel stronger. *Kali bromatum* have numerous 'delusions of abandonment', 'delusions of persecution', 'delusions of original sin', and 'delusions of impending doom'. *Kali bromatum* are paranoid that everyone, including their family, is going to harm them. *Kali bromatum* fear that there is nothing for them to stand on in life – standing on and around emptiness.

When they are sick, *Kali bromatum* need hubristic visions of omnipotence so they can believe they will be saved.

Kali bromatum have the *Mind* rubric: *looking in all directions.* *Kali bromatum* are constantly checking for potential attackers and constantly checking for an exit. *Kali bromatum* blame their sins on God's vengeance and the devil's influence. Underneath their psychological delusions of omnipotence they are fearful that their illness is the object of God's vengeance because they have neglected their duty.

Kali bromatum have the *Delusion* rubric: *she is being watched.* *Kali bromatum* suffer from exaggerated psychological delusions of conscience and disproportionate 'delusions of original sin'. *Kali bromatum* have the *Delusion* rubric: *her brother fell overboard in her sight.* [1] 1. This rubric should not be interpreted literally; rather it indicates a guilty conscience. *Kali bromatum* feel annihilated when they have to face illness. When *Kali bromatum* are sick they abandon themselves because they believe their illness is God's punishment. *Kali bromatum* have the *Mind* rubric: *suicidal disposition to throw himself under a car.* *Kali bromatum* have the *Delusion* rubric: *thought everything had been experienced before.* This *Delusion* rubric pertains to the degree to which Kali bromatum feel undermined and defeated: their own life has no relevance to them. Kübler-Ross identified denial as the first stage in her model of grief. *Kali bromatum* similarly start their story from the assumption of immortality i.e. the denial of mortality. A patient who is struggling to come out of denial, or who refuses to believe they are sick, is suffering psychological 'delusions of grandeur'. *Kali bromatum* will not present at the start of an illness with the psychological delusions of persecutory guilt which are commonly associated with *Kali bromatum* in the repertory. *Kali bromatum* are experts at dissociation – *floating in air*.

Kali bromatum believe they are omnipotent; they deny they are sick. *Kali bromatum* believe they are influenced by a powerful force that is able to cure them of all illnesses.

To say that *Kali bromatum* have an internalized conflict between their morality and immorality is an incorrect assumption derived from the *Mind* rubric: *anxiety of conscience*. To have a psychological delusional conflict there has to be a conflict between the Denial process in Stage one and the Resignation process in Stage five. On the one hand *Kali bromatum* have pretensions of power, and on the other hand they have psychological 'delusions of annihilation'. *Kali bromatum* need to psychologically maintain their 'delusions of grandeur' otherwise they fear destruction. If *Kali bromatum* acknowledge that they are sick they will sink into a depressive doom and believe that their life is threatened.

In the case of *Kali bromatum* the stark inconsistency between Stage one and Stage five is not an internalized moral conflict, but an anxiety that they will become a victim of God's vengeance because they wish to keep being influenced by powerful forces.

Kali bromatum have anxieties of conscience and wring their hands because they fear God's vengeance *and* because they are aware that they identify with murderous rage [*devil*]. *Kali bromatum* have the *Mind* rubric: *desire to kill loved ones*, and the *Delusion* rubric: *she is about to murder her husband and child*. *Kali bromatum* have numerous *Mind* rubrics pertaining to *omitting words, unconsciousness and semi-consciousness*, and *disconnected answering*. *Kali bromatum* prefer to self-delude and suppress awareness of their own rages. *Kali bromatum* have 'transference neuroses'. *Kali bromatum* are vulnerable to believing that God has instructed them to murder. Believing you are controlled by someone else can be a pretentious and obviously dangerous psychological 'delusion of grandeur' which allows for the redirection of responsibility on to another person. *Kali bromatum* fear that they will be found to identify with powerful influences which are God and/or the devil. (This brings on their anxieties of conscience.)

1. Denial: *Delusion* rubric: *influence; one is under a powerful*: kali-br. *Delusion* rubric: *superhuman; is*: *control; is under superhuman*: kali-br. [This rubric can be interpreted as

God or the devil.] *Delusion* rubric: *floating*: *air, in*: kali-br. *Delusion* rubric: *enlarged*: kali-br. *Delusion* rubric: *fancy, illusions of*: *Kali-br*. *Delusion* rubric: *wealth, of*: kali-br. *Delusion* rubric: *religious*: *Kali-br*.

2. Forsaken: *Delusion* rubric: *forsaken; is*: *God; by*: kali-br. [1] 1. *Delusion* rubric: *God*: *vengeance; he is the object of God's*: **KALI-BR**. *Delusion* rubric: *conspiracies*: *against him; there are conspiracies*: kali-br. *Delusion* rubric: *danger, impression of*: kali-br. *Delusion* rubric: *life*: *threatened; life is*: kali-br. [1] 1. *Delusion* rubric: *persecuted*: *he is persecuted*: **KALI-BR**. *Delusion* rubric: *poisoned*: *he*: *about to be poisoned; he is*: *Kali-br*. *Delusion* rubric: *pursued; he was*: *Kali-br*. *Delusion* rubric: *watched, she is being*: *Kali-br*. *Delusion* rubric: *danger, impression of*: *family, from his*: kali-br. [1] 1. *Delusion* rubric: *injury*: *being injured; is*: kali-br. *Delusion* rubric: *money*: *sewed*[14] *up in clothing; is*: kali-br. [1] 1.

3. Causation: *Delusion* rubric: *murdering; he is*: *husband and child; she is about to murder her*: kali-br. [1] 1. *Delusion* rubric: *neglected*: *duty; he has neglected his*: kali-br. *Delusion* rubric: *devil, he is a devil*: *Kali-br*. *Delusion* rubric: *superhuman; is*: *control; is under superhuman*: kali-br. [This rubric can be interpreted as God or the devil.] *Delusion* rubric: *thieves*: *accused of robbing; he has been*: kali-br. [1] 1.

4. Depression: *Delusion* rubric: *ground*: *gave way beneath his feet*: *Kali-br*. *Delusion* rubric: *melancholy*: **KALI-BR**. *Delusion* rubric: *painful, with sadness*: kali-br. [1] 1. *Delusion* rubric: *mind*: *out of his mind; he would go*: *Kali-br*. *Delusion* rubric: *doomed, being*: *Kali-br*. *Delusion* rubric: *depressive*: **KALI-BR**. *Delusion* rubric: *wrong*: *everything goes wrong*: kali-br. [2] 1. *Delusion* rubric: *destruction of all near her; impending*: *Kali-br*. [2] 1.

5. Resignation: *Delusion* rubric: *life*: *threatened; life is*: kali-br. [1] 1. *Delusion* rubric: *emptiness; of*: *around and under*

one on standing; emptiness: kali-br. [1] 1. *Delusion* rubric: *destruction of all near her; impending*: *Kali-br*. [2] 1. [These rubrics pertain to 'delusions of annihilation'.]

Lachesis need the hubristic *Delusion* rubric: *one is under a powerful influence* so they can delude themselves that they are always one-up on everyone else. The 'persecution complexes' are crucial to the understanding of *Lachesis.* The *Delusion* rubrics listed below reveal the extent of their ability to side-step responsibility.

Even though *Lachesis* have the rubrics allocating blame, *committed a crime,* they will for the most part attribute their sins to the influence of a higher power. *Lachesis* have the *Delusion* rubric: *hearing a voice commanding him to commit a crime.* [1]1. *Lachesis* have a strong need to maintain their hubristic visionary view of themselves and their 'hubristic denial'.

Underpinning their 'delusions of grandeur' are numerous 'delusions of abandonment', 'delusions of persecution', 'delusions of impending doom', and 'delusions of hypochondria'. *Lachesis* fear any exposure of their weaknesses. *Lachesis* have the *Delusion* rubric: *sent to a mental asylum* [1] 1., which alludes to a conflict in their psyche. *Lachesis* have the *Delusion* rubric: *a great person* opposing the *Delusion* rubric: *he is friendless.* If a remedy profile has a weakened 'ego' then their psyche is under threat. Psychoses are a conflict between the 'ego' and the external world. A psychosis is a severe mental derangement of the whole personality. The *Delusion* rubrics which cover psychoses are the *Delusion* rubrics: forsaken, depression and resignation. These *Delusion* rubrics emphasize the threat that the world poses to the self or 'ego'. They contain the 'delusions of abandonment', 'delusions of persecution', 'delusions of impending doom', and the 'delusions of hypochondria', in that order. *Lachesis* struggle to secure their own 'ego' in the world, which is why they are *so* jealous of others' self-assuredness. *Lachesis* have the *Delusion* rubric:

with jealousy, and the *Mind* rubric: *irresistible jealousy as foolish as it is*. [2] 1. *Lachesis* need to transfer their responsibilities to others to avoid acknowledging that they are weakened by their own psychoses. *Lachesis* have the *Mind* rubrics: *desire to be magnetized*, and *easily magnetized*. Both rubrics pertain to the illusion and desire that they are influenced by a powerful force, or under the superhuman power of someone else. *Lachesis* have the *Delusion* rubric: *hearing a voice that she must confess things she never did*. [1]1. *Lachesis* are particularly skilled at projecting and transferring the responsibility for their illness on to the homoeopath. *Lachesis* transfer responsibility for their life and death to other people. *Lachesis* have the *Delusion* rubric: *one was about to die and wishes someone would help her off*. [1]1. The psychodynamic consequence of their weakened 'ego' means that *Lachesis* cannot afford to move out of the psychological stage of denial. Kübler-Ross identified denial as the first stage in her model of grief.

Lachesis will not acknowledge that they are sick. If they did they would have to acknowledge that they are not *charmed and powerful*. *Lachesis* fear disease because they suffer from paranoid fears that their illness will *disintegrate* their *beautiful* body and destroy their looks.

Lachesis have the *Delusion* rubric: *beautiful*, opposing the *Delusion* rubric: *body disintegrating*. *Lachesis* have the *Mind* rubrics: *fear of impending contagious epidemic diseases*, and *lamenting about his sickness*. [3] 4.

1. Denial: *Delusion rubric: superhuman; is: control; is under superhuman: Lach. Delusion* rubric: *someone else: she was someone else: power; and in the hands of a strong*: lach. [1]1. *Delusion* rubric: *charmed and cannot break the spell: Lach* [2]1. *Delusion* rubric: *influence; one is under a powerful: Lach. Delusion* rubric: *voices: hearing: follow, that he must*: lach. [Although these rubrics can be interpreted as God or the devil, with *Lachesis* they pertain to God and are reflective of their 'delusions of grandeur'.] *Delusion*

rubric: *possessed; being*: lach. *Delusion* rubric: *identity*: *someone else, she is*: Lach. *Delusion* rubric: *person*: *other person; she is some*: Lach. *Delusion* rubric: *journey; he is on a*: lach. *Delusion* rubric: *visions, has: beautiful*: lach. *Delusion* rubric: *beautiful*: Lach. *Delusion* rubric: *beautiful*: *landscape; of*. Lach. *Delusion* rubric: *enlarged*: lach. *Delusion* rubric: *religious*: lach. *Delusion* rubric: *great person, is a*: Lach. *Delusion* rubric: *proud*: lach.

2. Forsaken: *Delusion* rubric: *talking*: *friends are talking about her*. lach. [1] 1. *Delusion* rubric: *laughed at and mocked at; being*: lach. *Delusion* rubric: *wrong: suffered wrong; he has*: lach. *Delusion* rubric: *friendless, he is*: lach. *Delusion* rubric: *lost; she is: salvation*; *for. predestination, from*: Lach [2]1. *Delusion* rubric: *poisoned: medicine; being poisoned by*: lach. *Delusion* rubric: *poisoned: he: about to be poisoned; he is*: lach. *Delusion* rubric: *pursued; he was*: lach. *Delusion* rubric: *injury: about to receive injury; is: friends; from his*: lach. *Delusion* rubric: *asylum: mental asylum; sent to*: lach. [1] 1. *Delusion* rubric: *criticized, she is*: lach. *Delusion* rubric: *hated; by others*: lach. *Delusion* rubric: *home: away from home; he is*: lach. *Delusion* rubric: *wrong: suffered wrong; he has*: lach. *Delusion* rubric: *snakes: in and around her*. lach.

3. Causation: *Delusion* rubric: *crime: committed a crime; he had*: lach. *Delusion* rubric: *wrong: done wrong; he has*: Lach.

4. Depression: *Delusion* rubric: *doomed, being*: lach.

5. Resignation: *Delusion* rubric: *die: about to die*; *one was*: Lach. *Delusion* rubric: *disease: incurable disease*; *he has an*: Lach. *Delusion* rubric: *body: disintegrating*: Lach. *Delusion* rubric: *die: about to die; one was: exhaustion; she would die from*: lach.

Naja is a homoeopathic remedy derived from the venom of the Indian cobra snake. *Naja* suffer paranoid psychological delusions that they are being deceived or taken over by powerful forces. *Naja* have the *Delusion* rubrics: *he has suffered wrong, someone is behind him, trapped, injured,* and *being deceived.* It is widely believed that the cobra snake responds to the music of the snake charmer. This is false. The cobra rises when it follows the smell of the food that the snake charmer hides in his hand. The snake is controlled by the snake charmer because it has been starved. *Naja* have the *Delusion* rubric: *being starved,* and *deceived.* The cobra eventually starves to death and the snake charmer then traps and deceives another snake. *Naja,* similarly to *Lachesis,* suffer from 'persecution complexes' when they fall ill. *Naja* feel extremely wronged by circumstances in their lives, and believe they are extremely unfortunate because of the choices they have made. *Naja* have the *Mind* rubric: *sadness, as if having done everything in the wrong way.* [2] 2. When they are faced with disease and death they do not move into the same 'hubristic denial' as *Kali bromatum* or *Lachesis,* in which blame is transferred on to someone else. In relation to the constitutional remedy profile of *Naja,* the *Delusion* rubric: *is under superhuman control,* is more reflective of their 'delusions of persecution' and their 'delusions of impending doom'. *Naja* sink into depressive predictions of failure when they become sick. *Naja* have the *Delusion* rubrics: *everything goes wrong,* and *he does everything wrong he cannot succeed.*

Although *Naja* are listed in the hubristic rubrics, *visions* and *illusions of hearing,* both of these along with *under superhuman control,* pertain to paranoid predictions of being *persecuted* and *controlled* and *trapped.*

Naja have the *Mind* rubric: *sensation as if he had two wills. Naja* feel trapped inside of themselves as well as feeling trapped on the outside. This *Mind* rubric reflects an internal battle. The battle inside of *Naja* involves deciding whether they are worthy of life. *Naja* will defeat themselves and feel defeated when they are sick. *Naja* embrace death. *Naja* have the *Mind* rubric: *loss of will.*

Naja submissively embrace death when they are sick. Whether this is an act of suicide or Santhara[15] is contentious.

Sankaran makes a note in *The Soul of Remedies* that *Naja* have a "make of nobility about them", and that his *Naja* patients have "an intense spiritual orientation". *Naja* have the *Mind* rubric: *exaltation of fancies*, and the *Delusion* rubric: *has visions*. Both of these rubrics justify and allude to the glorification of Santhara. I have noted in *Naja* a marked lack of confidence and an intense self-deprecating need to annihilate themselves. I have also noted that they nobly choose to *waste away* when they realize that they are dying. *Naja* also have the *Mind* rubric: *weary of life, unworthy of the gift of life*, which is a rubric which alludes to a spiritual assessment of the worthiness of one's soul. Whether their self-annihilation is spiritually aligned or pertains to depressive tendencies is debatable. *Naja* have the *Mind* rubrics: *want of self-confidence, self-depreciation*, and *suicidal disposition from sadness*. *Naja* have the *Delusion* rubrics: *wasted away*, and *starved*. *Naja* have the *Delusion* rubric: *body is smaller*, and the *Mind* rubric: *bulimia nervosa*.

A patient who has hubristic visions of exaltation glorifies the abdication of life.

1. Denial: *Delusion* rubric: *superhuman; is; control; is under superhuman*: *Naja*. *Delusion* rubric: *hearing: illusions of*: naja. *Delusion* rubric: *visions, has*: naja. [In relation to *Naja*, these rubrics can pertain more persecution.]

2. Forsaken: *Delusion* rubric: *neglected: he or she is neglected*: naja. *Delusion* rubric: *deceived; being*: naja. *Delusion* rubric: *trapped; he is*: naja. *Delusion* rubric: *poisoned: he; has been*: naja. *Delusion* rubric: *injury: being injured; is; surroundings; by his*: *Naja*. *Delusion* rubric: *people: behind him; someone is*: naja. *Delusion* rubric: *wrong: suffered wrong; he has*: naja. *Delusion* rubric: *injury: being injured; is*: naja.

3. Causation: *Delusion* rubric: *neglected*: *duty*; *he has neglected his*: naja.

4. Depression: *Delusion* rubric: *wrong*: *everything goes wrong*: naja. *Delusion* rubric: *succeed, he does everything wrong; he cannot*: naja.

5. Resignation: *Delusion* rubric: *wasting away*: naja. [1] 1. *Delusion* rubric: *starve*: *being starved*: naja. *Delusion* rubric: *sick*: *being*: naja.

Thuja are listed in the *Delusion* rubric: *under superhuman control*, but they have self-conflicting denial about who is influencing them. *Thuja* have the *Delusion* rubric: *being at war*. *Thuja* choose to abdicate personal responsibility for their power because they fear that the powerful influence is coming from 'the evil side', and not 'the good side'. This secret will be the underlying self-denial in every *Thuja* case. Another rubric to consider in a *Thuja* case would be the *Delusion* rubric: *someone calls*. The homoeopath needs to ask *who* is influencing them.

All *Thuja* cases will have a divided self which they are trying to keep secret; this conflict will always cause eventual destruction of either the mind or body.

Thuja are significantly the only remedy listed in the *Delusion* rubric: *divided into two parts, and which part he has possession of when he wakes he does not know*. *Thuja* have a strongly developed defense which manifest in their obsessive need for religion – *Mind* rubric: *fanaticism, too occupied with religious affections*. *Thuja* need to believe they are being controlled by God or a 'good' higher being, otherwise they are overwhelmed by their own fears of immoral behavior. The *Thuja* (case) in the *Case Companion* to *Homoeopathic Psychiatry* feared that the higher power with which he was in contact was the devil, and not Jesus. It was this fear which drove him to become a Christian pastor and give up his previous 'unconventional' spiritual life. If he had stayed in the alternative world of spirituality, the power influencing him could have been the devil. In the Christian ministry he felt he would be protected, and more assured that Jesus would influence him, and not the devil.

1. Denial: *Delusion* rubric: *influence; one is under a powerful*: thuj. *Delusion* rubric: *divided: two parts; into: which part he has possession on waking; and could not tell*: thuj. [1] 1. *Delusion* rubric: *superhuman; is: control; is under superhuman: Thuj.* [These previous three rubrics can refer to illusions that one is under the control of God or the devil.] *Delusion* rubric: *power: all-powerful; she is*: thuj. *Delusion* rubric: *fancy, illusions of*: thuj. *Delusion* rubric: *floating: air, in*: thuj. *Delusion* rubric: *feet: touch scarcely the ground: walking; when*: thuj.

2. Forsaken: *Delusion* rubric: *appreciated, she is not: Thuj. Delusion* rubric: *forsaken; is*: thuj. *Delusion* rubric: *outcast; she were an*: thuj. *Delusion* rubric: *friend: affection of; has lost the: Thuj.* [This rubric can pertain to abandonment or guilt.]

3. Causation: *Delusion* rubric: *criminal, he is a*: thuj. *Delusion* rubric: *dirty: he is*: thuj. *Delusion* rubric: *sinned; one has*: thuj. *Delusion* rubric: *divided: two parts; into: which part he has possession on waking; and could not tell*: thuj. [1] 1. *Delusion* rubric: *influence; one is under a powerful*: thuj. *Delusion* rubric: *superhuman; is: control; is under superhuman: Thuj.* [These rubrics can refer to illusions that one is under the control of God or the devil.] *Delusion* rubric: *friend: affection of; has lost the: Thuj.*

4. Depression: *Delusion* rubric: *worthless; he is*: thuj.

5. Resignation: *Delusion* rubric: *body*: delicate, is: *Thuj.* [2] 1. *Delusion* rubric: *existence: longer; she cannot exist any*: thuj. [1] 1. *Delusion* rubric: *body: immaterial, is*: thuj. *Delusion* rubric: *die: about to die; one was: Thuj.*

If a constitutional remedy has two opposing forces they will be evident in the *Delusion* rubrics. *Thuja* have the *Delusion* rubric: *she is all powerful* versus the *Delusion* rubric: *he is worthless* in Stage four. A person with such extreme conflicting polarities will move into a psychological process of self-denial; it is too painful to live with the self-realizations.

The rubric-repertorisation using the above model is extremely worthwhile because it will always reveal the psychodynamic crisis within each remedy. The self-denial in *Thuja* is the precursor for their secrecy. *Thuja* have the *Mind* rubric: *secretive*.

• *Delusions: martyr; of being a*: carc.[1] 1.

Avoidance: There is no greater hubristic goal than sacrificing oneself to a higher being. Martyrdom is fueled by 'hubristic visions' of a grand persona. Being willing to become a martyr and suffer death for the advancement of a righteous cause can be analyzed as visionary or self-destructive.

All psychological delusions of martyrdom are a complex mixture of self-deceit fueled by paranoid fears of impotence.

Carcinosin use martyrdom self-righteously to excuse themselves for not taking personal power and control over their own lives. I have a *Carcinosin* patient who had to end her medical studies in her third year of medicine because she was suffering from extreme anorexia. She gave up medical studies because the pressure from her mother to succeed and become a doctor was too much pressure for her. She freely admitted that when she became anorexic her mother finally allowed her to leave her medical studies. She is still anorexic, but she does not acknowledge this; it is cleverly hidden under the veil of being sensitive to particular foods. She is now working as a dietitian in a hospital. She came to have a consultation with me because she felt overwhelmed by, and exhausted with her work. She has a tendency to overwork, see too many patients, and not be able to put any protective boundaries in place. (*Carcinosin* have the *Delusion* rubric: *has no defense mechanism*.) In her second consultation with me she told me in great detail how she helps 'lost souls' leave this 'plane' and move on and acknowledge their death. She said: *I can just be* *in the dispensary at the hospital and then I realize I am not feeling good, and I realize I have managed to attach a lost soul to myself. Every morning when I get up I clear my house of all the lost souls who have visited in the night or who have come attached to patients the previous day.* I asked her why she attracts them. She replied: *I don't actually mind this, they need me. Because without people like me they would not be able to leave this plane and they would stay confused. I get very weary sometimes, having all these souls influencing my energy and mood. When I get tired I then have to restrict my food intact, and I can then only eat certain foods. All my food sensitivities then become worse, but I don't mind because I am helping these lost souls. They know they can attach themselves to me because I am sensitive. Who else would do this? I have to offer myself to these lost souls.*

A *Delusion* rubric is used in a case only when you can see that it is psychologically advantageous to the patient to maintain the avoidance or self-deluding. This particular *Carcinosin* patient needs to believe she is influenced by external agents who make her tired. It is difficult for her to acknowledge that *she* overworks and is not able to put time restrictions into place to prevent exhaustion. If the 'lost souls' make her feel tired and exhausted, and if they cause her extreme food sensitivities (which she uses to justify her incredibly restricted diet and calorie intake) then she does not have to take personal responsibility for her obsessive eating problem or for her inability to deal with work pressure. This is evidence of denial and is the meaning of the *Delusion* rubric: *is under superhuman control*, and the *Delusion* rubric: *one is under a powerful influence*. The problem in her story is not her exhaustion, nor her inability to put boundaries into place to prevent overworking; the problem is her *glorification* of martyrdom. The story (regardless of whether it is real or not), is not what I prescribe on. It is also not my role as a homoeopath to point out patients' delusions. The action of the simillimum will provide her with a stronger sense of her own 'boundaries' so she can resist 'lost souls'. The action of the simillimum will also give her the ability to be able to say *no* to picking up the 'lost souls'. The insight gained from doing the five stage rubric-repertorisation in the case of *Carcinosin* is that it explains why they struggle intensely with self-ownership and personal responsibility.

Carcinosin use martyrdom to avoid facing their fear of failure. *Carcinosin* use martyrdom self-righteously so they can avoid feeling crippled by fears that they are not important.

The *Delusion* rubrics: *she is not appreciated*, and *she is friendless* highlight this. Martyrdom is far more advantageous to maintain than having to face the fact that she feels unappreciated and unneeded. If a patient needs to believe that they pick up 'lost souls' then the *Delusion* rubrics one uses are: *she did not belong to anyone*, *she is always alone*, and *friendless*. If a patient needs to believe that the 'lost souls' are what causes them to feel weak and tired and it is not the fact that they do not eat, then this is a need for denial. Martyrdom for *Carcinosin* is far more advantageous to maintain than having to face personal responsibility, which comes with an all consuming fear of *failure* and *annihilation*.

In the rubric-repertorisation, *Carcinosin* do not take responsibility for personal blame. *Carcinosin* are martyred to powerful forces outside of themselves. This is the psychodynamic meaning of the *Delusion* rubric: *hand does not belong to her*, and the *Delusion* rubric: *feet do not belong to her*.

Carcinosin will not be responsible for controlling their own motivation; they abdicate responsibility for what their hands or feet decide to do, or who they are influenced by. The action of the simillimum will provide her with a stronger sense of her own 'boundaries' so she can feel connected[16] to herself. As soon as personal responsibility or 'ownership' develops inside *Carcinosin* the glorification of martyrdom diminishes. As soon as the glorification of martyrdom diminishes, *Carcinosin* will stop depleting their energy.

1. Denial: *Delusion* rubric: *martyr; of being a*: carc. [1]1. *Delusion* rubric: *superhuman; is; control; is under superhuman*: carc. *Delusion* rubric: *influence; one is under a powerful*: Carc. *Delusion* rubric: *visions; has*: carc. [These rubrics can refer to illusions that one is under the control of God or the devil.]

2. Forsaken: *Delusion* rubric: *appreciated, she is not*: Carc. *Delusion* rubric: *separated*: *world; from the*: *he is separated*: carc. *Delusion* rubric: *wrong*: *suffered wrong*; *he has*: carc. *Delusion* rubric: *poisoned*: *he*; *about to be poisoned*; *he is*: carc. *Delusion* rubric: *criticized, she is*: carc. *Delusion* rubric: *murdered*: *will be murdered; he*: carc. *Delusion* rubric: *pursued; he was*: carc. *Delusion* rubric: *alone, being*: *belong to anyone; she did not*: carc. *Delusion* rubric: *alone, being*: *always alone; she is*: carc. *Delusion* rubric: *friendless, he is*: carc.

3. Causation: *Delusion* rubric: *wrong*: *doing something wrong; he is*: Carc. *Delusion* rubric: *influence; one is under a powerful*: Carc. *Delusion* rubric: *superhuman; is; control; is under superhuman*: carc. [These two rubrics can refer to illusions that one is under the control of the devil.]

4. Depression: *Delusion* rubric: *fail, everything will*: carc. *Delusion* rubric: *annihilation; about to sink into*: Carc. *Delusion* rubric: *protection, defense; has no*: carc.

5. Resignation: *Delusion* rubric: *cancer, has a*: carc. *Delusion* rubric: *hand*: *belong to her, does not*: carc. [1]1. *Delusion* rubric: *feet*: *belong to her, does not*: carc. [1]1. *Delusion* rubric: *protection, defense; has no*: carc. [This rubric can pertain to emotional sensitivity or physical sensitivity.]

- *Delusions*: *messenger: she is a*: irid-met.[1] 1.
- *Delusions*: *messages; hears*: irid-met.[1] 1.
- *Delusions*: *mystic hallucinations*: aether. irid-met.
- *Delusions*: *mission: one has a*: ignis-alc. *Plat.*
- *Delusions*: *awakened; he is*: *just been awakened; he has*: cycl. irid-met. mang.

Self-Deluding: It is important in the case-management and case analysis to fully understand the *exact* nature of the psychodynamic crisis your patient needs to protect. If you believe you are on a 'mission from God' then 'God is on your side' to *protect* you.

Iridium metallicum have the *Delusion* rubric: *being the goddess Iris*. In Greek mythology, Iris was a messenger, she linked the Gods to humanity. *Iridium metallicum* have pretentious 'delusions of grandeur' that they are elevated above the world. *Iridium metallicum* have the *Delusion* rubric: *he is separated, floating in his inner self*. [1] 1. *Iridium metallicum* have 'hubristic visions' of grandeur that they are a messenger from the Gods – *she is a messenger*.

Iridium metallicum feel pure, as if they have come from a 'God-like' state. *Iridium metallicum* have the *Delusion* rubric: *he was newly born in the world and he was overwhelmed in wonder at the novelty of his surroundings*.

Iridium sits next to Platinum and Gold in the Periodic table. Jan Scholten notes, in *Homoeopathy and The Elements*, Radar™, the following profile of *Iridium metallicum*: "Picture of Iridium Metallicum: They always feel they have to extend their business, to go into it in more depth, to do more. They haven't nearly finished what they set out to do and they do their best to get the business to the very top. Their potential hasn't been fully exploited yet. And that which remains outside their reach is seen as a sign that they have failed to be a super power. They tend to be quite single minded, they are always preoccupied with what is yet to be done. The people around are usually several steps behind and blame them for being unrealistic or irresponsible. They may seem irresponsible but this is only because they see everything from the point of unexplored possibilities."

Iridium metallicum are narcissistic.

Iridium metallicum have such huge pretensions of grandeur that they suffer from a narcissistic crisis of their 'super-ego'.

The 'super-ego' aims for perfection. A narcissist puts their own needs in front of anyone else's. The narcissist exaggerates their own superiority. The narcissist seeks constant attention, has unreasonable expectations of importance, and has unreasonable expectations of favorable treatment. The narcissist uses rationalization to justify self-centered behavior.

The narcissist uses denial to downplay their own inadequacies or failings. *Iridium metallicum* believe they are enlightened – *he has just been awakened*. Energy which is disproportionately redirected into a narcissist persona cause 'delusions of grandeur'.

'Narcissistic neurosis' is a pre-emptive causation for manic-depressive psychosis insofar as it is characterized by the withdrawal of energy from the realistic and rational 'ego'.

Iridium metallicum are prone to manic-depressive psychosis because their narcissist pretensions are so unrealistic that they can't fulfill them.

Bipolar disorder, also known as manic depression, is a psychiatric diagnosis that describes a category of mood disorders defined by the presence of one or more episodes of abnormally elevated mood, clinically referred to as mania. Individuals who experience manic episodes also commonly experience depressive episodes. Extreme manic episodes can sometimes lead to psychotic symptoms such as delusions and hallucinations. In some cases it can be a long-lasting disorder; in others, it has been associated with creativity, and extraordinary achievements. *Iridium metallicum* have the *Delusion* rubrics: *weight pressing down from above,* and *as if suffocating. Iridium metallicum* have the *Delusion* rubric: *a heavy black cloud enveloped her.*

When *Iridium metallicum* are in a manic episode they are inspired by *mystical hallucinations from angels.* When *Iridium metallicum* are in a depressive episode they are enveloped by heavy black clouds of suffocating depression.

When *Iridium metallicum* are physically sick they alternate between manic episodes of delusional belief in cure and all enveloping depression. *Iridium metallicum* suffer from psychosomatic conditions which arise from their 'narcissistic neuroses'. Clarke notes, in *A Dictionary of Practical Materia Medica*: "weariness in back and limbs followed by favorable reaction; feeling of aplomb and self-confidence." *Iridium metallicum* is an excellent homoeopathic remedy for neuralgic weakness followed by increased strength. This *peculiar* alternation of neurotic symptoms of weakness followed by increased narcissistic self-confidence, is consistent with the polarities of psychotic mania and the neurotic depression. *Iridium metallicum* have the *Delusion* rubrics: *he seems to reach the clouds,* and *a heavy black cloud enveloped her.* ('Neuroses', relate to physical psychosomatic conditions, and 'psychoses', relate to mental conflict between the 'ego' and the external world.)

The simillimum will *not* be *Iridium metallicum* if the patient acknowledges that they have contributed to their disease. *Iridium metallicum* have no *Delusion* rubrics pertaining to self-blame. *Iridium metallicum* maintain their delusional belief in their hubristic role because it reinforces their narcissistic self-confidence. When *Iridium metallicum* are physically sick they are forced to acknowledge their depressive episodes because they feel as if they are *diminishing*. When *Iridium metallicum* are sick they feel as if they are being compressed into a narrow space.

Iridium metallicum maintain their delusional belief in their hubristic role because it elevates them above their depression. *Iridium metallicum* maintain their delusional belief in their hubristic role as a messenger from God because they need to believe they are floating above the mundane.

1. Denial: *Delusion* rubric: *messenger; she is*: irid-met. [1]
   1. *Delusion* rubric: *awakened; he is*: *just been awakened; he has*: irid-met. *Delusion* rubric: *angels, seeing*: irid-met. *Delusion* rubric: *beautiful: landscape; of*: irid-met. *Delusion* rubric: *elevated: air, elevated in the*: irid-met. *Delusion*

rubric: *clouds*: *reach the clouds; he seems to*: irid-met. [1] 1. *Delusion* rubric: *enlarged*: irid-met. *Delusion* rubric: *influence; one is under a powerful*: irid-met. *Delusion* rubric: *iris; being the goddess*: irid-met. [1] 1. *Delusion* rubric: *mystic hallucinations*: irid-met. *Delusion* rubric: *separated*: *floating in his inner self; he is*: irid-met. [1] 1. *Delusion* rubric: *born into the world; he was newly*: *wonder at the novelty of his surroundings; and was overwhelmed with*: irid-met. *Delusion* rubric: *separated*: *world; from the*: *he is separated*: irid-met. [This rubric normally pertains to 'delusions of abandonment', but in relation to *Iridium metallicum* it indicates that they are elevated from the world.]

2. Forsaken: *Delusion* rubric: *strangers*: *surrounded by*: irid-met. *Delusion* rubric: *alone, being*: *world; alone in the*: irid-met. *Delusion* rubric: *injury*: *about to receive injury; is*: irid-met.

3. Causation: NONE.

4. Depression: *Delusion* rubric: *clouds*: *black cloud enveloped her*: *a heavy*: irid-met. *Delusion* rubric: *weight*: *pressing down from above*: irid-met. [1] 1. *Delusion* rubric: *diminished*: *all is*: irid-met.

5. Resignation: *Delusion* rubric: *suffocating; as if*: irid-met. *Delusion* rubric: *narrow; everything seems too*: irid-met. *Delusion* rubric: *space*: *contraction of*: irid-met. [1] 1. [When *Iridium metallicum* are sick they suffer from claustrophobia.]

Platina are listed in more of the *Delusion* rubrics pertaining to 'delusions of grandeur' than any other remedy profile. The underlying motive behind the belief that they are *on a mission* is the need to believe their *noble religious superiority*. *Platina*, like *Iridium metallicum*, have the *Delusion* rubric: *being alone in the world*.

Platina think they are superior to everyone else and that no one can possibly be as great as them; their superiority is why they are alone in a strange land, and their aloneness is also what undermines them.

Platina when they are sick go into a deep psychosis of self-denial because they are extremely fearful of the illness inside themselves, which they equate with being *possessed by the devil*. Alignment to God is extremely important to *Platina*. This is why they have so many *Delusion* rubrics of religiosity. *Platina* also have the *Mind* rubric: *religious affections, too occupied with religion, desires religious penance.* [2] 1., and the *Mind* rubric: *religious affections, too occupied with religion, alternating with sexual desire. Platina* call and *talk to spirits* (God) to save themselves from the devil inside themselves and outside of themselves.

When *Platina* are sick, they move into and stay in 'hubristic denial' to avoid their numerous 'delusions of abandonment'. *Platina* equate illness with proof that they have been abandoned because they are not good enough. The simillimum will only be *Platina* if the patient admits or asks you if the reason why they are sick is because God has abandoned them because they have been bad.

Denial: "I will be cured": *Delusion rubrics: in communication with God.*

- *Delusions: help: calling for:* plat. [1] 1.
- *Delusions: talking: spirits, with:* Plat.
- *Delusions: superhuman; is; control; is under superhuman:* plat.
- *Delusions: diminished: everything in room is diminished; while she is tall and elevated:* plat. [1] 1.
- *Delusions: better than others; he is:* plat.
- *Delusions: body: greatness of, as to:* Plat.
- *Delusions: exalted; as if:* plat.
- *Delusions: fancy, illusions of:* Plat.
- *Delusions: great person, is a:* Plat.

- *Delusions: humility and lowness of others; while he is great:* plat.
- *Delusions: inferior, people seem mentally and physically: entering the house after a walk; when:* plat. [1] 1.
- *Delusions: mission; one has a: Plat.*
- *Delusions: noble; being:* plat.
- *Delusions: proud:* plat.
- *Delusions: religious:* plat.
- *Delusions: superiority, of: Plat.*
- *Delusions: wealth, of: Plat.*
- *Delusions: looking: down; he was looking: high place; from a:* **PLAT**.
- *Delusions: grow: larger and longer; he grew:* plat.
- *Delusions: strong; he is:* plat.
- *Delusions: tall: he or she is tall:* plat.

Forsaken: "I have been abandoned": ***Delusion* rubrics: forsaken.**

- *Delusions: alone, being: world; alone in the: Plat.*
- *Delusions: belong to her own family; she does not: Plat.*
- *Delusions: appreciated, she is not:* plat.
- *Delusions: disgraced: she is:* plat.
- *Delusions: disgraced: family or friends; he has disgraced his:* plat.
- *Delusions: enemy: everyone is an:* plat.
- *Delusions: family, does not belong to her own:* plat. [1] 1.
- *Delusions: forsaken; is: Plat.*
- *Delusions: place: no place in the world; she has: Plat.*
- *Delusions: strange: land; as if in strange:* plat.
- *Delusions: neglected: he or she is neglected:* plat.
- *Delusions: place: strange place; he was in a:* plat.

- *Delusions: devil: all persons are devils:* **PLAT**.
- *Delusions: choked: he is about to be: night: waking; on:* *Plat.*

1. Denial: *Delusion* rubric: *mission; one has a:* *Plat. Delusion* rubric: *superhuman; is; control; is under superhuman:* plat. *Delusion* rubric: *looking: down; he was looking: high place; from a:* **PLAT**.

2. Forsaken: *Delusion* rubric: *alone, being: world; alone in the:* *Plat. Delusion* rubric: *belong to her own family; she does not:* *Plat. Delusion* rubric: *appreciated, she is not:* plat. *Delusion* rubric: *disgraced: she is:* plat. *Delusion* rubric: *enemy: everyone is an:* plat. *Delusion* rubric: *family, does not belong to her own:* plat. [1] 1. *Delusion* rubric: *forsaken; is:* *Plat. Delusion* rubric: *place: no place in the world; she has:* *Plat. Delusion* rubric: *strange: land; as if in strange:* plat.

3. Causation: *Delusion* rubric: *devil: possessed of a devil: he is:* plat.

4. Depression: *Delusion* rubric: *depressive:* plat. *Delusion* rubric: *doomed, being:* *Plat. Delusion* rubric: *insane: become insane; one will:* plat. *Delusion* rubric: *melancholy:* plat. *Delusion* rubric: *terrible; everything seems:* plat.

5. Resignation: *Delusion* rubric: *dead: he himself was:* plat. *Delusion* rubric: *die: about to die; one was:* *Plat. Delusion* rubric: *body: cut though; he is: two; in:* plat.

- *Delusions: people: conversing with absent people:* agar. aur. bell. calc. cham. crot-c. dig. hyos. lach. op. *Stram.* thuj. *Verat.*
- *Delusions: mushroom: he is commanded by a: confess his sins; to fall on his knees and to:* agar.[1] 1.

Self-deluding: The need behind each remedy listed in this rubric is a delusional need to deny both the weakness felt when sick and the finality of death. The remedies listed in the rubric *conversing with absent people*, have a psychological need to deny the powerlessness inherent in illness and death.

It is not unusual for patients to be visited by lost relatives in their dreams who assure them they are so special that they have been chosen by God to be saved or blessed.

Agaricus have exalted 'delusions of grandeur' which cover up their fears of becoming so small and helpless that they will diminish in all importance. *Agaricus* psychologically need to *converse with absent people* to maintain an illusion that they are powerful.

1. Denial: *Delusion* rubric: *people: conversing with absent people*: agar. *Delusions: mushroom: he is commanded by a: confess his sins; to fall on his knees and to*: agar. [1] 1. *Delusion* rubric: *great person, is a: Agar. Delusion* rubric: *body: out of body: enjoy to provoke out of body experiences*: agar. [1] 1. *Delusion* rubric: *fancy, illusions of*: agar. *Delusion* rubric: *hearing: illusions of*. agar. *Delusion* rubric: *large: everything looks larger*. agar. *Delusion* rubric: *superhuman; is: control; is under superhuman*: agar.

2. Forsaken: *Delusion* rubric: *arms: belongs to her; arms do not*: agar. *Delusion* rubric: *legs: belong to her; her legs don't. Agar.* [These rubrics in relation to *Agaricus* pertain to fears of self-abandonment.] *Delusion* rubric: *poisoned: he; has been*: agar.

3. Causation: *Delusion* rubric: *hell; confess his sins at gate of; obliged to*: agar [1] 1.

4. Depression: *Delusion* rubric: *paralyzed; he is*: agar.

5. Resignation: *Delusion* rubric: *body, diminished; is*: agar. *Delusion* rubric: *arms: belongs to her; arms do not*: agar. *Delusion* rubric: *legs: belong to her; her legs don't. Agar. Delusion* rubric: *paralyzed; he is*: agar.

Agaricus need to view themselves as great; this is reflected in the *Mind* rubric: *egotism, reciting their exploits*: agar. [1] 1. *Agaricus* have a strong need for materialistic proof of their grandeur and worldly success; this is not only reflected in the *Delusion* rubric: *is a great person*, but also in the *Mind* rubric:

incorrect judgement of size. However, *Agaricus* feel threatened with any illness; this is the meaning and significance of all the rubrics pertaining to the loss of arms and legs.

> If the homoeopath recognizes and understands the importance of rubric-analysis, and understands the rubrics associated with a remedy, they will know that when sick, *Agaricus* will present in the first consultation in a very depressed and paralyzed state. The grandness of the egotistical *Agaricus* is not what you will see; *Agaricus* will be in a very small and diminished state.

If they feel threatened or shamed by failure they immediately feel as if they are diminishing in size and losing all power. This is reflected in the *Mind* rubric: *looking down when looked at.* [1] 1. If challenged they feel as if they are losing their arms and legs in the world and they compensate for their feeling of vulnerability by being extremely nasty. *Agaricus* have the *Mind* rubric: *hatred of persons who have offended him,* and the *Delusion* rubric: *vindictive.* [1] 1. Their psychological need to connect to a metaphysical power outside of themselves is paramount to their ability to find their power in the world. *Agaricus* have the *Delusion* rubrics: *conversing with absent people, objects are enlarged, is under superhuman control,* and *enjoy to provoke out of body experiences.* [1] 1. The psychodynamic polarity of expanding greatness and diminishing smallness is extreme in *Agaricus.* In the *Case Companion* to *Homoeopathic Psychiatry,* the *Agaricus* (case) solves her psychological dilemma of expanding and diminishing potency by creating two worlds. In each world she has a boyfriend; having two partners makes her feel strong. *Agaricus* have hubristic visions of grandeur which they maintain because they need to avoid their underlying fear that they will be diminished.

1. Denial: *Delusion* rubric: *great person, is a*: *Agar.*

    Versus

5. Resignation: *Delusion* rubric: *body, diminished; is*: agar.

The *Delusion* rubric: *he is commanded by a mushroom to fall on his knees and confess his sins* is a fascinating *Delusion* rubric which is *peculiar* to *Agaricus* since it is the only remedy listed. Until I understood the self-denial within *Agaricus* I had previously assumed that this rubric resonated with the source of the remedy, which is a hallucinogenic fungi. *Agaricus* have the *Mind* rubrics: *weakness of memory for what he has just done*, and *revealing secrets*. *Agaricus* are very happy to reveal *others' secrets* but they are extremely selective about remembering or revealing things about themselves. *Agaricus* have the *Mind* rubrics: *refusing to answer*, and *aversion to answer, sings, talks, but will not answer questions.* [1] 1. *Agaricus* never tell the whole truth about their sins to anyone, except to the mushroom who is able to have power of command over them. This *Delusion* rubric: *he is commanded by a mushroom to fall on his knees and confess his sins*, reinforces what I have written in the section above. *Agaricus* need to connect to a metaphysical power outside of themselves to be able to find their own power in the world. This is why *Agaricus* have the *Delusion* rubric: *conversing with absent people*. The *Delusion* rubric: *he is commanded by a mushroom to fall on his knees and confess his sins*, can obviously not be taken literally. The psychodynamic meaning is that *Agaricus* would rather transfer control to a mushroom than allow anyone to have control over them.

Agaricus are extremely attached to not allowing 'the right hand to see what the left hand is doing'.

Agaricus also have the *Delusion* rubric: *obliged to confess his sins at the gate of hell.* [1] 1. The psychological denial inherent within this *Delusion* rubric alludes to the fact that unless *Agaricus* are forced by someone else, they do not want to acknowledge their 'dark-side' [*sins*]. *Agaricus* have the *Delusion* rubric: *enjoy out of body experiences.* [1] 1. It is a mistake to assume that this *Delusion* rubric resonates with the energy of the hallucinogenic fungi.

Agaricus have the *Mind* rubric: *self-denial.* [1] 2. [staph.] *Agaricus* have a strong psychotic split within their persona which allows them to dissociate from their body and indulge their personality in exalted hubristic visions.

Agaricus have the *Delusion* rubric: *illusions of fancy*, and the *Mind* rubrics: *euphoria*, and *egotism, reciting their exploits.* [1] 1. Conversely, *Agaricus* have the *Delusion* rubric: *body is diminished*, and the *Mind* rubric: *biting himself.* The latter two rubrics reinforce the need within *Agaricus* to maintain hubristic visions of grandeur because they need to avoid their underlying fear that they will be diminished not only from outside themselves but also from within. *Agaricus* have several *Mind* rubrics which collaborate: not only do they struggle to assert themselves, they are also involved in a self-punishing battle. Not only do *Agaricus* want to be out of their body [*Delusion* rubric: *out of body*] they want to self-destruct. The *Mind* rubric: *self-denial* will always indicate psychotic, self-destructive addictive behavior. *Agaricus* have several *Mind* rubrics which corroborate this: *ailments from alcoholism – ailments from debauchery – ailments from punishment – ailments from sexual excesses – anger with himself – biting himself – bulimia – frenzy causing him to injure himself.* *Agaricus* have the *Delusion* rubrics: *he is intoxicated*, and *he is drunk.* Both of these *Delusion* rubrics indicate a strong psychodynamic need to split from their conscious mind. Not only do *Agaricus* transfer their metaphysical power outside of themselves, [*to a mushroom*], they also hand over control of their body. *Agaricus* have the *Delusion* rubric: *he is commanded by a mushroom to rip up his bowels.* [1] 1.

Agaricus displays on the one hand, 'delusions of grandeur' – *is a great person* – and on the other hand, self-diminishing needs to dissociate themselves from their body – *legs don't belong to her.* This polarity indicates self-destructive tendencies.

This psychological understanding of *Agaricus* has always been in our *Mind* and *Delusion* rubrics, but my aim in this rubric-analysis is to apply psychological labels to what is already in our repertories.

The purpose in identifying psychological behavioral patterning inherent within the remedy profile is that this understanding can then be applied to identifying the simillimum in case analysis.

Aurum metallicum believe they can converse with God – *Delusion* rubric: *religious*. *Aurum metallicum* fear they have *neglected their duty*. Conversing with *absent people*, (God or spirits) reinstates righteousness which protects them from their own feeling of doom.

When they are sick *Aurum metallicum* present with the two polarities of sinking depressive hopelessness and religious fervor.

The underlying fear is that their psyche will feel empty of all salvation – *hollow*. *Aurum metallicum* have the *Delusion* rubric: *emptiness of internal*: aur. [1] 1. *Aurum metallicum* also have the *Delusion* rubric: *she is lost for salvation*. This profound religious fear of being lost indicates why *Aurum metallicum* will hang on to their fundamentalist need for God and religion.

1. Denial: *Delusion* rubric: *people: conversing with absent people*: aur. *Delusion* rubric: *religious*: aur.
2. Forsaken· *Delusion* rubric: *forsaken; is*: Aur. *Delusion* rubric: *lost; she is; salvation; for.* Aur.
3. Causation: *Delusion* rubric: *sinned; one has; unpardonable sin; he had committed the*: aur.
4. Depression: *Delusion* rubric: *succeed, he does everything wrong; he cannot*: Aur.
5. Resignation: *Delusion* rubric: *hollow: body is hollow; whole*: aur.

Crotalus cascavella is a homoeopathic remedy derived from the South American rattlesnake. *Crotalus cascavella* suffer exaggerated 'persecution complexes'. *Crotalus cascavella* use their clairvoyant and clairaudient ability to hear voices and converse with spirits and ghosts who warn *Crotalus cascavella* of any impending attacks. *Crotalus cascavella* have the *Mind* rubrics: *clairvoyance,* and *déjà vu. Crotalus cascavella* have the *Delusion* rubrics: *conversing with absent people, hearing voices, specters, ghosts, spirits,* and *hearing voices that he must follow.* Underpinning their hubristic connections with the spirits are numerous paranoid 'persecution complexes' and numerous rubrics pertaining to 'delusions of persecution'. *Crotalus cascavella* have the *Delusion* rubrics: *being attacked, deceived, persecuted,* and *surrounded by snakes.*

Crotalus cascavella maintain their 'delusions of superiority' because underpinning their hubristic visions is the fear that they will be looked down upon.

When they are looked down upon they feel vulnerable to being attacked. *Crotalus cascavella* have the *Delusion* rubric: *he is insulted and looked down upon. Crotalus cascavella* will maintain their hyper-vigilance because their fears of being attacked from behind rule their every waking moment. *Crotalus cascavella* have the *Delusion* rubrics: *someone is behind him,* and *hearing footsteps behind him.*

The 'never-well-since-event' in *Crotalus cascavella* will always have its origins in physical abuse in their childhood. *Crotalus cascavella* are trapped in a cycle of abuse. They alternate between the one who is being abused, self-abuse, and becoming the abuser. *Crotalus cascavella* self-mutilate. *Crotalus cascavella* have the *Mind* rubrics: *antagonism with herself,* and *destructiveness alternating with fear of being harmed.* [1] 1. *Crotalus cascavella* have the *Mind* rubric: *desire to cut, mutilate or slit with a sharp knife.* [1] 1. *Crotalus cascavella* maintain the illusion that they are *superior* to overcome feeling *small. Crotalus cascavella* disproportionately fear that they are *insulted and looked down upon. Crotalus cascavella* suffer exaggerated fears of retaliation. This undermining paranoia creates pent up anger. *Crotalus cascavella* are preoccupied with impending death. *Crotalus cascavella* have the *Delusion* rubrics: *death appears as a gigantic black skeleton,* and *sees skeletons. Crotalus cascavella* suffer psychological delusional fears of once again being abused. *Crotalus cascavella* is a good homoeopathic remedy to use for all psychosomatic illusions that the body is being constricted, strangulated, constrained, or choked. *Crotalus cascavella* have the *Mind* rubric: *violent anger. Crotalus cascavella* somatically strangle themselves with their own pent up anger. *Crotalus cascavella* have the *Delusion* rubric: *that she is forced. Crotalus cascavella* need to maintain their hyper-vigilant reliance on their conversations with absent people and their hyper-vigilant anger because it is the only weapon they have to protect themselves from being abused.

1. Denial: *Delusion* rubric: *people: conversing with absent people*: crot-c. *Delusion* rubric: *fancy, illusions of: Crot-c. Delusion* rubric: *visions, has: Crot-c. Delusion* rubric: *great person, is a*: crot-c. *Delusion* rubric: *superiority, of:* crot-c. *Delusion* rubric: *tall: he or she is tall*: crot-c.

2. Forsaken: *Delusion* rubric: *attacked; being*: crot-c. *Delusion* rubric: *deceived; being*: crot-c. *Delusion* rubric: *forsaken; is*: crot-c. *Delusion* rubric: *insulted, he is: looked down upon*: crot-c. [1] 1. *Delusion* rubric: *neglected: he or she is neglected*: crot-c. *Delusion* rubric: *outcast; she were an*: crot-c. *Delusion* rubric: *persecuted: he is persecuted*: crot-c. *Delusion* rubric: *snakes: in and around her*: crot-c. *Delusion* rubric: *skeletons, sees*: crot-c. [1] 2. [op.] *Delusion* rubric: *people: behind him; someone is*: crot-c. *Delusion* rubric: *footsteps; hearing*: crot-c. *Delusion* rubric: *talking: people talk about her*: crot-c. *Delusion* rubric: *forced; that she is*: crot-c. [1] 1.

3. Causation: *Delusion* rubric: *criminal, he is a*: crot-c. *Delusion* rubric: *neglected: duty; he has neglected his*: crot-c. *Delusion* rubric: *wrong: done wrong; he has*: crot-c.

4. Depression: *Delusion* rubric: *insulted, he is: looked down upon*: crot-c. [1] 1. [This rubric is descriptive of their self-deprecation as well as pertaining to persecution rubrics of abandonment.] *Delusion* rubric: *forced; that she is*: crot-c. [1] 1.

5. Resignation: *Delusion* rubric: *small: body is smaller.* crot-c.

Digitalis is a homoeopathic remedy commonly used for angina pectoris, auricular fibrillation and cardiac muscular failure. *Digitalis* have the *Mind* rubric: *fear of death during heart symptoms* [3]. I have consulted with only one *Digitalis* patient. She was an elderly woman, aged eighty-two years. Since her marriage at nineteen she had suffered intense fears of dying from a heart attack in her sleep. Her fear was that *she would not be there* (conscious) *and not be able to stop death*. She had several keynote symptoms of *Digitalis*: swelling of her feet, waking with a start in her sleep, jaundice, nausea after eating, and hypertrophy of her heart. She had an irregular beat because of ventricle valve failure, as well as early signs of cyanosis. She had been anxious her whole life that she would not be *awake at her time of death*. Her daughter was a homoeopath who had given her every remedy one would consider such as: *Aconite, Arsenicum album, Calcarea carbonica, Kali carbonica, Sulphur,* etc. The list was extensive. The specific peculiarity which unlocked her case, and the remedy profile of *Digitalis,* was the *Delusion* rubric: *brain is made of glass.* Phatak, in *Materia Medica of Homeopathic Medicines,* notes that *Digitalis* "feels as if he would fly to pieces. Great anxiety like from troubled conscience." *Digitalis* have psychological delusions of having failed. They fear that others will perceive their failure. *Digitalis* expect at any moment to be *reproved* because of their accumulated 'delusions of original sin'. It is important never to dismiss a patient's seemingly irrational fear or illogical statement. I asked her, "why is it important that you are awake if you are going to have a heart attack at night?" She replied: *if God was going to come when I am asleep I wouldn't be able to hide my sins. God will be able to see right through my brain and see everything I have done. If I am awake I will be able to make sure that I am also in contact with my dear mother who will guide me to the light.*

Regardless of how bizarre a *Delusion* rubric might appear, it will always have a significant and *specific* meaning. The *Delusion* rubric: *brain is made of glass*, indicates that the brain can be looked through. *Digitalis* fear being exposed.

Digitalis specifically fear they will fall to pieces if someone sees the sins which they feel they have committed. I gave the patient *Digitalis* 200 c x 3 doses in a 24 hour period. She defied medical expectations and lived for another two years. She died having resolved her guilt. She had been disappointed in her marriage and felt very guilty because she had actively hated and punished her husband for years. Ironically, she died in her sleep of a heart attack. *Digitalis* have the *Mind* rubric: *ailments from disappointed love.* Her husband had turned out to be "a gambler and a drunk". She felt that shortly after their marriage she began to spend her life *terrorizing him* for not being what she had hoped for. She felt that she had spent her life lamenting her situation. *Digitalis* have the *Mind* rubric: *tearful, morose.* [1] 1. *Digitalis* suffer from sadness over failures in their life, especially failure in love. This overwhelming sense of having made wrong decisions causes them to not want to be in their conscious mind.

Digitalis converse with absent people to create a bridge between their own consciousness and 'the world of ghosts'. *Digitalis* set up a subconscious psychodynamic struggle because they want to live in a semi-conscious state aligned with *specters, ghosts,* and *spirits. Digitalis* have the *Delusion* rubrics: *it was time for rising*, [1] 1., *he had not slept enough*, and *he would faint.* All three rubrics indicate that *Digitalis* have a tentative hold on conscious wakefulness; they want to live in a semi-awake state. *Digitalis* prefer to live in a semi-conscious state to avoid the pain of what the future will hold. *Digitalis* is a remedy profile of grief from disappointed love. *Digitalis* continue to live out their lives, but part of their mind has left and no longer has a hold on consciousness. *Digitalis* have the *Mind* rubric: *confusion of mind, as after being intoxicated*. *Digitalis* have the psychological expectation that they will be scolded and rebuked for their part in their failed love. *Digitalis* have the *Delusion* rubric: *expects to be reproved*. [1] 1. *Digitalis* have the *Delusion* rubric: *he has done wrong*. *Digitalis* choose to escape into confusion so they can avoid being scolded. *Digitalis* have the *Mind* rubric: *attempts to escape*. The *Delusion* rubric: *brain is made of glass*, also indicates that at any moment they could be broken and *lose consciousness*. *Digitalis* suffer from crippling anxiety about the future.

Their *illusions of fancy* create an imaginary world in which they have assured confidence over life. *Digitalis* struggle to get over the sense that they have failed and that it is their fault.

1. Denial: *Delusion* rubric: *people: conversing with absent people*: dig. *Delusion* rubric: *visions, has*: dig. *Delusion* rubric: *fancy illusions, of*: dig.

2. Forsaken: *Delusion* rubric: *reproved: expects to be reproved; he*: dig. [1] 1.

3. Causation: *Delusion* rubric: *criminal, he is a*: dig. *Delusion* rubric: *wrong: done wrong; he has*: dig.

4. Depression: *Delusion* rubric: *consciousness: lose consciousness; he would*: dig.

5. Resignation: *Delusion* rubric: *brain: glass; made of*: Dig. [2] 1. *Delusion* rubric: *light: is light; he*: dig. *Delusion* rubric: *faint; he would: standing; while*: dig. [1] 1.

Opium have persecution paranoia based upon a guilty conscience. *Opium* are *pursued* as if they are a *criminal* by *devils*, *scorpions*, *rats*, and *people wanting to execute them*. *Opium* have numerous *Delusion* rubrics, all pertaining to 'delusions of abandonment', and 'delusions of persecution'. Their 'never-well since-event', or causation, will always have its origins in real or perceived crimes committed. It should be noted that in *Opium* the 'hubristic denial' is so extreme that often, their 'delusions of original sin' are not only hidden from the practitioner, they are also hidden from the patient's conscious mind. *Opium* have the *Mind* rubrics: *blissful feeling,* and the *Delusion* rubric: *is in heaven.*

The visionary illusions allow *Opium* to escape from the reality and harshness of life.

Opium are listed in all the *Mind* rubrics: *ailments from fright, grief, homelessness, reprimands, mental shock,* and even *sudden joy. Opium* choose to delude themselves that they are in a beautiful heaven in order to avoid feeling. *Opium* are fearful of feeling.

Opium need to maintain their illusions because they have an intense 'persecution complex'. *Opium* are pursued by their own guilty conscience. *Opium* is a homoeopathic remedy derived from the hallucinogenic opium poppy. *Opium,* as a constitutional remedy profile, carry with them a drug-like, euphoric need to create a vision of the world other than the one in their conscious mind.

I have discussed *Opium* in the chapter on Causation. In that chapter I emphasize their need to avoid reality. In this chapter, it is important to highlight the euphoric nature of *Opium. Opium* will stay in the denial stage of disease and death longer than any other constitutional remedy profile. If *Opium* are faced with the reality of their illness, they will be forced to face their numerous fears of abandonment and persecution from society. *Opium* will also have to face their own demons, and their guilty conscience. *Opium* create an inner world of illusions that their illness is a journey of delightful discovery.

Opium psychosomatically wish to distance themselves from feeling. *Opium* the drug acts as a sedative and analgesic. *Opium* the constitutional remedy profile similarly suppress their somatic responsiveness to themselves and to others in the world. The *Opium* patient lacks appropriate empathic responsiveness to their own pain.

Anyone who has nursed a cancer patient in the last weeks of the patient's life, when they are consuming huge amounts of the drug morphine, will be well aware of the surreal emotional hopefulness that the patient moves into. Although, the patient is clearly at the end of their life, they are convinced that they have complete control of their disease – *is under superhuman control*. Often, God and angels are visiting them to reassure them of immortality and cure, and their semi-conscious mind is filled with delightful images of beautiful visions of themselves cured. In the chapter on Causation I make the comment that *Opium* are attracted to Tibetan Buddhism. They are also attracted to modalities like Neuro-Linguistic Programming, (NLP). The 'inspiritive'© promise within the philosophy of NLP is extremely attractive to *Opium*. *Opium* thrive on the illusion that they can create and have created a world of realized visions. *Opium* thrive on their 'delusions of hubristic visions'. Their 'hubristic denial' will *peculiarly* lack appropriate empathic responses to pain and/or illness because they have a delusional inconsistency in their psyche. *Opium* as a homoeopathic remedy is often used for the patient who is so constipated that they have no sensation of peristaltic movement. *Opium* deny they are sick because they do not wish to feel pain.

1. Denial: *Delusion* rubric: *well, he is*: op.

   Versus

5. *Delusion* rubric: *dying*: *he is*: op.

1. Denial: *Delusion* rubric: *people*: *conversing with absent people*: op. *Delusion* rubric: *beautiful*: op. *Delusion* rubric: *heaven, is in*: op. *Delusion* rubric: *visions, has beautiful*: **OP**. *Delusion* rubric: *fancy, illusions of*: *Op*. *Delusion* rubric: *journey; he is on*: op. *Delusion* rubric: *superhuman; is*: *control; is under superhuman*: op. *Delusion* rubric: *pleasing delusions*: op. *Delusion* rubric: *visions, has*: *fantastic*: op.

Delusion rubric: *well, he is*: op. *Delusion* rubric: *visions, has*: *delight; visions of: night; filled his brain all*: op. [1] 1.

2. Forsaken: *Delusion* rubric: *execute him; people want to*: **OP**. *Delusion* rubric: *poisoned: he, has been*: op. *Delusion* rubric: *criminal, he is a*: *executed, to be*: **OP**. *Delusion* rubric: *bed*: *surrounded by devils; is*: op.[1] 1. *Delusion* rubric: *home*: *away from home; he is*: *must get there*: Op. *Delusion* rubric: *pursued; he was*: op. *Delusion* rubric: *rats, sees*: op. *Delusion* rubric: *scorpions; sees*: **OP**. [3] 1. *Delusion* rubric: *skeletons, sees*: op. *Delusion* rubric: *snakes*: *in and around her*. op. *Delusion* rubric: *stabbed*: *somebody threatened to stab him; as if*: op. [1] 1. *Delusion* rubric: *visions, has*: *monsters, of*. op. *Delusion* rubric: *house*: *own house; not being in one's*: Op.

3. Causation: *Delusion* rubric: *criminal; he is a*: op. *Delusion* rubric: *criminal, he is a*: *executed, to be*: **OP**. [3] 1. *Delusion* rubric: *wrong*: *done wrong; he has*: *punished; and about to be*: op. [1] 1.

4. Depression: *Delusion* rubric: *doomed, being*: op.

5. Resignation: *Delusion* rubric: *weight*: *no weight; has*: op. *Delusion* rubric: *body*: *lighter than air; body is*: Op. *Delusion* rubric: *dying*: *he is*: op.

- *Delusions*: *friend*: *fantasy world of imaginary friends*: *lives in a*: calc. [1] 1.
- *Delusions*: *friend*: *surrounded by friends*: *being*: aids. bell. cann-i. germ-met.
- *Delusions*: *people*: *seeing people*: *Ars.* atro. **BELL**. *Bry. Calc.* chin. con. *Hyos.* kali-c. kola. lac-loxod-a. lyc. lyss. mag-c. mag-s. med. merc. nat-m. op. petr. plb. *Puls.* rheum. sep. *Stram.* sulph. thuj. valer. verat.
- *Delusions*: *caressed on head by someone*: *Med.* [2] 1.
- *Delusions*: *hand*: *smoothing her; felt a hand*: med. [1] 1.
- *Delusions*: *women*: *bedside; by*: med. [1] 1.

- *Delusions: touched; he is: head; someone touched her.* fic-m. **MED**.
- *Delusions: doctors come; three:* sep. [1] 1.
- *Delusions: witches; believes in:* sep. [1] 1.
- *Delusions: calls: someone calls: sleep; someone calls him during:* **SEP**. [3] 1.

Avoidance: Homoeopaths have traditionally applied, and interpreted the use of, these rubrics in case-taking to the patients suffering hallucinations from a high fever. The psychotherapeutic need behind why each remedy is listed in these rubrics are a far more accurate indicator of their meaning and relevance in case analysis. Believing you have a special friend in your life is a common delusional childhood fantasy which is most commonly seen in the remedy pictures of *Calcarea carbonica* and *Pulsatilla*. *Belladonna* can see people who are either friends or foes. *Magnesium carbonicum* need to connect with illusions and visions of their dead loved ones to reassure themselves they are not alone. On the one hand, *Medorrhinum* fear they are *seeing people* who are judging them, and on the other hand they believe that the people they see are proof that they are connected to a greater mystical force who is protecting them. *Lycopodium* often deludes themselves that they are surrounded by people to allay their fears of not being socially important. The *Delusion* rubric: *seeing people,* can pertain to 'delusions of grandeur' or it can indicate 'delusions of persecution'.

Belladonna choose to delude themselves that they are surrounded by friends to avoid feeling vulnerable. *Belladonna* suffer from severe and crippling imaginary fears of being attacked and possessed by the devil. The classical interpretation of why *Belladonna* is listed in the *Delusion* rubric: *seeing people*, has always been that *Belladonna* are visually delusional when they have a high fever. The psychotherapeutic application and explanation reveals that *Belladonna* are terrified of being sick. They will become crippled with psychological 'delusions of persecution' from the devil within, and from the devil outside.

Belladonna use their psyche to develop visions when they are sick because otherwise they will be distraught with fear of their own internal devil, and of the putrefying nature of disease.

Belladonna carry within the memory of their psyche the asphyxiating death associated with the plant's botanical history. *Belladonna* need the psychological 'delusion of grandeur' and their religiosity to protect themselves. *Belladonna* have the *Delusion* rubric: *about to receive injury*. *Belladonna* will always present as alternating between the extremes of grand religiosity and crippling terror when they are sick.

1. Denial: *Delusion* rubric: *friend; surrounded by friends: being*: bell. *Delusion* rubric: *religious*: bell. *Delusion* rubric: *great person, is a*: bell. *Delusion* rubric: *people: seeing people*: **BELL**. [This rubric can pertain to 'hubristic visions' or 'delusions of persecution'.

2. Forsaken: *Delusion* rubric: *devil: taken by the devil; he will be*: bell. *Delusion* rubric: *home: away from home; he is*: bell. *Delusion* rubric: *injury: about to receive injury; is*: bell. *Delusion* rubric: *people: seeing people*: **BELL**.

3. Causation: *Delusion* rubric: *devil*: *Bell*.

4. Depression: *Delusion* rubric: *devil: taken by the devil; he will* be: bell. [This rubric can pertain to persecutory fears or depressive fear of disease.] *Delusion* rubric: *caught; he will be*: bell.

5. Resignation: *Delusion* rubric: *body: putrefy, will*: bell. *Delusion* rubric: *sick; being*: bell.

Calcarea carbonica is a commonly prescribed remedy which homoeopathic students learn about early on in their studies. *Calcarea carbonica* is one of the first remedies homoeopathic students learn because it is noted as a good remedy for children suffering from nightmares, especially if they are away from home. *Calcarea carbonica* as a remedy profile are noted for worrying about their health, their family's health, and every unknown trifle which they can fixate upon to worry about. *Calcarea carbonica* manage their overwhelming stress by creating a strong focus on their job and family.

Calcarea carbonica need their *fanciful illusions* of a *fantasy world of imaginary friends* and money [*wealth*]. *Calcarea carbonica* have the *Delusion* rubric: *talks about money,* and the *Delusion* rubric: *lives in a fantasy world of imaginary friends.*

As adults, *Calcarea carbonica* develop obsessive, systematic and methodical work and life practices to create strong boundaries around them in which to contain their overwhelming anxiety. What is not commonly understood about *Calcarea carbonica* because it is assumed that it is 'a simple children's remedy', is the complexity of their delusional pathology.

Calcarea carbonica are significantly <u>not listed</u> in any of the *Delusion* rubrics pertaining to psychological 'delusions of original sin' or self-blame. *Calcarea carbonica* have the *Delusion* rubrics: *has horrible visions,* and *on closing eyes, sees images and phantoms. Calcarea carbonica* are the victims of, and are tormented by, projected visions of demons taking them away from their home and causing them harm. This vulnerability has been accepted as the cause of the anticipatory anxiety from which *Calcarea carbonica* suffer. *Calcarea carbonica* is often overlooked and subsequently under-prescribed as the simillimum for adults because the pathological inconsistencies have not been identified. *Calcarea carbonica* suffer from 'narcissistic neurosis'. 'Narcissism' describes the personality trait of excessive self-love. Narcissism is recognized as a personality disorder of excessive selfishness. *Calcarea carbonica* are notably stubborn and pompous. Energy which is disproportionately redirected on to a narcissist persona causes 'delusions of grandeur'. 'Neuroses' relate to psychosomatic conditions. ('Psychoses' relate to mental conflict and mental derangement.) If a remedy profile has stark inconsistencies within the personality profile, then there is underlying pathology within their psyche.

Calcarea carbonica create grandiose stability on the outer to deny their inner fragility.

Calcarea carbonica have the *Delusion* rubric: *body being dashed to pieces.* [1] 1. *Calcarea carbonica* suffer from numerous psychoses to do with their health because energy is redirected from their 'ego' to the 'id'. The 'id' is unrestrained selfish self-gratification. 'Narcissistic neurosis' is a pre-emptive cause for manic-depressive psychosis insofar as it is characterized by the withdrawal of energy from the realistic and rational 'ego'.

Calcarea carbonica is under-prescribed for adults because the delusional need for security has not been recognized as 'neurotic narcissism', which in turn is the cause of their manic-depressive psychoses.

Calcarea carbonica have the *Delusion* rubric: *he would go out of his mind.* Manic-depressive psychoses result in the patient alternating between grandiose delusions of stature and depressive periods of unreasoning despair. This is the pattern in *Calcarea carbonica.* Underpinning the psychoses are neurotic fears which preempt their numerous 'delusions of persecution' and 'delusions of abandonment'. *Calcarea carbonica* have the *Mind* rubrics: *important and pompous* versus, *fear of being laughed at and mocked.* [1] 1. 'Narcissistic neurosis' is the underlying cause of the pathology behind their desire to be controlled and their crippling lack of confidence from being over controlled. *Calcarea carbonica* have the *Mind* rubrics: *desire to be magnetized*[17], [3]., versus *ailments from long time domination.* *Calcarea carbonica* are narcissistic because they attribute no blame to themselves, this is why they have no psychological 'delusions of original sin'. *Calcarea carbonica* are neurotic because their narcissist 'delusions of grandeur' do not tally with their inner fragility. Their grandiose belief in *wealth* and *friends* protects them and assures them of security, but the need to maintain their grandiosity reinforces and perpetuates future insecurity and emotional collapse. *Calcarea carbonica* have the *Mind* rubric: *constant fear of everything.*

1. Denial: *Delusion* rubric: *friend: fantasy world of imaginary friends; lives in a*: calc. [1] 1. *Delusion* rubric: *wealth, of*: calc. *Delusion* rubric: *people: conversing with absent people*: calc. *Delusion* rubric: *fancy, illusions of*: calc. *Delusion* rubric: *visions, has wonderful*: calc. *Delusion* rubric: *faces, sees: closing eyes, on*: **CALC**. [This rubric can pertain to seeing friendly or evil faces. The interpretation should be specific to each remedy profile.]

2. Forsaken: *Delusion* rubric: *home: away from home; he is*: calc. *Delusion* rubric: *criticized, she is*: calc. *Delusion* rubric: *ruined: is ruined; he*: calc. *Delusion* rubric: *images, phantoms; sees: closing eyes, on*: **CALC**. *Delusion* rubric: *criticized, she is*: calc. *Delusion* rubric: *snakes: in and around her*. calc. *Delusion* rubric: *vermin: seeing vermin crawl about*: calc. *Delusion* rubric: *watched, she is being*: *Calc*. *Delusion* rubric: *murdered: will be murdered; he*: *Calc*. *Delusion* rubric: *persecuted: he is persecuted*: calc. *Delusion* rubric: *people: behind him; someone is*: calc. *Delusion* rubric: *specters, ghosts, spirits; seeing*: *Calc*.

3. Causation: NONE

4. Depression: *Delusion* rubric: *wrong: everything goes wrong*: calc. *Delusion* rubric: *anxious*: calc. *Delusion* rubric: *annihilation; about to sink into*: calc. *Delusion* rubric: *ruined: is ruined; he*: calc. *Delusion* rubric: *horrible: everything seems*: **CALC**. *Delusion* rubric: *insane: become insane; one will*: *Calc*. *Delusion* rubric: *confusion; others will observe her*. *Calc*. *Delusion* rubric: *brain: dissolving and she were going crazy; brain were*: calc. [1] 1. *Delusion* rubric: *mind: out of his mind; he would go*: calc.

5. Resignation: *Delusion* rubric: *body: dashed to pieces, being*: calc. [1] 1. *Delusion* rubric: *die: about to die; one was*: calc. *Delusion* rubric: *disease: incurable disease; he has an*: calc. *Delusion* rubric: *sick: being*: **CALC**.

(The *Delusion* rubrics: *seeing specters, ghosts, spirits*[18], should be assessed according to the individual remedy and how the visions are advantageous or injurious to each individual constitutional remedy.)

Magnesium carbonicum avoid feeling alone because they suffer from 'delusions of abandonment'. *Magnesium carbonicum* believe they can see people, especially members of their family, so as not to feel they have been deserted. The *Delusion* rubrics: *sees dead persons,* and *seeing people,* should always be interpreted according to the remedy profile.

Magnesium carbonicum need to connect with illusions and visions of their dead loved ones to reassure themselves they are not alone.

Magnesium carbonicum have the *Mind* rubrics: *forsaken feeling of not being beloved by his parents, wife and friends,* and *ailments from being neglected by one's father. Magnesium carbonicum* have the *Delusion* rubric: *seeing thieves.* The *Delusion* rubrics: *he is counting his money,* and *lumps in bed,* both confirm the depth of their need for security, and the intensity of their exaggerated fears of loss, especially financially. The *Delusion* rubric: *lumps in bed,* lists only two remedies: *Magnesium carbonicum* and *Arnica.* Within the remedy profile of *Arnica,* this rubric pertains to disproportionate sensitivity: emotionally, mentally, and physically. Within the remedy profile of *Magnesium carbonicum,* this rubric pertains to the need for security in their home and specifically in their bed. *Magnesium carbonicum* have the *Mind* rubric: *fear something will happen, the warmth of the bed ameliorates.*

Magnesium carbonicum are not listed in any of the *Delusion* rubrics pertaining to self-blame or 'delusions of original sin'. *Magnesium carbonicum* transfer all their neuroses outwards on to family and friends. A neurosis shows an inability to have a rational or realistic objective view of one's life. Transference is characterized by unconscious self-deluding denial which allows for the redirection of feelings on to another person. A 'transference neurosis' is typically transferred on to God or the devil. The 'never-well since-event' or causation in a *Magnesium carbonicum* case will have its origins in abandonment by family.

Magnesium carbonicum transfer all their neuroses on to their family because it is their family which has abandoned and forsaken them. *Magnesium carbonicum* maintain their psychological need for the illusions and delusions of *seeing dead people* because they feel insecure when their family leaves them.

Magnesium carbonicum are neurotically disturbed by any real or perceived abandonment as a result of discord within their family, or within their group of friends. *Magnesium carbonicum* have the *Mind* rubrics: *ailments from quarrelling*, and *unable to answer when hurt emotionally*, and the *Delusion* rubric: *is forsaken*. A 'transference neurosis' perpetuates insecurity because it reinforces the undermining belief that without support from, for example, one's family, one cannot feel secure inside of oneself. This neurosis is the reason behind the hysterical hypochondria which cripples *Magnesium carbonicum*. *Magnesium carbonicum* are hysterically worried that they have an incurable disease when they are sick. It is not uncommon for them to allay these fears by becoming obsessive about money, family and friends, and their home when they are sick.

Conversely, the *Delusion* rubric: *illusions of fancy*, alludes to and indicates the degree to which *Magnesium carbonicum* can pretend they are not sick.

1. Denial: *Delusion* rubric: *people: seeing people*: mag-c. *Delusion* rubric: *fancy, illusions of*: mag-c. *Delusion* rubric: *dead: persons, sees: Mag-c.* [This rubric can be interpreted as pertaining to persecution or it can be interpreted as a false or deluded assurance of a connection with lost loved ones.]

2. Forsaken: *Delusion* rubric: *thieves: seeing*: mag-c. *Delusion* rubric: *forsaken; is*: **MAG-C**. *Delusion* rubric: *murdered*: *will be murdered; he*: mag-c.

3. Causation: NONE.

4. Depression: *Delusion* rubric: *anxious*: mag-c.

5. Resignation: *Delusion* rubric: *disease: incurable disease; he has an*: mag-c. *Delusion* rubric: *faint; he would*: mag-c.

Medorrhinum have the *Delusion* rubric: *seeing persons*. On the one hand *Medorrhinum* fear they are *seeing people* who are judging them, and on the other hand they believe the people they see are proof that they are connected to a greater mystical force that is protecting them. *Medorrhinum* are so intent on avoiding societal expectations that they are always paranoid about someone judging them. *Medorrhinum* have numerous *Delusion* rubrics which highlight their inner instability over real or perceived rejection. *Medorrhinum* have the *Delusion* rubrics: *persecuted, watched, spied on, poisoned,* and *pursued*. *Medorrhinum* withdraw into an inner world in which they are able to align themselves with a mystical inner conviction that God is *a delicate hand that has smoothed* their psyche. *Medorrhinum* have the *Delusion* rubric: *she was smoothed by a delicate hand*.

Medorrhinum do not have any hubristic delusions of personal grandeur.

God for *Medorrhinum* is a mystical *woman standing beside their bed whispering guidance*. *Medorrhinum* have the *Delusion* rubric: *talking with dead persons*, and the *Delusion* rubric: *caressed on head by someone*. [2] 1. *Medorrhinum* have the *Delusion* rubric: *women by the bedside*. Transference is characterized by unconscious redirection of feelings on to another person.

All the *Delusion* rubrics for *Medorrhinum* which pertain to communication with God transfer hubristic power on to spirits.

Medorrhinum quite often create sculptural representations

of their 'spirit guides'. *Medorrhinum* have the *Delusion* rubric: *delusions about imaginary objects.* The *Medorrhinum* (case) in the *Case Companion* to *Homoeopathic Psychiatry* is a sculptor who concentrates her work around the imagery of women. *Medorrhinum* have the *Delusion* rubric: *women by the bedside.* The dead women who are *talking* and *whispering* and *smoothing the head* of *Medorrhinum* are their ancestral guides.

With no hubristic 'delusions of grandeur' allocated to their own persona, *Medorrhinum* struggle with self-actualization[19].

Medorrhinum transfer inner knowledge and personal power to the dead.

1. Denial: *Delusion* rubric: *people: seeing people*: med. *Delusion* rubric: *touched; he is: head; someone touched her.* **MED**. [3] 2. *Delusion* rubric: *caressed on head by someone: Med.* [2] 1. *Delusion* rubric: *women: bedside; by:* med. [1] 1. *Delusion* rubric: *smoothed by a delicate hand; she was*: med. [1] 1. *Delusion* rubric: *hand: smoothing her; felt a hand*: med. [1] 1. *Delusion* rubric: *religious*: med. *Delusion* rubric: *talking: dead people; with*: med. *Delusion* rubric: *voices: hearing*: med. *Delusion* rubric: *faces, sees: wherever he turns his eyes, or looking out from corners*: med. *Delusion* rubric: *watched, she is being*: med. *Delusion* rubric: *whispering to him; someone is*: med. [These last three rubrics can pertain to 'delusions of persecution' or to delusions of hubristic visions.

2. Forsaken: *Delusion* rubric: *persecuted: he is persecuted*: med. *Delusion* rubric: *footsteps; hearing: behind him: Med.* *Delusion* rubric: *watched, she is being*: med. *Delusion* rubric: *spied; being*: med. *Delusion* rubric: *walking: behind him; someone walks*: med. *Delusion* rubric: *poisoned: he: has been*: med. *Delusion* rubric: *pursued; he was*: med.

3. Causation: *Delusion* rubric: *hell: going to hell because he had committed an unpardonable crime*: med. [1] 1.

4. Depression: *Delusion* rubric: *anxious*: med. *Delusion* rubric: *happened; something has: dreadful has happened; something*: med. [1] 1. *Delusion* rubric: *torture: rid her mind of the torture; she must do something to*: med. [1] 1.

5. Resignation: *Delusion* rubric: *die: time has come to*: med. *Delusion* rubric: *legs: cut off; legs are*: med.

Mercurius suffer with paranoid delusions that they are being attacked. *Mercurius* have the *Delusion* rubric: *surrounded by enemies*. In a *Mercurius* case, the *Delusion* rubric: *seeing persons* reflects their paranoid delusions of a guilty conscience. *Mercurius* have numerous 'delusions of persecution' which underpin their persona. *Mercurius* have numerous *Mind* rubrics which also highlight their need to defend themselves from real or perceived attacks to their person. *Mercurius* have the *Mind* rubrics: *so angry he could have stabbed someone, hatred of persons who have offended him*, and *desire to kill the person who contradicts her*. *Mercurius* cannot take a joke. *Mercurius* have the *Mind* rubrics: *cannot take a joke, sensitive to reproaches*, and *suspicious insulted*. [1] 1. Psychoses are a conflict between the 'ego' and the external world. A psychosis is a mental derangement or over-reaction. The *Delusion* rubrics which cover psychoses are the *Delusion* rubrics: Forsaken, Depression and Resignation. These *Delusion* rubrics emphasize the threat that the world poses to the self or 'ego'. They contain the 'delusions of abandonment', 'delusions of persecution', 'delusions of impending doom', and the 'delusions of hypochondria', in that order. *Mercurius* have a psychotic split within their psyche. The consequences of this fragmentation[20] are that they are unable to hold on to their own stature in the world. *Mercurius* continually exaggerate, and disproportionately over-react to, real or perceived attacks to their persona.

Mercurius don't like to 'lose face'. *Mercurius* do not like to be made aware of their internal rage. *Mercurius* have such an intense need to be seen in a good light that they will say they are well when they are sick.

Mercurius have the *Mind* rubric: *says he is well when very sick*. *Mercurius* have the *Mind* rubric: *disgust with oneself, has no courage to live with himself*. [2] 2. *Mercurius* lack courage to be able to face themselves. They are crippled by fear of their own rage. *Mercurius* have the *Mind* rubric: *fear of committing something wrong*. [2] 1. *Mercurius* self-deflect their rage by creating a *peculiar* 'delusion of grandeur' which paints a picture of themselves as being sweet. The two *Delusion* rubrics: *is made of sweets*, and *body is made of sweets*, should not be interpreted literally. The psychodynamic meaning of those rubrics alludes to the ability *Mercurius* have to entice and charm – *Mercurius take people by the nose*. *Mercurius* also take themselves by the nose. They need to believe the picture which they have painted of themselves because they lack courage to be able to face the true picture which contains evidence of their reactive rage. *Mercurius* have the *Mind* rubric: *attempts to escape for fear of having committed a crime*. [2] 1. *Mercurius* escape from others confronting them and they also escape from confronting themselves. This is why they are so attracted to all suppressive drugs. When confronted with themselves *Mercurius* need to suppress what they see by either taking medically prescribed anti-depressants or drugs such as cocaine which increase their hubristic visions of persona.

Mercurius have hubristic visions of persona – they will only want to work with the homoeopathic practitioner who they feel they have been able to charm, and to convince that they are *made of sweets*.

This need to charm will apply to every communication and interaction in their lives. The 'never-well-since-event' or causation in any *Mercurius* case will always have its foundation in the humiliation of their hubristic persona. The rubrics which pertain to 'hubristic denial' or 'delusions of grandeur' for *Mercurius* highlight the need within their psyche to maintain the delusional belief in their sweetness. *Mercurius* have the *Delusion* rubric: *suffers the torments of hell without being able to explain why*. *Mercurius* know they have murderous rage inside them, but they the lack the courage to be able to face, or even own up to, that rage. This is why they are confused as about why they have been thrown into the torments of hell. The need to maintain the 'hubristic denial' is the reason why they obsessively take all the people in their life, including their health practitioners, by the nose and charm them.

Mercurius do not transfer any of their 'hubristic denial' on to God or the devil. *Mercurius* have self-actualized their own hubristic visions of their own grandiose persona.

The inconsistency between Stage one and Stage five preempts their undermining belief that everything they do will fail. It is this undermining psychological delusion which in turn fuels their hyper-vigilance to real or perceived attacks on their person. On the one hand *Mercurius* need to see people surrounding them who love and adore them, and on the other hand, the people they see around them can undermine and threaten them.

1. Denial: *Delusion* rubric: *well, he is*: merc.

   Versus

5. Resignation: *Delusion* rubric: *sick: being*: merc.

1. Denial: *Delusion* rubric: *people: seeing people*: merc. *Delusion* rubric: *sweets; is made of sweets*: merc. [1] 1. *Delusion* rubric: *body: sweets, is made of*: merc. [1] 1. *Delusion* rubric: *nose: takes people by the nose*: merc. [1] 1. *Delusion* rubric: *fancy, illusions of*: *Merc*. *Delusion* rubric: *well, he is*: merc. *Delusion* rubric: *religious*: merc. *Delusion* rubric: *hearing: illusions of*: merc.

2. Forsaken: *Delusion* rubric: *enemy: everyone is an*: *Merc*. *Delusion* rubric: *criminals, about*: merc. *Delusion* rubric: *persecuted: he is persecuted*: merc. *Delusion* rubric: *injury: about to receive injury; is*: merc. *Delusion* rubric: *murdered: will be murdered; he*: merc. *Delusion* rubric: *people: seeing people*: merc. [In relation to *Mercurius* this rubric can pertain to 'delusions of grandeur' or 'delusions of persecution'.]

3. Causation: *Delusion* rubric: *crime: committed a crime; he had*: merc. *Delusion* rubric: *wrong: done wrong; he has*: merc.

4. Depression: *Delusion* rubric: *fail, everything will*: merc. *Delusion* rubric: *hell: in; is*: merc.

5. Resignation: *Delusion* rubric: *sick: being*: merc.

Pulsatilla need constant consolation and reassurance. *Pulsatilla* have the *Delusion* rubric: *seeing people*, because it reassures them they are not alone. Students of homoeopathy learn early on in their studies that one of the *Mind* keynotes of *Pulsatilla* is the child needing to be carried and caressed – *Pulsatilla* have the *Mind* rubric: *the child always clings on to the hand of the mother*. I can remember learning this image of *Pulsatilla* and then jumping from that image to the other *Mind* keynote of *Pulsatilla* – *aversion to women/men*, and *aversion to marriage*. I was not able to reconcile the jump because psychologically it appeared on the surface to be a contradiction in behavior. *Pulsatilla* are listed in bold [3] in the *Delusion* rubric: *she is always alone*, and is the only remedy listed in the *Delusion* rubric: *being alone, she did not belong to anyone*. One would assume *Pulsatilla* would transfer their neediness of reassurance and continual company on to their partner. *Pulsatilla* instead transfer their neediness of reassurance and continual company on to ill health. Changeability[21] and inconsistency are keynotes of the remedy profile of *Pulsatilla,* but the delusional need to maintain the inconsistency is reflective of a deeper, more problematic pathology. *Pulsatilla* become attached to ill health. *Pulsatilla* have the *Mind* rubric: *actions are contradictory to intentions*. *Pulsatilla* have a pathological need to psychosomatically *cling to the hand* of their hypochondria. *Pulsatilla* have the *Mind* rubrics: *charlatan, feigning sickness,* and *hysterical hypochondriasis*. *Pulsatilla* maintain their hysteria because it reinforces that they need protection. *Pulsatilla* have the *Mind* rubric: *hypochondriacal mania to read medical books*.

Pulsatilla also struggle to live alone, without God. (It is important to remind the reader that 'God' is a generic term which can be applied to any fanatical belief which is transferred on to any person, or group, or philosophy, outside of oneself.)

Pulsatilla have a strong need to believe in religion. *Pulsatilla* need God to reassure them because they are undermined by 'delusions of hypochondria'.

Pulsatilla will abandon their partners and abstain for religious reasons whenever they have to confront their own ineffectual power over their life. *Pulsatilla* have the *Delusion* rubrics: *she is not appreciated,* and *delusions of emptiness.* [3]. *Pulsatilla* will also abandon their partner when their partner is not able to show strong God-like direction and guidance. There is no inconsistency between *the child hanging on to the mother not wanting to let go of her hand,* and the adult hanging on to God's hand. *Pulsatilla* have the *Mind* rubrics: *religious aversion in women/men to men/women,* and *fanaticism too occupied with religion.* *Pulsatilla* often delude even themselves. If there is an inconsistency between Stage one ('delusions of grandeur') and Stage five ('delusions of hypochondria') then there has to be evidence of internal discord which will precipitate pathology.

Pulsatilla need to delude themselves that they are well, even when sick. Conversely, *Pulsatilla* need to delude themselves that they are sick, even when well. *Pulsatilla* have the *Delusion* rubric: *she is some other person.* The psychodynamic interpretation and implication of this means that *Pulsatilla* not only feel abandoned by others, they also abandon themselves. It is to their advantage to feel abandoned because this reinforces the pathological need for illness. *Pulsatilla* struggle to live alone, without illness.

Pulsatilla develop co-dependency; they struggle to live independently[22]. In the subconscious or unconscious, *Pulsatilla* have a disproportionate pathological need to hang on to, and believe in, their illness. The role of the homoeopath working with this need is to help the patient feel like they can live as a self-actualized person – that is, without the need to hang on to anyone's hand.

1. Denial: *Delusion* rubric: *well, he is*: puls.
   Versus
5. Resignation: *Delusion* rubric: *sick: being*: **PULS**.
1. Denial: *Delusion* rubric: *people: seeing people*: *Puls*.
   Delusion rubric: *religious*: *Puls*. *Delusion* rubric: *well, he is*:
   puls. *Delusion* rubric: *fancy, illusions of*: puls.
2. Forsaken: *Delusion* rubric: *alone, being: belong to anyone;
   she did not*: puls. [1] 1. *Delusion* rubric: *alone, being: world;
   alone in the*: *Puls*. *Delusion* rubric: *devil: taken by the devil;
   he will be*: *Puls*. *Delusion* rubric: *forsaken; is*: **PULS**. *Delusion*
   rubric: *persecuted: he is persecuted*: puls. *Delusion* rubric:
   conspiracies: against him; there are conspiracies: puls.
   Delusion rubric: *poisoned: he: has been*: puls. *Delusion*
   rubric: *abused, being*: puls. *Delusion* rubric: *appreciated,
   she is not*: puls. *Delusion* rubric: *enemy: everyone is an*:
   puls. *Delusion* rubric: *insulted, he is*: puls. *Delusion* rubric:
   women: evil and will injure his soul; women are: puls. [1] 1.
3. Causation: *Delusion* rubric: *sinned; one has*: puls. *Delusion*
   rubric: *sinned; one has: day of grace; sinned away his*:
   puls.
4. Depression: *Delusion* rubric: *anxious*: *Puls*. *Delusion*
   rubric: *ruined: will be ruined; he*: puls. [1] 1. *Delusion*
   rubric: *person: other person; she is some*: puls. [This rubric
   pertains to abandonment of the self.] *Delusion* rubric:
   clouds: black cloud enveloped her: a heavy: puls. *Delusion*
   rubric: *doomed, being*: puls. *Delusion* rubric: *emptiness; of*:
   PULS.
5. Resignation: *Delusion* rubric: *sick: being*: **PULS**. *Delusion*
   rubric: *die: about to die; one was*: puls.

Sepia[23] is a homoeopathic remedy derived from a sea
creature. The *Delusion* rubric: *seeing people*, can be interpreted
as one's feelings of persecution and potential threat, or it can
be interpreted as a sign that one will be saved. *Sepia* fear

being exposed. They feel they need to protect themselves from potential threat. *Sepia* fear being looked at and mocked. *Sepia* alternate between illusions or idealized perceptions of hope that they will be saved, and psychological 'delusions of persecution' that they will be attacked or persecuted. The differing interpretation of the *Delusion* rubric: *seeing people* highlights an inherent polarity within their psyche. The theme is dependence versus independence. When *Sepia* are sick it is easy for them to feel anxious and ungrounded and unable *to understand anything*. *Sepia* appear extremely foggy and confused when they are sick. This is indicative of their psyche somatically mirroring the murky ink of the cuttlefish.

The homoeopathic practitioner will be viewed as their 'God' who is able to save them. This is the psychodynamic application and relevance of the *Delusion* rubric: *three doctors come*. *Sepia* disproportionately over-react to their illness; this is why they need not one, but *three doctors* to attend to them. *Sepia* are also listed in the *Mind* rubrics: *fear doctors,* and *aversion to homoeopathy*. It is normal to struggle with the acceptance of disease and death, but *Sepia* struggle with their *dependence* on their health practitioner. *Sepia* disproportionately depend on their health practitioner and conversely react negatively to becoming dependant on their practitioner. The essence is the internal struggle for independence. *Sepia* are listed in the *Mind* rubric: *antagonism with self*.

Sepia struggle to survive unsupported in their life in general. Conversely, they struggle to *allow* themselves to be supported.

A *Delusion* rubric is only used if you can see a misinterpretation of reality which prevents the person from making a correct assessment of reality. The *Delusion* rubrics of the psychological 'delusions of grandeur' become relevant in case-taking when the patient presents with an unrealistic belief that they can depend on someone else to save them. The psychodynamic relevance of the *Delusion* rubric: *three doctors come*, and the *Delusion* rubric: *illusions of fancy*, is that it indicates an exaggerated belief in cure, as well as an exaggerated assessment of the gravity of their illness. If there is an exaggerated belief in cure or need, then underneath it are numerous *Delusion* rubrics of being forsaken. If there is an exaggerated assessment of the gravity of their illness then the fear of losing support will also be exaggerated. This is why *Sepia* have numerous rubrics pertaining to persecution and abandonment. The most potent is the *Delusion* rubric: *he or she is neglected*. *Sepia* feel ungrounded and unsupported in life, particularly around their inability to survive financially in the world. *Sepia* have the *Delusion* rubrics: *he is poor*, and *family will starve*. The *Delusion* rubrics: *family will starve, going to be robbed*, and *he or she is neglected*, are *Delusion* rubrics which indicate psychological 'delusions of deprivation'. In *Sepia* the psychodynamic struggle to survive in the world and become a self-actualized person has its causation in neglect and starvation as a baby. *Sepia* struggle their whole life to be able to have their needs met. The psychodynamic trauma inside *Sepia* which undermines them, or leaves them floundering in *starving emptiness,* is that they do not believe they can have their needs met in a relationship, or in life, because they literally do not know how to verbalize or understand those needs. *Sepia* have the *Delusion* rubrics: *she would have to learn anew everything she wished to do*, and *she could not understand anything*. Both of these *Delusion* rubrics indicate that the 'never-well-since-event' in a *Sepia* case has its foundation in the early, pre-verbal years of their life. If the first needs of the infant are not met then the infant presumes that their needs will remain unmet for the rest of their lives.

Sepia are confused and unrealized in their emotional independence[24] and in particular in their financial independence. The *Mind* rubric: *antagonism with self*, indicates the degree to which *Sepia* feel unsupported, even within themselves and towards themselves. Interestingly, *Sepia* do not have any psychological 'delusions of original sin'. Their internal battle is about whether to accept and trust the support offered from the world, not about whether *they* have personally caused the unsupported dilemma they find themselves in. *Sepia* struggle to acknowledge any wrong doing. The biggest undermining fear which causes *Sepia* pain is the fear that others will laugh at them particularly when they are unable to know how to do something. *Sepia* have the *Delusion* rubric: *being laughed and mocked at,* and *she could not understand anything.* [1] 1. *Sepia* have the *Delusion* rubric: *suspended in the air.* This rubric should not be taken literally, rather it is indicative of the psychodynamic trauma within *Sepia* which is caused by lack of support. *Sepia* often appear unable to enact effective change. *Sepia* have the *Delusion* rubric: *he was chased and had to run backwards.* [1] 1. The psychodynamic interpretation of this rubric indicates that *Sepia* feel as if they can always be potentially defeated. Furthermore, all effort to enact change [*escape*] is self-defeating because it is ineffective [*backwards*]. *Sepia* are often noted for their confusion and inactivity if they are depressed. Their depression is not the cause of their confusion. Their depression arises as a result of feeling defeated in their attempts to enact change. *Sepia* have the *Delusion* rubric: *delusions of emptiness. Sepia,* aside from feeling empty and unsupported, literally feel crushed if they are over-controlled. *Sepia* have the *Delusion* rubric: *something else from above which is pressing the chest.* [1] 1. My *Sepia* (case) in the *Case Companion* to *Homoeopathic Psychiatry* reflected on the following dream, which highlights the conflict between the need to be dependent versus the need for independence: *It is interesting when I think back about that dolphin dream. The dolphin landed on me like that, but the dream I was having when the dolphin landed on me was I was in the Garden of Eden. It was all happy, beautiful fruit trees all covered in fruit and then bang there it was. The dolphin was jumping from one level to another, then it landed on me.* This dream is a good example of the paradox of *Sepia* relationships and of their life in general. Dependency in relationship is associated with being smothered, like when the dolphin landed on her. Dependency on the homoeopathic practitioner brings to the surface the same dilemma; this is why *Sepia* have the conflicting *Mind* rubrics: *fear doctors,* and *aversion to homoeopathy*, versus the *Delusion* rubrics: *three doctors come,* and *believes in witches*. Dependency on the homoeopathic practitioner brings to the surface their 'delusions of hypochondria'. The underlying, psychodynamic, somatic feedback loop that *Sepia* are embroiled in is a negative reinforcement and it is self-deprecating. *Sepia* undermine their power to support themselves financially in this world. *Sepia* were undermined as infants; they in turn, then undermine themselves by not taking their own energy seriously. *Sepia* have been unsupported and they, in turn, struggle to believe their own body will support them. This is why *Sepia* have numerous hypochondriac *Delusion* rubrics alluding to not being strong enough to work. *Sepia* have the *Delusion* rubric: *he would faint*, and the *Delusion* rubric: *she could easily strain herself*, and the *Delusion* rubric: *being sick and for this reason will not work.*

The *Delusion* rubric: *seeing people* highlights an inherent polarity within their psyche. The simillimum will only be *Sepia* if the patient has a need to create dependency and a need to create independence.

1. Denial: *Delusion* rubric: *people: seeing people*: sep. *Delusion* rubric: *doctors come; three*: sep. [1] 1. *Delusion* rubric: *witches; believes in*: sep. [1] 1. *Delusion* rubric: *calls: someone calls: sleep; someone calls him during*: **SEP**. [3] 1. [These rubrics can pertain to *doctors* or *witches* or *specters and ghosts* coming to save them, or illusions of people coming to *mock* them.] *Delusion* rubric: *fancy, illusions of*: sep. *Delusion* rubric: *visions, has*: sep.

2. Forsaken: *Delusion* rubric: *laughed at and mocked at; being*: sep. *Delusion* rubric: *poor; he is*: Sep. *Delusion*

rubric: *robbed, is going to be*: sep. *Delusion* rubric: *starve: family will*: Sep. *Delusion* rubric: *unfortunate, he is*: sep. [This rubric can pertain to feeling abandoned, or feelings of depression and failure.] *Delusion* rubric: *air: suspended in the air*: sep. [1] 1. *Delusion* rubric: *alone, being: graveyard; alone in a*: sep. *Delusion* rubric: *neglected: he or she is neglected*: sep. *Delusion* rubric: *poisoned: he: has been*: sep.

3. Causation: NONE.

4. Depression: *Delusion* rubric: *anxious*: sep. *Delusion* rubric: *understand: not understand anything; she could*: sep. [1] 1. *Delusion* rubric: *unfortunate, he is*: sep. *Delusion* rubric: *emptiness; of*: **SEP**. *Delusion* rubric: *learn: anew everything she wished to do; she would have to learn*: sep. [1] 1. *Delusion* rubric: *run: backward; he was chased and had to run*: sep. [1] 1. [This rubric pertains to ineffectual actions.]

5. Resignation: *Delusion* rubric: *sick: being*: sep. *Delusion* rubric: *strain herself, she could easily*: sep. [1] 1. *Delusion* rubric: *faint; he would*: sep. *Delusion* rubric: *sick: being: work; and for this reason will not*: sep.

- *Delusions: voices, hearing*: abrot. acon. agar. anac. anh. aster. bell. benz-ac. calc-sil. calc. cann-i. *Cann-s.* cann-xyz. canth. carb-v. carbn-s. cench. **CHAM**. chlol. coca coff. con. *Crot-c.* crot-h. *Cupr-act.* dros. *Elaps.* germ-met. hyos. ign. *Kali-br. Kola.* lac-c. lach. lyc. mag-m. manc. med. nat-m. nit-ac. petr. ph-ac. *Phos.* plb. rhus-t. spong. sol-ni. stram. tarent. thal-xyz. verat. *Zinc.*

- *Delusions: hearing, illusions of*: absin. agar. am-c. *Anac.* anh. *Antip.* ars. atro-s. atro. bell. bold. calc. *Cann-i.* canth. carb-v. carbn-o. carbn-s. **CHAM**. cocain. colch. con. conin. corv-cor. elaps. eup-pur. hyos. iodof. kali-ar. lyss. mag-m. med. merc. naja. nat-p. nux-m. ph-ac. puls. rhodi-o-n. stram. streptoc. thea. thres-a.

- *Delusions: voices: hearing; follow, that he must*: anac. crot-c. lach. thuj.

- *Delusions*: *voices*: *hearing*: *absent persons; of*: anac. cham. germ-met.
- *Delusions*: *people*: *conversing with absent people*: agar. aur. bell. calc. cham. crot-c. dig. hyos. lach. op. *Stram*. thuj. *Verat*.
- *Delusions*: *calls*: *someone calls*: *absent mother or sister call his name*: anac. [1] 1.
- *Delusions*: *sounds*: *listens to imaginary sounds*: hyos. [1] 1.
- *Delusions*: *voices*: *hearing*: *calling*: *his name*: anac. [1] 1.
- *Delusions*: *voices*: *hearing*: *dead people, of*: anac. *Bell*. calc-sil. hyper. nat-m. stram.
- *Delusions*: *sight and hearing, of*: anac. bell. carc. eup-pur. kali-br.
- *Delusions*: *calls*: *someone calls*: anac. ant-c. bell. brass-n-o. cann-i. dros. hyos. kali-c. med. plat. *Plb*. rhod. rosm. ruta. *Sep*. stram. sulph. taosc. thuj. verat.
- *Delusions*: *music*: *thinks he hears*: anh. **CANN-I**. croc. ign. *Lach*. lyc. merc. nat-c. plb. puls. sal-ac. sarr. *Stram*. thuj.

Self-Deluding: It is a mistake to assume that these rubrics apply only to psychologically unwell patients who hear voices. A *Delusion* rubric is used when the patient has a perception of reality which is disproportionate to the truth. I have used this rubric category for patients who believe in divine intervention when they are dealing with an incurable disease. Our desire to live, and our hope of deliverance, supersedes all rational thought processes when we have to face our death. If you look at the list of remedies in the *Delusion* rubric: *hearing voices,* you will notice that remedies such as *Natrum muriaticum*, *Calcarea carbonica*, *Magnesium carbonica*, or *Lycopodium* are not those one would normally associate with clairvoyance or clairaudience or, most importantly, delusional psychosis which is associated with hearing voices.

It is essential to acknowledge that a patient who is in denial of their ill health will often hear and believe in the supernatural powers of a greater force who will save them from death. Illness and impending death are the ultimate loss of our control.

The most common remedies in this rubric category are those I have prescribed for older women struggling to fall pregnant. This group of rubrics is applicable to the patient who tells you in a consultation that she will be blessed with a child when in fact it is highly improbable because she is forty-eight years old with high Follicle Stimulating Hormonal [FSH] levels. (The high FSH could indicate that she is pre-menopausal.) *Lycopodium* and *Natrum muriaticum* and *Calcarea carbonica* are remedies which I use in my fertility work specifically because they are so relevant to the emotional denial women can move into when they realize they are no longer in control of their own fertility. Hearing voices or hearing messages should not be interpreted literally. In case-taking this rubric is applicable to the patient who tells you they have had a message from God or that a lost relative has come to them in a dream and told them everything is going to work out for the best, and not to worry because they will get pregnant. The remedies *Ignatia* and *Natrum muriaticum* are remedies used for 'hysterical grief'. It is not uncommon for an *Ignatia* patient to tell you their loved one is still with them in the room, talking to them daily.

If the patient presents with a disproportionate need to believe in the presence of their loved one's ghost then it is applicable in the case to consider that the rubric is not just the *Mind* rubric: *grief*, but also the *Delusion* rubric: *hearing voices*.

The remedies *Ignatia* and *Natrum muriaticum* are in the Mind rubrics: *inconsolable* and *grief* as well as in the above *Delusion* rubric, so it will not make a difference to the rubric selection in the case analysis but it will make a difference to your understanding of the depth of your patient's grief.

Each remedy listed above has a secret agenda behind the belief that they are able to hear voices (God's voice). (In using the word God, I am not assuming personage. God is used liberally and is a generic terminology pertaining to any belief in any supernatural power, spiritual power, ghosts, or personal clairaudience or clairvoyance which connects one to a divine power which one believes is greater than oneself.) The role of a homoeopath in case analysis is to understand the patient's *peculiar* agenda or need to connect to a 'hubristic vision'. The *specific* underlying psychotherapeutic delusional need behind this belief will indicate the next rubric which will often be the decisive rubric to confirm the simillimum.

Anacardium suffer loss of memory with any sort of performance anxiety. If their failure is observed they feel exposed to criticism and rejection.

Anacardium avoid facing their fear of being criticized and avoid feeling vulnerable to their own lack of self-confidence by aligning themselves and relying on their 'divine' (whether it be devil or angel) auditory intervention. Anacardium are clairaudient and clairvoyant.

Anacardium have the *Delusion* rubric: *of sight and hearing,* and the *Delusion* rubric: *hearing voices of dead people. Anacardium* also have the *Delusion* rubric: *someone is whispering to him.* [1] 1. It is extremely important to *Anacardium* that they do not show their weaknesses. Illness is viewed by *Anacardium* as proof of failure. *Anacardium* is a constitutional remedy profile which historically has not been associated with 'delusions of grandeur'. However, *Anacardium* more than any other remedy have profound 'hubristic denial' around illness. Illness threatens their perfectionist hubristic vision of themselves as being 'one who is aligned with God'. If *Anacardium* fail by becoming sick, they believe this to be proof that they are aligned with the devil. In using the word devil, I am not assuming personage. The devil is used liberally and is a generic terminology pertaining to any belief in a supernatural power which is evil. Unless a patient is suffering from psychosis, they will not walk into your consulting room and declare they are the devil. *Anacardium* allude in the consultation to an internal struggle between the good part of themselves and the bad part of themselves. *Anacardium* rarely act on their 'evil' instincts. *Anacardium* are in conflict between the two sides of themselves which is why they are always alluding to their guilt over feeling aligned with the 'devil' inside of themselves. *Anacardium* have the *Delusion* rubric: *divided into two parts*.

The aim of the *Rubric-categories* is to identify the psychological delusions that each constitutional remedy profile will present with when they are sick, as opposed to when they are well.

Anacardium have the *Delusion* rubric: *he is three persons*. Once again, this rubric should not be translated literally. The underlying psychodynamic meaning of this rubric is far more accurate and descriptive of the dilemma within their psyche. *Anacardium* believe they *are* God, the devil and a person with hubristic visionary powers because they are in visual and auditory communication with both God, and the devil. Hubris is an insolent pride or alignment with the Gods leading to nemesis. 'Hubristic denial' is the belief that God has bestowed upon one great powers of omnipotence. A patient suffering with 'hubristic denial' refuses to believe that they are sick or could die. In relation to disease, and impending death, a patient believes they will be cured by God. Often, they believe that they are so powerful they can cure themselves. 'Hubristic denial' is the denial of illness or impending death because one believes one *is* an omnipotent God. *Anacardium* believe that they are so powerful they can cure themselves. *Anacardium* also believe that God will cure them.

If the patient does not continually allude to an urgent need to connect with a 'greater spiritual power' to overcome their shortfalls then the simillimum is not *Anacardium*.

The underlying dilemma which undermines *Anacardium* if they move out of denial, is having to face their psychological 'delusions of original sin'. *Anacardium* are divided into two contradictory sides. *Anacardium* believe that the devil within has caused their illness. *Anacardium* display an urgent need for a 'higher spiritual connection', but this need is motivated by an ulterior motive to gain a 'free get-out-of-hell card'. Sankaran, writes in *The Soul of Remedies*, "Whereas Anacardium is known for its hard-heartedness, cruelty, want of moral feeling, a compensated Anacardium cannot be cruel even when the situation demands. He will, perhaps, be unable to kill even an irritating mosquito.' The reason Sankaran refers to a "compensated *Anacardium*" is that *Anacardium* are motivated by a desire to be good in order to assure themselves of a passage into heaven. Sankaran also refers to the fact that *Anacardium* are not able to be confident of themselves. *Anacardium* fear that they cannot succeed without the power of either God or the devil (God or the devil is synonymous with any dominant[25] power). *Anacardium* have the *Delusion* rubric: *he does everything wrong, he cannot succeed*. *Anacardium* self-sacrifice to others to deny their rage [*devil*]. To sacrifice your life to save others is akin to an assured passage into heaven. Self-sacrifice is the best way to wipe clean your slate of crimes or sins committed. Self-sacrifice contains an ulterior motive for *Anacardium*, it assures them they are not the devil. *Anacardium* wish to be seen in a good light. *Anacardium* have 'hubristic visions' of persona. *Anacardium* have the *Delusion* rubric: *devil speaking in one ear, prompting to murder and an angel in the other ear prompting to do acts of benevolence*, [2] 1. *Anacardium* need to maintain their psychological delusions of 'hubristic denial' to be able to feel assured that they *are* God and not the devil. The "compensated *Anacardium*" who allows themselves to be dominated by God-like acts of *benevolence* is compelled to martyr themselves to a greater cause because they are trying to avoid and deny their own devil-like rage. The "compensated *Anacardium*" trying to avoid their rage by self-sacrificing themselves can't help but fall victim to self-perpetuating rage. As *Anacardium* become more aware of the fact that they have allowed themselves to be tied to the *bier*[26], their vengeful, devil-like rage is overwhelmingly violent, and malicious. This is why *Anacardium* are trapped between two contradictory wills. *Anacardium* have the *Delusion* rubric: *body is separated from the mind*, and the *Delusion* rubric: *soul is separated from the body*.

Anacardium alternate between 'hubristic denial' and devil-like rage which they feel victim to because they have fallen into a seductive trap and sold their soul to God and the devil for clairaudience and clairvoyance. Their 'hubristic denial' perpetuates self-sacrifice, and the self-sacrifice in turn perpetuates rage at allowing themselves to be self-sacrificed.

1. Denial: *Delusion* rubric: *voices: hearing: follow, that he must*: anac. *Delusion* rubric: *calls: someone calls: absent mother or sister call his name*: anac. [1] 1. *Delusion* rubric: *voices: hearing: calling: his name*: anac. [1] 1. *Delusion* rubric: *hearing: illusions of*. Anac. *Delusion* rubric: *voices: hearing: distant*: anac. *Delusion* rubric: *voices: hearing: dead people, of*: anac. *Delusion* rubric: *sight and hearing, of*. anac. *Delusion* rubric: *three persons, he is*: Anac. [Another interpretation of this rubric is that it reflects the belief that *Anacardium* assume they can achieve the work of three people]. *Delusion* rubric: *fancy, illusions of*. anac. *Delusion* rubric: *religious*: Anac. *Delusion* rubric: *superhuman; is: control; is under superhuman*: anac. *Delusion* rubric: *air: go into the air and busy himself; he must*: anac. [1] 1. *Delusion* rubric: *walking: behind him; someone walks*: anac. *Delusion* rubric: *whispering to him; someone is*: anac. *Delusion* rubric: *calls: someone calls*: anac. *Delusion* rubric: *touched; he is*: anac. *Delusion* rubric: *visions, has*: anac. *Delusion* rubric: *person: room; another person is in the*: anac. *Delusion* rubric: *people: beside him; people are*: anac. *Delusion* rubric: *people: behind him; someone is*: anac. [The *Delusion* rubrics: *people beside*, and *behind*, in relation to *Anacardium* are not reflective of a 'persecution complex'. They pertain to the many ghosts or 'spiritual guides' that *Anacardium* are in communication with.]

2. Forsaken: *Delusion* rubric: *outcast; she were an*: anac. *Delusion* rubric: *enemy: surrounded by enemies*: Anac.

Delusion rubric: *separated: world; from the: he is separated:* *Anac.* [This rubric in relation to *Anacardium* does not necessarily pertain to separation or abandonment – it can pertain to 'delusions of grandeur'. *Anacardium* have a hubristic vision of persona: they believe themselves to be set apart from mere mortals who do not have clairaudience or clairvoyance.]

3. Causation: *Delusion* rubric: *devil: he is a devil:* **ANAC**. *Delusion* rubric: *devil: sits in his neck; devil: prompting to offensive things:* anac. [1] 1. *Delusion* rubric: *whispering to him; someone is: blasphemy:* anac. [1] 1. *Delusion* rubric: *crime: committed a crime; he had:* anac.

4. Depression: *Delusion* rubric: *anxious: Anac. Delusion* rubric: *succeed, he does everything wrong; he cannot:* *Anac. Delusion* rubric: *worthless; he is:* anac. *Delusion* rubric: *troubles: impending; troubles were: trifle would lead into great troubles; every:* anac. [1] 1.

5. Resignation: *Delusion* rubric: *grave, he is in his:* anac. *Delusion* rubric: *dead: he himself was:* anac. *Delusion* rubric: *dead: corpse: bier; on a:* anac.

Anhalonium want to escape identifying with the external world by involving themselves in their inner spiritual clairvoyance and clairaudience. *Anhalonium* use divine auditory intervention to avoid emotional, mental, or physical interaction with the worldly plane. *Anhalonium* have the *Delusion* rubric: *merged with present eternity.* [1] 1. *Anhalonium* only experience conflict if they are *hindered*. *Anhalonium* experience all illness as a *hindrance* because they do not want to identify with their emotions, their mind, or their physical body. *Anhalonium* do not want to identify with their 'ego'. The 'ego' is the realistic rational part of the psyche. If a remedy profile has a weakened 'ego' then their psyche is under threat. *Anhalonium* choose to abandon their psyche, preferring *transparency* of the self. *Anhalonium* do not want to identify with their somatic 'id'. *Anhalonium* abandon their unconscious instinctual 'id', preferring an *out of body decomposition*. *Anhalonium* have the *Delusion* rubric: *body is immaterial*. *Anhalonium* do not want to be ruled by the conscience of the 'super-ego'.

Anhalonium do not want to identify with the inspirational ideals and spiritual goals and conscience of the 'super-ego' which criticizes or prohibits any feelings or actions. *Anhalonium* identifies entirely with their *immortal* ethereal body. Their spiritual goal is to *merge in eternity* and not to strengthen their 'super-ego' on this earthly plane. *Anhalonium* have the *Delusion* rubric: *of immortality*. *Anhalonium* are in tune with the psychical energies of the soul.

Because *Anhalonium* are in tune with the psychical energies of their soul they have no fear of death. *Anhalonium* know that their soul goes with them when they die. Disease is viewed as a *hindrance* because it forces them to become aware of their somatic body. *Anhalonium* will always be very agitated when they are sick because it forces them to re-enter their somatic consciousness. *Anhalonium* have the *Delusion* rubric: *parts of the body seem too large*. *Anhalonium* do not want to 'live in their body'. When they are sick they often complain that their body is cumbersome and irritating. If *Anhalonium* are forced by illness to 'live in their body' they often experience a *peculiar* 'persecution complex'. *Anhalonium* patients have often said to me: *I hate it when I am sick, it forces me to become aware of my body. People around me love it when I am sick because it makes them think I am just like them. I don't want to be like them. I think they all sit around looking at me, willing me to be sick so that I have to come back to this earthly plane. I feel surrounded and attacked*. This is the *Delusion* rubric: *sees faces scheming*, and the *Delusion* rubric: *snakes in and around her*. It is crucial that the *Delusion* rubrics are used in case analysis to psychosomatically mirror any emotive theme which is disproportionately paranoid. When *Anhalonium* are forced by illness to 'live in their body' they imagine that their body is forcing them to become aware of a somatic consciousness which they wish to discard. This is the psychodynamic meaning of the *Delusion* rubric: *parts of the body seem to large*.

1. Denial: *Delusion* rubric: *hearing: illusions of*: anh. *Delusion* rubric: *voices: hearing*: anh. *Delusion* rubric: *music: thinks he hears*: anh. *Delusion* rubric: *visions, has: wonderful*: anh. *Delusion* rubric: *visions, has: colorful*: anh. [1] 1. *Delusion* rubric: *sounds: color; are like*: anh. [1] 1. *Delusion* rubric: *transparent: everything is*: Ành. [2] 1. *Delusion* rubric: *seeing: herself*: anh. *Delusion* rubric: *space: decomposition of space and shape*: anh. *Delusion* rubric: *visions, has: beautiful: kaleidoscope changes; varied*: anh. *Delusion* rubric: *figures: seeing figures*: anh. *Delusion* rubric: *floating: air, in*: anh.

2. Forsaken: *Delusion* rubric: *faces, sees: scheming*: anh. *Delusion* rubric: *snakes: in and around her*. anh.

3. Causation: NONE.

4. Depression: *Delusion* rubric: *hindered; he is*: anh.

5. Resignation: *Delusion* rubric: *body: out of the body*: Anh. *Delusion* rubric: *transparent: he is*: anh. [These rubrics can pertain to hubristic visions of clairvoyance or to physical disassociation.] *Delusion* rubric: *large: parts of the body seem too large*: anh.

Chamomilla are capriciously agitated with themselves and by everyone else, as well. *Chamomilla* are in a continual internal debate [*council*] with themselves, as well as continually being *vexed* by everyone else. Their mind and body are agitated. *Chamomilla* have the *Delusion* rubrics: *body looks ugly*, and *unable to collect senses*. *Chamomilla* are paranoid that they have been *insulted* and in turn feel guilt over their own counter-offensive *vexations*. *Chamomilla* is commonly used as a homoeopathic remedy for infants who are in so much frustrated pain from teething that they don't know whether they want to be picked up or left alone. *Chamomilla* is well known as an excellent remedy for an inconsolable screaming baby who will only settle once it is picked up and carried. The keynote associated with the need for the homoeopathic remedy *Chamomilla* is that the child stiffens their body, and arches back and screams when they are picked up. *Chamomilla* have the *Mind* rubrics: *capriciousness, when offered he rejects the things he has been longing for*, and *desire to be carried*, and conversely the *Mind* rubric: *aversion to being carried*. *Chamomilla* have the *Mind* rubric: *disposition to contradict*, and, ironically, *intolerant of contradiction*. This capriciousness is also reflected in their management of illness. *Chamomilla* have the *Mind* rubric: *irritability: sends doctor home, says he is not sick*, and the *Mind* rubric: *says he is well, when he is sick*. *Chamomilla* is commonly used as a homoeopathic remedy for the person who is oversensitive to all external influences, whether it be environmental allergens or food allergens. As a remedy profile *Chamomilla* have the same psychodynamic confusion, they don't know whether they want to be involved in life with others or not. On the one hand people irritate them, and on the other hand they irritate themselves.

The theme within the persona of the constitutional remedy profile is a desire to over-dramatize reactions to everything. *Chamomilla* maintain their capricious agitation with themselves and with everyone else because it is to their advantage psychologically.

The 'never-well-since-event' or causation in a *Chamomilla* case always has its origins in physical trauma and shock. *Chamomilla* are uncertain and untrusting of support. They are angry with themselves for needing support, and angry with others for offering their support. *Chamomilla* find protection in religion. *Chamomilla* have the *Mind* rubric: *too occupied with religion*. *Chamomilla* need their conversations with God to carry them through this life. Without 'God on their side' *Chamomilla* feel defenseless. God does not necessarily refer to a religious concept. God is synonymous with an internal need to believe that one is connecting to an energy outside of oneself whose sole purpose is to protect us from outside attacks or internal self-attack. This analysis of God is particularly applicable to the remedy profile of *Chamomilla*.

Chamomilla rely on their hubristic visions and clairaudience to warn them of potential attacks. *Chamomilla* are extremely traumatized by, and fearful of, being touched.

This is why they have numerous *Mind* rubrics all pertaining to fear of being touched, and to fear of doctors. Their need to counter-attack was originally created within their psyche when they were an infant as a way to protect themselves. As an infant, and as an adult, the need to counter-attack is obviously self-destructive and counter-productive because *Chamomilla* can never allow themselves to trust enough to be touched by others, or to be supported [*carried*] by anyone in their life. This is a typical psychological aversion associated with victims of physical trauma, and it explains why *Chamomilla* often choose to live alone. The only people *Chamomilla* trust are the dead, with whom they have conversations, who can't physically abuse them. Their psychological delusions that their own body is a source of pain [*groans*] and that their *body is ugly* is reflective of the self-hate that victims of abuse often experience. This is another counter-productive pattern which reinforces their aversion to being touched by living beings.

1. Denial: *Delusion* rubric: *hearing, illusions of:* **CHAM**. *Delusion* rubric: *people: conversing with absent people:* cham. *Delusion* rubric: *voices: hearing: absent persons; of:* cham. *Delusion* rubric: *fancy, illusions of:* cham.

2. Forsaken: *Delusion* rubric: *insulted, he is:* cham. *Delusion* rubric: *animals: bed: under it:* cham. [1] 1. *Delusion* rubric: *animals: frightful:* cham. *Delusion* rubric: *images, phantoms; sees:* cham. *Delusion* rubric: *voices: hearing: strangers, of:* Cham.

3. Causation: *Delusion* rubric: *vexation: offenses; of vexations and:* cham.

4. Depression: *Delusion* rubric: *collect senses; unable to*: cham. *Delusion* rubric: *insane: become insane; one will*: cham. *Delusion* rubric: *council; holding a*: cham. *Delusion* rubric: *obstacles: wants them to be removed*: cham. [1] 1.

5. Resignation: *Delusion* rubric: *body: ugly: body looks*: cham. *Delusion* rubric: *sick: being*: cham. *Delusion* rubric: *groans: with*: Cham.

Elaps corallinus is a homoeopathic remedy derived from the Brazilian coral snake. Similarly to other snake remedy profiles, their hubristic visions allude to possible attack. *Elaps corallinus* are not listed in the *Delusion* rubrics pertaining to self-blame for sins. *Elaps corallinus* feel persecuted and hunted by others, they do not attribute blame to themselves. *Elaps corallinus*, in contrast to *Crotalus cascavella, Lachesis,* or *Naja*, lack the grandiosity or the exaggerated guilt normally associated with the psychological profile of a snake remedy.

Elaps corallinus are not listed in any of the *Delusion* rubrics pertaining to psychological 'hubristic denial' or 'delusions of grandeur', other than *hearing voices*. The psychological significance of having no delusions of exaggerated guilt in a snake remedy profile is that it indicates that their grandiose stature does not need to be compensated for by 'delusions of original sin'. It also indicates that they do not have enough grandiose belief in themselves to be able to enact change in their lives.

When *Elaps corallinus* find out that they are seriously sick they give up any struggle to fight for their life. *Elaps corallinus* have the *Mind* rubrics: *hiding himself in a corner*, and *inclination to sit as if wrapped in deep, sad thoughts and notices nothing*. *Elaps corallinus* is a homoeopathic remedy which is commonly used for aphasia. *Elaps corallinus* have the *Mind* rubric: *aphasia, comprehension of speech lost, but can speak oneself*. [1] 1. *Elaps corallinus* abandon any fight for their life, nor in fact do they appear to comprehend the severity of the situation when they are faced with a life threatening disease. The Brazilian coral snake is found in South America. It is a shy and timid reptile that is easily captured in comparison to other snakes. If gently tapped on the head with a stick it will coil itself up and lie still, only raising its tail and rattling. It is then easily captured. *Elaps corallinus* have the *Delusion* rubric: *standing on head*. *Elaps corallinus* are not able to motivate themselves. *Elaps corallinus* behave as if they are *being beaten* into submissiveness. *Elaps corallinus* in the face of adversity immediately surrender, they lack the 'hubristic denial' of the other snake remedy profiles.

1. Denial: *Delusion* rubric: *voices*: *hearing*: *Elaps*. *Delusion* rubric: *talking*: *hears talking*: *he*: elaps. [These rubrics in relation to *Elaps corallinus* are more reflective of a 'persecution complex'.]

2. Forsaken: *Delusion* rubric: *beaten, he is being*: elaps. *Delusion* rubric: *rowdies would break in if she was alone*: elaps. [1] 1. *Delusion* rubric: *injury*: *being injured; is*: elaps. *Delusion* rubric: *talking*: *hears talking*: *he*: elaps.

3. Causation: NONE.

4. Depression: *Delusion* rubric: *beaten, he is being*: elaps. [This rubric can pertain to physical persecution or mental and emotional persecution leading to depression and predictions of failure.] *Delusion* rubric: *standing*: *head; standing on*: elaps. [This rubric pertains to an inability to enact positive change.]

5. Resignation: *Delusion* rubric: *falling*: *forward*: *is falling forward; she*: elaps.

Hyoscyamus delude themselves that they *hear the voices* of God and the devil. *Hyoscyamus* have numerous psychological 'delusions of persecution', and a notable number of *Mind* rubrics all pertaining to perceived persecution which reinforce their diabolism. *Hyoscyamus* have the *Mind* rubrics: *delirious delusions of persecution, megalomaniac insanity, religious insanity, demonic mania*, and *delirious imagined wrongs*. [1] 1. These *Mind* rubrics are applicable in the case analysis to describe paranoia and diabolical guilt. *Hyoscyamus* also have the *Mind* rubrics: *temper tantrums, abusive, sudden desire to kill, sardonic laughing, anger alternating with cheerfulness,* and *behaves like a crazy person,* all of which refer to their diabolical unpredictability. *Hyoscyamus* have the *Mind* rubrics: *fits of amorousness, lewd talking,* and the keynote *peculiarity: manic running about naked. Hyoscyamus* have a strong delusional need to exaggerate their 'persecution complex' and an equally strong need to nurture their extrovert mania and *lewdness.*

It is common nowadays, especially with the onset of 'New-Age' language, for a patient to say that they are tempted by the 'dark-side', but it is rare for a patient to refer to themselves as the victim of the 'devil' (Satan). *Hyoscyamus* are the exception to this. They will often refer to the devil in their everyday language. *Hyoscyamus* exaggerate the threat of the devil because they need to deny the 'devil' within who possesses them. *Hyoscyamus* alternate between demonic rage and demonstrative God-like *amorous* affection.

Hyoscyamus have the *Delusion* rubrics: *the devil is after her,* and *possessed of a devil. Hyoscyamus* have a strong need to delude themselves that they are possessed by a *powerful,* superhuman being. The problem for *Hyoscyamus* is that they are undecided as to whom the powerful force is. *Hyoscyamus* have the *Delusion* rubric: *being in debate.* [1] 1. *Hyoscyamus* are devoutly religious because they need to protect themselves from the devil, and because they believe they are in direct auditory communication with God – *hearing voices. Hyoscyamus* maintain their delusions and illusions of *hearing voices* because the voices tell them of others' deceit. If 'God is on your side', telling you others are going to attack you, it absolves you of all guilt over attacking others first. *Hyoscyamus* obsessively nurture their exaggerated paranoia about others' devilry because they need to deny their own devilry. *Hyoscyamus* are the only remedy in the *Mind* rubric: *talking on religious subjects.* [2] 1. *Hyoscyamus* obsessively nurture their religiousness because they need to know they will not be abandoned by God. *Hyoscyamus* are constantly needing to check in with God because they know they are being diabolical – *Delusion* rubric: *religious*.

Hyoscyamus are constantly needing to charm their way into your good-books to make up for whatever transgressions of devilish conduct they have just subjected you to. *Hyoscyamus* nurture their exaggerated 'persecution complexes' and delude themselves about being abandoned because they need to cover up the fact that they are devilish, obsessive, and childishly jealous. The parents of a *Hyoscyamus* child can come to doubt their own version of events or their own sanity because their child can alternate between murderous devil-like rage and God-like *fits of amorousness*. I have watched a *Hyoscyamus* child viciously bite their mother when she was conversing with me, and literally seconds later turn around and cuddle and comfort their mother and sooth the bitten area of skin. *Hyoscyamus* are obsessively jealous. *Hyoscyamus* have the *Mind* rubric: *bites everyone who disturbs him* [1] 1., and the *Mind* rubric: *meddlesome children, disturbing parents when they are conversing* [1] 1. *Hyoscyamus* have the *Mind* rubrics: *animus possession*, and *ailments from jealousy*. *Hyoscyamus* are narcissistic. 'Narcissism' describes the personality trait of excessive vanity or self-love. *Hyoscyamus* are the only remedy in the *Mind* rubrics: *rage from disappointed love* [2] 1., and *suicidal disposition to drowning from disappointed love*. [2] 1. *Hyoscyamus* have the *Delusion* rubric: *is going to be married*. [1] 1. *Hyoscyamus* also have the *Delusion* rubric: *his wife is faithless*. [1] 2. [stram.] The most profound of the Forsaken rubrics for *Hyoscyamus* is the *Delusion* rubric: *being sold*. [1] 1. The delusions of 'hubristic denial' are maintained by *Hyoscyamus* to reinforce their belief that they are being overlooked or discarded [*sold*]. This is why *Hyoscyamus* have the keynote *peculiarities* of *lewd talking*, and *manic running about naked*; they need to maintain their obsessive mania to be the centre of attention. *Hyoscyamus* obsessively nurture their 'persecution complexes' so they can feel justified in obsessively seeking attention. Energy which is disproportionately redirected on to a narcissist persona causes 'delusions of grandeur'. 'Neuroses' relate to psychosomatic conditions, and 'psychoses', relate to mental conflict. Psychoses are a result of difficulties in the relationship between the 'ego' and the external world. *Hyoscyamus* are neurotically and disproportionately obsessed and undermined by psychotic fears that they will be attacked by animals. *Hyoscyamus* have the *Delusion* rubrics: *people are animals,* and *men are swine.* [1] 1. *Hyoscyamus* have the *Delusion* rubrics: *will be bitten,* and *devoured by animals.* [2] 1. *Hyoscyamus* have numerous *Delusion* rubrics pertaining to persecutory fears of animals, and in the majority of the rubrics *Hyoscyamus* are the only remedy listed. *Hyoscyamus* have the *Delusion* rubrics: *beetles, worms, ants, crabs, chasing peacocks, insects, geese, mice, rats, snakes,* and *picking feathers from a bird.* [1] 1.'Neuroses' relate to functional psychosomatic disorders of the nervous system which affect one's ability to be able to have a rational, objective view of life. 'Narcissistic neurosis' is a pre-emptive cause for manic-depressive psychosis insofar as it is characterized by the withdrawal of energy from the realistic and rational 'ego'.

Hyoscyamus alternate between heightened narcissistic mania in which they believe they are attuned to God, and suicidal depression in which they believe they are attuned to the devil. *Hyoscyamus* have seventy-nine *Mind* rubrics pertaining to psychosis [*Delirium*] and fourteen *Mind* rubrics pertaining to mania.

1. Denial: *Delusion* rubric: *hearing: illusions of:* hyos. *Delusion* rubric: *voices: hearing:* hyos. *Delusion* rubric: *people: conversing with absent people:* hyos. *Delusion* rubric: *sounds: listens to imaginary sounds:* hyos. [1] 1. *Delusion* rubric: *fancy, illusions of:* **HYOS**. *Delusion* rubric: *religious:* hyos. *Delusion* rubric: *well, he is:* hyos. *Delusion* rubric: *influence; one is under a powerful:* Hyos. [This rubric can pertain to God or the devil.]

2. Forsaken: *Delusion* rubric: *sold: being*: hyos. [1] 1. *Delusion*
    rubric: *wrong: suffered wrong; he has*: **HYOS**. *Delusion*
    rubric: *criticized, she is*: hyos. *Delusion* rubric: *abused
    being*: hyos. *Delusion* rubric: *forsaken; is*: hyos. *Delusion*
    rubric: *friend: affection of; has lost the*: Hyos. *Delusion*
    rubric: *devil: after her; is*: Hyos. *Delusion* rubric: *home:
    away from home; he is*: Hyos. *Delusion* rubric: *poisoned:
    he: about to be poisoned; he is*: Hyos. *Delusion* rubric:
    watched, she is being: Hyos. *Delusion* rubric: *animals:
    devoured by: had been*: Hyos. [2] 1. *Delusion* rubric: *bitten,
    will be*: Hyos.

3. Causation: *Delusion* rubric: *devil: possessed of a devil:
    he is*: Hyos. *Delusion* rubric: *wrong: done wrong; he has*:
    hyos.

4. Depression: *Delusion* rubric: *suicide; compelled to commit*:
    hyos. *Delusion* rubric: *doomed, being*: hyos. *Delusion*
    rubric: *collect senses; unable to*: hyos. *Delusion* rubric:
    hand: bound: chains; with: hyos. [1] 1.

5. Resignation: *Delusion* rubric: *weight: no weight; has*:
    hyos.

- *Delusions: depending on him; everything is*: lac-lup. lil-t.
- *Delusions: irresistible, he is*: Kola. [2] 1.
- *Delusions: superhuman, is*: cann-i. ignis-alc. psil.
- *Delusions: superiority, of*: crot-c. germ-met. granit-m. *Kola.
  Plat.* polys.
- *Delusions: rank: he is a person of*: cupr. phos. verat.
- *Delusions: distinguished, he is*: marb-w. phos. stram. verat.
- *Delusions: great person, is a*: aeth. *Agar.* alum. bell. *Cann-i.*
  cic. *Coca.* crot-c. cupr. cur. glon. graph. ignis-alc. iod. *Kola.*
  lac-leo. *Lach.* lyc. *Lycpr.* lyss. marb-w. phos. *Plat.* sal-fr.
  stram. sulph. *Syph.* taosc. verat-v. *Verat.*
- *Delusions: presumptuous*: lyc. [1] 1.

- *Delusions: insulting; with:* lyc. [1] 1.
- *Delusions: general, he is a:* cupr. [1] 1.
- *Delusions: commander; being a:* cann-i. cupr.
- *Delusions: officer, he is an:* agar. bell. cann-i. cupr-act. Cupr.

Self-Deluding: You have to ask why each constitutional remedy needs to believe they are *irresistible*, or *a great person*, or *distinguished*.

You have to know how, and why, each constitutional remedy is using the psychological delusion, and what would happen if they did not put the psychological energy into believing they were so *great*.

All remedies will have an 'Achilles heel', the homoeopath needs to know why the delusional denial is in place. Psychological delusions of being abandoned are the underlying need to reinforce 'delusions of grandeur'; this is why Forsaken is the next Stage after Denial. Each remedy profile will be undermined by a *specific* and *peculiar* fear of abandonment. *Coca* need to believe they are a *great person* because they alternate between exalted hubristic visions of persona and crippling paranoia ('delusions of persecution'). *Cuprum* have 'delusions of narcissistic superiority' [*a person of rank*] because they need to deny that they are crippled with fear and paranoia about losing their social status. *Graphites* maintain their 'delusions of superiority' because they are undermined by crippling 'delusions of hypochondria'. Underpinning the 'delusions of grandeur' in *Lycopodium* are crippling fears of being *persecuted* for things *they believe* they have *done wrong*. *Syphilinum* need their psychological 'delusions of *greatness*' to protect their fear of *paralyzed* powerlessness.

Coca resonate with the same energy as the drug cocaine. *Coca* is a homoeopathic remedy derived from *Erythroxylaceae coca*. The *Erythroxylaceae coca* plant contains the alkaloid cocaine. When I have asked patients what they like about doing a line of cocaine (the drug) they tell me it makes them think they are powerful and wonderful people; they tell me everyone loves them and thinks they are fantastic. *Coca* are narcissistic.

Coca need to delude themselves that they are wonderful people because they have fear of abandonment and 'delusions of persecution'.

Coca have the *Delusion* rubric: *separated from the world* and the *Delusion* rubric: *hearing unpleasant voices about himself.* Underlying 'delusions of grandeur' is fear of abandonment. Underlying fear of abandonment is fear and guilt for sins. *Coca* have *no* delusions of self-blame. Having no 'delusions of original sin' allows *Coca* to continue with their addictive need to reinforce their narcissism because they have no guilt. Patients report that what they like about 'doing' the drug cocaine is that it allows them to be completely self-absorbed and self-interested and guilt free. They don't have any guilt, or any social conscience or concern for anyone else's needs other than their own. Patients report that what they don't like about 'doing' cocaine (the drug) is the paranoia which makes them want to *run away* on the Monday and not go to work. The other aspect they don't like is the paranoid 'persecution complex' which undermines them on the Tuesday following their weekend indulgences. This is commonly known as the 'Tuesday blues'. The symptoms of the 'Tuesday blues' are exhaustion, inability to think, and extreme paranoia that everyone is talking negatively about them, all of which are reflected in the rubrics below.

Coca have 'delusions of grandeur' and hubristic visions because they need to deny that they are crippled with fear and paranoia about others seeing them fall from grace. The psychological delusion that they are *separated from the world* is maintained because they need to be invulnerable to *hearing unpleasant things* said about themselves. The psychological delusion that they are *separated from the world* is maintained because they need to elevate themselves from the mundane. *Coca* have 'delusions of grandeur' that they are *beautiful*. *Coca* have the *Mind* rubrics: *full of desires for grandeur*, and *feeling of ease in business*. [1] 1.

Coca need to maintain their narcissistic grandeur because, like the drug, it boosts their confidence about worldly performance.

In a case analysis, the homoeopath needs to determine the psychological advantage that the patient maintains by keeping their psychological delusions. The reason for using my five-stage process is so that the fragility and 'hubristic denial' of the patient can be fully understood.

Coca need to maintain the belief that they are a *great person* because they cannot face the truth about their life. *Coca* *expect* themselves to be *beautiful*, and they narcissistically reinforce that belief.

People consume cocaine (the drug) so they can escape their 'delusions of inadequacy' and their paranoia about being self-defective. People also consume cocaine (the drug) because it gives them an experience of guilt-free narcissism. *Coca* expect themselves to perform, and strive to achieve *exalted euphoria*. When *Coca* are sick they can alternate between delusional ecstasy: their *body is so great* that they will be able to cure themselves, and extreme fear, that they need to isolate themselves from others and themselves from themselves.

Their 'hubristic denial' will often result in *Coca* refusing treatment because they do not believe they need it.

Coca when sick behave in the opposite manner to the extroverted persona normally associated with the high achievement, performance orientated personality remedy profile. *Coca* have the *Mind* rubrics: *desire to remain in bed*, and *bashful timidity*. [3]. *Coca* have the *Mind* rubrics: *exaltation of fancies, pleasant fancies ecstasy, excitement, elated, exhilaration, abundant ideas, nymphomania, desire physical exertion, night industrious,* [1] 1., *morning industrious,* 7-9 h.

[1] 1. *Coca* are conversely extremely shy. This polarity within the persona resonates with the neurotic need of the cocaine (drug) user. Consumption of cocaine (the drug) allows the user to cover up their social inadequacies. *Coca* is an excellent homoeopathic remedy to use for the patient who is suffering from 'social anxiety' [*stage fright*]. *Coca* have the *Mind* rubrics: *anticipation, stage fright,* and *blushing.*

Energy which is disproportionately redirected on to a narcissist persona causes 'delusions of grandeur'. In psychology and psychiatry, narcissism is recognized as a personality disorder of excessive selfishness. 'Narcissistic neurosis' is a pre-emptive cause of manic-depressive psychosis insofar as it is characterized by the withdrawal of energy from the realistic and rational 'ego'.

Coca maintain their personal power at the expense of everyone else. Their desire is not malicious, (they have no *Delusion* rubrics pertaining to wrongs committed) rather it is a need which is maintained to protect a fragile 'ego'.

Freud used the word 'ego' to mean the *realistic* rational part of the mind. The simillimum will not be *Coca* if the patient does not have manic-depressive denial. *Coca* alternate between exalted hubristic visions of persona and crippling paranoia which causes them to hide from themselves and society. *Coca* have 'delusions of grandeur' and hubristic visions because they need to deny that they are crippled with fear and paranoia about others seeing them fall from grace. The psychological delusion that they are *separated from the world* is maintained because they need to be invulnerable to *hearing unpleasant things* said about themselves. *Coca* alternate between heightened manic hubristic power and crippling social paranoia which causes them to run away from themselves, and society, and hide. *Coca* have the *Delusion* rubric: *while lying he was carried into space.* *Coca* have a strong need to deny reality by *running away into space* and *separating themselves from the world* so they can reside in a world of *beautiful visions* of hubristic grandeur. *Coca* have the *Mind* rubric: *lies, never speaks the truth, does not know what she is saying.* *Coca* never tell the truth, especially not to themselves and *especially* not when they are sick. The denial *specific* and *peculiar* to *Coca* is fueled by a strong narcissist desire to maintain their delusion of *beauty*. *Coca* are very attracted to the idea of dying with their body intact and unspoiled by decay. *Coca* are not suicidal and they have no rubrics pertaining to suicide, but when they are sick and dying they do not wish to face decay or the realities of dying. *Coca* have the *Mind* rubric: *unconsciousness, semi-consciousness.* *Coca* will choose a highly medicated, drug-induced exit rather than have to face the reality of their body decaying.

1. Denial: *Delusion* rubric: *great person, is a*: *Coca*. *Delusion* rubric: *beautiful*: coca. *Delusion* rubric: *body*: *greatness of, as to*: *Coca*. *Delusion* rubric: *expectant; he is*: coca. [1] 1. *Delusion* rubric: *visions, has beautiful*: coca. *Delusion* rubric: *space*: *carried into space; he was*: *lying; while*: coca. *Delusion* rubric: *separated*: *world; from the, he is separated*: coca. [This rubric in relation to *Coca* can pertain to 'delusions of grandeur' that they are separate from others, and separate from the mundane.]

2. Forsaken: *Delusion* rubric: *separated*: *world; from the, he is separated*: coca. [This rubric can pertain to 'delusions of grandeur' or 'delusions of abandonment'.] *Delusion* rubric: *voices: hearing, unpleasant voices about himself*: coca. [1] 1.

3. Causation: NONE.

4. Depression: *Delusion* rubric: *run: long way; he could run a*: coca. [1] 1. [*Coca* do not want to remain in their conscious mind, they abandon conscientiousness.]

5. Resignation: *Delusion* rubric: *exhausted; he was*: coca. [1] 1. *Delusion* rubric: *brain: confused; brain were*: coca. [1] 1.

Cuprum need to believe that they are important to avoid facing their fears of social and financial destruction [*misfortune*].

Cuprum suffer from psychotic paranoia about their standing in the world. Psychosis relates to mental conflict between the 'ego' and the external world. The *Delusion* rubrics which cover psychoses are the *Delusion* rubrics: forsaken, depression and resignation. *Cuprum* deny their feelings of social inadequacy. Their denial is maintained to avoid fears of being forsaken [*persecution*], feelings of guilt [*devil*], fear of failure [*misfortune*], and fears of disease [*unfit for work*]. *Cuprum* suffer fears of loss of social standing. Cuprum have two *Delusion* rubrics which reveal their fear that they will not become a person of social *rank*: *he is repairing old chairs*, and *he is selling green vegetables*. I do not wish to make disparaging remarks about green grocers, but my mother used to say to me: "If you don't study hard and do well in school you'll just end up selling vegetables in the local greengrocers". The inference is obvious. *Cuprum* have 'delusions of superiority'. A 'delusion of superiority' is a delusion that one is superior to others.

Cuprum have 'delusions of narcissistic superiority' [*a person of rank*] because they need to deny that they are crippled with fear and paranoia about losing their social status.

Narcissism is recognized as a personality disorder of excessive self-interest and self-preservation. The more *Cuprum* intimidate others, the more they can boast of their standing and position in the world. *Cuprum* alternate between manic social extroversion and depressive social introversion. *Cuprum* are single-minded in their pursuit of success. *Cuprum* have the *Mind* rubrics: *increased competitive ambition, joy at the misfortune of others*, and *increased ambition he will be the best*, [1] 1. *Cuprum* have the *Mind* rubrics: *hardhearted to himself* and *hardhearted to others*. [1] 1. 'Delusions of superiority' emphasize the threat that the world poses to the self or 'ego'. The converse of their fastidious push to achieve is the depressive, psychotic paranoia around their social anxiety. *Cuprum* have the *Mind* rubrics: *antisocial*, and *evading the look of other persons*. 'Narcissistic neurosis' is a pre-emptive cause of manic-depressive psychosis. The simillimum will not be *Cuprum* unless you can see mania to succeed on the one hand, and depressive persecutory fears of loss of work security on the other.

1. Denial: *Delusion* rubric: *rank; he is a person of:* cupr. *Delusion* rubric: *general, he is a:* cupr. [1] 1. *Delusion* rubric: *commander; being a:* cupr. *Delusion* rubric: *officer, he is an: Cupr.* *Delusion* rubric: *fancy, illusions of:* cupr. *Delusion* rubric: *business: doing business; is:* cupr. *Delusion* rubric: *engaged: occupation; he is engaged in some:* cupr.

2. Forsaken: *Delusion* rubric: *pursued; he was: enemies by:* cupr. *Delusion* rubric: *persecuted: he is persecuted:* cupr. *Delusion* rubric: *arrested, is about to be:* cupr.

3. Causation: *Delusion* rubric: *devil:* cupr.

4. Depression: *Delusion* rubric: *insane: become insane; one will:* cupr. *Delusion* rubric: *misfortune: approaching; as if some misfortune were:* cupr. *Delusion* rubric: *vegetable: green vegetables, he is selling:* cupr. [1] 2. [cupr-act.] *Delusion* rubric: *chair: repairing old chairs; he is:* cupr. [1] 2. [cupr-act.]

5. Resignation: *Delusion* rubric: *die: about to die; one was:* cupr. *Delusion* rubric: *unfit: work; for:* cupr.

Graphites are not a constitutional remedy profile that one would normally associate with 'delusions of grandeur' or 'delusions of superiority', yet they have the *Delusion* rubric: *is a great person.* Graphites are supposedly traumatized by all assertive acts. They have the following *Mind* rubrics, all of which pertain to a fragile persona. *Graphites* have the *Mind* rubrics: *ailments from discords between one's parents*, and *ailments from discords between one's friends.* [3]. Graphites also have the *Mind* rubrics: *cowardice, without courage to express one's opinion,* and *anguish* so profound they *cannot sit still.*

All the remedy profiles within this group of *Delusion* rubrics: *distinguished, great person, superior, superhuman*, are all narcissistic in an individualistic way and are all *peculiarly* neurotically obsessed with needing to maintain denial for self-preservation. The neurotic need to maintain narcissistic self-interest pre-empts manic-depressive psychosis.

Graphites alternate between manic *haughtiness* and *cowardice*. This is why *Graphites* have the keynote characteristic of *alternating cheerfulness* and *causeless weeping*. *Graphites* have the *Mind* rubrics: *exaltation of fancies, increased ambition for fame* and *haughty mania*. *Graphites* need to deny turmoil. They cannot understand the emotional turmoil of life. *Graphites* have the *Delusion* rubric: *he is drunk on rising*, and *everything is strange* – both are indicative of their inner confusion. *Graphites* need to maintain delusional narcissistic self-preservation because they are so fragile. Underpinning their fragile 'ego' are persecutory fears that their inner sanctuary has been infiltrated. *Graphites* feel their psyche is threatened. If a remedy profile has a weakened 'ego', then their psyche is under threat. *Graphites* have the *Delusion* rubric: *as if someone is with him in bed*. This *Delusion* rubric should not be interpreted literally; the somatic interpretation indicates that *Graphites* feel threatened in the inner sanctuary of their psyche.

There is an inconsistency between the delusion that they are *great* and the delusion of impotency that their *body is smaller* and that they are *about to die*. *Graphites* cannot face the turmoil[27] of illness. *Graphites* maintain their 'delusions of superiority' because they are undermined by crippling 'delusions of hypochondria'. The simillimum will not be *Graphites* unless the patient alternates between delusional greatness and deprecating littleness.

1. Denial: *Delusion* rubric: *great person, is a*: graph. *Delusion* rubric: *visions, has*: graph.

2. Forsaken: *Delusion* rubric: *assembled things, swarms, crowds etc.*: graph. *Delusion* rubric: *bed: someone: in the bed; as if someone is: with him*: graph.

3. Causation: *Delusion* rubric: *criminal, he is a*: graph.
4. Depression: *Delusion* rubric: *drunk*: *is drunk*; *he*: *rising; on*: graph. [1] 1. *Delusion* rubric: *strange*: *everything is*: *Graph*. *Delusion* rubric: *unfortunate, he is*: graph.
5. Resignation: *Delusion* rubric: *die*: *about to die; one was*: graph. *Delusion* rubric: *dead*: *he himself was*: graph. *Delusion* rubric: *sick*: *being*: graph. *Delusion* rubric: *small*: *body is smaller*: graph.

Lycopodium[28] need to believe they are a *great person* because they have underlying fears of personal destruction. *Lycopodium* are not afraid of failure, they are afraid they cannot succeed. Failure and not succeeding might seem synonymous, but the difference, which is *peculiar* to *Lycopodium,* is 'ego' fragility. Underpinning *Graphites* 'ego' fragility are persecutory fears that their inner sanctuary has been infiltrated. This is because *Graphites* feel threatened from outside. *Lycopodium* have crippling fears of being *persecuted* for things *they believe they have done wrong*. Their 'ego' is not in conflict with the external world, it is under threat from their own self-deprecating nature. If a remedy profile has a weakened 'ego' then their psyche is under threat from the world.

Lycopodium are under threat from within their own persona. The keynote characteristic[29] of *Lycopodium* is their *presumptuous* need to boast about their indispensability. *Lycopodium* delude themselves that they are surrounded by people who look up to them in order to allay their fears of not being important.

Lycopodium have the *Mind* rubric: *spying on everything.* *Lycopodium* also have the *Delusion* rubric: *being in two places at the same time.* *Lycopodium* need to believe they have complete control of their position in life and that they have a 'finger in every pie'. The need to constantly remind themselves and others of their position or standing in life comes from self-doubt, but their self-doubt is fueled from within. *Lycopodium* diminish themselves in their own eyes. *Lycopodium* have the failure *Delusion* rubrics: *to be sinking, he is unfortunate,* and *being doomed. Lycopodium* are undermined by numerous 'delusions of persecution' which are based on disproportionate reactions to their 'delusions of original sin'. *Lycopodium* diminish their own standing because they over-react to psychological delusions of exaggerated guilt specifically centered around fear that they have *neglected their duty. Lycopodium* have forty-six *Mind* rubrics pertaining to weeping. Their self-criticism and self-deprecation because of exaggerated psychological delusions of guilt cause emotional pain and a disproportionate need to be appreciated. *Lycopodium* are the only remedy listed in the *Mind* rubric: *weeping when thanked.* [3] 1. The 'never-well-since-event' or causation in any *Lycopodium* (case) will always come from an exaggerated sense of guilt over fear and hate of the father. *Lycopodium* have been dominated by their father. The fact that *Lycopodium* grow up and need to assert their authority is reflective of learned behavior, but more importantly it is reflective of the need to establish their own potent 'ego'. *Lycopodium* and *Coca* are both in the same *Delusion* rubric: *is a great person,* but *Lycopodium* (in contrast to the narcissistic *Coca*) have exaggerated guilt which causes self-betrayal. *Lycopodium* need to maintain their 'delusions of grandeur' to avoid their own persecutory guilt.

Lycopodium have the following *Mind* rubrics which map the psychodynamic crisis within their psyche. Domination of the child by the father results in emotional insecurity, which in turn creates a need for the mother, and finally a need to find their own people to dominate. This psychological analysis of the 'never-well-since-event' has always been in the *Mind* and *Delusion* rubrics attached to *Lycopodium.* My aim here is to highlight the psychological behavioral patterning which has developed within the psyche of *Lycopodium* as a result of over-domination.

Lycopodium have the *Delusion* rubric: *childish fantasies*. The reason I have allocated this *Delusion* rubric in Denial is that *Lycopodium* have fairytale imaginings and 'hubristic visions' of being recognized. *Lycopodium* are the child prince or princess who never found favor with the king. Their father has banished them into the woods, but fate and destiny intervene and finally their royal blood is recognized and they take their rightful place on the throne. The psychological understanding of the 'never-well-since-event' can then be used to identify the simillimum.

- *Mind: ailments from: domination: children; in: Lyc.*
- *Mind: ailments from: domination: long time; for a:* lyc.
- *Mind: ailments from: neglected; being: father; by one's:* lyc.
- *Mind: clinging: children; in: mother; child clings to the: hand of the mother; child will always take the:* lyc.
- *Mind: holding: mother's hand; child constantly holding:* lyc.
- *Mind: confidence: want of self-confidence: self-depreciation: Lyc.*
- *Mind: dictatorial: talking with air of command: Lyc.*
- *Mind: respected: desire to be:* lyc.

Lycopodium react very strongly to feeling vulnerable. They have the *Mind* rubric: *aversion to homoeopathy*, not because they react to homoeopathy per sé, rather they react to *dependency* on medicine because they are terrified of illness. *Lycopodium* have the *Mind* rubric: *hypochondriasis with hysteria*, and are the only remedy in the *Mind* rubric: *hysteria with white discoloration of the tongue.* [2] 1. *Lycopodium* feel *peculiarly* threatened by any signs of illness specifically and *peculiarly* on their tongue. *Lycopodium* have the *Mind* rubric: *feeling of helplessness.* [3]. It is invaluable to consider the *Delusion* rubrics of 'hubristic denial' for the patient struggling to realistically acknowledge or assess the gravity of the situation regarding their health. *Lycopodium* are hysterical when confronted with their own illness and immediately assume they are going to die. *Lycopodium* have the *Delusion* rubric: *one would die from weakness*. *Lycopodium* maintain their 'delusions of grandeur', they constantly remind themselves and others of their position, they need to be needed. Their need to maintain psychological delusions that they are *great* are related to self-preservation. *Lycopodium* feel their life is threatened if they allow themselves to become a weak link in any situation.

Lycopodium need to maintain their domination of others so they can avoid the feeling that they do not exist. *Lycopodium* have the *Delusion* rubric: *everything will vanish*. [1] 1. *Lycopodium* need to insure that others remain weak so they can reinforce their strength. The simillimum will only be *Lycopodium* if the patient is threatened and undermined by any loss of stature.

1. Denial: *Delusion* rubric: *great person, is a*: lyc. *Delusion* rubric: *presumptuous*: lyc. [1] 1. *Delusion* rubric: *insulting; with*: lyc. [1] 1. *Delusion* rubric: *place: two places at the same time; of being in*: Lyc. *Delusion* rubric: *childish fantasies, has*: lyc. *Delusion* rubric: *religious*: lyc. *Delusion* rubric: *fancy, illusions of*: lyc.

2. Forsaken: *Delusion* rubric: *persecuted: he is persecuted*: lyc. *Delusion* rubric: *injury: about to receive injury; is*: lyc. *Delusion* rubric: *pursued; he was: enemies, by*: lyc.

3. Causation: *Delusion* rubric: *wrong: done wrong; he has*: lyc. *Delusion* rubric: *neglected: duty; he neglected his*: Lyc.

4. Depression: *Delusion* rubric: *succeed, he does everything wrong; he cannot*: lyc. *Delusion* rubric: *unfortunate, he is*: lyc. *Delusion* rubric: *doomed, being*: lyc. *Delusion* rubric: *sinking; to be*: lyc. *Delusion* rubric: *vanish: everything will*: lyc. [1] 1.

5. Resignation: *Delusion* rubric: *die: about to die; one was*: lyc. *Delusion* rubric: *die: about to die; one was: weakness; one would die from*: lyc. *Delusion* rubric: *sick: being*: Lyc.

Syphilinum have the opposing *Delusion* rubrics: *is a great person* and *about to be paralyzed*. [1] 1. Their psychological 'delusions of grandeur' protect their fear of *paralyzed* powerlessness. *Syphilinum* need to deny their self-destructive deprecation [*dirty*] by believing they are invincible [*great*]. Underpinning their psyche is guilt over their 'delusions of original sin'. *Syphilinum* believe that they are *dirty*, and this undermines their 'ego'. *Syphilinum* need to reinforce their greatness because they feel undermined by everything, from within themselves and outside of themselves, and this is the cause behind their neurotic obsession with cleanliness. *Syphilinum* suffer from obsessive-compulsive disorder (OCD) specifically centered around cleanliness. *Syphilinum* have the *Delusion* rubric: *washing*, and the *Mind* rubrics: *mania for cleanliness*, and *desire to always wash her hands*, and the *Mind* rubric: *must check twice or more*, and *verifying the doors are locked*. [1] 1. Underpinning the behavioral peculiarities of the OCD sufferer is a need to reinforce the belief that they are in control. Sufferers obsessively clean everything in the hope of achieving control over their environment. The more in control they feel, the less their anxiety. The need to create security comes from a belief that they are not in control. This in turn becomes self-punishing as it fuels continual doubt over whether they have cleaned their hands well enough, or checked that the iron is off, or checked that the door is shut, etc. Their doubt *paralyzes* them with crippling anxiety and they are forced to wash their hands again or check the door again, in the hope of regaining power and control. The delusion which ignites their behavior is the belief that once they have checked everything again they will achieve complete control over their environment. *Syphilinum* have the *Delusion* rubric: *he would lose consciousness after confusion*. [1] 1. The OCD sufferer can often become so anxious and confused that they faint. In treating an OCD sufferer, one slowly reinforces confidence that even if they haven't got control over everything they are still going to be okay. The OCD sufferer believes that their life is threatened if they don't have control over all disorder, in particular any dirt. Slowly, the OCD sufferer learns that they can cope with disorder.

The hubristic need to create an illusion of omnipotent control is a 'delusion of grandeur' which traps the OCD sufferer and reinforces the belief that they will be in danger [*insane*] if there is any evidence of imperfection [*dirty*].

Syphilinum have the same delusional need to create control [*great person*] so they can allay their fears of powerlessness [*he is about to be paralyzed*]. This is why *Syphilinum* can appear fanatical if they are threatened. Their *insanity* is fuelled by a fanatical need to protect their hubristic visions of themselves. This is why *Syphilinum* have the *Mind* rubric: *megalomania insanity*. Megalomania is an insanity of self-exaltation, a passion for grandiose perfection. It is a mistake to assume that a *Syphilinum* patient will present in a consultation as a fragile troubled soul. *Syphilinum* are megalomaniacs[30]. They seek grandiose self-exaltation. Family members of OCD sufferers often feel dominated and controlled. *Syphilinum* is a profile of a cripple who refuses to acknowledge his predicament. He feels persecuted by his illness. He becomes abusive and controlling of the people who are caring for him. As a result of becoming tyrannical he is then able to boost his opinion of himself enough to believe he is powerful. Family members and partners who are looking after patients in this predicament have often relayed to me that they feel as if they are living with a tyrant. The wife of a man suffering from multiple sclerosis told she could never do anything right: *The more I try, the more obsessive he becomes about everything. He is aggressive and abusive towards me in front of the children. Every day the rules around his food and hygiene are becoming more obsessive. He now won't go out of the house in case he can't have control over everything and this means I am totally confined to the house. He insists everyone must come to him and really he is not that bad with his condition yet. It is like he is already paralyzed in his head now.*

This psychological analysis of *megalomania* has always been in the *Mind* and *Delusion* rubrics attached to *Syphilinum*, but my aim here is to label psychological behavioral patterning. This psychological label can then be applied to identifying the simillimum in case analysis.

1. Denial: *Delusion* rubric: *great person, is a*: Syph.
2. Forsaken: *Delusion* rubric: *persecuted: he is persecuted*: syph.
3. Causation: *Delusion* rubric: *dirty, he is*: Syph.
4. Depression: *Delusion* rubric: *insane: become insane; one will*: Syph.
5. Resignation: *Delusion* rubric: *disease: incurable disease; he has an*: Syph. *Delusion* rubric: *consciousness: lose consciousness; he would: confusion; after*: syph. [1] 1. *Delusion* rubric: *paralyzed; he is*: *about to be paralyzed*: syph. [1] 1.

- *Delusions: power. diseases: he had power over all: Stram.* [2] 1.
- *Delusions: body: greatness of, as to: Cann-i. Coca. Hell. Plat.* staph. taosc.
- *Delusions: strong; he is*: aids. androc. coff. dendr-pol. hydrog. lac-leo. plat.
- *Delusions: adolescent; he was again an*: androc. [1] 1.
- *Delusions: insane: everyone is*: androc. [1] 1.
- *Delusions: enlarged*: acon. alum. apis. *Aran.* arg-met. *Arg-n. Bapt.* bell. berb. *Bov.* caj. **CANN-I.** coc-c. con. euph. ferr. *Gels.* glon. hydrog. *Hyos.* irid-met. kali-ar. kali-bi. kali-br. kola. lach. laur. limest-b. loxo-recl. mang. nat-c. nux-m. nux-v. *Op.* ox-ac. *Par.* phos. pic-ac. pip-m. *Plat.* puls. rhus-t. sabad. spig. stram. zinc.
- *Delusions: enlarged: tall: he is very*: aur. hydrog. *Irid-met.* op. pall. plat. pyrog. staph. stram.
- *Delusions: tall: he or she is tall*: arizon-l. cob. cop. crot-c. eos. fic-m. hydrog. iodof. *Irid-met.* limest-b. ol-eur. oncor-t. op. pall. plat. plut-n. staph. **STRAM.** *Sulph.* tung-met.

Self-deluding: It would be incorrect to translate these rubrics literally and to imply that one's patient believes that their body is *large* or *tall* or *great*. Psychotherapeutically, the application in case analysis is relevant to the patient who needs to delude themselves about their invincibility.

Believing you are *strong* and that your body is *great* and powerful allays fears of failure, or fears of potential attack. The most obvious form of attack is illness. The group of *Delusion* rubrics above is invaluable to consider for patients who move into delusional denial about their illness and who believe they are so powerful and strong that they will beat everything thrown in their path.

Each constitutional remedy will express their abandonment of health, and potentially of life, in an individualistic and *peculiar* way which will indicate not only the next *Delusion* rubric but also the simillimum. If one's patient is notably convinced of their invincibility and assured in their belief of cure (contrary to medical evidence) this is indicative of the first stage: Denial. Each constitutional remedy will need to maintain their denial because of a *peculiar* and specific need which they wish to avoid.

Psychotherapeutically, it is invaluable to know why each constitutional remedy chooses to believe they are invincible [*body is great, strong, tall, power over all disease*].

Androctonus is a homoeopathic remedy derived from a scorpion. The somatic theme of the scorpion, predator and victim, resonates within *Androctonus*. *Androctonus* have the *Mind* rubrics: *malicious desire to injure someone,* and the *desire to feel and crawl behind rocks.* [1] 1. *Androctonus* have the *Delusion* rubric: *he is going to be assaulted. Androctonus* need to delude themselves that they are *strong* because they fear being attacked by larger predators. *Androctonus* also need to delude themselves that they are *strong* so they have the confidence to become a predator. *Androctonus* have the same emotive approach to illness. *Androctonus* have no *Delusion* rubrics which pertain to Resignation.

Androctonus will *never* admit they are sick. The simillimum is not *Androctonus* if the patient admits they are sick; admitting you are sick is synonymous with admitting you are not *strong*.

Androctonus have the *Mind* rubric: *says he is well when very sick*. *Androctonus* have the *Delusion* rubric: *views the world through a hole*. [1] 1. *Androctonus* deflect responsibility, self-blame, and guilt and see only what they wish to see. *Androctonus* have no *Delusion* rubrics which pertain to 'original sin'. *Androctonus* are akin to a self-centered teenager [*adolescent*] who believes everyone else is crazy [*insane*] for accusing them of misdemeanors. *Androctonus* need to maintain the belief that everything is a *terrifying mystery* because it allows them to emotionally distance themselves from their part in the trauma.

Androctonus deflect responsibility. Everything will always be someone else's fault, while they remain invincible [*strong*].

1. Denial: *Delusion* rubric: *strong; he is*: androc. *Delusion* rubric: *adolescent; he was again an*: androc. [1] 1. *Delusion* rubric: *insane*: *everyone is*: androc. [1] 1.

2. Forsaken: *Delusion* rubric: *umbrella was a knife*: androc. [1] 1. [This rubric indicates threat.] *Delusion* rubric: *persecuted*: *he is persecuted*: androc. *Delusion* rubric: *appreciated, she is not*: Androc. *Delusion* rubric: *outcast; she was an*: androc. *Delusion* rubric: *alone, being*: *world; alone in the*: Androc. *Delusion* rubric: *separated*: *world; from the*: *he is separated*: Androc. [In relation to *Androctonus*, the last three rubrics can pertain to 'delusions of persecution', or 'delusions of superiority' which reinforce their feeling of safety.]

3. Causation: NONE.

4. Depression: *Delusion* rubric: *wrong*: *everything goes wrong*: androc. *Delusion* rubric: *mystery; everything around*

seems a terrifying: androc. *Delusion* rubric: *identity: errors of personal identity*: androc.

5. Resignation: NONE.

Baptisia tinctoria delude themselves that they are powerful [*enlarged*] to cover up their inner vulnerability and weakness. *Baptisia tinctoria* overreact with disproportionate fear and believe that their illness will cripple them emotionally, mentally and physically. *Baptisia tinctoria* suffer psychological fears which relate to abandonment of the body – *Delusion* rubric: *legs don't belong to her,* and *arms don't belong to her.*

The *Delusion* rubric: *enlarged* and the *Delusion* rubric: *parts of body are enlarged* can pertain to exaggerated assumptions of wellness or exaggerated presumptions of illness.

Baptisia tinctoria are in perpetual self-conflict. *Baptisia tinctoria* as a homoeopathic remedy is excellent for sudden weakness from influenza or diarrhoea, which affects the use of one's legs. *Baptisia tinctoria* as a homoeopathic remedy is also an excellent remedy for threatened miscarriage. *Baptisia tinctoria* have the *Delusion* rubric: *one part of the body is talking to another part,* and the *Delusion* rubric: *legs are conversing.* [1] 1. Instead of assuming that these rubrics mean "erroneous ideas as to the state of his body" (Vermeulen), one could consider their psychosomatic meaning. *Baptisia tinctoria* as a constitutional remedy profile reflect the psychological duality of exaggerated psychosomatic fear of destruction and exaggerated delusions of power.

I had a *Baptisia tinctoria* patient relay this story: *Really Liz, the homoeopathic remedy did nothing to alleviate my terrible fear that I would die. What happened was, I did die and then I came back, and now I am not afraid of dying anymore* [*Baptisia tinctoria* have the *Mind* rubric: *conviction of death*]. *I experienced being outside of my body. I could see that I was falling* [*sinking*] *into death and that I was leaving behind my body which I no longer needed. Then I decided that all I needed to do was to tell my body that it would survive and it would. I was then overcome with a vision that I was going to fight and win this battle. At that point I re-entered my body and have felt empowered [enlarged] ever since.*

The simillimum will not be *Baptisia tinctoria* unless the patient is rattled about being sick. *Baptisia tinctoria* have the *Mind* rubric: *taciturn about sickness or injuries.* [3] 1. *Baptisia tinctoria* are also listed in the *Dream* rubric: *always fights, always conquers,* indicating a delusional belief that they will triumph in disputes.

1. Denial: *Delusion* rubric: *enlarged: Bapt. Delusion* rubric: *enlarged: body is: parts of body:* bapt. [These rubrics can pertain to exaggerated assumptions of cure or exaggerated presumptions of disease and death.] *Delusion* rubric: *double: being: outside of patient; there was a second self: Bapt. Delusion* rubric: *three persons, he is:* bapt.

2. Forsaken: *Delusion* rubric: *arms: cut off; arms are:* bapt. [1] 1. *Delusion* rubric: *body: parts: taken away; parts of body have been: Bapt.* [2] 2. *Delusion* rubric: *legs: cut off; legs are:* bapt.

3. Causation: *Delusion* rubric: *succeed, he does everything wrong; he cannot:* bapt. [This rubric can pertain to fault ('delusions of original sin') or assumptions of failure ('delusions of impending doom').]

4. Depression: *Delusion* rubric: *succeed, he does everything wrong; he cannot:* bapt. *Delusion* rubric: *sinking; to be:* bapt.

5. Resignation: *Delusion* rubric: *arms: belong to her; arms do not:* bapt. *Delusion* rubric: *body: scattered about; body was: tossed about to get pieces together. Bapt. Delusion* rubric: *legs: belong to her; her legs don't:* bapt.

Helleborus is a homoeopathic remedy often used for physical swellings as a result of injury. *Helleborus* is derived from *Helleborus niger* which is a toxic plant. Contact with the plant causes an allergic skin reaction and swelling. Ingestion of the plant causes gastrointestinal inflammation and severe emesis. Its toxicity is fatal only if consumed in large quantities. *Helleborus* have the *Skin* rubric: *dropsical swelling* [3]., *swelling on affected parts*, and the *Stomach* rubric: *distention epigastrium*. The belief in the *greatness of one's body* somatically mirrors the psychodynamic memory of the inflammatory reactions of the body when it comes into contact with the poison. The belief in the *greatness of one's body* reflects their inflammatory response to the poison. *Helleborus* as a remedy profile overreact emotionally, mentally and physically. They are over-sensitized to all environmental stressors. The theme inherent in the plant remedies is hypersensitivity to all environmental influences. *Helleborus* emotionally overreact to stress with crippling anxiety: *Mind* rubric: *shuddering with anxiety* [3] 14. *Helleborus* mentally overreact to stress with paralyzing confusion: *Mind* rubric: *dullness, does not understand what is happening* [1] 1., and *Mind* rubric: *concentration difficult, rubbing forehead when trying to concentrate.* [1] 1. *Helleborus* physically overreact to stress with immobilizing physical and mental confusion: *Mind* rubric: *confusion of mind, muscles refuse to obey the will when attention is turned away.* *Helleborus* is particularly relevant to consider for the patient who is so overwhelmed by the fact that they are sick that they withdraw into a comatose depression. *Helleborus* have the *Mind* rubric: *indifference, has no desire nor action of will.* *Helleborus* have the *Delusion* rubrics: *being doomed*, and *to be sinking*.

Helleborus have a conflict between Stage one: Denial, and Stage five: Resignation. If there is a contradiction between psychological 'delusions of grandeur' and psychological 'delusions of hypochondria' then this is indicative of self-perpetuating punishment. The psychological profile of the remedy must contain evidence of the denial being injurious to the self in order to justify the use of a *Delusion* rubric in the rubric-repertorisation.

Helleborus is relevant for the patient who is in denial about their physical illness or physical disability. *Helleborus* physically hurt themselves through an inability to realistically assess their emotional, mental and/or physical dysfunction. *Helleborus* have the *Delusion* rubric: *greatness of body* because they are in denial about their disabilities. Despair overwhelms them, which then gives rise to the need to break out of their own restrictions. As soon as they start to move they repeat their injuries; it is at this point that *Helleborus* give up and sink into oblivion. Their psychological 'delusions of grandeur' manifest in the belief that their *body is so great* it can overcome all injuries.

These are psychological delusions of denial which are self-punishing because they perpetuate injuries. *Helleborus* have the *Delusion* rubric: *he cannot walk, he must run or hop.* *Helleborus* have a psychodynamic need to cause injury within their psyche. *Helleborus* need to punish themselves for *something they have done which is wrong.* Their psychological 'delusions of original sin' perpetuate their psychological delusions of self-punishment. *Helleborus* is for the patient who causes injury to themselves under the guise of hubristic righteousness. The image which comes to mind is the fundamentalist religious person who feels *doomed, they have lost their salvation* but they are able to redeem their *greatness* and make themselves *new* again by lashing their body. *Helleborus* have the *Mind* rubric: *sensation as if he could do great deeds.* [2] 3.

1. Denial: *Delusion* rubric: *body: greatness of, as to: Hell.* *Delusion* rubric: *fancy, illusions of:* hell. *Delusion* rubric: *new; everything is:* hell. *Delusion* rubric: *visions, has:* hell.

2. Forsaken: *Delusion* rubric: *persecuted: he is persecuted:* hell.

3. Causation: *Delusion* rubric: *neglected: duty; he has neglected his:* hell. *Delusion* rubric: *wrong: doing something wrong; he is:* hell. [1] 2.

4. Depression: *Delusion* rubric: *doomed, being*: hell. *Delusion* rubric: *sinking; to be: Hell. Delusion* rubric: *lost; she is: salvation; for:* hell.

5. Resignation: *Delusion* rubric: *die: about to die; one was:* hell. *Delusion* rubric: *sick: being:* hell.

- *Delusions: clothes: beautiful; clothes are:* aeth. olib-sac. *Sulph.*
- *Delusions: rags are as fine as silk; old:* **SULPH**. [4] 1.
- *Delusions: beautiful: rags seem, even: Sulph.* [2] 1.
- *Delusions: wealth, of:* adam. agn. alco. bell. calc. cann-i. cann-xyz. kali-br. nit-ac. phos. *Plat. Pyrog. Sulph.* verat.
- *Delusions: person: other person; she is some: existed in another person; she:* pyrog. [1] 1.
- *Delusions: abundance of everything, she has an:* adam. sulph.
- *Delusions: harmony: order and clarity of everything:* adam. [1] 1.
- *Delusions: prince; he is a: Indian prince; an:* adam. [1] 1.
- *Delusions: sparkling, everything is:* adam. [1] 1.
- *Delusions: arms: four arms; she has:* adam. sulfon.
- *Delusions: face: four faces; she has:* adam. [1] 1.
- *Delusions: hand: four hands; she has:* adam. [1] 1.
- *Delusions: galaxies spiraling:* adam. [1] 1.
- *Delusions: deity; huge Tibetan:* adam. [1] 1.

Self-deluding: When analyzing a case, I systematically construct rubric after rubric. The meaning and relevance of particular rubrics which form the simillimum will often be explained by other rubrics attached to the remedy profile.

The application and relevance of the *Delusion* rubrics of abundance and wealth to illness is very interesting. I have had several extremely wealthy patients over the years who cannot believe they could ever become sick because they have always been blessed with everything they have ever wanted.

I have had several patients tell me: *I can't possibly be sick Liz, do you know how much I have achieved in life? I have never had anything wrong with me. I have always had the best doctors and health practitioners looking after me, I simply cannot believe that this is the situation. I have been blessed with ease all my life. I have had no stress to do with money, I have been completely happy. There is absolutely no reason why it should be me who is sick because I have had the best of everything and the best life.*

Cancer affects one in three people. The assumption that one will not get cancer because one is wealthy and famous is a 'delusion of grandeur'. (The assumption that one will not get cancer because one is a homoeopath is also a 'delusion of grandeur'.)

The psychological 'delusions of grandeur' to do with wealth have traditionally been applied in case analysis to the patient who is avoiding responsibility by exaggerating their wealth, or for the patient who believes they are entitled to special significance. For example, both the remedies *Adamas* and *Sulphur* appear in the *Delusion* rubric: *abundance of everything* and the *Delusion* rubric: *wealth*, but each will be motivated by a different need behind their avoidance of, or glorification of, fiscal reality. *Adamas need* money and power to prove to others and themselves that they are worthy, therefore they maintain their delusions of exaggerated wealth. *Sulphur* on the other hand choose *to believe* that they are wealthy so they can avoid fiscal reality, therefore they also maintain their 'delusions of abundance'.

Adamas is a homoeopathic remedy derived from a diamond. My aim in the *Rubric-categories* is to provide a psychological profile which is synonymous with the constitutional remedy profile. A psychological diagnosis can contextualize what can often appear to be countless confusing keynotes attached to a remedy profile.

Peter Tumminello notes in his book, *Twelve Jewels,* that the positive keywords for *Diamond* are: "Balance; Calm; Centred; Clarity; Clear; Command; Confident; Destiny; Detachment; Focused; Freedom; Genius; Golden; Greatness; Goodness; Harmony; Indomitable; Intelligent; Joy; Magic key; Magnanimity; Manifestation; Mastery; Positive; Perfection; Pure; Shining; Serene; Straight; Strong; Successful; Transformation; Universal/Unity; Victory; Virtuosity; White; Will; Old wisdom."

The negative keywords for *Diamond* are: "Alone; Black hole; Darkness; Depression; Despair; Ego-destruction; Egotism, Existential agony; Failure; Fatal flaws; In a fog; Hate; Hopeless; Imperfect; Loss of faith; Madness; Meaningless; Mutilation; Negative; Perfection, relentless drive for; Self-abuse; Self-blame; Self-criticism; Self-destruction; Self-hate; Suicide; Selfish wrong; Shame and guilt; Tunnel worthless."

The psychological profile of *Adamas* is consistent with the psychological profile of the mental disorder, bipolar. A patient suffering with bipolar alternates between heightened states of awareness [*clarity*], which give them spurts of extraordinary creativity (mania), and crippling depression. *Adamas* strive for perfection.

The paradox of perfection – that imperfection is perfect – is the paradox that exists within the creative arts. The creative genius has always been recognized for their work which has managed to capture the paradox of perfection in life – that imperfection is perfect. It is therefore not surprising to find that sufferers of bipolar are prevalent within the creative arts. The self-perpetuating fluctuation between striving for creative perfection and the failure to achieve that ideal is synonymous with the manic-depressive artistic persona.

A psychological diagnosis means that the homoeopath has a framework which illuminates the apparent personality polarities. The psychological framework explains why *Diamond* have contrasting and conflicting personality polarities: *greatness* and *failure*. Although a psychological prognosis provides verification of the bipolar polarities, this prognosis must in turn be confirmed in the rubric-repertorisation.

If one's patient is convinced of their invincibility and assured of their belief in a cure (contrary to medical evidence) this is indicative of the first stage: Denial. If one's patient is, on the other hand convinced that they are *hopeless* and that their life is *meaningless* this is evidence of the fourth stage: Depression.

Below are the five stages of the rubric-repertorisation for *Adamas* confirming the psychological profile of the mental disorder, bipolar.

1. Denial: *Delusion* rubric: *abundance of everything, she has an*: adam. *Delusion* rubric: *harmony: order and clarity of everything*: adam. [1] 1. *Delusion* rubric: *prince; he is a: Indian prince; an*: adam. [1] 1. *Delusion* rubric: *sparkling, everything is*: adam. [1] 1. *Delusion* rubric: *arms: four arms; she has*: adam. *Delusion* rubric: *face: four faces; she has*: adam. [1] 1. *Delusion* rubric: *hand: four hands; she has*: adam. [1] 1. *Delusion* rubric: *galaxies spiraling*: adam. [1] 1. *Delusion* rubric: *deity; huge Tibetan*: adam. [1] 1. *Delusion* rubric: *flying: could fly; as if he*: adam. *Delusion* rubric: *power: all powerful; she is*: adam.

2. Forsaken: *Delusion* rubric: *hated; by others*: adam. *Delusion* rubric: *watched, she is being*: adam. *Delusion* rubric: *laughed at and mocked at; being*: adam. *Delusion* rubric: *wrong: suffered wrong; he has*: adam.

3. Causation: *Delusion* rubric: *worthless; he is*: adam. [This rubric can pertain to self-blame and guilt or it can pertain to feelings of depression.]

4. Depression: *Delusion* rubric: *succeed, he does everything wrong; he cannot*: adam. *Delusion* rubric: *hard; everything*

is: adam. *Delusion* rubric: *driving a car: uphill though the road is flat*: adam. [1] 1. [This rubric pertains to feelings of never succeeding.] *Delusion* rubric: *old*: *feels old*: adam. *Delusion* rubric: *clouds*: *black cloud enveloped her; a heavy: Adam.*

5. Resignation: *Delusion* rubric: *disease*: *incurable disease; he has an*: adam. *Delusion* rubric: *old*: *feels old*: adam. [This rubric can pertain to depression or fear of disease and death.]

One day *Adamas* can feel as if they are *flying*, and the next day they can feel as if they *are driving a car uphill even though the road is flat*. On the one hand *Adamas* have the *Delusion* rubric: *harmony order and clarity of everything,* and on the other hand they also have the *Delusion* rubric: *heavy black clouds enveloped her*. When *Adamas* are in a manic state they believe they are *all powerful* and that everything is *sparkling* and wonderful. *Adamas* seek perfection in the manic stage. Whilst in the manic phase, bipolar patients believe they have such incredible clarity that they are able to see and understand everything. This mania has been associated with creative genius precisely because it is so productive and illuminating. Alternatively, when *Adamas* are in their depressive phase they feel everything is so *hard* that they *will never be able to succeed*. In their depressive phase, bipolar patients believe they are so *worthless* that they are *being laughed at*. In their depressive phase, bipolar patients also believe they are dying *of an incurable disease*. *Adamas* seek perfection in the mania stage, but they also seek perfection in the depressive stage.

A *Delusion* rubric can only be used in case analysis when there is evidence of psychological patterning which perpetuates self-destruction. Within the remedy profile of *Adamas* there is evidence of a psychological delusional state which perpetuates future pathology. Tumminello has noted *perfection* in the positive and negative keywords. Patients suffering bipolar perpetuate self-destruction because regardless of which stage they are in, mania or depression, the need to strive for perfection throws them into the opposite phase of the psychological disorder. Perfection is a 'delusion of grandeur' which perpetuates self-destruction because it is not attainable.

Adamas have numerous psychological 'delusions of grandeur' all alluding to the real or perceived allure of a *perfect* diamond. The remedies *Adamas* and *Sulphur* appear in the same *Delusion* rubric: *abundance of everything*, but the rubric which distinguishes *Adamas* from *Sulphur* is the *Delusion* rubric: *she has four arms*. The psychological metaphor is that *Adamas,* which is derived from a diamond, believe that they have much more than everyone else. *Adamas* have *four faces, four arms* and *four hands,* they have an *abundance of everything.* It is in their manic phase that *Adamas* will believe and create the *Delusion* rubrics: *four faces, four arms* and *four hands.* This is the psychotherapeutic meaning of these rubrics. Within the psyche of *Adamas* are all the multi-facets of one of the most expensive of gems. The mistake is to take the meaning of these rubrics literally. Such misunderstanding has meant that homoeopaths have thought that a patient would literally relay in a consultation, *I have four arms. Adamas* will despair: *I have all the wealth in the world and it is no use to me now I am dying. I look so foolish. All the wealth in the world now is meaningless and I might as well have nothing. I am worth nothing without my health. It is not fair that I have this disease and there is no way I can ever even get well. Everyone will think I deserve this, they will look at me and gloat over my misfortune. Adamas* think money will make people love them. *Adamas* also think money will make people respect them. *Adamas* fear they will be abandoned if they are not abundantly wealthy. This is why they have so many *Delusion* rubrics of grandeur and self-importance. *Adamas* have 'delusions of superiority'. They believe they are as important as an *Indian prince*, and as special as a *huge Tibetan deity.*

Adamas think they need wealth to make people love them; their Achilles heel is that they think they are hated *because they are not perfect. Adamas* need to believe they have an *abundance of everything* because, ironically, they feel *worthless.*

Sulphur. Similarly to *Adamas, Sulphur* are trapped in a self-perpetuating dilemma involving the need to achieve perfection. In *Adamas* perfection is a 'delusion of grandeur' which perpetuates self-destruction because it is not attainable.

In *Sulphur,* perfection is a 'delusion of grandeur' which perpetuates self-denial. Because perfection is not attainable, and *Sulphur* cannot afford to contemplate failure, the only solution is to perpetuate self-denial. The self-perpetuating fluctuation between striving for creative perfection and the failure to achieve that ideal is synonymous with the manic-depressive personality patterning in *Adamas.* In *Sulphur,* the self-perpetuating fluctuation between striving for creative perfection and the failure to achieve that ideal is synonymous with delusional denial of reality.

Sulphur choose *to believe* that they are wealthy so they can avoid fiscal reality. *Sulphur* transpose their 'delusions of deprivation' into 'delusions of grandeur' that their *rags are as fine as silk.* This is how *Sulphur* manage to side-step practicalities. *Sulphur* believe they are wealthy so they can avoid being bored by the mundane nature of work. *Sulphur* believe they are inspired by loftier creative goals. *Sulphur* need their psychological delusions of *wealth* and *abundance of everything* to protect themselves from their exaggerated fears of poverty. The psychological 'delusion of abandonment' which underpin their 'delusions of grandeur' is their fear of poverty. *Sulphur* have the *Delusion* rubric: *he will come to want. Sulphur* deny this fear and transform it into the psychological delusional belief that they will be *abundant.* Furthermore, the psychological 'delusions of abandonment' for *Sulphur* which underpin their 'delusions of grandeur' are their fears of being abandoned and *not appreciated* as a creative genius: *Delusion* rubric: *she is not appreciated.*

Sulphur need to maintain their 'delusions of grandeur' to avoid sinking into their psychological delusions of self-blame for their lack of success: *Delusion* rubric: *she is disgraced*. *Sulphur* are hypochondriacally stressed about their health for the very reason that if they get sick they will feel like they can no longer achieve greatness which will be recognized. *Sulphur* are terrified of dying unrecognized.

It is this fear which underpins their 'delusions of impending doom'. *Sulphur* will declare: *I will need to stay healthy and well and I cannot die until I am at least in my eighties. I don't want to live to be in my nineties, because then I will be too old and decrepit; it would not be good to look that old. When I am in my early eighties I will have achieved the recognition and fame I have been working towards. When I am dead I will achieve even greater fame for the works that I will leave behind.* *Sulphur* are a constitutional remedy profile with many psychological 'delusions of grandeur'. If their ego and need for greatness is undermined by either failure or illness then *Sulphur* sink into crippling depression[31] and hypochondria. An emotionally, mentally or physically sick *Sulphur* will always move through the psychological 'delusions of impending doom' listed below. A *Sulphur* patient will literally be buoyant and robust one week, whilst the next week they will be crippled with presentiments of impending doom. *Sulphur* need their psychological delusions of *wealth* and *abundance of everything* to protect themselves from their crippling fear that they have not succeeded and will never be able to succeed.

1. Denial: *Delusion* rubric: *abundance of everything, she has an*: adam. *Delusion* rubric: *rags are as fine as silk; old*: **SULPH**. [4] 1. *Delusion* rubric: *beautiful: rags seem, even*: Sulph. [2] 1. *Delusion* rubric: *clothes: beautiful; clothes are*: Sulph. *Delusion* rubric: *great person; is a*: sulph.

2. Forsaken: *Delusion* rubric: *appreciated, she is not*: sulph. *Delusion* rubric: *want: he will come to*: sulph.

3. Causation: *Delusion* rubric: *sinned; one has, day of grace;*

sinned away his: sulph. *Delusion* rubric: *disgraced*: *she is*: sulph.

4. Depression: *Delusion* rubric: *succeed, he does everything wrong; he cannot*: sulph.

5. Resignation: *Delusion* rubric: *die: about to die; one was*: sulph.

Pyrogenium as a homoeopathic remedy is used for delirious visions associated with very high feverish temperatures which accompany severe infections. *Pyrogenium* is a homoeopathic remedy which is derived[32] from 'artificial sepsin' (a product of decomposed lean beef). *Pyrogenium* have the *Delusion* rubrics: *too many legs*, and *too many arms*. It is a mistake to assume that the unusual *Delusion* rubrics of having *too many arms and legs* are only clinical and therefore their application is to a patient experiencing delirium from a high fever. Although *Pyrogenium* have the *Mind* rubric: *delirium from sepsis,* it is important to understand and incorporate the meaning and application of the *Delusion* rubrics. When looking at a remedy profile, it is important that the psychotherapeutic themes in the *Delusion* rubrics are assessed in terms of how they can best be applied to their constitution. Sepsis is the bacterial contamination of blood from a festering wound.

Sepsis is the essence of the psychodynamic theme within the action of the homoeopathic remedy *Pyrogenium*. Constitutionally, *Pyrogenium* have the psychic, emotional, mental and physical need to expand and *pervade*.

Pyrogenium feel threatened and undermined if they are not expanding into and pervading all surrounding areas (tissue). *Pyrogenium* have the *Delusion* rubrics: *she is some other person and has existed in another person.* [1] 1. *Pyrogenium* have no *Delusion* rubrics pertaining to self-blame. *Pyrogenium* have no guilt over who they inhabit or control. This is why it is a mistake to assume that the use of *Pyrogenium* as a homoeopathic remedy is only clinical.

As well as having the *Delusion* rubrics: *too many legs*, and *too many arms, Pyrogenium* have the *Delusion* rubric: *wealth*. Believing you are wealthy is synonymous with psychological 'delusions of superiority'. Delusions of wealth indicate a delusional need to feel powerful and important; wealth opens all doors and allows one access to all areas. *Pyrogenium* is a constitutional remedy with 'delusions of grandeur' which are maintained to deny powerlessness. *Pyrogenium* have the *Delusion* rubric: *she would break if she lay in one position too long. Pyrogenium* have an identity restlessness across all levels, even psychically – this is the meaning of the *Delusion* rubric: *she is someone else. Pyrogenium* suffer 'identity confusion'. My aim here is to provide a psychological profile which is synonymous with the constitutional remedy profile. A psychological diagnosis can provide a psychotherapeutic framework which offers an explanation of the *Delusion* rubrics. The clinical diagnosis of identity confusion is applicable to the patient who is suffering from post-traumatic stress disorder (PTSD). PTSD is an anxiety disorder which develops as a result of the patient experiencing a traumatic event. PTSD is also known as 'shell shock', or 'battle fatigue'. The shock may involve physical injury or threat to the patient's life, or witnessing trauma involving other people. As a result of experiencing trauma, the patient suffering from PTSD feels that their defenses can always be undermined in the future. Diagnostic symptoms include the patient experiencing flashbacks which are triggered by any psychosomatic stimuli. Patients will often go through periods of identity confusion after they have experienced trauma. It is normal for a patient to feel like they don't know who they are after the trauma of a serious illness. The underlying psychodynamic crisis in *Pyrogenium* will become most obvious when the patient is faced with physical illness. *Pyrogenium* have the *Mind* rubric: *says he is well when very sick*. If the practitioner forces a *Pyrogenium* patient to stop denying or avoiding the seriousness of their illness, the confrontation will fracture an already fractured and unstable psyche.

Pyrogenium carry the somatic memory of the trauma of sepsis within their psyche, just as the patient suffering PTSD carries the memory of their trauma in their psychological defenses or somatic body.

Pyrogenium have several *Mind* rubrics which confirm the profile of a patient experiencing PTSD. *Pyrogenium* have the *Mind* rubrics: *desire for being rocked, whispering to herself,* and *causeless weeping without knowing why.* Confusing rubrics attached to a remedy profile have their meanings become clear if the homoeopath understands the psychotherapeutic relationship between the substance which the homoeopathic remedy was derived from, and the psychodynamic behavior of the patient. *Pyrogenium* maintain their delusional belief that they can *exist in another person* so they can deny the destructive effect that the trauma of being sick has had on their psyche. *Pyrogenium* is applicable to the patient who believes that their life is threatened. *Pyrogenium* maintain their delusional body expansiveness [*he is very tall*] and their delusions of *wealth* so they can feel potent in the face of future traumatic attacks to their psyche.

1. Denial: *Delusion* rubric: *wealth, of: Pyrog. Delusion* rubric: *person: other person; she is some: existed in another person; she:* pyrog. [1] 1. *Delusion* rubric: *identity: someone else, she is:* pyrog. *Delusion* rubric: *enlarged; tall; he is very:* pyrog. *Delusion* rubric: *visions, has: closing the eyes, on:* pyrog. [This rubric can pertain to hubristic visions or illusions of disease and destruction.]

2. Forsaken: *Delusion* rubric: *identity: errors of personal identity:* pyrog. *Delusion* rubric: *identity: someone else, she is:* pyrog. *Delusion* rubric: *body: scattered about; body was:* pyrog. [This rubric can pertain to self-abandonment or delusions of disease and destruction.]

3. Causation: NONE.

4. Depression: *Delusion* rubric: *identity: someone else, she is*: pyrog. [This rubric can also pertain to 'delusions of superiority'.]

5. Resignation: *Delusion* rubric: *arms: many arms; she has too*: pyrog. [1] 1. *Delusion* rubric: *arms: many arms; she has too: legs; and*: pyrog. [1] 1. *Delusion* rubric: *body: scattered about; body was*: pyrog. *Delusion* rubric: *break: she would break; lay too long in one position; if she*: pyrog. [1] 1. *Delusion* rubric: *large: he himself seems too*: pyrog. *Delusion* rubric: *crowded with arms and legs*: Pyrog. *Delusion* rubric: *double: being: fever would not run alike in both; and*: pyrog. [1] 1. [All of these rubrics can also pertain to 'delusions of superiority'. *Pyrogenium* need to feel expansive.]

- *Delusions: proud*: lach. plat. stram. verat.
- *Delusions: exalted; as if*: cann-i. lac-c. plat.
- *Delusions: beautiful*: anh. bell. *Cann-i.* coca. *Lach.* op. petr-ra. positr. *Sulph.* taosc.
- *Delusions: noble: being*: marb-w. phos. plat.
- *Delusions: business: success; is a*: phos. [1] 1.
- *Delusions: pleasing delusions*: aeth. atro. cann-i. nitro-o. op. phos. psil. stram.
- *Delusions: sensual fancies*: phos. tritic-vg. verb.
- *Delusions: honest: is honest; she*: marb-w. olib-sac.
- *Delusions: distinguished; he is*: marb-w. phos. stram. verat.
- *Delusions: fairies; searching for*: marb-w. [1] 1.
- *Delusions: jumping: safely; she can jump from a height and land*: marb-w. [1] 1.
- *Delusions: cats: he is a cat: kitten; he is a newly born*: marb-w. [1] 1.
- *Delusions: cats: he is a cat*: marb-w. [1] 1.

Self-deluding: These *Delusion* rubrics should be used when the patient refuses to acknowledge the ugly side of themselves or the world.

The psychological 'delusions of grandeur' of nobility are applicable to the patient who is deluding themselves about their negative behaviors. All the *Delusion* rubrics of exalted beauty and pride become relevant to consider in case-taking when the patient is struggling to realistically assess the gravity of the situation with their health.

Rather than face our human frailty, which we have to acknowledge when we face disease and death, we commonly choose to believe we can be cured of our fatal diseases and we delude ourselves that we will be young and beautiful forever.

Marble deceive themselves and others about their self-indulgent nature. *Marble* need to feel very important and distinguished. They spend a lot of money on themselves while all the time pretending to others they have no money. *Marble* have the *Mind* rubrics: *thoughts about her own beauty* [1] 1. – *desire to have servants* [1] 1. – *desire to be rich* [1] 1. – *desire for magnetizing others* [1] 1. – *desire to be watched* – *deceitful* – *secretive* – and *self-indulgent*. A *Delusion* rubric is used when the patient is misinterpreting reality. *Marble* deceive others about their wealth. They also deceive themselves about their illness.

The simillimum will *not* be *Marble* unless the patient is in *total denial* about their body *disintegrating*.

When *Marble* are faced with illness they move into intense self-disorganization [*as if drugged*], and believe they are losing everything [*body disintegrating*]. *Marble* refuse to acknowledge the ugly side of themselves and consequently the ugly side of their illness. In the numerous *Mind* rubrics listed above, it is easy to see that *Marble* have an enormous amount of self-importance invested in looking beautiful and rich. *Marble* have numerous *Delusion* rubrics pertaining to being abandoned and neglected. Their fear of being neglected is projected entirely on to their looks; they *desire to be watched. Marble* have the *Delusion* rubrics: *she can jump from a height and land safely,* and *he is a cat.* Jocelyn Wildenstein is a wealthy socialite who is said to have spent millions on plastic surgery to transform her face into a 'feline-like' beauty. On Google there are lots of photos listed by people who are fascinated with her looks. People have even commented that they are confused about their own desire to continue to look at her photos. Cats have a very hedonistic nature, they love being admired and looked at. I have only ever had one patient who was a *Marble* constitution. She had had extensive plastic surgery which caused her to become unwell. She did not take the remedy *Marble* and did not come back to see me for a second consultation. She didn't like my suggestion that more plastic surgery would cause her more exhaustion, and would exacerbate the damage to her muscular structure. *Marble* acknowledges no self-blame – *Mind* rubric: *aversion responsibility* – nor are they listed in any of the *Delusion* rubrics of sin. *Marble* have the *Delusion* rubric: *searching for fairies. Marble* need to continue to believe in a fantasy world in which they are able to live in fantasy. I have since realized that I made a terrible mistake by confronting a *Marble* constitution with the consequences of her actions. Furthermore, I did not truly appreciate the intensity of her need to maintain her youth, nor did I understand how much *Marble desire to be watched* and how much they think obsessively about their own beauty. The irony is that I could not stop looking at her face in the consultation because she had had so much plastic surgery that her face appeared strangely marble and 'feline-like'. A *Delusion* rubric is used when there is notable inner conflict and evidence of self-destruction and pathology. The pathological need to lust after her youth was self-destructive because she could not acknowledge that the obsession was causing her permanent damage.

When they are sick, the first fear which consumes *Marble* is the fear that they are losing their looks – *Delusion* rubric: *body disintegrating.*

It is good for a homoeopath to note unusual feelings or thoughts they may have about a patient during a consultation. When I was studying homoeopathy, I was taught that one should never note how one feels with a patient. If a patient has a strong psychological delusion they will project and transfer that psychosis on to the homoeopath.

Marble have the *Mind* rubric: *desire to be watched* and by obsessively needing to look at her [*as if drugged* and *magnetized*] I was falling into counter-transference. *Marble* have the *Mind* rubric: *desire for magnetizing others* [1] 1.

In psychotherapy, counter-transference refers to the therapist's emotional reactions to a patient that are not the patient's mental and emotional delusions, but rather the therapists. Counter-transference is defined as the body of feelings, empathic or hostile, that the therapist has toward the patient. In psychotherapy and homoeopathy these feelings, regardless of whether they are empathic or hostile, obstruct the treatment of the patient. Counter-transference, commonly involves taking on the suffering and the psychological delusions of the patient. Counter-transference for the homoeopathic therapist can involve taking on the symptoms of the constitutional remedy profile; this can be labeled 'a proving of the patient'. In the *Marble* case the counter-transference meant that on the one hand, I fell into being *magnetized* by the patient's *need to be looked at*, and on the other hand I projected hostile feelings of needing to *criticize* her actions. *Marble* have the *Delusion* rubric: *she is criticized*. I had never criticized a patient's actions before, even actions which I have viewed as self-destructive. Rather, I would constructively support the patient so they could move out of their self-destructive behavior. *Marble* draw one in to being fixated upon their beauty, just as one is fixated upon the beauty of Michelangelo's marble statue of David. Their self-destructive pathology of self-deceit means that when they are sick they deflect all fault onto the therapist. *Marble* will trap the therapist into counter-transference. *Marble* will justify and reinforce their own *distinguished* position by projecting their delusions of being abandoned [*surrounded by enemies*].

The homoeopathic therapist has to be careful with *Marble* not to fall in to the trap of either being *magnetized* by them or feeling like one needs to *criticize* them.

The irony of their transference behavior is, of course, that it reinforces their belief that they need to spend huge amounts of money on themselves to make themselves more desirable [*noble*]. In order to apply a *Delusion* rubric in case-taking, the homoeopath seeks to understand why the patient has set up their delusional state and why they need to maintain the misrepresentation of reality. Underlying psychological 'delusions of grandeur' are fears of abandonment. The lesson learnt from this *Marble* case highlighted for me the need to understand that the patient maintains an avoidance, or psychological delusion, because it is to their advantage.

If I had previously done the five step rubric-repertorisation I would have had insight into *Marble,* and I would not have confronted a *Marble* with the obvious consequences of her self-destructive behavior. I would have known that *Marble* have no *Delusion* rubrics pertaining to acknowledgment of sin, so they will never acknowledge the error of their ways even if it is injurious to their health.

1. Denial: *Delusion* rubric: *noble: being*: marb-w. *Delusion* rubric: *fairies; searching for:* marb-w. [1] 1. *Delusion* rubric: *jumping: safely; she can jump from a height and land:* marb-w. [1] 1. *Delusion* rubric: *cats: he is a cat: kitten; he is a newly born*: marb-w. [1] 1. *Delusion* rubric: *cats: he is a cat*: marb-w. [1] 1. *Delusion* rubric: *honest: is honest; she*: marb-w. *Delusion* rubric: *distinguished; he is*: marb-w. *Delusion* rubric: *great person, is a*: marb-w.

2. Forsaken: *Delusion* rubric: *criticized, she is*: marb-w.
   Delusion rubric: *neglected: he or she is neglected*: marb-w.
   Delusion rubric: *enemy: surrounded by enemies*: marb-w.
3. Causation: NONE.
4. Depression: *Delusion* rubric: *drugged; as if*: marb-w.
5. Resignation: *Delusion* rubric: *body: disintegrating*: marb-w.
   Delusion rubric: *mutilated bodies; sees*: marb-w. *Delusion*
   rubric: *penis: cut off penis; sees a*: marb-w. [The last two
   rubrics pertain to fear of their body disintegrating.]

Phosphorus delude themselves about the potentially destructive nature of their illness[33] to the extent that they believe they are (emotionally) dealing with it in such a *noble and distinguished* manner that it is unnecessary for them to discuss it (with you).

Phosphorus not only deny that they are sick, they arrogantly [*a person of rank*] refuse to believe that they could be sick.

Phosphorus have the *Delusion* rubric: *being choked by forms*. [1] 1. The psychosomatic meaning of this *Delusion* rubric is that *Phosphorus* will feel restrained or choked or suppressed as soon as any constraints or responsibilities or expectations are inflicted upon them. *Phosphorus* use this perception to reinforce that they cannot afford to acknowledge reality. When sick, *Phosphorus* implode and present in a very shut-down state; the direct opposite to their normal effervescent persona.

In *Phosphorus* illness is viewed as, and brings about, an extreme feeling of entrapment; they can literally feel like they are being consumed and choked.

Phosphorus are listed as the only remedy in the *Delusion* rubric: *body in several pieces; he could not get them adjusted*. *Phosphorus* create, and maintain, their implosion into themselves because it helps them try to reassemble the parts of themselves which they feel are being scattered.

Their containment then becomes a self-fulfilling prophecy of doom because the more inward *Phosphorus* become the more they feel like they are being choked and controlled by their disease. *Phosphorus* is a homoeopathic remedy which is often used for the treatment of cancers. (In many parts of the world homoeopaths are legally restricted when treating patients with cancer. Homoeopathic treatment is directed towards treatment of the patient as a whole. As a consequence, homoeopaths treat the symptoms of presentation of cancer in the *individual* patient rather than treating the disease.) Cancer arises from the abnormal and uncontrolled division and overgrowth of undifferentiated, or poorly differentiated cells. The undifferentiated cells divide and duplicate quickly. As the cancer grows the malignant cells invade surrounding tissues and begins to compete with the surrounding organs for space. Eventually the tumor metastasizes and invades the surrounding body cavities. Within the psyche of the remedy profile of *Phosphorus* I have observed that the consequences of social responsibilities can cause suppressive depression. The long term consequences for *Phosphorus* if they allow themselves to be restrained by expectations is that they will literally feel choked. *Phosphorus* avoid acknowledging that they are sick, which is what makes the remedy a powerful one to use in the treatment of the psychological delusions of denial associated with a fatal disease. *Phosphorus* chose to maintain *pleasing delusions* to avoid their own depressive resignation and fear that they *have an incurable disease.*

The internal crisis within the psyche of *Phosphorus* is synonymous with the psychodynamic energy of the ever expanding control and entrapment of the cancerous tumor inside a body. *Phosphorus* go into self-imploding denial about any illness, which then builds up like a crescendo inside of them to the point that they feel choked by anxiety and fear. Underpinning their denial are their 'delusions of abandonment'; *Phosphorus* believe they will be *despised* if they are sick.

Phosphorus reject and despise themselves when they are sick and this is part of their psychological need to go into self-denial about illness. They also project the fear of being rejected and despised on to others; this is why they feel they will be despised and forsaken when they are sick. *Phosphorus* literally feel under internal and external attack. The *Delusion* rubrics: *things creeping out of every corner*, and the *Delusion* rubrics: *about to die*, exemplify the intensity to which they feel compromised and under attack.

If the homoeopath does not fully appreciate the intensity of the need *Phosphorus* have for self-denial, and confronts them with their 'delusions of grandeur', they will fracture a fragile psyche and cause *Phosphorus* to implode further.

Homoeopathic psychiatry and the understanding of the meaning of the *Delusion* rubrics is crucial to the protection and nurturing of patients. *Phosphorus* need to believe they are *nobly* in control of any illness.

1. Denial: *Delusion* rubric: *pleasing delusions*: phos.
    Versus
5. Resignation: *Delusion* rubric: *disease: incurable disease; he has an*: phos.
1. Denial: *Delusion* rubric: *noble: being*: phos. *Delusion* rubric: *distinguished; he is*: phos. *Delusion* rubric: *pleasing delusions*: phos. *Delusion* rubric: *sensual fancies*: phos. *Delusion* rubric: *business: success; is a*: phos. [1] 1. *Delusion* rubric: *great person, is a*: phos. *Delusion* rubric: *rank; he is a person of*: phos.
2. Forsaken: *Delusion* rubric: *despised, is*: phos. *Delusion* rubrics: *creeping things; full of: corner; out of every*: phos. [1] 1. *Delusion* rubrics: *devil: present, is*: phos. *Delusion* rubric: *murdered: will be murdered; he*: phos.
3. Causation: *Delusion* rubric: *criminal, he is a*: phos. *Delusion* rubric: *obscene: action of which she had not been guilty; accuses herself of an obscene*: Phos. [2] 1.

4. Depression: *Delusion* rubric: *anxious*: Phos. *Delusion* rubric: *choked*: *forms*; *being choked by*: phos. [1] 1. [This rubric pertains to suppressive depression and denial.] *Delusion* rubric: *succeed, he does everything wrong; he cannot*: phos.

5. Resignation: *Delusion* rubric: *sick*: *being*: phos. *Delusion* rubric: *disease*: *incurable disease; he has an*: phos. *Delusion* rubric: *body*: *pieces*: *were in several pieces; he: adjusted; and could not get them*: phos. [1] 1. *Delusion* rubrics: *die*: *about to die; one was*: phos.

- *Delusions*: *elevated*: *air; elevated in the*: falco-pe. irid-met. nit-ac. nitro-o. phos. rhus-t. sil.

- *Delusions*: *elevated*: *air; elevated in the*: *looking down on a cesspool of ignorance and vulgarity; and*: ignis-alc. [1] 1.

- *Delusions*: *humility and lowness of others; while he is great*: germ-met. ignis-alc. plat. staph.

- *Delusions*: *enlightened; is*: ignis-alc. [1] 1.

- *Delusions*: *superhuman; is*: cann-i. ignis-alc. psil.

- *Delusions*: *creative power; has*: agath-a. cann-i. ignis-alc. psil.

- *Delusions*: *spirit, he is a*: cann-i. ignis-alc.

- *Delusions*: *pure; she is*: ignis-alc. stram.

- *Delusions*: *floating*: *air, in*: Acon. agar. agath-a. *Aids*. *Ambr*. anh. ara-maca. *Arg-met*. arge-pl. arn. asar. bell. brass-n-o. bry. calc-ar. calc. cann-i. canth. chir-fl. chlf. cocain. cygn-be. cypra-eg. dat-a. euon-a. *Euon*. fic-m. galla-q-r. germ-met. haliae-lc. hippoc-k. hura. hyos. hyper. irid-met. jug-r. kali-br. *Lac-c*. lac-f. *Lac-loxod-a*. *Lach*. lact-v. lact. lat-h. loxo-recl. luna. m-aust. manc. moni. mosch. mucs-nas. nat-ar. nat-m. nat-ox. *Nux-m*. ol-eur. olib-sac. *Op*. ozone passi. pen. *Ph-ac*. phos. phys. pieri-b. pin-con. pip-m. rhus-g. sep. **SPIG**. *Stach*. stict. stroph-h. suis-em. suprar. *Tarent*. tell. tep. ter. thuj. tung-met. urol-h. valer. visc. xan.

- *Delusions*: *flying*: anh. asar. bell. calc-ar. camph. *Cann-i*. cygn-be. dendr-pol. euon. falco-pe. galla-q-r. haliae-lc. irid-met. jug-r. lach.

lact. manc. nitro-o. oena. olib-sac. op. sal-fr. thiam. valer.

- *Delusions*: *walking*: *air. on air; walks*: asar. chin. coff. lac-c. merc-i-f. nat-m. nux-v. op. ph-ac. phos. rhus-t. spig. stict. stram. thuj.

Self-deluding: The above group of rubrics reflect a unique hubristic ability to deny reality by dissociating oneself from this world.

The remedy profiles above all contain within their persona an ability to dissociate themselves from reality and elevate themselves above any situation. The above group of Denial *Delusion* rubrics becomes relevant to consider in case-taking for the patient who is avoiding *acknowledging* that they are sick.

These rubrics indicate a condition called 'depersonalization disorder'. All 'depersonalization disorders' are dissociative because they allow the patient to live outside of themselves. There are four major dissociative disorders: Dissociative amnesia, Dissociative identity disorder, Dissociative fugue, and Depersonalization disorder. Depersonalization disorder is characterized by a sense of being outside yourself, observing your actions from a distance as though watching a movie. It may be accompanied by a perceived distortion of the size and shape of your body or of other people and objects around you. The patient is able to create distance between themselves and the world, or between themselves and their trauma which they are not able to integrate into their conscious mind.

When a patient is first told that they have a serious disease or a fatal disease it is normal for them to distance themselves from that news for a period of time, and pretend that news is not true. If the patient stays in shock and continues to remain in a consciousness outside or above themselves, then it is indicative of a condition called 'depersonalization disorder'. Patients have often described this state as being a blissful relief because they cannot be touched or affected by the trauma of their illness.

They believe that if they remain above and outside of their body then they will be able to cure themselves; this is a psychological delusion of 'hubristic denial'. Patients have described this state as similar to a drug induced state in which everything seems distorted or unreal, and even their own body seems to be a long way away from them. All the *Delusion* rubrics: *flying out of his skin* and *body is tall, body is small, head is divided, body shrunken, body diminished, body thin,* reflect someone experiencing 'depersonalization disorder'. In case-taking the homoeopath must consider *why* the patient needs to distance themselves from their trauma or their body. Most importantly, if the patient maintains the dissociative processing the homoeopath must understand the patient's *peculiar* 'hubristic denial' because this will indicate the simillimum.

Ignis alcholis have numerous hubristic *Delusion* rubrics indicating purity. *Ignis alcholis* have the *Delusion* rubrics: *he is pure, he is a spirit,* and *being divine. Ignis alcholis* have the *Delusion* rubric: *he was newly born into the world and was overwhelmed with wonder at the novelty of his surroundings. Ignis alcholis* is a remedy derived from the burning of pure alcohol. Fire is associated with *purification* of the spirit. Conversely, it is symbolic of banishment into the fires of *hell.* Fire, once it is unleashed, can be uncontrollable and destructive. 'Pyromania' is an impulse to deliberately start fires. A pyromaniac feels immediate relief and distance from any tension or stress in their lives once they light the fire. Pyromaniacs start fires to induce euphoria. They love to watch the fire burning from a distance and take great hubristic delight in the power they feel after unleashing the fire. Pyromaniacs are often fire fighters who need to be part of the rescue team that helps put out the fire.

Pyromaniacs need to believe they are heroes. *Ignis alcholis* have hubristic 'delusions of grandeur' that they are *superhuman* and on a *mission. Ignis alcholis* have the *Delusion* rubrics: *has creative power,* and *one has a mission. Ignis alcholis* have hubristic arrogance that they are *elevated in the air looking down on a cesspool of ignorance and vulgarity.* Pyromaniacs believe they are purifying the earth by lighting the fire.

Ignis alcholis have the *Mind* rubric: *yearning for beautiful things.* Pyromaniacs, especially children, believe that they have been instructed to light the fire by the devil within themselves. *Ignis alcholis* have the *Delusion* rubric: *possessed by evil forces. Ignis alcholis* have the *Mind* rubric: *love of power,* and the *Mind* rubric: *contemptuous of people who she believes are unfortunate and beyond redemption.*

Ignis alcholis present with opposing polarities. If there are contradictions and inconsistencies in the rubrics pertaining to 'hubristic denial' or Stage one, and the rubrics pertaining to disease and death, or Stage five, then there is evidence of suppression which will either accelerate present pathology or precede future pathology. When *Ignis alcholis* are confronted with illness, which they equate with impurity, they immediately disassociate from themselves. *Ignis alcholis* have the *Delusion* rubric: *evil power had control of the whole of him.* [1] 1. On the one hand they believe their illness will lead them to *enlightenment,* and on the other hand they believe their illness has *possessed* them and is *contaminating* their pure *spirit. Ignis alcholis* have a 'depersonalization disorder' which allows them to stand outside of themselves. *Ignis alcholis* have psychological delusions of being a highly *enlightened* being who has come to earth and is able to look down upon the lowly mortals who are in Saṃsāra[34] [*hell*]. *Ignis alcholis* have the *Delusion* rubrics: *is superhuman,* and *is enlightened.* [1] 1. They have the hubristic *Delusion* rubric: *elevated in the air looking down on a cesspool of ignorance and vulgarity.*

The simillimum will not be *Ignis alcholis* unless the patient presents with the same ability to dissociate themselves from their 'evil' acts.

Pyromaniacs start fires to purify the world. The simillimum will not be *Ignis alcholis* unless the patient believes that they are bringing a new enlightened perspective to the world.

1.   Denial: *Delusion* rubric: *pure; she is*: ignis-alc.
      Versus

5. Resignation: *Delusion* rubric: *contaminated*: *being contaminated; she is*: ignis-alc.

"Throughout history, fire has been associated with transformation, purification, the giving of life, power and strength, enlightenment and inspiration, the spirit, the invisible energy in life, illumination and divinity. Fire has been used as a means of sending messages and offerings to heaven. It was believed that, at death, a flame left the body. Fire and flame were associated with the heart. Fire can be either divine or demonic, creative or destructive. Fire represents truth; it consumes deceit and ignorance. Baptism by fire restores purity by burning away the dross. Passing through fire is necessary for the regaining of Paradise which, since it was lost, was surrounded by fire and protected by Guardians armed with swords of flame. These Guardians symbolize understanding, preventing entrance to the ignorant and the unenlightened. Buddhists consider fire to be the wisdom which burns all ignorance. Christians have the 'Tongues of fire' which represent the advent of the Holy Spirit, divine revelation and the voice of God. Of course, Christians also have the fires of hell." Proving of *Ignis alcholis* by N. Eising. Encyclopaedia Homeopathica. Radar™.

1. Denial: *Delusion* rubric: *elevated*: *air; elevated in the*: *looking down on a cesspool of ignorance and vulgarity; and*: ignis-alc. [1] 1. *Delusion* rubric: *humility and lowness of others; while he is great*: ignis-alc. *Delusion* rubric: *enlightened; is*: ignis-alc. [1] 1. *Delusion* rubric: *creative power; has*: ignis-alc. *Delusion* rubric: *spirit, he is a*: ignis-alc. *Delusion* rubric: *pure; she is*: ignis-alc. *Delusion* rubric: *superhuman; is*: ignis-alc. *Delusion* rubric: *divine, being*: ignis-alc. *Delusion* rubric: *great person, is a*: ignis-alc. *Delusion* rubric: *mission; one has a*: ignis-alc.

2. Forsaken: *Delusion* rubric: *separated: world; from the: he is separated*: ignis-alc.

3. Causation: *Delusion* rubric: *possessed; being*: *evil forces;*

by: ignis-alc. [1] 2. [manc]. *Delusion* rubric: *power: evil power had control of the whole of him*: ignis-alc. [1] 1.

4. Depression: *Delusion* rubric: *suffocating; as if*: ignis-alc. *Delusion* rubric: *hell*: *in*; *is*: ignis-alc.

5. Resignation: *Delusion* rubric: *contaminated*: *being contaminated; she is*: ignis-alc.

Spigelia are graded a three in the *Delusion* rubric: *floating in the air*. *Spigelia* self-delude. They believe that if they remain above their body then they will be able to cure themselves; this is a psychological delusion of 'hubristic denial'. This state can easily be identified as being similar to a drug[35] induced state in which everything seems at an unreal distance. However, this state of mind or approach is also a common 'New-Age' 'avoidance technique' which I have noticed in patients.

Within the 'New-Age' philosophy, any illness can be directly attributed to your own negative state of mind. I have noticed that if a patient is strongly entrenched in this belief system then they are more than likely, when confronted with illness, to move into a state of dissociative denial. *Spigelia* have an ability to dissociate. This deludes them into believing that they are not affected by this world, or consequently their illness.

Spigelia distance themselves from their own diseased body. This is a defense mechanism which allows them to be elevated above all of their troubles. If *Spigelia* acknowledge reality they feel overwhelmed. *Spigelia* have the *Delusion* rubrics: *sidewalk is rising up before him,* and *he was reeling*. These rubrics should not be interpreted literally. *Spigelia* believe illness will overwhelm them. All inner conflicts over reality have to form the basis of future pathology because the suppression of reality will eventually undermine the patient's psyche.

'Dissociative disorders' allows the patient to distance themselves from their trauma. The homoeopath should be alerted to this tendency within the followers of 'New-Age' philosophies.

Spigelia have the *Mind* rubric: *absorbed about future.* [1] 1. This dissociative suppression of the now, allows the patient distance from having to live in the daily world with their trauma. All suppression eventually has to erupt. *Spigelia* as a homoeopathic remedy is used for extreme neuralgic pains, especially for intolerably painful migraines. *Spigelia* have the following *Mind* rubrics, of which all indicate the severity of the neuralgic pain – *Mind* rubrics: *anxiety from pains from the eyes – anxiety from pains from the abdomen – anxiety from pains from the heart – anxiety from pains from the face.*

The *Delusion* rubrics: *floating in the air,* and *walking on air,* should be analyzed in terms of the psychological delusional advantage they allow the patient to maintain or nurture in their psyche. It is important to reemphasize that a patient will not literally say in a consultation, *I am floating in the air.* A patient will say, *I have been completely unaffected by finding out I have cancer. I am not concentrating on it at all, in fact it has been the most extraordinary time because I am filled with the most exquisite heightened sense of spiritual hope. I feel like I have been lifted above the whole thing. I do not want to go and have radiotherapy though because I believe I do not need it, and I also know that it will poison my body. I do not want to be attacked by all their needles. I have had one session and I immediately had the most terrible reaction and ended up with an excruciating migraine all down the side of my face. I am concentrating on the future. Every day, I am doing lots of visualizations of myself elevated above the horribleness of this disease. I do not think it is wise to concentrate on the 'now' of this disease. If I do then I feel like my whole head is going around and around.* This is the remedy profile of *Spigelia.*

The simillimum will not be *Spigelia* unless the patient dissociates from their own body to avoid acknowledging that they are in pain or sick.

1. Denial: *Delusion* rubric: *floating: air; in:* **SPIG**. *Delusion* rubric: *walking: air: on air; walks:* spig.

2. Forsake*n: Delusion* rubric: *poisoned: he: has been*: spig.

3. Causation: NONE.

4. Depression: *Delusion* rubric: *sidewalk: rising up before him; sidewalk is*: spig. [1] 1. *Delusion* rubric: *falling: he is*: spig. *Delusion* rubric: *falling: forward: is falling forward; she*: spig. *Delusion* rubric: *insane: become insane; one will: headache, from*: spig. [1] 1. *Delusion* rubric: *reel: she was reeling*: spig. [1] 1.

5. Resignation: *Delusion* rubric: *sick: being*: spig. *Delusion* rubric: *pins; about*: spig. [*Spigelia* also have the *Mind* rubric: *fear. pins; of*: **SPIG**.]

    •   Delusions: *walking: cotton; he walks on*: **ALUM**. apis. calc. carb-v. onos. phos. *Sulph.* zinc.

Avoidance: This rubric reflects the unique hubristic ability each remedy profile has of denying reality by dissociating from the harshness of this world. This *Delusion* rubric becomes relevant to consider in case-taking when the patient presents with an *unrealistic belief* that they can walk though life without having to let their feet touch the ground.

Sulphur elevate themselves above any situation in life which threatens their hubristic 'delusions of grandeur'. *Sulphur* have the *Delusion* rubric: *he is naked*. This *Delusion* rubric should not be interpreted literally, rather it is reflective of the fear *Sulphur* have when they have to face reality. *Sulphur* have the *Delusion* rubric: *the ground was wavering*. [1] 1., and the *Delusion* rubric: *everything on him was trembling*. [1] 1. *Sulphur* have numerous *Delusion* rubrics pertaining to 'delusions of grandeur' because they need to elevate themselves to a world in which everything looks *beautiful*. *Sulphur* are caught in a conflicting bind of self-denial. On the one hand they believe they have *beautiful abundance* in the world, and on the other hand is their fear that the abundance will *not succeed* and that they will *sink into the ground* and into *grotesque diminished* oblivion. *Sulphur* have the *Delusion* rubric: *they have given people something wrong which they die from.* [1] 1. The psychodynamic meaning of this rubric implies that *Sulphur* judge themselves by the effect they have on others. Boger, in *Synoptic Key to Materia medica,* Radar™, notes on *Sulphur:* "hopeful dreamers; ecstatic, religious, philosophic, etc. Peevish, mean, prying or easily excited. Melancholic. Tired of life."

Sulphur maintain their 'delusions of grandeur' and their belief that they are not touching the ground or that they are not touched by the ground because it helps to convince them that they have hope.

Sulphur maintain their 'delusions of grandeur' that the world is *beautiful* because they need to dissociate from their own 'delusions of impending doom'. *Sulphur* need to dissociate and elevate themselves above their melancholic despair of the *reality* of life. *Sulphur* are always the "hopeful dreamers".

1. Denial: *Delusion* rubric: *walking: cotton; he walks on: Sulph. Delusion* rubric: *beautiful:* sulph. *Delusion* rubric: *beautiful: things look:* sulph. *Delusion* rubric: *clothes: beautiful; clothes are:* **SULPH**. *Delusion* rubric: *tall: he or she is tall: Sulph. Delusion* rubric: *abundance of everything, she has an:* sulph.

2. Forsaken: *Delusion* rubric: *grotesque:* sulph. *Delusion* rubric: *faces, sees: ugly:* sulph. *Delusion* rubric: *diminished: all is:* sulph.

3. Causation: *Delusion* rubric: *wrong: gives people something wrong from which they die; she:* sulph. [1] 1.

4. Depression: *Delusion* rubric: *happened; something has:* sulph. *Delusion* rubric: *sinking; to be: Sulph.*

5. Resignation: *Delusion* rubric: *ground: wavering; the ground were: stood was wavering; the ground on which he:* sulph. [1] 1. *Delusion* rubric: *trembling: everything was trembling: on him was trembling; everything:* sulph. [1] 1.

Forsaken

"My body has let me down." (abandonment).

"My illness has been caused by others." (persecution).

"I have been cheated of my life." (abandonment and persecution).

"I have been singled out for punishment." (abandonment and persecution).

I have allocated all the *Delusion* rubrics which pertain to psychological 'delusions of abandonment' or 'delusions of persecution' into Forsaken. If the trauma inside your patient starts with them feeling alone and abandoned, or singled out for punishment by their illness then the simillimum is listed in all the *Delusion* rubrics: *forsaken* or *persecution*.

In my practice I have found that when a patient is dealing with the loss of their health, or with their impending death, they will feel overwhelmed with feelings of aloneness and abandonment. Feeling alone and abandoned and thinking that no one understands how one feels is a normal response to one's loss of health. A need to be with others who have experienced similar traumas is usually the inspiration behind survivors' groups. Alternatively, feeling alone and wanting to be alone to face one's illness and impending death is also normal and often preferred by some patients. A need to be with family and friends to have the strength to face one's illness and impending death is also normal. Alternatively, feeling that one should be alone and not embarrass other people with one's disease or decaying body is also normal. Every patient will react differently to illness, and the above scenarios are all normal, appropriate responses to the grief of illness or decay and death. We all think we will live to a ripe old age, so feeling emotionally distraught is a normal response to finding out one is sick. Feeling angry and cheated is the second stage of grief (called 'anger') in Doctor Elisabeth Kübler-Ross's model.

With the emergence of 'New-Age' philosophies the patient has also become a victim of the belief that they should always be blessed with good health if they are 'being true to oneself', or they are 'being here now'. What I notice is that patients today are angry that the promises of the 'New-Age' philosophies have not been delivered and that they are left feeling distraught and alone without a philosophy to believe in which will deliver good health. A patient will often say to me, *I am left with nothing to believe in anymore. Why has this happened to me? I have been meditating for years.* If the patient is angry that they are sick then the rubric used in the rubric-repertorisation should be the *Mind* rubric: *anger.*

Feeling that one has abandoned one's health by leading an unhealthy lifestyle is normal. Appropriate blaming of oneself is a normal response if, for example, one gets emphysema or lung cancer and has been a smoker all one's life. Developing late onset diabetes from allowing oneself to become obese is another example where it is normal to face the abandonment of one's health by regretting all the chocolates one has indulged in. Reforming one's health practices or trying to be a 'good' person to reverse the scales of fate or God's punishment is the third stage (called 'bargaining') of grief in Doctor Elisabeth Kübler-Ross's model. Feeling that one's body has unfairly abandoned one is normal. It is normal if one has led a healthy life to feel cheated and abandoned by one's own body if one becomes unwell. The rubric which applies in the case-repertorisation for all of the normal, appropriate responses to the loss of health is the *Mind* rubric: *forsaken.*

It is crucial for the homoeopathic practitioner to determine if the case justifies the use of a *Delusion* rubric. Stage one of psychological delusional pathology starts with 'hubristic denial'.

If the patient is suffering with psychological 'delusions of grandeur' and they are *incredulously overcome* with feelings of having been abandoned by what they believed was always going to be there for them, then the rubric should be the *Delusion* rubric: *forsaken*.

When a patient moves out of their 'delusions of grandeur' or 'hubristic denial' and admits to themselves they are sick, or that they have a serious illness which could be life threatening, they may feel that God or the world has personally abandoned them. Feeling abandoned by God is a normal response and so is feeling punishment by God. In psychiatry this is referred to as a 'persecution complex'. A 'persecution complex' is psychological terminology used to describe the feeling of being persecuted and abandoned.

Feelings of rage at being personally singled out for illness are covered in all the *Delusion* rubrics of being *persecuted*. 'Delusions of persecution' is applied to the patient who believes that the whole world is against them and that the whole world has abandoned them. 'Delusions of persecution' can justify reactive unfriendliness or pre-emptive acts of hostility, all of which are excused under the guise of presumed abandonment and rejection. The pre-emptive attacks then become a self-fulfilling prophecy because the patient is rejected and abandoned for their aggressive behavior. The *Delusion* rubrics of *persecution* and the *Delusion* rubrics of *forsaken* cover all the imagined or perceived feelings of rejection and acts of self-imposed exile, and all the psychological delusions of imagined self-inflicted abandonment.

The *Delusion* rubric: *forsaken* will be used by each constitutional remedy profile as an emotional avoidance or self-deluding denial, which will be adopted and destructively nurtured by the patient to justify *continually* feeling hurt and abandoned by friends or family.

The *Delusion* rubric: *separated from the world* is a misrepresentation of reality which is used as an excuse to actively separate from the world to either avoid future hurt and rejection or as an excuse to justify one's own desire to separate oneself emotionally. The *Delusion* rubrics: *he is friendless* or *alone in the world, neglected*, or *outcast*, indicate a psychological delusional stance which is used to justify feeling hurt and rejected as a consequence of a 'persecution complex'. A delusional stance is maintained because it is advantageous, and it will be maintained regardless of whether the stance has a negative outcome.

The reasons behind why someone needs to stay in a position of believing they are abandoned will be *peculiar* to each remedy profile. Each patient whose constitutional remedy is listed in the abandonment rubrics will concoct an individual story explaining why it is to their advantage to remain abandoned, *friendless*, *persecuted* and *alone*.

In the case-taking it is important to understand, firstly, how the patient has used the psychological delusion in a disproportionate way to misinterpret reality. Secondly, it is crucial to understand why the delusional stance is maintained by the patient and why and how it is advantageous to the patient to delude themselves that they are alone. Thirdly, it is essential to understand the conflict *specific* to the constitutional remedy profile which explains both the disproportionate need to maintain a misinterpretation of reality. Fourthly it is important to understand why that remedy profile needs to maintain the psychological delusion of being abandoned.

The psychological delusions of being *forsaken* are always maintained to help the constitutional remedy profile avoid exaggerated self-blame or 'delusions of original sin'. This is the reason why Causation, or the disproportionate guilt for sins committed follows the *Delusion* rubrics of being *forsaken* in the five step rubric-repertorisation model that I am proposing. When a patient moves out of their 'hubristic denial' and acknowledges that they are sick, they may feel that God, or the world, or their body has abandoned them. If God, or the world, or their body, or fate has abandoned them they must be evil or they must have *done wrong*. Exaggerated delusions of self-blame are psychological delusions which each patient wants to avoid. The best way to avoid self-blame is to redirect blame on to the world, your body (yourself), or God for abandoning you. This is why a particular remedy profile will need to maintain their 'delusions of persecution' or their 'delusions of abandonment'; they wish to avoid acknowledgment of sins committed.

All the remedies have a conflicting interpretation of reality, but it is important to understand the nature of what each individual remedy profile needs to avoid. If you understand the psychological delusional need to avoid and self-delude it will help you understand each homoeopathic remedy profile.

Understanding the five psychological processing steps in relation to the use of *Delusion* rubrics in case analysis will not only guide in the treatment of your patient, it will help you identify all the delusional inconsistencies that the remedy profile presents with. Identifying delusional inconsistencies is synonymous with identifying the simillimum in the case.

Delusion Rubrics in Forsaken

In this section I analyze and explain the meaning of each individual *Delusion* rubric. I offer previously unexplored explanations of the psychological delusional state inherent in each *Delusion* rubric. Furthermore, I explain their psychotherapeutic meaning and application by analyzing how each remedy listed under the rubric heading has utilized the delusional stance to its advantage. The reasons why each constitutional remedy is listed under a rubric will often be vastly different. Understanding the need for the psychological delusions within each of the constitutional remedy profiles will aid in remedy recognition.

Each selection of *Delusion* rubrics discussed are shaded. Analyses of the remedy profiles follow each sub-section. The psychological development of *Delusion* rubrics for each constitutional remedy profile is analyzed according to either **avoidance** or **self-deluding** need.

- *Delusions: forsaken; is*: agath-a. aids. **ARG-N**. *Aur-m-n. Aur.* bamb-a. bar-c. bit-ar. brass-n-o. camph. cann-i. carb-an. carb-v. chin. crot-c. *Cycl.* cygn-be. cypra-eg. *Dendr-pol.* dream-p. hura. hyos. *Kali-br. Kola. lil-t.* limest-b. lyss. **MAG-C**. marb-w. nat-c. *Ol-eur.* ozone. pall. phasco-ci. *Plat.* positr. **PULS**. sal-al. sanic. *Stram.* thuj.

- *Delusions: separated: world; from the; he is separated*: adam. aids. *Anac. Androc. Anh.* arge-pl. arizon-l. bit-ar. brass-n-o. carc. choc. coca dioxi. dream-p. falco-pe. galla-q-r. germ-met. haliae-lc. hippoc-k. **HYDROG**. ignis-alc. irid-met. lac-del. lavand-a. loxo-recl. mang-p.

moni. ol-eur. pin-con. plac. plut-n. polys. positr. sal-fr. sanguis-s. taosc. thiop. thuj. tung-met. ven-m.

- *Delusions*: *neglected*: *he or she is neglected*: *Arg-n*. aur-m-n. crot-c. kola. *Lac-h*. mag-m. marb-w. naja. nat-m. nicc-met. oci-sa. **PALL**. petr-ra. plat. positr. puls. rad-br. sacch. sep. staph. stront-c.

- *Delusions*: *friend; affection of; has lost the*: agath-a. ars. aur-m-n. *Aur*. hura. hydrog. hyos. rhus-t. *Thuj*.

- *Delusions*: *friendless, he is*: aids. alum. cygn-be. falco-pe. lac-h. lach. mag-m. oci-sa. phasco-ci. positr. sars. *Thuj*.

- *Delusions*: *outcast; she was an*: anac. androc. atra-r. crot-c. crot-h. germ-met. haliae-lc. hura. thuj.

- *Delusions*: *home: away from home; he is*: acon. *Aster*. bell. **BRY**. calc. cic. *Coff*. des-ac. germ-met. *Hyos*. lach. limest-b. meli. merc. *Nux-v*. *Op*. par. plb. puls. *Rhus-t*. valer. verat. vip.

Avoidance: If the patient demonstrates exaggerated hyper-vigilant fears and predictions of being abandoned then these psychological delusions indicate 'delusions of persecution'.

The psychological delusions of being forsaken are often maintained by the patient to avoid what they might have contributed to the situation.

This is why the psychological 'delusions of original sin' always follow on from the psychological delusions of being forsaken in the five stage rubric-repertorisation process. Commonly, the patient will deflect blame outwards on to society or their family for abandoning them rather than face or acknowledge the real or perceived sins committed which have caused them to feel overcome with inner shame. The *Delusion* rubrics of abandonment reflect a complex collection of self-fulfilling prophecies which are maintained because the patient believes it will protect them from feelings of future hurt and abandonment.

If the *Delusion* rubric is relevant to the case-taking, the homoeopath must see that the patient believes it is advantageous to continue with the psychological delusion. The homoeopath must question why each patient continues to exaggerate and/or continue a particular mental or emotional pattern in their lives.

Argentum nitricum have no sins, other than the failure to achieve, so therefore they cannot understand why they have been abandoned. *Argentum nitricum* have numerous persecutory *Delusion* rubrics: *he is repudiated by relatives, not appreciated, neglected*, and *despised*. Stage one of psychological delusional pathology starts with 'hubristic denial'. Underneath 'hubristic denial' are the over-exaggerated, hyper-vigilant fears and predictions of being forsaken and abandoned.

Because *Argentum nitricum* have no delusions of 'hubristic denial', their ability to not feel repudiated is greatly diminished.

A self-imposed 'persecution complex' is applied to the patient who deliberately instigates pre-emptive abandonment. 'Delusions of persecution' is applied to the patient who believes that the whole world is against them and that the whole world has abandoned them.

Argentum nitricum feel they have been personally singled out for punishment. *Argentum nitricum* feel persecuted walking along the street.

Argentum nitricum have numerous *Delusion* rubrics: *walls will crush him, he cannot pass a certain place, crushed by the houses,* and *corners of the houses project while he is walking in the street so that he fears he will run against them.* [2] 1. *Argentum nitricum* also have numerous *Delusion* rubrics of self-destructive depression and predictions of failure. *Argentum nitricum* believe that they will never be *appreciated*. Because *Argentum nitricum* have no rubrics of self-blame for 'original sins' committed, their feeling of being singled out for abandonment by the world will feel unjustified. If someone knows they have done wrong, they are not as despairing as *Argentum nitricum.*

Argentum nitricum have the *Delusion* rubric: *jumping off a high place*.[1] 1. *Argentum nitricum* are *lost for salvation*, they have *no hope*. The simillimum will only be *Argentum nitricum* if the patient feels that they will always be alone.

1. Denial: NONE. [*Delusion* rubric: *visions, has*: arg-n. *Delusion* rubric: *enlarged*: *Arg-n*. It is highly debatable whether these rubric are an indicator of 'delusions of grandeur' because *Argentum nitricum* have so many *Delusion* rubrics of being haunted by *visions of phantoms*, especially when they are trying to go to sleep.]

2. Forsaken: *Delusion* rubric: *forsaken; is*: **ARG-N**. *Delusion* rubric: *appreciated, she is not*: arg-n. *Delusion* rubric: *despised; is*: **ARG-N**. *Delusion* rubric: *neglected*: *he or she is neglected*: *Arg-n*. *Delusion* rubric: *home*: *changed; everything at home has*: arg-n. [1] 1. *Delusion* rubric: *repudiated; he is*: *relatives; by his*: arg-n. *Delusion* rubric: *images, phantoms; sees*: *sleep preventing*: arg-n. *Delusion* rubric: *dead*: *persons, sees*: arg-n. *Delusion* rubric: *faces, sees; closing eyes, on*: *Arg-n*. *Delusion* rubric: *walls*: *crush him; walls will*: *Arg-n*. [2] 1. *Delusion* rubric: *lost; she is*: *salvation; for*: *world, to the, beyond hope*: arg-n. [1] 1. *Delusion* rubric: *world*: *lost to the world, beyond hope; he is*: *Arg-n*. [2] 1. [The last two rubrics pertain to abandonment of the soul, beyond help or redemption. These rubrics can also pertain to predictions of doom and depression.]

3. Causation: NONE. [*Argentium nitricum* have the *Delusion* rubric: *right*: *doing nothing right; he is*: arg-n. This rubric is usually allocated into Depression. *Argentium nitricum* feel they have failed and sinned because they can doing nothing right.]

4. Depression: *Delusion* rubric: *clouds*: *black cloud enveloped her; a heavy*: arg-n. *Delusion* rubric: *insane*: *become insane; one will*: arg-n. *Delusion* rubric: *fail, everything*

will: *Arg-n*. *Delusion* rubric: *right*: *doing nothing right; he is*: arg-n. *Delusion* rubric: *lost; she is: salvation; for: world, to the, beyond hope*: arg-n. [1] 1. *Delusion* rubric: *world*: *lost to the world, beyond hope; he is*: *Arg-n*. [2] 1.

5. Resignation: *Delusion* rubrics: *die: about to die; one was*: *Arg-n*. *Delusion* rubric: *disease*: *incurable disease; he has an*: *Arg-n*. *Delusion* rubric: *sick*: *being*: arg-n. *Delusion* rubric: *enlarged*: *body is*: arg-n.

Aurum muriaticum natronatum assume they will be abandoned. All of the ten *Delusion* rubrics for *Aurum muriaticum natronatum* resonate with self-deserving punishment and self-blame. *Aurum muriaticum natronatum* disproportionately delegate punishment for their sins by assuming they are *unfit for the world*. *Aurum muriaticum natronatum* have been abandoned by the *world*, their *friends*, and their *mother*.

Aurum muriaticum natronatum assume disproportionate punishment for *wrongs* they have committed because they have no rubrics of 'delusions of grandeur' with which to delude themselves about their grandeur.

When sick, *Aurum muriaticum natronatum* feel undeserving of treatment and are convinced they will never be cured. *Aurum muriaticum natronatum* will project or transfer 'delusions of abandonment' on to the homoeopathic practitioner. 'Transference' is a psychological term which explains the projection process that can take place in all helping professions, including a homoeopathic consultation. In 'transference' the patient pressures the homoeopath into playing a role that mirrors their own delusional internal world. Because *Aurum muriaticum natronatum* do not feel worthy of love, they will transfer this projection of *disappointed love* on to the homoeopathic practitioner. *Aurum muriaticum natronatum* will delude themselves that there is discord between their practitioner and themselves and that the homoeopathic practitioner is not the right person to treat them. They will also delude themselves that their practitioner has deceived them. *Aurum muriaticum natronatum* have the *Mind* rubric: *love with the wrong person*, and the *Mind* rubric: *deceived friendship*. *Aurum muriaticum natronatum* have the *Delusion* rubric: *unfit for the world*. This psychological delusion permeates their response to *presumed* abandonment. They tend to maintain the status quo because they are terrified of creating discord or of being abandoned by the world. *Aurum muriaticum natronatum* also stay in unsuitable relationships because they fear being alone. *Aurum muriaticum natronatum* do not feel worthy of love. *Aurum muriaticum natronatum* demonstrate exaggerated hyper-vigilant fears and predictions of being abandoned and they base these 'delusions of persecution' on their 'delusions of original sin'. *Aurum muriaticum natronatum* punish themselves and exile themselves from love. Because *Aurum muriaticum natronatum* have no hubristic illusions they over-exaggerate their delusions of unworthiness.

The simillimum will only be *Aurum muriaticum natronatum* if the patient believes that they can't, or don't deserve to be treated or cured.

- *Mind: ailments from: disappointment: Aur-m-n.*
- *Mind: ailments from: friendship; deceived:* aur-m-n.
- *Mind: ailments from: discords: friends; between one's:* aur-m-n.
- *Mind: ailments from: discords: parents; between one's:* aur-m-n.
- *Mind: ailments from: love; disappointed:* aur-m-n.
- *Mind: quarrelling: aversion to:* aur-m-n.
- *Mind: sadness: love; from disappointed: Aur-m-n.*
- *Mind: love: wrong person; with the:* aur-m-n.
1. Denial: NONE.
2. Forsaken: *Delusion* rubric: *forsaken; is: Aur-m-n. Delusion*

rubric: *friend: affection of; he has lost the*: aur-m-n. *Delusion* rubric: *unfit: world; he is unfit for the*: aur-m-n. *Delusion* rubric: *dead: mother is, his*: aur-m-n. [This rubric should be used when the patient feels alone, regardless of whether their mother is dead in reality or not.]

3. Causation: *Delusion* rubric: *wrong: done wrong; he has*: Aur-m-n. *Delusion* rubric: *unfit: world; he is unfit for the*: aur-m-n.

4. Depression: *Delusion* rubric: *succeed, he does everything wrong; he cannot*: Aur-m-n. *Delusion* rubric: *unfit: world; he is unfit for the*: aur-m-n.

5. Resignation: *Delusion* rubric: *unfit: world; he is unfit for the*: aur-m-n. [This rubric can be proof of abandonment, or sins, or can reflect a fatalistic doom which permeates their state of mind when they are sick. *Aurum muriaticum natronatum* when they are sick are convinced they will never be cured.]

Aurum metallicum fear they have *neglected their duty* and specifically feel they have *neglected their friends.*

Aurum metallicum have an intensely exaggerated sense of guilt and self-reproach over rejecting people.

Aurum metallicum believe they have lost their friend. The underlying fear is that their psyche will feel bereft of internal substance.

Aurum metallicum fear they are *lost for salvation.* This profound religious fear of being lost and abandoned by the world explains why *Aurum metallicum* hang on to their fundamentalist need for God and religion.

The sense of guilt inside *Aurum metallicum* is so heightened that they fear being punished and abandoned by their friends. *Aurum metallicum* have the Delusion rubric: *lost the affection of his friends*, and his *friends have lost confidence in him. Aurum metallicum* have the *Delusion* rubric: *internal emptiness.* [1]

1. Without the support of God [*religious*], and without support

from the world [*friends*], *Aurum metallicum* feel bereft of all internal worthiness. When *Aurum metallicum* are sick they are overwhelmed by these same feelings of abandonment. The 'never-well-since-event' with *Aurum metallicum* often involves overwhelming fears of being abandoned because they believe they have abandoned their friend. *Aurum metallicum* will often give up all hope of cure and they will also often give up homoeopathic treatment when they are sick. On the one hand they feel assured that they are worthy of punishment and that their disease is evidence of God's retribution. And on the other hand they presume that the homoeopathic practitioner will abandon them, so they leave treatment before they can be rejected. Without assurance of support, *Aurum metallicum* sink into depressive melancholy and feelings of worthlessness. *Aurum metallicum* have thirty-four *Mind* rubrics relating to suicide[36].

Aurum metallicum not only feel abandoned, they also abandon their right to their own life.

1. Denial: *Delusion* rubric: *fancy, illusions of*. Aur. *Delusion* rubric: *religious*: aur.
2. Forsaken: *Delusion* rubric: *forsaken; is*: *Aur*. *Delusion* rubric: *lost; she is; salvation; for*. Aur. *Delusion* rubric: *friend*: *affection of; has lost the*: Aur. *Delusion* rubric: *appreciated, she is not*: aur. *Delusion* rubric: *confidence in him*; *his friends have lost all*: aur. *Delusion* rubric: *persecuted*: *he is persecuted*: aur. *Delusion* rubric: *unfit*: *world; he is unfit for the*: Aur. *Delusion* rubric: *pursued; he was*: aur. *Delusion* rubric: *poisoned*: *he*: *has been*: aur. *Delusion* rubric: *pursued; he was*: *enemies, by*: aur.
3. Causation: *Delusion* rubric: *neglected*: *duty; he has neglected his*: **AUR**. *Delusion* rubric: *neglected*: *friends, his*: *Aur*. [2] 1. *Delusion* rubric: *sinned*; *one has*: *unpardonable sin; he had committed the*: aur.
4. Depression: *Delusion* rubric: *depressive*: *Aur*. *Delusion* rubric: *worthless; he is*: aur. *Delusion* rubric: *doomed,*

being: aur. *Delusion* rubric: *obstacles*: *in his way*: aur. [1]
1. *Delusion* rubric: *emptiness; of: internal*: aur. [1] 1. [This
rubric pertains to depression and despair.]

5. Resignation: *Delusion* rubric: *hollow*: *body is hollow; whole*:
   aur.

Magnesium carbonicum suffer from intense
'delusions of abandonment'. *Magnesium carbonicum,* similarly
to *Bryonia,* focus their fears of abandonment on monetary
security. *Magnesium carbonicum* have the *Delusion* rubric:
he is counting his money and *seeing thieves. Magnesium
carbonicum* suffer from fear of something being taken away
from them. *Magnesium carbonicum* are the abandoned children
who have grown up with fear of future loss. It is common for
abandoned[37] children to grow up with a burning desire to
accumulate wealth so that they can feel more secure internally
and externally.

Psychological 'delusions of deprivation' will continue in the profile of
Magnesium carbonicum regardless of their existing wealth. The 'never-
well-since-event' or causation in any *Magnesium carbonicum* case
will always be 'delusions of deprivation' which have arisen from real or
perceived abandonment.

Magnesium carbonicum have the *Delusion* rubric: *sees
dead people because they continually need to be assured that
all of their dead ancestors and parents are still caring for them
and are still with them. Magnesium carbonicum* do not want to be
left alone without the support from friends and family. Similarly,
they also need financial security. *Magnesium carbonicum* are
extremely overwhelmed by anxiety and exaggerated 'delusions
of hypochondria' when they are sick. The simillimum will only
be *Magnesium carbonicum* if the patient indicates that they
need the practitioner for emotional support.

1. Denial: *Delusion* rubric: *fancy, illusions of*: mag-c. *Delusion*
   rubric: *people*: *seeing people*: mag-c. *Delusion* rubric:

dead: *persons, sees*: *Mag-c*. [These last two rubrics can pertain to Denial because *Magnesium carbonicum* need to believe their lost family is still with them for support.]

2. Forsaken: *Delusion* rubric: *forsaken; is*: **MAG-C**. *Delusion* rubric: *murdered*: *will be murdered; he*: mag-c. *Delusion* rubric: *thieves*: *seeing*: mag-c. *Delusion* rubric: *bed*: *lumps in bed*: mag. [1] 2. [arn.] [*Magnesium carbonicum* need their home and specifically their bed to be secure when they are sick. They fear losing the security and safeness of their own bed.]

3. Causation: NONE.

4. Depression: *Delusion* rubric: *anxious*[38]: mag-c.

5. Resignation: *Delusion* rubric: *disease*: *incurable disease; he has an*: mag-c. *Delusion* rubric: *faint; he would*: mag-c.

Palladium have numerous 'delusions of persecution'. *Palladium* are disproportionately hyper-sensitive to all real or perceived rejection. *Palladium* have 'delusions of superiority'; they believe they are greater than everyone else. *Palladium* have the *Delusion* rubric: *tall, he is very enlarged*. Their 'delusions of superiority' preempt their heightened sensitivity to being rejected. The 'never-well-since-event' or causation in any *Palladium* case will always be 'delusions of paranoia' which have arisen from real or perceived rejection of their personage or worldly status. *Palladium* have an obsessive compulsive need to remain the centre of attention. *Palladium* have the *Mind* rubric: *haughty, wounded self-esteem; wishes to be flattered*. [3] 4. They also have the *Mind* rubrics: *ailments from being rejected*, *ailments from being rejected by the mother*, *offended easily*, and *desire to be flattered*. *Palladium* display a contradiction between their Denial in Stage one and Resignation in Stage five. Consequently, *Palladium* feel extremely compromised and undermined by their own internal self-deprecation. *Palladium* suffer from internal doubt that they do not have any substance [hollow]. *Palladium* need to believe they are enlarged and tall in the world.

When *Palladium* are attacked they feel like they are being decimated. *Palladium* have the *Delusion* rubric: *dogs attack him gnawing flesh and bones*. *Palladium* are demanding (haughty) and hysterical if they do not remain the centre of everyone's attention. *Palladium* have the *Mind* rubric: *hysteria* and the *Mind* rubric: *vanity*.

Because *Palladium* do not have any 'delusions of original sin', or no *Delusion* rubrics pertaining to personal wrongs, they are able to project and transfer all blame on to others for upsetting them.

Palladium have an 'id' which is uncontrolled by their 'ego' or their 'super-ego'. The perfectionist critical function of all our moralistic and inspirational ideals and spiritual goals and conscience is the 'super-ego'. The organized realistic part of the psyche is the 'ego'. The instinctual and unstructured inspirations in our somatic behavior is the 'id'. The 'id' is unconscious and is not restricted by social conventionality and is unrestrained selfish self-gratification synonymous with the unfettered impulses of a child who demands instant gratification. The 'id' is in opposition to the 'super-ego' which moderates behavior by being moralistically principled. The 'ego' is the mediator between the childish and selfish 'id', and the principled 'super-ego'. Our 'ego' is the reasonable part of our conscious mind which develops with age and maturity. A child is not expected to have developed a strong 'ego'. The 'id' is egocentric and infantile. The 'id' has no appropriate social conscientiousness. *Palladium* are egocentric and infantile. *Palladium* have no appropriate social awareness. The 'id' is equivalent to a demanding and petulant child who refuses to take *no* for an answer. *Palladium* are unrelenting in their need and demand to be the centre of attention.

Palladium have an 'ego' which is *hollow* and haunted by insanity; they feel undermined by their own ability to be able to achieve stability. It is this weakness in their 'ego' which causes them to be so hyper-sensitive to rejection. *Palladium* have an 'id' which grows with attention. *Palladium* have the *Delusion* rubric: *he or she has grown tall while walking*. *Palladium* childishly demand constant praise because their 'ego' and 'super-ego' is so weakened that they are under the illusion that they need to protect themselves from perceived attacks and criticisms. *Palladium* have the *Mind* rubric: *self-deprecation, want of self-confidence* and *suspicious people are talking about her*. The simillimum will only be *Palladium* if the patient is obsessively demanding of your attention. The simillimum will also only be *Palladium* if the patient is hypersensitive to perceived neglect.

1. Denial: *Delusion* rubric: *enlarged: tall; he is very:* pall.
    Versus
5. Resignation: *Delusion* rubric: *hollow: body is hollow; whole:* pall.

1. Denial: *Delusion* rubric: *enlarged: tall; he is very:* pall. *Delusion* rubric: *tall: he or she is tall: walking; had grown while:* pall. [1] 1.
2. Forsaken: *Delusion* rubric: *forsaken; is:* pall. *Delusion* rubric: *appreciated, she is not:* Pall. *Delusion* rubric: *abused, being:* pall. *Delusion* rubric: *criticized, she is:* pall. *Delusion* rubric: *dogs: attack him: gnawing flesh and bones:* pall. *Delusion* rubric: *insulted, he is:* Pall. *Delusion* rubric: *neglected: he or she is neglected:* **PALL**. *Delusion* rubric: *touching: anything; she could not touch:* pall. [1] 1.
3. Causation: NONE.
4. Depression: *Delusion* rubric: *insane: he is insane:* pall. *Delusion* rubric: *insane: become insane; one will:* pall.
5. Resignation: *Delusion* rubric: *hollow: body is hollow; whole:* pall.

•   *Delusions: persecuted; he is persecuted:* abrot. absin. aids. allox. ambr. anac. androc. ars. aur. bell. brom. calc. canth. *Cench.* **CHIN**. choc. *Cocain.* con. crot-c. crot-h. cupr. *Cycl.* dendr-pol. dream-p.

DROS. falco-pe. hell. hydrog. *Hyos. Ign.* iodof. **KALI-BR.** lac-leo. *Lach.* lyc. manc. med. meli. merc. moni. nat-c. nat-m. nux-v. petr-ra. positr. puls. rhus-t. sal-fr. sil. spong. staph. stram. stry. *Sulph.* syph. tarent. thyr. urol-h. verat-v. verat. *Vesp. Zinc.*

* *Delusions: persecuted: he is persecuted: everyone; by: Cycl.* [2] 1.

* *Delusions: strangers; control of; under:* aster. bry.

* *Delusions: strangers; surrounded by:* androc. aster. irid-met. nit-ac. *Puls.*

* *Delusions: spied; being:* aq-mar. lach. med. olib-sac. positr.

* *Delusions: watched, she is being:* adam. aids. aq-mar. **ARS.** *Bar-c. Calc.* choc. dream-p. falco-pe. *Hyos. Kali-br. Kola.* med. meli. musca-d. nat-pyru. olib-sac. petr-ra. rhus-t. sanguis-s.

* *Delusions: looking: everyone is looking at her:* meli. petr-ra. rhus-t. sanguis-s.

* *Delusions: people: beside him; people are:* anac. apis. *Ars.* atro. bell. calc. camph. carb-v. cench. hyos. *Med.* nux-v. petr. pyrog. thuj. valer.

* *Delusions: people; behind him; someone is:* anac. bell. brom. calc. casc. cench. crot-c. crot-h. dendr-pol. ephe-si. lach. led. mag-m. *Med.* naja. ozone. psil. ruta. sacch-l. sal-fr. sanic. sil. staph. stront-c. thuj. tub.

* *Delusions: person: present; someone is:* arizon-l. hyos. lyc. olib-sac. thuj.

* *Delusions: devil: after her; is: Hyos. Manc. Zinc.*

* *Delusions: criminals, about:* alum. am-c. *Ars.* bell. carb-v. caust. *Chel.* cina. *Cocc.* coff. dig. *Ferr.* graph. *Hyos.* merc. nat-c. nit-ac. nux-v. puls. ruta sil. stront-c. sulph. verat.

* *Delusions: enemy; everyone is an:* granit-m. *Merc.* plat. puls.

* *Delusions: enemy: surrounded by enemies:* ambr. *Anac.* carbn-s. *Crot-h.* dros. lac-del. marb-w. *Merc.* moni. verat.

* *Delusions: footsteps; hearing:* canth. carb-v. crot-c. nat-p. taosc.

- *Delusions*: *footsteps; hearing; behind him*: crot-c. *Med.*

- *Delusions*: *people*: *beside him; people are*: anac. apis *Ars.* atro. bell. calc. camph. carb-v. cench. hyos. *Med.* nux-v. petr. pyrog. thuj. valer.

- *Delusions*: *pursued; he was*: absin. aids. ambr. *Anac.* ars. aur. bell. brom. bry. carc. choc. con. cycl. dros. hydrog. *Hyos. Kali-br.* lach. manc. med. merc. moni. nux-v. op. plat. plb. positr. rhus-t. sanguis-s. sil. staph. stram. thuj. verat-v. verat.

- *Delusions*: *pursued*: *he was*: *enemies, by*: absin. anac. ars. aur. *Bell.* carneg-g. *Chin.* cic. *Cocain.* con. crot-h. cupr. cycl. dros. hell. *Hyos. Kali-br. Lach.* lepi. lyc. med. meli. merc. nat-c. nux-v. plb. positr. *Puls.* rhus-t. sil. stram. stry. zinc.

- *Delusions*: *specters, ghosts, spirits*: ars. *Atro-s.* bell. camph. *Cann-xyz.* carb-an. carb-v. caust. cimic. *Crot-c.* dros. dulc. hell. hyos. kali-br. kali-c. lach. mag-m. merc. nat-c. *Nux-v. Op.* orot-ac. ph-ac. phos. plat. rhus-t. ruta. sep. sil. sinus. stram. verat.

- *Delusions*: *specters, ghosts, spirits*: *pursued by, is*: lepi. plat. stram. stry.

- *Delusions*: *specters, ghosts, spirits*: *seeing*: acon. agar. alum. am-c. ambr. ant-t. ars-met. *Ars.* atro. aur. **BELL.** bov. brom. *Calc. Camph.* carb-v. cocc. *Croc. Cupr-act. Cupr.* dig. dulc. hell. hep. hura *Hyos.* hyper. ign. *Kali-br.* kali-c. kali-i. kali-sil. lach. lepi. lyc. merc. *Nat-c. Nat-m.* nit-ac. *Op.* phos. phys. plat. psor. puls. ran-b. sal-fr. sars. sep. sil. spig. *Stram. Sulph.* tarent. thuj. verb. visc. zinc.

- *Delusions*: *faces, sees*: *diabolical faces crowd upon him*: *Ambr.* carb-an. caust. tarent.

- *Delusions*: *insulted, he is*: adam. alco. aur-ar. aur-m-n. bell. cham. cocc. cygn-be. granit-m. haliae-lc. ign. ilx-a. kali-br. lac-c. *Lac-e.* lyss. nat-m. nux-v. oci-sa. *Pall.* puls. staph. sulph. tarent.

- *Delusions*: *conspiracies*: *against him; there are conspiracies*: ars. cygn-be. kali-br. lach. plb. puls. sal-fr.

- *Delusions*: *criticized, she is*: arizon-l. bar-act. *Bar-c.* calc. carc.

carneg-g. cocain. *Dys.* germ-met. hydrog. hyos. ign. lac-ac. lac-leo. *Lac-lup.* lach. laur. loxo-recl. lyss. marb-w. nat-m. pall. pin-con. plb. positr. prot. rad-br. rhus-r. sacch. sal-fr. staph. toxi.

- *Delusions: betrayed; that she is*: adam. dros. falco-pe. hydrog. lac-h. ol-eur. petr-ra. rad-br. *Rhus-g.* urol-h.

- *Delusions: deceived; being*: bamb-a. crot-c. dros. *Ign.* lyss. naja. *Nat-ar.* nicc-met. nicc. ozone. ruta. spong. *Staph.* stront-c.

- *Delusions: life: burdened by my life*: aloe. des-ac.

- *Delusions: life: threatened; life is*: kali-br.[1] 1.

- *Delusions: poisoned: he: about to be poisoned; he is*: carc. falco-pe. *Hyos. Kali-br.* lach. meli. plb. **RHUS-T**. verat-v.

- *Delusions: poisoned: he: has been*: agar. ang. aur. bufo caj. carb-ac. chinin-s. chlor. cic. cimic. cocc. cor-r. croc. culx. cur. cypra-eg. euph. ferr. gels. glon. hydr. hydrog. *Hyos.* iodof. jug-r. kali-br. kali-c. kali-i. lac-c. lac-h. *Lach.* lact. lil-t. lina. lyc. m-aust. mag-p. marb-w. med. merl. mez. mill. naja. nicc. nux-m. nux-v. olnd. op. petr. ph-ac. phos. pip-m. plat-m. psor. ptel. puls. ran-b. raph. rat. rheum. rhod. **RHUS-T**. sabad. sec. sep. spig. squil. staph. stram. sul-ac. sulph. tab. tarax. thuj. valer. vip. zinc.

- *Delusions: poisoned: medicine; being poisoned by*: cimic. cypra-eg. hyos. lach. lina. rhus-t.

- *Delusions: injury: about to receive injury; is*: aq-mar. ars. bell. cann-i. carbn-s. con. dendr-pol. galeoc-c-h. hyos. irid-met. lac-h. lach. lyc. merc. nux-v. oci-sa. *Op.* polys. rad-br. sil. stram. sulph.

- *Delusions: injury: about to receive injury: is: friends; from his*: fum. lach.

- *Delusions: people: pranks with him; people carry on all sorts of*: hydrog. **NUX-V**. *Delusions: injury: being injured; is*: bry. cact. canth. elaps kali-br. lach. lyss. naja phos. rhus-g. rhus-t. **STRAM**. sulph.

- *Delusions: murdered: being murdered; he is*: absin. bell. kali-br. plb. sulph.

- *Delusions: murdered: will be murdered; he*: absin. am-m. *Bell.*

Calc. camph. carc. cimic. hep. *Hyos.* ign. kali-c. lac-c. lact. lyc. mag-c. merc. *Op.* phos. plb. positr. *Rhus-t.* staph. *Stram.* verat. zinc.

- *Delusions: murdered: will be murdered; he: conspire to murder him; others*: ars. hydrog. plb. tab.
- *Delusions: criminals, about*: alum. am-c. *Ars.* bell. carb-v. caust. *Chel.* cina *Cocc.* coff. dig. *Ferr.* graph. *Hyos.* merc. nat-c. nit-ac. nux-v. puls. ruta sil. stront-c. sulph. verat.

Avoidance: This group of *Delusion* rubrics indicate paranoid 'delusions of persecution'. *Surrounded by enemies, strangers, watched, pursued by the devil, criminals,* and *enemies, haunted by specters, ghosts and spirits, insulted, persecuted, criticized, betrayed, threatened, deceived, poisoned, murdered* and *choked,* are all psychological delusions of predicted persecution.

It is quite common, especially when one is sick for the first time in one's life, for a patient to feel they have been singled out for punishment.

'Delusions of persecution' can also be projected on to the homoeopathic practitioner. It is quite common, especially when sick for the first time, for patient's to be nervous about what the practitioner is prescribing for them. Only the practitioner can judge, at the time of the consultation, if their patient's nervousness is in proportion, or over-exaggerated and indicative of paranoid psychological delusions. It is important for practitioners to remember that although *we* are familiar with homoeopathic remedies, our patients are new to homoeopathy, so they can be unsure. It is also important for the homoeopathic practitioner not to over-react to a patient's appropriate hesitant response. Their hesitancy is often a response to feeling terrified about being sick. A patient can often transfer their hesitancy on to the practitioner.

Paranoid delusions about being *poisoned* or *betrayed* or *cheated* are often projected on to the practitioner so the vulnerable (abandoned) patient can reinforce their illusions and delusions that they are *not sick*.

This group of persecution rubrics are important to use when it is obvious that the patient is avoiding the fact that they need treatment. Avoidance and self-deluding denial enables a person to justify their misrepresentation of reality. These *Delusion* rubrics are of great benefit when a patient is absolutely sure that chemotherapy or radiotherapy treatment for their cancer would kill them rather than save them. Transference is characterized by unconscious self-deluding denial which allows for the redirection of feelings of insecurity on to another person. A 'transference neuroses' in this case allows the patient to believe that they are under threat from the practitioner poisoning them.

Blaming others and projecting abandonment on to the world is the best defense mechanism to cover up intense self-punishing blame for 'delusions of original sin'. A 'persecution complex' is developed to deflect guilt.

A 'persecution complex' is also maintained to cover up personal failings and inadequacies. It is much easier to blame others for hindering one in one's pursuits than it is to acknowledge one's own lack of achievement.

Four different remedy profiles are discussed below: *China, Cyclamen,* and *Drosera* and *Spongia*. *China* maintain their 'delusions of persecution' so that their unfortunate state is not their doing. *Cyclamen* blame others to cover up their own guilt for sins committed. *Drosera* maintain their paranoid 'persecution complex' because it helps to cover up their own suicidal tendencies. *Spongia,* in contrast, maintain their 'delusions of persecution' because they feel trapped and persecuted by their own somatic memories of trauma.

China maintain their 'persecution complexes' because they need to avoid their own anger. Sankaran, in *The Soul of Remedies* writes: "The feeling in *China* is: "I am weak and so people attack, trouble and torture me", a feeling of being persecuted. The patient feels he is weak, not good enough, that he is persecuted and hindered at his work by other people, that he is obstructed from achieving his ambition. So he fantasizes and in these fantasies he makes himself worthy and achieves his ambitions, and in this way uses fantasies to cover up the inherent feeling of not being good enough." *China* over-exaggerate and attribute blame for their lack of success on to everyone else who is *hindering them in their work*. It is true that the simillimum will not be *China* unless the patient indicates that they feel persecuted. However, it is important to know *why* each constitutional remedy profile *needs* to continue feeling like a victim. If the homoeopath does not understand the psychological processes within each remedy profile the homoeopath could make the mistake of counselling the patient to confront their 'persecution complexes'.

China need to maintain their 'delusions of persecution' to avoid their own *vexations*.

China do not feel able to empower themselves because when they feel angry they are overcome with guilt.

China fantasies about beautiful things to avoid their own anger. *China* have the *Delusion* rubric: *offences of vexations*. All *Delusion* rubrics are an indication of the patient disproportionately assessing their own mental or emotional perceptions. 'Delusions of original sin' are extremely important to consider in understanding the self-deluding and avoidances in each constitutional remedy profile because the patient will often organize their life so that they avoid facing their own 'dark-side'.

The homoeopath working with *China* needs to counsel the patient that they should not feel crippled by their own anger. As soon as *China* feel angry they dissociate.

Anger is an emotion which can be used positively to enact change; all patients who are trapped in a 'victim mentality' need anger to be able to enact change in their lives. *China* have the *Delusion* rubric: *walking on air*. *China* believe the world is hostile. 'Dissociation' is a normal response to real or perceived threats. A 'Disassociation disorder' is far more complex in that the patient creates another reality or a more attractive world which allows their psyche protection from what they perceive to be a potentially injurious situation, either within or outside of themselves. *China* are *tormented* within by their own *vexations*, as well as being tormented by the outside world. Their dissociative process becomes a self-fulfilling prophecy because it reinforces their belief in their inability to succeed.

China have the *Mind* rubric: *heightened awareness of beautiful things. China* dissociate by making plans about *beautiful things.*

China have the *Mind* rubric: *making many plans at night.* [3] 1. It is hard to connect and make contact with *China* emotionally, and it is also hard for *China* to connect and make contact with themselves. By dissociating, *China* render themselves unable to enact change, which would overturn their sense of being *hindered in their work.* The simillimum will not be *China* unless the patient shows signs of choosing to dissociate from stark realities within their life. The simillimum will not be *China* unless the patient also shows signs of choosing to dissociate from feeling anger. Sankaran, in *The Soul of Remedies* writes: "He achieves his ambition by building castles in the air. He feels what he possesses is not good enough and that he would have possessed better things if he had not been obstructed and hindered. Therefore he fantasies and imagines that he possesses finer and more expensive things than he actually does. He never really put his plans into action. It is mere armchair planning." *China* will choose to stay an armchair dreamer and choose to believe they are a victim because they do not want to face their fear of their own *vexations*. *China* feel persecuted from within and outside of themselves.

The simillimum will also not be *China* unless the patient feels fragile and vulnerable in the world. The theme of hypochondria in Stage five is *exaggerated* fragility and weakness. *China* avoid the stark realities of life because they feel too fragile [*light*].

1. Denial: *Delusion* rubric: *fancy, illusions of:* chin. *Delusion* rubric: *walking: air: on air; walks:* chin. [This rubric should not be interpreted literally, it pertains to 'disassociation'.]

2. Forsaken: *Delusion* rubric: *persecuted: he is persecuted:* **CHIN**. *Delusion* rubric: *forsaken; is:* chin. *Delusion* rubric: *hindered; he is: everyone; by: Chin. Delusion* rubric: *pursued; he was: enemies, by: Chin. Delusion* rubric: *people: seeing people:* chin. *Delusion* rubric: *wrong: suffered wrong; he has:* chin. *Delusion* rubric: *faces, sees: dark, in the:* chin. [1] 2. *Delusion* rubric: *figures: seeing figures:* chin. *Delusion* rubric: *images, phantoms; sees:* chin.

3. Causation: *Delusion* rubric: *vexation: offences; of vexations and:* chin.

4. Depression: *Delusion* rubric: *tormented; he is: Chin. Delusion* rubric: *unfortunate, he is: Chin. Delusion* rubric: *work: hindered at work; is: Chin.* [2] 1.

5. Resignation: *Delusion* rubric: *light: is light; he:* chin.

Cyclamen are listed in numerous *Delusion* rubrics of abandonment and numerous *Delusion* rubrics pertaining to 'delusions of original sin'. *Cyclamen* want to remain in their solitude because they are overwhelmed by real or perceived imaginings of 'original sin'. *Cyclamen* are not listed significantly in the rubrics pertaining to 'delusions of grandeur'.

The reason why *Cyclamen* brood in persecuted doom is that they lack the delusional strength associated with psychological 'hubristic denial'. The only denial rubric in which they are listed is the *Delusion* rubric: *illusions of fancy.* Fanciful illusions predisposes them to becoming a victim to their own idealism which they can't live up to.

Cyclamen easily fall into the habit of predicting their own failure. *Cyclamen* remain *paralyzed* by gloom and doom about their fate. *Cyclamen* have the *Delusion* rubric: *great troubles had just come over him.* [1] 1. *Cyclamen* have the *Delusion* rubric: *he is persecuted by everyone.* [2] 1. *Cyclamen* are undermined by their belief that they have been bad. They also believe they should remain *alone* and isolated from the rest of humanity. Sankaran, in *The Soul of Remedies* writes the following about *Cyclamen*: "The situation of Cyclamen is that of a woman who feels that she has done something wrong, or that she hasn't done her duty and something bad has occurred as a result. She feels solely responsible for what has happened and feels like a criminal. She cannot reveal the crime to anyone, keeps everything within herself and tries to rectify things as much as possible. She avoids all social contact, does not talk to anyone and feels totally alone." Sankaran has written exactly what I have repertorised. Students and homoeopaths learning to use rubric-repertorisation in case-taking, and apply it within a psychotherapeutic model, will find they have much more depth of understanding in the treatment of a *Cyclamen* patient. *Cyclamen* resist and avoid treatment, and self-sabotage homoeopathic treatment, because as soon as their prominent layer of abandonment lifts inside of themselves they are swamped with their feelings of self-deprecating guilt. Their feelings of abandonment cover up their guilt. Homoeopathic practitioners must predict this.

The ability to predict the course of your patient's treatment will be achieved only through studying the rubrics attached to each remedy and understanding the psychological processing all patients progress through in illness. If you predict the avoidance, self-sabotage, and self-fulfilling prophecies which *Cyclamen* need to maintain, then you can counsel them about forgiveness, and about understanding the real or perceived sins which they have committed. This is the counselling responsibility you have in your role as a homoeopath. *Cyclamen* need help to forgive themselves for the sins they have committed.

Cyclamen have the *Delusion* rubric: *deprived of his senses*. *Cyclamen* lose all connection to their own psyche when they are overwhelmed by their 'delusions of original sin'. They also abandon their own intuition and practical sensibilities when they try to work out how to overcome their troubles. *Cyclamen* have the *Delusion* rubric: *as if two persons lay in the bed and the body of the other overlapped hers by half.* [1] 1. This rubric indicates that *Cyclamen* struggle to hold on to their own psyche. *Cyclamen* have to be encouraged to fight for their right to exist. They need to be encouraged not to give up and sink into psychological 'delusions of impending doom'. *Cyclamen* feel alone and abandoned and also abandon themselves.

1. Denial: *Delusion* rubric: *fancy illusions, of:* cycl.
2. Forsaken: *Delusion* rubric: *persecuted: he is persecuted: Cycl. Delusion* rubric: *persecuted: he is persecuted: everyone; by: Cycl.* [2] 1. *Delusion* rubric: *forsaken; is: Cycl. Delusion* rubric: *alone, being: world; alone in the:* cycl. *Delusion* rubric: *animals: surrounded by ugly animals:* cycl. *Delusion* rubric: *pursued; he was:* cycl. *Delusion* rubric: *pursued; he was: enemies, by:* cycl. *Delusion* rubric: *animals: large animal is running over her whole body:* cycl. [1] 1.
3. Causation: *Delusion* rubric: *evil: done some evil; had:* cycl. *Delusion* rubric: *crime: committed a crime; he had:* cycl. *Delusion* rubric: *neglected: duty; he has neglected his:* cycl.
4. Depression: *Delusion* rubric: *troubles: great troubles had just come over him:* cycl. [1] 1. *Delusion* rubric: *doomed, being:* cycl.
5. Resignation: *Delusion* rubric: *paralyzed; he is:* cycl. *Delusion* rubric: *senses: deprived of his senses:* cycl. [1] 1.

Drosera as a homoeopathic remedy was the principle remedy used by Hahnemann for whooping cough (Boericke). The theme running through *Drosera* is violent reactivity, followed by ineffectual action or paralysis. Physically, the cough which needs the homoeopathic remedy *Drosera* is noted for its violent coughing followed by ineffectual spasms of the larynx. These symptoms are mirrored in the constitutional remedy profile. *Drosera* are easily angered by people who they suspect of deceiving them. Conversely, however, *Drosera* are completely ineffectual in carrying through their anger and they give up and are inclined to self-denigrate themselves to the point where they suicide.

Drosera maintain their paranoid 'persecution complex' because it helps cover up their own suicidal ineffectualness.

Drosera have hubristic rubrics of heightened clairaudience and clairvoyance which reinforce their paranoia about being deceived or pursued rather than reinforce their 'delusions of grandeur'. *Drosera* are anxious and paranoid, easily undermined and full of 'persecution complexes'. The simillimum will not be *Drosera* unless the homoeopath is able to perceive the extreme polarities evident within all plant remedies: sensitivity to real or perceived persecution, and reactivity to real or perceived persecution. *Drosera* have the *Mind* rubrics: *discouraged about the future,* and *suspicious of his best friends. Drosera* have the *Mind* rubrics: *rage at trifles,* and *beside oneself with anger at trifles.* The self-defeating ineffectual tendencies within *Drosera* are fueled by guilt over their *vexations.* All their anger is oppressed and undermined by strong suicidal tendencies.

The psychosomatic symptoms associated with the homoeopathic use of the remedy *Drosera* is an irritated throat followed by ineffectual coughing and spasms. *Peculiar* to the constitutional remedy profile of *Drosera* is that they do not enact effective or productive change in their lives.

1. Denial: *Delusion* rubric: *fancy illusions, of:* dros. *Delusion* rubric: *voices: hearing:* dros. *Delusion* rubric: *visions, has*: dros. [These hubristic rubrics of heightened clairaudience and clairvoyance can be seen to re-enforce their 'delusions of paranoia' about being deceived or pursued.] *Delusion* rubric: *tall: things grow taller:* dros. [Normally this rubric would pertain to 'delusions of grandeur'. Within *Drosera* it contributes to exaggerate persecutory fears.]

2. Forsaken: *Delusion* rubric: *persecuted: he is persecuted*:
    DROS. *Delusion* rubric: *betrayed; that she is*: dros.
    Delusion rubric: *pursued; he was*: dros. *Delusion* rubric:
    deceived; being: dros. *Delusion* rubric: *enemy: surrounded
    by enemies*: dros. *Delusion* rubric: *enemy: rest; enemy
    allowed him no*: dros. [1] 1. *Delusion* rubric: *specters,
    ghosts, spirits*: dros. *Delusion* rubric: *images, phantoms;
    sees*: dros. *Delusion* rubric: *calls: someone calls*: dros.
    [This rubric can be allocated into 'delusions of grandeur';
    pertaining to God calling. Alternatively, this rubric can be
    allocated into 'delusions of persecution'; pertaining to the
    devil chasing someone for sins committed.]

3. Causation: *Delusion* rubric: *vexation: offenses; of vexations
    and*: dros.

4. Depression: *Delusion* rubric: *news: expecting news:
    unpleasant news*: dros. *Delusion* rubric: *suicide; impelled
    to commit: drowning; by*: dros. [1] 1.

5. Resignation: *Delusion* rubric: *enemy: rest; enemy allowed
    him no*: dros. [1] 1. [This rubric can pertain to 'delusions of
    persecution' or to persecutory illusions when the patient is
    sick. When *Drosera* are sick they feel unable to rest until
    they can "expel" the sickness from their body.]

Spongia maintain their 'delusions of persecution'
because they feel trapped and persecuted by their own somatic
memories of trauma. *Spongia* is a homoeopathic remedy
derived from the genus Euspongia officinalis or the common
bath sponge. The theme, within the sea remedies as a group,
is survival and the need to find a hiding place from predators.
Sea creatures feel like they are being spied upon and they
only feel safe when they are alone and hiding in a safe place
[*home*]. Although these are common themes within the group
of sea remedies as a whole, each constitutional remedy profile
within that group will have a *peculiar* survival strategy. The

genus *Euspongia* is attached by the under surface to the sea-bottom. *Spongia* have the *Mind* rubric: *desires to go home,* and *ailments from fright*. *Spongia* have the *Mind* rubric: *fear of suffocation*. Somatically, their fear of being crowded and suffocated means that they have a specific dislike of being looked at. *Spongia* feel suffocated[39] by living with people.

Spongia have the *Mind* rubric: *dictatorial talking with an air of command*. *Spongia* initially appear dictatorial. Their need to dictate comes from a inner need to protect their vulnerability.

The outer surface of the genus *Euspongia*, is covered by a skin or dermal membrane. *Spongia* similarly feel fearful if they are exposed. *Spongia* have the *Mind* rubric: *cannot bear to be looked at*. *Spongia* peculiarly feel spied upon by their own memories of the past which crowd in on them. *Spongia* psychosomatically feel suffocated by their own unhappiness. *Spongia* have the *Mind* rubric: *tormented by past disagreeable occurrences, dwells on a frightful scene of some mournful event of the past* [1] 1. They also have the *Mind* rubric: *on closing eyes thoughts intrude and crowd around each other.* [1] 1. *Spongia* feel enveloped by their own negative thoughts and fears. The *peculiar* theme within *Spongia* as a sea remedy is their need to be able to escape[40] from their own memories which constantly wash through them. *Spongia* feel persecuted by their own somatic memories of trauma. *Spongia* have the *Delusion* rubric: *has visions of past horrible events.* [1] 1, and *vivid delusions*. *Spongia* have the *Mind* rubric: *anger about past events*.

Spongia have the *Delusion* rubric: *delusion of a motion, up and down*. *Spongia* have a psychodynamic need to be able to move thoughts and emotions through their body. Sponges are perforated by miniscule canals trough which seawater is pumped by the action of thousands of flagellae. *Spongia* have a psychodynamic response to feeling trapped by any one view point or ideology. *Spongia* have the *Mind* rubrics: *brooding with suicidal thoughts*, and *brooding or moping in a corner*, and *brooding over one's condition*. Conversely, *Spongia* have the *Delusion* rubric: *when he sees something it seems as though he saw through someone else's eyes*[41]. [1] 3. *Spongia* struggle to hold on to their *own* perception of a situation, they tend to place another's perception or opinion over and above their own. *Spongia* also have the *Delusion* rubric: *errors of personal identity*. *Spongia* feel persecuted from outside of themselves, and persecute themselves inside by undermining their own perception. *Spongia* have the *Mind* rubric: *despair from the smallest criticism*. The homoeopath working with a *Spongia* patient needs to reinforce that the patient's perception of a particular situation was correct. Furthermore, the homoeopath then needs to help the *Spongia* patient move on from needing to hold [*brood*] on past trauma. The 'never-well-since-event' or causation in any *Spongia* case will always be 'delusions of persecution' which have arisen from a real or perceived threat to their psyche.

Spongia will always have a particular event or several events in their life in which their opinion was dismissed. *Spongia* have the *Delusion* rubrics: *being deceived*, and *not appreciated*.

Spongia as a homoeopathic remedy is commonly used for croup attacks in which the patient wakes at night feeling unable to breath because they feel like they are being suffocated. *Spongia* as a constitutional remedy profile will similarly feel suffocated; on the one hand, from their own memories of past traumas, and on the other hand from other's opinions [*persecutions*]. The simillimum will only be *Spongia* if the patient is literally choking from their memories of persecution. The unhealthy *Spongia* patient undermines themselves by abandoning their own opinion and dismissing everything they perceive as *meaningless*. *Spongia* have the *Delusion* rubric: *everything is meaningless*. [3] 2. The action of the simillimum in a *Spongia* case will be reflected in the patient no longer feeling undermined by other's opinions infiltrating their psyche.

A healthy *Spongia* patient will not abandon their own thoughts when they feel threatened [*persecuted*] by someone else's opinion.

1. Denial: *Delusion* rubric: *fancy illusions, of*: spong. [Because *Spongia* have so many *Delusion* rubrics of seeing ghosts it is debatable as to whether this rubric is a *Delusion* rubric of hubristic idealism or a *Delusion* rubric of persecution.]

2. Forsaken: *Delusion* rubric: *persecuted*: *he is persecuted*: spong. *Delusion* rubric: *deceived; being*: spong. *Delusion* rubric: *appreciated, she is not*: spong. *Delusion* rubric: *specters, ghosts, spirits: closing eyes, on*: spong. *Delusion* rubric: *images, phantoms; sees*: spong. *Delusion* rubric: *people: seeing people*: spong. *Delusion* rubric: *fire: visions of*: spong. *Delusion* rubric: *visions, has: horrible: events, of past*: spong. [1] 1. [This rubric can pertain to guilt over past events or to emotional trauma (persecution) as a result of past events.] *Delusion* rubric: *sees something; when he: someone else's eyes; seems as though he saw through*: spong.

3. Causation: *Delusion* rubric: *visions, has: horrible: events, of past*: spong. [1] 1. [This *Delusion* rubric can pertain to guilt. It can indicate that the patient is haunted by past sins.] *Delusion* rubric: *murdering; he is: has to murder someone; he*: spong.

4. Depression: *Delusion* rubric: *fail, everything will*: spong. *Delusion* rubric: *identity: errors of personal identity*: spong. *Delusion* rubric: *insane: he is insane*: spong. *Delusion* rubric: *falling: backward*: spong. [This rubric should not be interpreted literally. *Spongia* always feel that they are going backwards. *Spongia* presume that will always fail in everything they attempt.] *Delusion* rubric: *meaningless; everything is*: **SPONG**. [3] 2. [bamb-a.]

5. Resignation: *Delusion* rubric: *sick: being*: spong. *Delusion* rubric: *clothes: uncomfortable*: spong. [1] 1. [When *Spongia*

are sick they feel encroached upon by all restrictions, even their own clothes.]

• *Delusions: mirror; face; seeing everybody's face in the mirror except his own*: anac. [1] 1.

Avoidance: This rubric reveals two aspects about *Anacardium*. On the one hand their paranoia about not being recognized is so intense they expect to see everyone's face but their own. And on the other hand *Anacardium* avoid seeing their own face because they want to avoid self-reflection.

Anacardium believe they are outcasts and that no one will want them. The *Delusion* rubric: *sees everyone's face in mirror except his own* reflects internal paranoid fears about rejection from the outer world as well as self-rejection.

Their paranoia about being rejected is so intense that they believe everyone will be noticed except them: *everyone's face in mirror except his own*.

Anacardium also has the *Delusion* rubric, *he must go into the air and busy himself*. [1] 1. This rubric allows *Anacardium* to avoid inner reflection and self-confrontation. *Anacardium* have an intense fear of their own hate and devil-like rage which flares intensely if they are contradicted or criticized. *Anacardium* spend an enormous amount of time berating themselves for their devil-like rage and hate, which they try to make up for by overcompensating with God-like generosity. *Anacardium* have the *Delusion* rubric: *devil; speaking in one ear, prompting to murder and an angel in the other ear, prompting to acts of benevolence*. Guilt over their reactivity keeps them separate from the world – *Delusion* rubric: *separated from the world*. Separating themselves from the world allows them protection from being criticized and contradicted. *Anacardium* have the *Delusion* rubric: *his mother is dead*. *Anacardium* will in particular separate themselves from their mother. *Anacardium* have no peace because of their internalized dilemma of the *devil speaking in one ear, prompting to murder; and angel in the other ear, prompting to acts of benevolence.* They solve the debate by avoiding the world. This avoidance becomes a self-fulfilling prophecy for *Anacardium* as they then believe they have been forsaken because they are evil. Self-destructive behavior and self-blame will be maintained and nurtured because they help protect the *Anacardium* patient from their innermost dark secrets about themselves.

> Their dark secret is their innermost fear that they will not be recognized and that they are *worthless: seeing everybody's face in the mirror except his own.* Their self-destructive behavior is separating themselves from the world and remaining in self-inflicted exile – *she was an outcast.*

1. Denial: *Delusion* rubric: *religious*: Anac. *Delusion* rubric: *superhuman; is: control; is under superhuman*: anac. *Delusion* rubric: *air: go into the air and busy himself; he must*: anac. [1] 1.

2. Forsaken: *Delusion* rubric: *mirror; face; seeing everybody's face in the mirror except his own*: anac. [1] 1. *Delusion* rubric: *outcast; she were an*: anac. *Delusion* rubric: *enemy: surrounded by enemies*: Anac. *Delusion* rubric: *worthless; he is*: anac. *Delusion* rubric: *separated: world; from the: he is separated*: Anac.

3. Causation: *Delusion* rubric: *devil: he is a devil*: **ANAC**.

4. Depression: *Delusion* rubric: *anxious*: Anac. *Delusion* rubric: *succeed, he does everything wrong; he cannot*: Anac.

5. Resignation: *Delusion* rubric: *grave, he is in his*: anac.

> • *Delusions: mask; is behind a mask*: plut-n.[1] 1.

Avoidance: This rubric reveals two aspects about *Plutonium nitricum*. On the one hand they wish to avoid being exposed, and on the other hand they are separated from others. Like *Anacardium, Plutonium nitricum* are also listed in the *Delusion* rubric: *separated from the world*. *Anacardium* feel separated and abandoned from the world. *Plutonium nitricum,* in contrast, are not only separated and abandoned from the world, they are also separated from themselves and from their own spirit and soul.

Plutonium nitricum is a homoeopathic remedy derived from plutonium. Plutonium is a radioactive material that is produced in nuclear reactors. It was found to cause lung, liver, and bone cancer in the people who were directly in the fall out area of the atomic bomb testing sites. Trace levels of plutonium can be still be found in the environment from past nuclear bomb tests. The simillimum will not be *Plutonium nitricum* unless the patient feels threatened and destroyed from the inside and from outside themselves. *Plutonium nitricum* are as destructive as the substance plutonium to their own psyche. The abandonment is from within and also from outside themselves. *Plutonium nitricum* don't have *Delusion* rubrics of loss of identity or disassociation rubrics pertaining to psychological Dissociative Disorders. They have rubrics which pertain to *loss of identification with themselves*. The difference might appear subtle however in a psychological framework the difference is marked. Vermeulen in *Synoptic Materia Medica 2* notes: "The prover felt clearly that he changed identity depending on where he was and whom he was with." If one translates that into the *Delusion* rubric: *changing one's identity depending on circumstances*, it could imply Multiple Personality Disorders or Dissociative Disorders. If that rubric was applicable then the remedy *Plutonium nitricum* would be comparable to *Alumina*. *Alumina* have the *Delusion* rubric: *he transferred himself into another and only then he could see*. *Alumina* will transform and morph themselves into *another consciousness*. *Plutonium nitricum* in contrast are *separated* from knowing *who* they are. Their *body is separated from their soul and spirit*, and they are *separated from the world* and *from their body*.

Plutonium nitricum are a constitutional remedy suffering from *destruction of persona* as opposed to a *transformation of a persona* or identity according to circumstances.

It is extremely important when analyzing specific rubrics attached to a remedy that the *exact* wording is correct. If it is not *exact* then there is a tendency to misinterpret the psychological disorder associated with the constitutional remedy. *Plutonium nitricum* are an abandonment remedy. They are lost and *fallen from grace*. They are a *dirty dog trapped in the underworld*; they have lost connection with their soul. Their 'delusions of grandeur' are that they will be lifted out of the dark into the light. *Plutonium nitricum* are abandoned – they have *been walking for years – elbowing their way through the crowds of their past generations*. *Plutonium nitricum* carries the destructive nature of Plutonium within their somatic psyche. The psychosomatic destruction must be evident across all levels – emotionally in their inability to emotionally connect to loved ones, mentally in their confusion, and physically in their inability to be able to maintain their own structure in the world. *Plutonium nitricum* have the *Back* rubric: *weakness of back, standing almost impossible*.

Plutonium nitricum are also threatened from the outside and feel threatened and insecure about their continual existence. *Plutonium nitricum* have the *Mind* rubric: *confusion of mind, lost feeling,* and the *Delusion* rubric: *seeing the earth exploding.* [1] 1. Furthermore, *Plutonium nitricum* have the *Mind* rubrics: *anger internalized, sensation of being detached, withdrawal from reality, indifference to the suffering of others, exalted love of family,* and *unsympathetic to family*. Their anger is internalized. They are detached from themselves. They alternate between *exalted* love for others and family, and indifference, lack of sympathy and withdrawal. *Exalted love* is love which is unrealistically 'hyped-up' and disconnected from real empathic and compassionate connection. Their ability to love is corroded from within. Plutonium, the substance, corrodes and destroys the internal organs. *Plutonium nitricum* have the *Delusion* rubrics: *he is a child and acts like a child* and *he was newly born into the world*. *Olibanum sacrum* are also listed in the *Delusion* rubric: *he was newly born into the world. Olibanum sacrum* believe that they are pure (God) and as yet untouched by the world. In relation to *Olibanum sacrum* I allocated the *Delusion* rubric: *he was newly born into the world* in the *Delusion* rubrics which pertain to communication to God. *Plutonium nitricum,* in contrast, are listed in the *Delusion* rubric: *he was newly born into the world* because they are emotionally retentive and immature (baby-like); they are unable to live emotionally connected to the world. In relation to *Plutonium nitricum,* I have allocated this rubric to the Forsaken section because they are disconnected (abandoned) from an adult or mature ability to love.

The simillimum will not be *Plutonium nitricum* unless the patient displays a marked lack of empathic connection to firstly themselves, as well as to others.

Plutonium nitricum will *put on a mask* and play a role somewhat like an actor will play a role. It is important to note that in playing the role they have not *changed their identity,* they have just conveniently adjusted their personality to match the required role. Underneath and behind the mask, *Plutonium nitricum* have *not changed* their identity or consciousness into another identity. *Plutonium nitricum* have no emotional body left to change it has been destroyed. *Their spirit has separated from their body* – their *soul is separated from their body* and they have no compassion. *Plutonium nitricum* are full of emptiness. *Plutonium nitricum* have the *Mind* rubric: *detached as if observing from the outside.* [1] 1. The difference may appear to be a case of semantics, however when analyzing the psychological delusions and psychological disorders associated with a remedy profile it is crucial to be *exacting* in the interpretation of rubrics.

The homoeopath in a specific case analysis needs to be able to make a distinction between the *destruction* of a *Plutonium nitricum* patient's emotional identity, and personality disorders in which the patient *changes* identity.

1. Denial: *Delusion* rubric: *lifted; she was being*: plut-n. *Delusion* rubric: *dark: balancing with the light*: plut-n. [1] 1. *Delusion* rubric: *visions, has: shadows of light*: plut-n. [1] 1. *Delusion* rubric: *objects; about: shining*: plut-n. *Delusion* rubric: *dancing: revolving, twirling and spiraling dancers; of*: plut-n. [1] 1.

2. Forsaken: *Delusion* rubric: *mask; is behind a mask*: plut-n.[1] 1. *Delusion* rubric: *separated: world; from the*: *he is separated*: plut-n. *Delusion* rubric: *separated: body: spirit had separated from body*: *Plut-n*. *Delusion* rubric: *separated: body: soul; body is separated from*: plut-n. *Delusion* rubric: *hunted, he is*: plut-n. *Delusion* rubric: *past: generations; elbowing way through crowd of past*: plut-n. [1] 1. *Delusion* rubric: *born into the world; he was newly*: plut-n.

3. Causation: *Delusion* rubric: *paradise: lost; the fall from grace*: plut-n. [1] 1. *Delusion* rubric: *dirty: he is*: plut-n. *Delusion* rubric: *dogs: he is a dog*: plut-n. [1] 1.

4. Depression: *Delusion* rubric: *clouds: black cloud enveloped her; a heavy*: plut-n. *Delusion* rubric: *emptiness; of*: plut-n. *Delusion* rubric: *walking: he has been walking: years; for*: plut-n. [1] 1. *Delusion* rubric: *trapped; he is: underworld; in the*: plut-n.

5. Resignation: *Delusion* rubric: *die: waiting to die; being old and*: plut-n. [1] 1. *Delusion* rubric: *body: out of the body*: *Plut-n*.

- *Delusions: abused, being*: Bar-c. cocain. cur. falco-pe. hyos. ign. lyss. pall. puls. *Rhus-g. Staph.*
- *Delusions: laughed at and mocked at; being*: adam. *Aq-mar.* arizon-l. **BAR-C**. des-ac. germ-met. haliae-lc. ign. lac-leo. lach. lyss. nux-v. oci-sa. ph-ac. psor. rhod. sep.
- *Delusions: despised; is*: **ARG-N**. arizon-l. cob. cygn-be. hura hydrog. lac-c. lach. moni. orig-v. *Orig.* phasco-ci. phos. positr. prots-m. pseuts-m. rhod. rhus-g.

Avoidance: The underlying issues behind delusional feelings of having been abused or despised or laughed at, are disproportionate perceptions of real or perceived persecution; this is labeled a 'persecution complex'.

Deflecting responsibility for one's actions and redirecting it on to society in the form of a 'persecution complex' allows one to avoid taking responsibility for what one might be doing to contribute to being despised, or abused.

Alternatively, the patient who believes they will always be despised is suffering from an over-developed 'persecution complex'. In compiling the rubric-repertorisation the homoeopath needs to ask how a patient feels when they are abused by others.

Argentium nitricum fear they will *despised* if they fail. In *Baryta carbonica* the theme would be: *she is laughed at*. In a *Rhus glabra* case the theme of abandonment is about being: *deceived* and *cheated, betrayed* and *attacked, tricked* and *stabbed in the back*. In a *Staphisagria* case the theme of abandonment or the 'persecution complex' would be: *deceived, abused, criticized, persecuted* and *poisoned*.

Argentium nitricum are highly successful but they are always afraid they will lose their success. *Argentium nitricum* fear they will fall from high places and fail – *Delusion* rubric: *everything will fail. Argentium nitricum* have the *Delusion* rubrics: *he could not pass a certain place without falling, he is lost to the world and beyond hope,* and the *wall will crush him. Argentium nitricum* fear they will be trapped and crushed. The underlying psychodynamic energy of feeling *despised* and beyond salvation is found in their feelings of inadequacy which have their emotional origin in the *Delusion* rubrics: *forsaken,* and *he is neglected.*

Argentium nitricum have highly developed feelings of inadequacy which reinforce their fears of failure and rejection. *Argentium nitricum* carry a tremendously heavy feeling that they will only be loved if they have met expectations and succeeded.

This fear of abandonment results in the ritualistic superstitious behaviors that they are well recognized for.

Fear of failure reinforces their sudden anxiety attacks. *Argentium nitricum* have the *Mind* rubric: *undertake nothing, lest it fail*: all failure will result in *Argentium nitricum* feeling they are *lost to the world for salvation, and beyond hope*. *Argentium nitricum* avoid acknowledging they are wrong and despised by others by developing exacting obsessive compulsive superstitions to protect themselves. *Argentium nitricum* have the *Delusion* rubric: *he cannot pass a certain place*. [2] 2.

Illness is viewed as proof of failure, this is why *Argentium nitricum*, similarly to *Arsenicum album* are listed in so many of the rubrics pertaining to anxiety about illness and failure.

1. Denial: *Delusion* rubric: *visions, has*: arg-n. [The visions *Argentium nitricum* have reinforce superstitious doom; the visions are not hubristic visions of success.]

2. Forsaken: *Delusion* rubric: *despised; is*: **ARG-N**. *Delusion* rubric: *appreciated, she is not*: arg-n. *Delusion* rubric: *forsaken; is*: **ARG-N**. *Delusion* rubric: *lost: she is: salvation: for: world, to the, beyond hope*: arg-n. [1] 1. *Delusion* rubric: *home: changed; everything at home has*: arg-n. [1] 1. *Delusion* rubric: *house: crush him; houses on each side would approach and*: arg-n. [1] 1. *Delusion* rubric: *corners: project; corners of the houses: walking in the street; so that he fears he will run against then while*: Arg-n. [2] 1.

3. Causation: NONE. [*Argentium nitricum* have the *Delusion* rubric: *right: doing nothing right; he is*: arg-n. This rubric is usually allocated into Depression. *Argentium nitricum* feel they have failed and sinned because they can doing nothing right.]

4. Depression: *Delusion* rubric: *succeed, he does everything wrong; he cannot*: Arg-n. *Delusion* rubric: *fail, everything will*: Arg-n. *Delusion* rubric: *fail, everything will*: *his understanding*: arg-n. [1] 1. *Delusion* rubric: *world: lost to*

the world, beyond hope; he is: *Arg-n.* [2] 1. *Delusion* rubric: *walls*: *crush him; walls will*: *Arg-n.* [2] 1. [This rubric can pertain to fears of persecution or depression.] *Delusion* rubric: *clouds*: *black clouds enveloped her; a heavy*: arg-n.

5. Resignation: *Delusion* rubric: *sick*: *being*: arg-n. *Delusion* rubric: *disease*: *incurable disease; he has an*: *Arg-n.*

Baryta carbonica: The *Baryta carbonica* (case) in the *Case Companion* to *Homoeopathic Psychiatry* was abandoned in hospital as a child but it was not until very recently, after a long time of taking her constitutional remedy, that she realized her obesity was the tool she used to reinforce societal rejection of her as an 'obese person'. *Baryta carbonica* blame themselves and hate themselves because they believe their *body looks ugly*.

All the psychological delusions of being forsaken and neglected in *Baryta carbonica* are complicated, enmeshed psychological avoidance techniques which become self-fulfilling prophecies of self-inflicted abandonment.

With my *Baryta carbonica* (case), what I am particularly interested in is the patient's delusional stance and how she sets herself up to be repeatedly abandoned because of her obesity. She stays obese so that people will abandon her as her mother and father did when she was young. In the consultation, she tells me: *I need to be overweight to get people to abandon me*; *it is also proof they will abandon me*. This is the *Delusion* rubric: *forsaken*; in particular, the *Delusion* rubric: *being laughed at and mocked*. Although it is true that society rejects obese people, she has used her body as self-fulfilling proof of future abandonment. *Baryta carbonica* are weighted heavily in all the rubrics of being forsaken; I have listed ten of them below in Forsaken.

Baryta carbonica are the only remedy listed in the *Delusion* rubric: *beloved friend is dying*. *Baryta carbonica* fear that everyone they become close to will abandon them.

The world is a particularly unsafe place for *Baryta carbonica*; they have the *Delusion* rubric: *every noise is a cry of fire and she trembles.* [1] 1.

1. Denial: *Delusion* rubric: *fancy, illusions of*: bar-c. [This rubric pertains to idealism. In relation to *Baryta carbonica* it reinforces what they have *not* achieved as distinct from what they *have* achieved.]

2. Forsaken: *Delusion* rubric: *abused, being*: Bar-c. *Delusion* rubric: *laughed at and mocked at*; *being*: **BAR-C**. *Delusion* rubric: *forsaken; is*: bar-c. *Delusion* rubric: *criticized, she is*: *Bar-c. Delusion* rubric: *dying: friend is*; *beloved*: bar-c. [1] 1. *Delusion* rubric: *robbed, is going to be*: bar-c. *Delusion* rubric: *laughed at and mocked at*; *being*: *street*; *whenever she goes into the*: bar-c. [1] 1. *Delusion* rubric: *people*: *seeing people*: *looking at him*: bar-c. *Delusion* rubric: *wrong*: *suffered wrong; he has*: bar-c. *Delusion* rubric: *watched, she is being*: *Bar-c.*

3. Causation: NONE. [*Delusion* rubric: *body*: *ugly; body looks*: bar-c. This rubric is allocated into 'delusions of original sin' because *Baryta carbonica* blame themselves over their looks.]

4. Depression: *Delusion* rubric: *succeed, he does everything wrong; he cannot*: *Bar-c. Delusion* rubric: *walking*: *knees, he walks on his*: *Bar-c. Delusion* rubric: *small*: *body is smaller*: *Bar-c.* [The last two rubrics can be allocated to depression and failure, or resignation to illness and death. They indicate feelings of helplessness or inability to do anything about one's situation.]

5. Resignation: *Delusion* rubric: *die: about to die; one was*: bar-c. *Delusion* rubric: *legs: cut off; legs are*: bar-c. *Delusion* rubric: *sick*: *being*: bar-c. *Delusion* rubric: *walking*: *knees, he walks on his*: *Bar-c. Delusion* rubric: *body*: *ugly; body looks*: bar-c. *Delusion* rubric: *small*: *body is smaller*: *Bar-c.*

Baryta carbonica lack self-confidence to the extent that if they are sick, it adds to their fear of being looked at; therefore they view illness as a threat. *Baryta carbonica* are not listed in any significant 'delusions of grandeur', or 'hubristic denial' rubrics. If you have a patient who is presenting with psychological delusions of denial about their illness the constitutional remedy cannot be *Baryta carbonica.* When sick, *Baryta carbonica* do not fall into psychological denial; they instead collapse into the stages of projected abandonment and self-abandoning predictions of failure and decline. *Baryta carbonica* feel mocked and hopelessly wronged and unable to enact change of any kind – *Delusion* rubric: *walking on his knees.* Their only psychological delusion and perceived sin is that their body looks ugly; hence their fear of ridicule. The *Delusion* rubric: *being laughed and mocked at,* is a self-fulfilling prophecy of self-condemnation and expected abandonment. *Baryta carbonica* feel self-defeated because they feel guilty for their *body looking ugly.* Over-reacting is self-deprecating and self-deluding.

Rhus glabra is one of the remedies in the *Anacardiaceae* family. *Anacardium* have the *Delusion* rubric: *devil; speaking in one ear, prompting to murder and an angel in the other ear, prompting to acts of benevolence. Anacardium* overcompensate for their alternating moods with God-like generosity. The guilt from their reactivity keeps them separate from the world – *Delusion* rubrics: *separated from the world,* and *she was outcast from the world.* They also separate themselves from the world and remain in self-inflicted exile to protect themselves from being criticized and protect themselves, and others, from their reactivity. *Rhus glabra* similarly don't like being criticized. Their mood can alternate from *hatred* of those who have *offended* them to *exalted love* and *desires to be embraced and please. Rhus glabra* are noted for their distaste for society. Their distaste is based on real and perceived issues to do with abandonment. Below are listed ten *Delusion* rubrics of persecution in Forsaken for *Rhus glabra.*

The theme of being forsaken in *Anacardium* is one of being *outcast* and *separated from the world.* In *Rhus glabra* the theme of abandonment is about being *deceived* and *cheated, betrayed* and *attacked, tricked* and *stabbed in the back.*

Rhus glabra have the *Delusion* rubrics: *heart is like a rock* and *hole in his chest.* The psychological 'delusions of persecution' are disproportionately exaggerated within *Rhus glabra. Rhus glabra harden their heart like a rock* to protect themselves from being *stabbed in the back* and *betrayed. Anacardium* have the *Delusion* rubric: *surrounded by enemies.* This delusional, paranoiac feeling of being surrounded by enemies leaves them open to being hypersensitive about all real or perceived criticisms. *Anacardium* consequently over-react when they are criticized. This is why *Anacardium* are listed so prominently in the rubrics for the devil in one ear, and the angel in the other. *Anacardium* have the *Mind* rubric: *antagonism with self. Rhus glabra* similarly have the *Delusion* rubric: *war inside her.*

The profound difference between the two remedy profiles is that *Anacardium* have psychological 'delusions of original sin'; they believe they *are* the devil. *Rhus glabra* have *no Delusion* rubrics of sin.

If *Rhus glabra* had psychological 'delusions of original sin' they would be less likely to have exaggerated delusions of being *deceived* and *cheated, betrayed* and *attacked, tricked* and *stabbed in the back.* Because *Rhus glabra* do not have the exaggerated self-blame of *Anacardium* they are more likely to over-exaggerate their 'persecution complexes' and project these outwards on to society rather than inwards, which is what *Anacardium* tend to do.

Anacardium have intense self-loathing. They align themselves to God to feel worthy – *religious. Rhus glabra* do not have the self-loathing of *Anacardium. Rhus glabra* have the *Delusion* rubric: *authority in his work. Rhus glabra* have strong hubristic belief in *themselves* whereas *Anacardium* believe their hubristic powers come from being under the influence of a higher *superhuman power,* God or the devil. Although *Rhus glabra* have the *Mind* rubrics: *want of self-confidence,* and *anger with himself,* neither of these rubrics have the intensity of self-loathing evident within *Anacardium.*

- *Mind*: *power: sensation of*: rhus-g.
- *Mind*: *betrayed; from being*: rhus-g. [1] 1.
- *Mind*: *ailments from: friendship; deceived*: rhus-g.
- *Mind*: *hatred: persons: abusing him*: rhus-g. [1] 1.
- *Mind*: *kill; desire to*: *offended him; those who*: rhus-g. [1] 1. [Compare *Anac.*]
- *Mind*: *mood: changeable: quickly*: rhus-g. [Compare *Anac.*]
- *Mind*: *desire for: relax; of those she can*: rhus-g. [1] 1.
- *Mind*: *embraces: desire to be embraced*: rhus-g.
- *Mind*: *pleasing: desire to please others*: rhus-g.
- *Mind*: *love: exalted love*: rhus-g.
- *Mind*: *thoughts: stagnation of: examination; during*: rhus-g. [1] 1. [Compare to *Anacardium* who have the Mind rubrics: *fear of failure in exams,* and *anticipation before exams.*]
- *Mind*: *withdrawal: from reality*: rhus-g. [*Delusion* rubric: *separated*: *body*: *soul*; *body is separated from*: Anac. rhus-g.]

1. Denial: *Delusion* rubric: *authority*: *work; in his*: rhus-g. [1] 1. *Delusion* rubric: *floating: air, in*: rhus-g.

2. Forsaken: *Delusion* rubric: *abused, being*: *Rhus-g. Delusion* rubric: *despised; is*: rhus-g. *Delusion* rubric: *betrayed; that she is*: *Rhus-g. Delusion* rubric: *cheated; being*: rhus-g. *Delusion* rubric: *danger, impression of: world is dangerous*: rhus-g. [1] 1. *Delusion* rubric: *injury*: *being injured; is*: rhus-g. *Delusion* rubric: *robbed, is going to be*: rhus-g.

Delusion rubric: *tricked; being*: rhus-g. [1] 1. *Delusion* rubric: *stabbed: back; in the*: rhus-g. [1] 1. *Delusion* rubric: *snakes: in and around her. cobra: stomach; in his*: rhus-g. [1] 1.

3. Causation: NONE.
4. Depression: *Delusion* rubric: *energy: scattered; his energy is*: rhus-g. [1] 1. *Delusion* rubric: *war. inside her.* rhus-g. [1] 1.
5. Resignation: *Delusion* rubric: *heart: rock; is like a*: rhus-g. [1] 1. *Delusion* rubric: *hole: chest; in his*: rhus-g. [1] 1. *Delusion* rubric: *light: is light; he*: rhus-g. *Delusion* rubric: *separated: body: soul; body is separated from*: rhus-g.

Rhus glabra, when they are faced with illness and impending death, choose to disassociate[42] from themselves – *soul separated from body. Anacardium* and *Rhus glabra* are both listed in the same rubric. *Rhus glabra* are not listed in the *Delusion* rubric: *he is separated from the world*, nor in the *Delusion rubric*: *spirit has separated from the body; Anacardium* are listed in both.

Rhus glabra dissociate *from themselves* not the world; *Anacardium* dissociate from themselves *and* the world.

Anacardium also give their spirit to God or the devil; *Rhus glabra* do not have religious 'hubristic denial'. Dissociation is a normal response to the trauma of facing one's illness. If the patient dissociates and allows themselves space [*Delusion* rubric: *floating in air*] their mind is able to distance themselves from the feelings which are overwhelming them. *Rhus glabra* are sensitive, they are the only remedy listed in the *Mind* rubric: *desire for company of those she can relax. Rhus glabra* are much more sensitive [*cowardice*] and vulnerable than *Anacardium*. They do not have 'God on their side', they need to dissociate as soon as their *authority* is threatened.

Illness undermines *Rhus glabra* because they have no God-like or devil-like authority over their illness; this is why they need to dissociate from being sick.

Staphisagria exaggerate real and/or perceived insults. The numerous rubrics below all attest to the fact that they are overwhelmed with 'delusions of persecution'. Psychological 'delusions of grandeur' or 'hubristic denial' are developed within the psyche to protect vulnerability. *Staphisagria* have overwhelming paranoiac feelings of being *deceived, abused, criticized, persecuted, poisoned* and *starved*. *Staphisagria* have numerous *Mind* rubrics: *ailments from indignation, with mortification* [4] 1., *fear about his social position, fear of losing self-control* and *egotism speaking about themselves in company* – which allude to their need to protect their *great* position. *Staphisagria* also have the *Mind* rubric: *scrupulous practices as to their religious salvation.* For all their greatness and egotism *Staphisagria* are prone to paranoiac 'delusions of persecution', especially when they are sick. *Staphisagria* have the *Mind* rubric: *fear of his own shadow.* When *Staphisagria* are sick they sink into feelings of deprivation – *Delusion* rubrics: *unfortunate, legs go from under him* [1] 1., and *he will lose his fortune. Staphisagria* are well known for their violent outbursts of passionate anger[43].

Staphisagria are listed as a grading of four in all the *Mind* rubrics: *ailments from anger*, and *ailments from anger with indignation.* The patient suffering from a 'persecution complex' justifies their actions and violent reactions because they presume the world is directing hostility towards them.

A 'persecution complex' can become a self-fulfilling prophecy because one is more likely to be rejected and criticized if one is angry and reactive. *Staphisagria* are caught in a cycle of persecutory abuse: the *Staphisagria* patient who feels wrongly abused becomes an abuser to defend themselves, and then often becomes the one who is abused for their abusive behavior. *Staphisagria* are self-punishing when they have reacted inappropriately: *he has neglected his duty*. *Staphisagria* disproportionately exaggerate their 'original sin'; it is this disproportionate self-blame which in turns feeds into their 'persecution complexes'. *Staphisagria* believe they *have committed a crime* and that *someone will come up from behind* to *persecute* and *murder* them. The persecutory underside of *Staphisagria* is often not emphasized in the Materia medica. After completing the rubric-repertorisation process below, I saw why *Staphisagria* need approval.

When *Staphisagria* are ill they become very insecure and they are easily overwhelmed by their own persecutory damnation.

1. Denial: *Delusion* rubric: *body: greatness of, as to*: staph. *Delusion* rubric: *humility and lowness of others; while he is great*: staph. *Delusion* rubric: *enlarged: tall; he is very*: staph.

2. Forsaken: *Delusion* rubric: *abused, being: Staph. Delusion* rubric: *deceived; being: Staph. Delusion* rubric: *criticized, she is*: staph. *Delusion* rubric: *disgraced: she is*: staph. *Delusion* rubric: *insulted, he is*: staph. *Delusion* rubric: *persecuted: he is persecuted*: staph. *Delusion* rubric: *persecuted: he is persecuted: backwards; and looks*: staph. [1] 1. *Delusion* rubric: *pursued; he was*: staph. *Delusion* rubric: *poisoned: he: has been*: staph. *Delusion* rubric: *people: behind him; someone is: coming up behind*: staph. *Delusion* rubric: *murdered: will be murdered; he*: staph.

3. Causation: *Delusion* rubric: *crime: committed a crime; he had*: staph. *Delusion* rubric: *neglected: duty; he has neglected his*: staph.

4. Depression: *Delusion* rubric: *unfortunate, he is: Staph. Delusion* rubric: *starve, family will*: staph. *Delusion* rubric: *fortune, he was going to lose his*: staph. *Delusion* rubric: *happened; something has: Staph. Delusion* rubric: *legs: go from under him; legs would*: staph. [1] 1. [This rubric pertains to the inability to cope with failure.] *Delusion* rubric:

wife: *run away from him; wife will*: staph. [1] 1.

5. Resignation: *Delusion* rubric: *sick*: *being*: *Staph*. *Delusion* rubric: *falling*: *backwards*: staph.

- *Delusions*: *misunderstood; she is*: brass-n-o. germ-met. limest-b. olib-sac. *Propr.* rad-br. sal-fr.

- *Delusion*: *appreciated, she is not*: acer-circ. *Aids. Androc.* arg-n. arge-pl. aur. caps. *Carc.* cygn-be. limest-b. musca-d. *Pall.* plat. polys. positr. puls. pycnop-sa. rad-br. seq-s. sulph. *Thuj.* urol-h.

Self deluding: Exaggerated psychological delusions of feeling misunderstood are a less severe form of 'persecution complex'.

The delusion behind the need to continue to believe that you are misunderstood is usually based on avoiding acknowledging the necessity of 'self-actualization'.

The patient who continues to blame their lack of success in life on others not understanding them needs to maintain the 'persecution complex' for a specific reason. The role of the homoeopath is to understand the *peculiar* reason behind the exaggerated feelings of perceived abandonment within each remedy profile in these rubrics. If the patient hangs on to the belief that they are misunderstood or not appreciated then it allows them to deflect blame from themselves. These *Delusion* rubrics should be considered when the patient blames their lack of recognition on others. These *Delusion* rubrics should also be considered when the patient uses rejection as an excuse to justify why they have not managed to be successful. 'Self-actualization' requires that the patient not abandon faith in themselves.

Limestone Burren is a homoeopathic remedy derived from limestone. Limestone is partially soluble, therefore it forms many eroded landforms and gorges. These include Burren in Co. Clare, Ireland which was the source of the limestone for the proving. Limestone is very reactive to acid solutions.

Many limestone statues suffer from severe damage due to acid rain. Within the remedy profile of *Limestone* is the same theme of somatic solubility and vulnerability. *Limestone* abandon themselves and feel they have been abandoned by others.

Limestone have the *Delusion* rubric: *had lost their ego.* [1] 1. *Limestone* have the *Delusion* rubric: *he is away from home* and the *Mind* rubrics: *estranged from society* and *estranged from his family.* When sick *Limestone* feel threatened and fear they will *disappear*. Lack of faith in personal success [*they have lost their ego*] is the underlying psychodynamic crisis behind the lack of 'self-actualization' in *Limestone*.

The need to maintain their social appearance is heightened because inherent in their somatic nature is evidence of destruction. *Limestone* have the *Delusion* rubrics: *she looks wretched when looking in a mirror,* and *others will observe her confusion.* The simillimum will only be *Limestone* if the patient needs to create an illusion that they are not sick.

Limestone will not acknowledge sickness because they don't want to face the reality that they are penetrable. *Limestone* need to maintain their belief that their *body is enlarged* to protect themselves from *disappearing* [*thinning*].

Limestone display an inconsistency between their hubristic 'delusions of grandeur' (in which they are *enlarged* like a great gorge), and their 'delusions of hypochondria' (in which they are *thinning* and vulnerable to destruction from the environment). Inherent in their somatic memory is the fear that they will *disappear* all together just as the great Sphinx in Egypt is disappearing. The *Delusion* rubrics: *she is misunderstood, she is not appreciated,* and *she will disappear* highlight their vulnerability. Illness is difficult for *Limestone* because illness is a material reality which they can't escape. Illness confronts their belief in unreal fancies; illness destroys their delusional believe that their *body is enlarged* and impenetrable. *Limestone* need to be admired and recognized. *Limestone* need to continue to believe they have been *misunderstood.* The perception that they are *misunderstood* and *not appreciated* by others allows *Limestone* to avoid 'self-actualization'. *Limestone* uses rejection from the world and their family in particular as an excuse to justify why they have not managed to be successful. *Limestone* blames their lack of recognition on others. Illness creates an interesting dilemma for *Limestone*. On the one hand, they receive attention when they are sick, (especially if it is a destructive disease which it is quite often with *Limestone*) and on the other hand, the disease creates a conflict. *Limestone* wish to hide the disease from themselves and others, which is often hard to do, especially if it is a destructive disease. *Limestone* have the *Delusion* rubric: *others will observe their confusion*.

Illness can allow *Limestone* an 'out' from having to prove they are successful.

Cure from the simillimum comes in *Limestone* being able to realistically assess reality without needing to create an unreal fanciful illusion or without needing to maintain their illness to avoid feelings of failure (having *lost their ego*). Cure in a *Limestone* case is when the patient doesn't rely on worldly recognition to maintain their 'ego' strength. The organized *realistic* part of the psyche is the 'ego'. If a remedy profile has a weakened 'ego' then their ability to perceive reality is under threat. No-one likes to be criticized. The role of the homoeopath is to identify the patient's *peculiar* response to criticism. *Limestone* feel eroded by criticism, they feel as if the criticism penetrates deep within their psyche and it is destroying the fabric of their whole structure [*ego*]. *Limestone* view illness as proof of failure. *Limestone* need to hide their illness to protect themselves from others' criticism.

When *Limestone* are ill they feel *trapped* and *enslaved* by their body and illness, and they feel *enslaved* by the person who is looking after them. *Limestone* escape the reality of their destruction by creating an illusion that their illness does not exist.

The simillimum will only be *Limestone* if the patient needs to create an illusion that their illness is not real. *Limestone* will literally say in a consultation that their illness is not real and that life as we see, and know it, *is not real.*

Limestone have the *Mind* rubric: *cannot tell what is unreal and what is real.* [1] 1. *Limestone* have the *Delusion* rubric: *everything seems unreal.* *Limestone* when sick need to create another [*unreal*] perception of their life and their illness. *Limestone* have the *Mind* rubrics: *absorbed in fancies* and *attempts to escape,* and the *Delusion* rubric: *body is lighter than air.*

On one hand they need to maintain the appearance or illusion they are well, and on the other hand they need to hide their illness because they are unable to cope with others' grief. *Limestone* have the *Mind* rubrics: *horrible things and sad stories affect her profoundly* and *weeping from thought of other's grief at her death.* [1] 1. *Limestone* have no ordinary defense mechanisms which are able to protect themselves from others' emotions. The simillimum will only be *Limestone* if the patient indicates that they are highly sensitive to others' emotions. *Limestone* feel as if *they* will *disappear* when others around them are negative or depressed.

The 'never-well-since-event' underpinning their belief in self-punishment is formulated around the perception that they believe they have, and will continue to, inflict injuries on others. *Limestone* have the *Delusion* rubric: *about to inflict injury on someone.* [1] 1. *Limestone* will hide their illness because they believe that, by doing so, they are protecting others from the reality of their illness. *Limestone* have the *Delusion* rubric: *she is poisoning people.*

Limestone believe that they have a corrosive effect on others around them.

1. Denial: *Delusion* rubric: *enlarged*: limest-b. *Delusion* rubric: *enlarged*: *body is*: *parts of body*: limest-b. *Delusion* rubric:

enlarged: *body is*: limest-b. *Delusion* rubric: *tall*: *he or she is tall*: limest-b. *Delusion* rubric: *body*: *lighter than air; body is*: limest-b. *Delusion* rubric: *unreal*: *everything seems unreal*: limest-b. [This rubric pertains to the need to create an illusion.] *Delusion* rubric: *boat*: *owns a boat; he/she*: limest-b. [1] 1. [*Limestone* need to believe they can float on water and escape their susceptibility to water (acid rain) corroding their psyche. They have a few *Delusion* rubrics about boats and seeing ships because they feel like they are drowning in water when they are sick.]

2. Forsaken: *Delusion* rubric: *misunderstood; she is*: limest-b. *Delusion* rubric: *appreciated, she is not*: limest-b. *Delusion* rubric: *home*: *away from home; he is*: limest-b. *Delusion* rubric: *forsaken; is*: limest-b. *Delusion* rubric: *disappear; she will*: limest-b. [1] 1. [This rubric pertains to self-abandonment or lack of self-confidence.]

3. Causation: *Delusion* rubric: *dirty*: *he is*: limest-b. *Delusion* rubric: *injury*: *someone; is about to inflict injury on*: limest-b. [1] 1. *Delusion* rubric: *poisoning people, she is*: limest-b.

4. Depression: *Delusion* rubric: *trapped; he is*: limest-b. *Delusion* rubric: *ego; had lost their*: limest-b. [1] 1. *Delusion* rubric: *enslaved; he is*: limest-b. [1] 1. *Delusion* rubric: *unreal*: *everything seems unreal*: limest-b. [This rubric reiterates how much *Limestone* struggle with holding on to their thoughts.] *Delusion* rubric: *confusion; others will observe her*: limest-b. *Delusion* rubric: *water*: *under water; he is*: limest-b. [This rubric indicates penetrability.]

5. Resignation: *Delusion* rubric: *thin*: *he is getting*: limest-b. *Delusion* rubric: *body*: *lighter than air; body is*: limest-b. [This rubric can pertain to 'delusions of grandeur' or 'delusions of hypochondria'.]

- *Delusions*: *body*: *one with his body*: *is; world*: *and at odds with the*: *positr.*[1] 1.

Avoidance: *Positronium* need to abandon the world, and in turn be rejected by the world in order to feel strong in their body.

Positronium is a homoeopathic remedy prepared[44] from Positronium which is a short-lived atomic system formed of an electron and a positron before they interact to annihilate each other. Positronium (Ps) is a system consisting of an electron and its anti-particle, a positron, bound together into an "exotic atom". The orbit of the two particles and the set of energy levels is similar to that of the hydrogen atom (electron and proton).

Positronium have a battle between matter and anti-matter. On the one hand *Positronium* have the *Delusion* rubric: *sees the completeness of its inner structure body.* [1] 1. This is a rubric which emphasizes structure and clarity. On the other hand *Positronium* have the *Delusion* rubric: *body is torn to pieces.* This is a rubric which emphasizes decay.

The same theme of not caring, or abandonment of the self, is evident in the *Delusion* rubric: *he is evil and doesn't care. Positronium* are in conflict over matter and anti-matter; over substance (matter) and lack of substance (anti-matter). *Positronium* have the *Delusion* rubric: *she cannot bend,* and the *Delusion* rubric: *hypnotized.* On the one hand, *Positronium* hang on to their structure; *Delusion* rubric: *a stone statue,* and on the other hand they let it go; *body torn to pieces. Positronium* are disturbingly fatalistic when sick: *about to die.* In fact, there is a relishing of destruction and embracing of death's final decay of matter. *Positronium* have the *Delusion* rubric: *final acceptance of being slaughtered like something innocent.* The theme of *Positronium* is weight and structure, versus isolation, indifference and final decay[45]. Their hubristic grandeur builds [*building stones*] structure while at the same time everything is *decayed, tarnished and impure.* Their abandonment is within and from outside themselves, "compression and oppression[46]".

What is most relevant to note with *Positronium* is that when sick, they are strangely fatalistic about their destruction. *Positronium* have the *Delusion* rubric: *God's works are ill made and ill done* as well as the above *Delusion* rubric: *one with his body, at odds with the world.*

Positronium enjoy the self-abandonment of illness. *Positronium* have the *Delusion* rubric: *she is squeezed dry in the devil's fist* [1] 1.

The self-abandoning depression in *Positronium* is particularly notable. This is discussed further in the chapter on Causation because the theme of self-abandonment is reinforced in the *Delusion* rubric: *he is evil and doesn't care.* The simillimum will only be *Positronium* if the patient has a similar need to maintain self-persecution, and perpetuate persecution from others. When *Positronium* feel abandoned by the world they feel powerful in their body. *Positronium* needs to build structure in their lives and they need to destroy structure in their lives. There is an Argentine crime fiction TV series called *Epitafios,* (English: Epitaphs). The character of the woman detective Marina (portrayed by Cecilia Roth), is a portrayal of *Positronium*. Her character has two obsessions: one is building structures out of playing cards, the other is playing Russian Roulette for money with live bullets. The simillimum will not be *Positronium* unless the patient *needs* to challenge life and death. The simillimum will only be *Positronium* if the patient feels stronger when they are faced with destruction and abandonment.

1. Denial: *Delusion* rubric: *ancestors*: *one with her ancestors; she is* positr. [1] 1. *Delusion* rubric: *value, she is*: positr. [1] 1. *Delusion rubric*: *gifts*; *she is showered with*: positr. [1] 1. *Delusion rubric*: *beautiful*: positr. *Delusion rubric*: *building stones, appearance of*: positr.

2. Forsaken: *Delusion* rubric: *body*: *one with his body*: *is; world*: *and at odds with the*: positr.[1] 1. *Delusion* rubric: *friendless, he is*: positr. *Delusion* rubric: *appreciated, she is*

not: positr. *Delusion* rubric: *attacked; being*: positr. *Delusion* rubric: *despised; is*: positr. *Delusion* rubric: *forsaken; is*: positr. *Delusion* rubric: *neglected*: *he or she is neglected*: positr. *Delusion* rubric: *murdered*: *will be murdered*; *he*: positr.

3. Causation: *Delusion* rubric: *evil*: *he is evil and does not care*: positr. [1] 1. *Delusion* rubric: *God*: *God's works are ill made and ill done*: positr. [1] 1.

4. Depression: *Delusion* rubric: *crushed*: *she is*: positr. *Delusion* rubric: *devil*: *squeezed dry in the devil's fist; she is*: positr. [1] 1. *Delusion* rubric: *oppressed; he were*: positr.

5. Resignation: *Delusion* rubric: *die*: *about to die one was*: positr. *Delusion* rubric: *decayed, tarnished and impure; everything is*: positr. [1] 1. *Delusion* rubric: *diminished*: *shrunken, parts are*: positr.

- *Delusions: alone: being: always alone; she is*: chir-fl *Lac-h*. petr-ra. **PULS**. stram.

- *Delusions: alone: being: belong to anyone; she did not*: puls. [1] 1.

- *Delusions: alone: being: world; alone in the*: Androc. bamb-a. camph. choc. cycl. germ-met. hura. irid-met. *Kola*. *Lac-h*. moni. *Plat*. *Puls*. tax-br.

Avoidance: Exaggerated feelings of aloneness can be a deliberate stance which is maintained by the patient to justify how needy they feel so they can continue to seek more attention and reassurance. On the other hand, it can also be an indication of over-exaggerated or disproportionate feelings of abandonment. Psychologically, the essential premise will be constructed differently for each remedy profile.

The key to understanding these *Delusion* rubrics is to ask the patient what happens if they are alone. Their answer will explain why their *particular* constitutional remedy profile needs to seek attention or reassurance.

Alternatively, their answer may also reveal extreme paranoia. A person who believes they have been rejected by society [*alone*], may have *disproportionate* feelings of abandonment; this is labeled a 'persecution complex'. Concentrating on feeling abandoned is often used psychologically to avoid taking responsibility for 'wrongs' committed. These crimes or sins more than likely may have caused the societal rejection in the first place, but instead of taking responsibility a person can project their feelings of persecution on to society. Each remedy profile follows the five psychological processes listed below. 'Delusions of original sin' perpetuate self-isolation. If the patient *continues to stay alone* or if they maintain the situation of being alone, then it is more than likely that the patient has an exaggerated, disproportionate feeling of being 'evil' or having committed 'wrongs'. Alternatively a patient will maintain their feeling of rejection to avoid facing their contribution ('original sins'), to their real or perceived feelings of abandonment. Once their 'wrongs' are acknowledged, a patient will display disproportionate, depressive reactions to their 'crimes'. Once depressive predictions of predetermined doom have descended upon the patient, they will sink into exaggerated hypochondria about their illness.

The reason for re-emphasizing the psychological stages is that it may help explain why a patient will maintain feelings of persecution and abandonment and why they will continue to maintain their psychological delusions of being alone. If the patient lets their feelings of being wrongly abandoned go, then they will have to face their own fears about themselves and their potential fate.

Below, I analyze the reactions of *Lac humanum,* a human mammal remedy profile; *Pulsatilla,* a plant remedy profile; and *Androctonus,* a spider remedy profile, in relation to the same *Delusion* rubrics of being alone. According to their nature, each constitutional remedy profile will react differently to the dilemma of being alone in the world. *Lac humanum* deals with the separation by over-mothering humanity. If your patient feels alone and separated from others and yet continues to care for others, then the simillimum could well be *Lac humanum. Pulsatilla* as a plant remedy profile feel alone and defenseless to the environment. If your patient feels sensitive and unprotected when they are left alone, then the simillimum could well be *Pulsatilla*. *Androctonus,* on the other hand, enjoy being alone because it strengthens their chance of survival. If your patient is needy of reassurance and comfort when they are sick, then the simillimum is *not Androctonus. Androctonus* are strategically strengthened by being alone.

Lac humanum: In my *Lac humanum* (case) in the *Case Companion* to *Homoeopathic Psychiatry* the patient needs to maintain her feelings of aloneness and being abandoned because they protect her from her overwhelmingly disproportionate feelings of guilt for not being able to save her sister in their last life together. The *Lac humanum* patient relays a past life story told to her by her clairvoyant guide and teacher. They were sisters in the second World War; their parents were arrested by the Nazis and they were left to fend for themselves. Her older sister died in her arms, and she died next. *I was not able to save her* (sister) *and take away her death. In this life my journey is to share in her* (sister's) *pain and help save her life.* She describes herself: *I am currently exhausted, my baby is sucking my life from me, and I cannot relate to him* (baby) *anymore, I feel nothing. I have no love to share with him* (baby) *or my husband; I feel nothing. I remember making a conscious decision to become my mother's friend and counsellor. I sacrificed myself to help her; she needed me; she would talk to me for hours, and unburden her heart to me. I now do that to my baby, and he* (baby) *is sucking the life out of me. I am here and my journey in this life is to save my sister's life, and to save my mother's life; to complete the Karmic lesson from the last life; to give myself. I am still there for my mother – now she shares all her burdens with me. I have nothing but hate for my father, and his lack of love and support for us.* She finds her husband irritating because he does not understand the support she needs with the baby. *He has no idea how it is for me*; (cries) *I am alone with my baby.* This *Lac humanum* patient alternates between martyring herself to save her mother and sister, and feelings of bewilderment as to why she has been abandoned and left alone with her baby. Her abandonment is reminiscent of Jesus declaring on the cross; *father my God why have you abandoned me*? This *Lac humanum* patient is trying to resolve her guilt by continuing to martyr herself. Her course of action is a self-fulfilling prophecy. The more she martyrs herself by looking after her mother, her sister, her husband and her baby, the less likely it is that she will receive the attention and care she needs as a new mother left alone with a baby. It is her 'duty' and 'fate' in this life to look after them and save them because she failed in her last life; this is the 'original sin'. *Lac humanum* has an inner conflict between living as a self-determined individual in a group and feeling beholden to the group. The theme in the remedy profile of *Lac humanum* is the group versus self. When the *Lac humanum* patient explains that she decided to abandon herself to looking after her mother because it was an act of love, she says: *I sacrificed myself to help her; she needed me. She would talk to me for hours, and unburden her heart to me. I love her dearly and I did it with love but it was at a cost; I know that now.* This reflects the importance of the group versus her self-importance. It also explains another crucial aspect of *Lac humanum*. *Lac humanum* have one rubric of grandeur, the *Delusion* rubric: *he was newly born into the world*. *Lac humanum* are the 'milk of human kindness'.

They have sacrificed themselves so that life will continue. *Lac humanum* are the only remedy listed in the *Delusion* rubric: *as if she is nesting*. *Lac humanum* are the savior and the mother and nurturer of the human race.

Lac humanum also have the *Mind* rubric: *Oedipus complex*[47]. *Lac humanum* will always develop an overprotective, symbiotic relationship with one parent, and a hate relationship with the other. *Lac humanum* project on to the parent whom they hate, all their psychological 'delusions of persecution'. *Lac humanum* will be convinced that the parent whom they hate is injurious to them and the rest of the family. In my *Lac humanum* (case) the woman says: *I have nothing but hate for my father, and his lack of love and support for us*. *Lac humanum* always equate all abandonment with *injury*, this is why the list of abandonment rubrics below are a mixture of being *alone*, *friendless* and *neglected* as well as being *poisoned* and about to receive *injury*. This association relates to the fact that they are *newly born to the world*; a baby themselves who needs to be protected. They will always hate the parent who has abandoned them, and they will always encourage a symbiotic love/mothering/ oedipal relationship with the other parent. It is possible to see the co-dependent symbiosis of an 'Oedipus complex' when the *Lac humanum* patient says of her relationship with her mother: *I sacrificed myself to help her; she needed me. She would talk to me for hours, and unburden her heart to me.*

Lac humanum continue to stay alone and maintain the situation of being alone, because they have exaggerated and disproportionate feelings of having committed 'wrongs'. Once *Lac humanum* acknowledge all 'wrongs' they sink into disproportionate depressive reactions to their 'crimes'.

Lac humanum have disproportionate feelings of being *worthless*. Saving humanity is more important than saving themselves. *Lac humanum* have the *Mind* rubric: *detached from ego*. [1] 1.

Lac humanum justify their predetermined martyrdom and self-actualized abandonment because they are *too ugly and fat* to be worthy of individualization. When *Lac humanum* are sick they question whether they are worthy enough to save. A *Lac humanum* patient will more than likely quibble over the cost of the consultation because they feel unworthy of spending the money on *their* welfare rather than their families. *Lac humanum* have the *Delusion* rubric: *face distorted*, as well as the *Delusion* rubric: *body looks fat and ugly*. *Lac humanum* have the *Mind* rubric: *anxiety about food*. [1] 1. *Lac humanum* believe that when they are sick they are too *ugly, fat* and *distorted* to be included in the human family. *Lac humanum* also have the *Mind* rubric: *aversion to being watched.* [1] 1. They will feel *unwanted by friends, alone,* and *friendless. Lac humanum* deals with the separation by over-mothering humanity. If your patient feels alone and separated from others and yet continues to care for others, then the simillimum could well be *Lac humanum.*

Lac humanum perpetuate being alone and abandoned because they struggle to ask for help in their lives.

1. Denial: *Delusion* rubric: *born into the world; he was newly*: lac-h.

2. Forsaken: *Delusion* rubric: *alone: being: always alone; she is: Lac-h. Delusion* rubric: *body: ugly; body looks: fat; too*: lac-h. *Delusion* rubric: *betrayed; that she is*: lac-h. *Delusion* rubric: *friend: unwanted by friends: Lac-h.* [2] 1. *Delusion* rubric: *friendless, he is*: lac-h. *Delusion* rubric: *neglected: he or she is neglected: Lac-h. Delusion* rubric: *poisoned: he has been*: lac-h. *Delusion* rubric: *violence, about*: lac-h. *Delusion* rubric: *injury: about to receive injury; is*: lac-h.

3. Causation: *Delusion* rubric: *crime: committed a crime*; *he had*: lac-h. *Delusion* rubric: *wrong: done wrong; he has*: lac-h.

4. Depression: *Delusion* rubric: *worthless; he is*: lac-h. *Delusion* rubric: *unreal: everything seems unreal*: lac-h. *Delusion* rubric: *body: ugly; body looks: fat; too*: lac-h. [This rubric pertains to being depressed with oneself or self-rejection.]

5. Resignation: *Delusion* rubric: *face: distorted*: lac-h. [1] 1.

Pulsatilla are noted for their jealousy, their tearfulness and their neediness for reassurance. *Pulsatilla* have inconsistencies between their 'hubristic denial' [*they are well*] and hypochondriac, psychological delusions that they are *sick*.

Pulsatilla over-exaggerate feelings of aloneness to justify how needy they feel so they can continue to receive more attention and reassurance.

The abandonment theme in *Pulsatilla* is that everything will be taken away from them; they will even be taken *away from their home*. *Pulsatilla* feel justifiably distraught and obsessively jealous because they are convinced that there are *conspiracies* against them. Their heightened fear of conspiracies are perceived as coming from outside, and from within their own body. *Pulsatilla* are fearful of their own body abandoning them. The following *Mind* rubrics indicate the intensity of their hypochondria. *Pulsatilla* are distraught when they are sick; their perversity and need to be capricious are reflected in the *Mind* rubrics: *feigning sickness* and conversely, *when sick says he is well*. The key to understanding the *Delusion* rubrics of conspiratorial abandonment for *Pulsatilla* is to understand what happens when they are alone. *Pulsatilla* suffer from extreme paranoia about their own survival when they are alone. *Pulsatilla* have the *Delusion* rubrics: *religious* and *will be taken by the devil*. Their fanaticism about religious matters is in direct proportion to their fear of being taken by the *devil* and illness when, and if, they are alone. Underpinning their internal insecurity is an overwhelming fear of *emptiness*. *Pulsatilla* have the *Delusion* rubric: *of emptiness*. [3]. *Pulsatilla* need company to avoid having to face their own internal void.

Pulsatilla need possessions to avoid having to face their own internal void. *Pulsatilla* significantly, need the company of sickness to avoid the emptiness. *Pulsatilla* have the *Delusion* rubric: *being sick*. [3].

If the homoeopath working with a *Pulsatilla* patient doesn't fully appreciate the need they have to maintain their hypochondriacal delusions then *Pulsatilla* will be left feeling distraught. If the *Pulsatilla* patient is stripped of their belief in themselves being sick then they are overcome with fear of being alone and defenseless. The capricious perversity demonstrated by *Pulsatilla* in relation to *feigning sickness,* or *saying they are well when they are sick* are attention seeking techniques which are maintained to insure they will never be left alone. *Pulsatilla* believes that they need illness to feel secure. The homoeopath working with a *Pulsatilla* patient should not confront them over their need for illness.

Pulsatilla have numerous conspiracy rubrics listed below. *Pulsatilla* have the potential to feel persecuted by everything: *devils, dogs, cats, bees* and *specters* and *ghosts.*

- *Delusions: black: objects and people, sees*: puls.
- *Delusions: bed: someone: in the bed; as if someone is: with him: Puls.*
- *Delusions: bees; sees*: puls.
- *Delusions: cats: sees: black*: puls.
- *Delusions: criminals, about*: puls.
- *Delusions: devil: sees: Puls.*
- *Delusions: devil: taken by the devil; he will be: Puls.*
- *Delusions: die: about to die; one was*: puls.
- *Delusions: dogs: sees*: puls.
- *Delusions: doomed, being*: puls.
- *Delusions: enemy: everyone is an*: puls.
- *Delusions: fire: world is on*: puls.
- *Delusions: fire: visions, of: Puls.*
- *Delusions: images, phantoms; sees: black*: puls.
- *Delusions: people: seeing people: Puls.*
- *Delusions: poisoned: he: has been*: puls.
- *Delusions: strangers: surrounded by: Puls.*
- *Delusions: specters, ghosts, spirits: seeing*: puls.
- *Delusions: women: evil and will injure his soul; women are*: puls. [1] 1.

Pulsatilla have the following *Mind* rubrics which highlight their teary and emotionally needy nature:

- *Mind: ailments from: jealousy:* **PULS**.
- *Mind: carried: desire to be carried: caressed; and: Puls.*
- *Mind: weeping: desire to weep: all the time: Puls.*
- *Mind: anxiety: hypochondriacal: read books; mania to: medical books: Puls.*
- *Mind: feigning: sick; to be: Puls.*
- *Mind: well: says he is well: sick; when very:* **PULS**.
- *Mind: weeping: telling: sickness; when telling of her:* **PULS**.

1. Denial: *Delusion* rubric: *well, he is*: puls. *Delusion* rubric: *religious: Puls.*

2. Forsaken: *Delusion* rubric: *alone, being: belong to anyone; she did not:* puls. [1] 1. *Delusion* rubric: *alone: being: always alone; she is:* **PULS**. *Delusion* rubric: *alone: being: world; alone in the: Puls. Delusion* rubric: *appreciated, she is not:* puls. *Delusion* rubric: *conspiracies: against him; there are conspiracies:* puls. *Delusion* rubric: *forsaken; is:* **PULS**. *Delusion* rubric: *home: away from home; he is:* puls.

3. Causation: *Delusion* rubric: *sinned; one has: day of grace; sinned away his:* puls.

4. Depression: *Delusion* rubric: *clouds: black cloud enveloped her; a heavy:* puls. *Delusion* rubric: *ruined: will be ruined; he:* puls. [1] 1. *Delusion* rubric: *emptiness; of:* **PULS**.

5. Resignation: *Delusion* rubric: *sick, being:* **PULS**.

Androctonus is a homoeopathic remedy derived from a scorpion. Scorpions need to be manipulative and cunning in order to be able to survive. They need to know how to trap and they also need to be very calculative about their own safety. *Androctonus* are extremely suspicious and have numerous 'persecution complexes'.

Spider remedy profiles have numerous paranoid 'delusions of persecution' which keep them on their guard against potential attackers, as well as on the lookout for prey.

Androctonus have a keynote rubric of grandeur; the *Delusion* rubric: *he was again an adolescent*. With assured adolescent omnipotence, and no *Delusion* rubrics of having committed sins, *Androctonus* are able to delude themselves about their strength. Because *Androctonus* have no rubrics pertaining to sins committed they have nothing to stop them from following their tunnel vision of 'attack and destroy'. *Androctonus* have the *Delusion* rubric: *views the world through a hole*. [1] 1. *Androctonus* have the *Mind* rubric: *want of moral feeling*. *Androctonus* have the capacity to deflect and deny feelings of guilt. They can immediately convince themselves that they are some other person and not the person who is being cunning and malicious. *Androctonus* have the 'hubristic denial' *Delusion* rubric: *she is some other person*. *Androctonus* also have the *Mind* rubric: *malicious desire to injure someone*. The remedy profile of *Androctonus* is consistent with the theme of a scorpion; they are expert at stalking their prey. *Androctonus* have the *Mind* rubric: *mocking sarcasm with great intuition concerning other people's weaknesses*. *Androctonus* have numerous persecution and abandonment *Delusion* rubrics but because they also have so many Denial rubrics of grandeur they are able to survive with their omnipotent adolescent ego intact. Their 'delusions of grandeur' are further enhanced by the fact that they have no *Delusion* rubrics of illness or death.

Androctonus will never admit to destruction from an illness.

The last psychological stage in the *Delusion* rubrics repertorisation is Resignation. Resignation means uncomplaining *endurance,* or *exaggerated* acceptance of defeat. *Androctonus* will never sink into any resignation of disease and death. *Androctonus* have the ability to pretend they are another person; *never* admit defeat. If the remedy profile has numerous 'hubristic denial' rubrics and no rubrics of *disease* and *death* then they are able to convince themselves that they will not be destroyed by whatever illness they have.

> If your patient is supremely confident about their survival, blames all attacks on the outer world, and has no sense of self-blame for their illness, then the remedy could well be *Androctonus*. *Androctonus* enjoy being alone because it strengthens their chance of survival. If your patient is needy of reassurance and comfort when they are sick then the simillimum is not *Androctonus*.

1. Denial: *Delusion* rubric: *strong; he is*: androc. *Delusion* rubric: *adolescent; he was again an*: androc. [1] 1. *Delusion* rubric: *objects; about: colored; brilliantly*: androc. *Delusion* rubric: *alone, being: world; alone in the*: *Androc.* [This rubric is normally an abandonment rubric but for *Androctonus* it can be allocated into 'delusions of grandeur'. *Androctonus* enjoys being alone because it strengthens their chance of survival.] *Delusion* rubric: *person: other person; she is some*: androc. [This rubric is normally associated with loss of identity. In relation to *Androctonus* it can be allocated into 'delusions of grandeur' because it reinforces subterfuge and camouflage.]

2. Forsaken: *Delusion* rubric: *alone, being: world; alone in the: Androc.* *Delusion* rubric: *separated: world; from the: he is separated: Androc.* *Delusion* rubric: *persecuted: he is persecuted*: androc. *Delusion* rubric: *appreciated, she is not: Androc.* *Delusion* rubric: *assaulted, is going to be*: androc. *Delusion* rubric: *strangers: surrounded by*: androc. *Delusion* rubric: *outcast; she was an*: androc. *Delusion* rubric: *umbrella was a knife*: androc. [1] 1. *Delusion* rubric: *insane: everyone is*: androc. [1] 1.

3. Causation: NONE.

4. Depression: *Delusion* rubric: *wrong: everything goes wrong*: androc. *Delusion* rubric: *mystery; everything around seems a terrifying*: androc.

5. Resignation: NONE.

  • *Delusions: lost: she is*: arge-pl. ars. cot. cygn-be. des-ac. hippoc-k.
    ol-eur. urol-h.

Avoidance: When a patient says to you, *help me I am lost*
it is reflective of someone who is uncertain, ungrounded and
unsure of themselves or unsure of the direction their life should
be taking. If a patient maintains the belief that they will *always*
be lost and *never* know where they are in their life or what
direction they should take in life then this is the *Delusion* rubric:
she is lost. If someone wants to maintain their feelings of being
lost, it is an indication that they wish, for whatever reason, to
avoid being found, i.e. they want to *remain* unsure.

Cotyledon are lost to the world and lost to themselves.
Cotyledon have the *Delusion* rubric: *parts of the body are
absent*. *Cotyledon* is a homoeopathic remedy derived from
the succulent plant, Wall Pennywort. As a herbal remedy it is
regarded as a good rejuvenating tonic for sensitive stomach
disorders. As an herbal ointment it was applied externally to
help relieve aggravated piles, and smarting burns and scalds.
As a homoeopathic remedy it is used for "hysterical joints"
(Boericke), all muscular aches in joints and fibrous tissue, and
oppressed breathing, and hysterical sensations of choking
in the throat. *Cotyledon* as a constitutional remedy profile
are emotionally sensitive and easily bought to tears if they
are overwhelmed. Hysteria is a theme running through the
emotional, mental and physical sphere of the remedy profile.
Cotyledon have the *Mind* rubrics: *lost, feeling confusion of mind*,
ailments from emotional excitement and *hysteria*. *Cotyledon*
have the *Delusion* rubrics: *he is intoxicated*, and *he is drunk*.
Neither of these rubrics should be interpreted literally.

Cotyledon use the belief that they are 'not quite conscious' [*intoxicated*] to
avoid taking responsibility.

Cotyledon have no psychological 'delusions of original sin' which force them to take responsibility for their actions. If your patient believes that they truly *deserve* their illness and this is why they are sick then the simillimum cannot be *Cotyledon*. *Cotyledon* have no psychological 'delusions of grandeur' or no *Delusion* rubrics listed in Denial. *Cotyledon* do not possess enough psychological denial processes to believe that they *can* be in control.

The simillimum will only be *Cotyledon* if the patient chooses, and *needs* to remain confused and hysterical.

1. Denial: NONE.

2. Forsaken: *Delusion* rubric: *lost; she is*: cot.

3. Causation: NONE.

4. Depression: *Delusion* rubric: *mind: out of his mind; he would go*: cot. *Delusion* rubric: *mind: out of his mind; he would go: waking on*: cot. [1] 1. *Delusion* rubric: *tears; he would burst into*: cot. [1] 1. *Delusion* rubric: *weep, he would*: cot. *Delusion* rubric: *drunk: is drunk; he*: cot. *Delusion* rubric: *intoxicated: is; he*: cot.

5. Resignation: *body: parts: absent; parts of body are*: cot.

    *   *Delusions: legs: belong to her; her legs don't*: Agar. Bapt. coll. ign kola. op. sumb.

Self Deluding: The above rubric reflects psychosomatic self-abandonment. I have included this *Delusion* rubrics: *legs don't belong to her*, in the rubrics of abandonment because when *Agaricus* are sick they feel like their own body is abandoning them.

Agaricus have exalted hubristic delusions which cover up their fears of diminishing. *Agaricus* need to view themselves as great; this is reflected in the *Mind* rubric: *egotism, reciting their exploits*: agar. [1] 1., as well as the *Delusion* rubric: *is a great person*. *Agaricus* have a strong need for materialistic proof of their grandeur and worldly success. This is not only reflected in the *Delusion* rubric: *is a great person*, but also in the *Mind* rubric: *incorrect judgement of size*.

Agaricus feel threatened when they are sick, they feel like they will diminish in size, and lose their height and importance and that their own body will abandon them.

If the homoeopath understands the rubrics associated with all the remedies and their importance, they will know that when *Agaricus* are sick they will present in the first consultation in a very depressed and *paralyzed* state. The grandness that is normally associated with the egotistical *Agaricus* is not what you will see. They will be in a very small and *diminished* state. If they feel threatened or shamed by failure they immediately feel as if they are diminishing and losing all power – *Mind* rubric: *looking down when looked at*. [1] 1. If challenged they feel as if they are losing their arms and legs in the world and they compensate for their feeling of vulnerability by being extremely nasty. *Agaricus* have the *Mind* rubric: *hatred of persons who have offended him*, and the *Delusion* rubric: *vindictive*. [1] 1. Their psychological need to connect to a metaphysical power outside themselves is paramount to finding their power in the world. *Agaricus* have the *Delusion* rubrics: *objects are enlarged*, *is under superhuman control*, and *enjoy provoking out of body experiences*. [1] 1. The psychodynamic polarity of expanding greatness and diminishing smallness is extreme in *Agaricus*. The *Agaricus* (case) which I present in the *Case Companion* to *Homoeopathic Psychiatry*, solves the psychological dilemma of expanding and diminishing potency by creating two worlds. In each world she has a boyfriend. By having two partners and two worlds she is able to feel strong and *enlarged*, or 'larger than life'. Understanding the psychological processes that apply to illness and understanding the rubric-analysis which I have outlined below, allows the homoeopathic practitioner to have more wisdom and understanding of the remedies and the *Agaricus* patient.

1. Denial: *Delusion* rubric: *great person, is a*: Agar.
2. Forsaken: *Delusion* rubric: *legs: belong to her; her legs don't*. *Agar*. *Delusion* rubric: *arms: belong to her; arms do not*: agar. [These rubrics can reflect self-abandonment or they can be rubrics of hypochondria and be allocated to Resignation.]
3. Causation: *Delusion* rubric: *hell; confess his sins at gate of; obliged to*: agar [1] 1.
4. Depression: *Delusion* rubric: *paralyzed; he is*: agar.
5. Resignation: *Delusion* rubric: *body, diminished; is*: agar. *Delusion* rubric: *arms: belong to her; arms do not*: agar. *Delusion* rubric: *legs: belong to her; her legs don't*. *Agar*.

   - *Delusions: standing; beside oneself*: anh. [1] 1.

Self Deluding: This rubric alludes to the unique ability *Anhalonium* have of questioning their motivations.

Anhalonium: The above rubric can be interpreted as: one is standing beside oneself to support oneself. It can also be analyzed as: one is standing beside oneself to scrutinize oneself. Since *Anhalonium* are the only remedy listed under this rubric it is important to analyze it specifically in relation to *Anhalonium*. *Anhalonium* have a unique ability to abandon themselves and this world, because they want to become an ethereal spirit. *Anhalonium* are separated from the world and separated from their own mortality and their own body. *Anhalonium* are in tune with the psychical energies of the soul. Death is not feared because they know they travel with their soul and not with their body. Physicality is viewed as a *hindrance* because it forces them to live in their somatic body.

Anhalonium want to abandon their somatic body, they want to stand beside themselves on the worldly plane but they do not want to be *in their own body*.

Anhalonium want to be *floating in air, transparent* and

merged with immortality. Anhalonium have the *Delusion* rubrics: *body is immaterial*, and *out of the body. Anhalonium* have the *Delusion* rubric: *of emaciation. Anhalonium* choose to abandon their own body by literally starving themselves because it enhances their ethereal connection to their clairaudience and clairvoyance. The thinner *Anhalonium* becomes the more heightened their experience of not 'being in their body'. *Anhalonium* always struggle with the day to day practicalities of looking after their physicality. If they don't starve themselves they will alternatively go for long periods of time not eating anything and then consume huge amounts of snack foods. The psychodynamic energy behind their behavior is a desire to dismiss their somatic awareness and body needs in preference for their ethereal spiritual connection to the soul. *Anhalonium* have the *Mind* rubrics: *merging of self with one's environment* and *in general being beside oneself*. These *Mind* rubrics can be interpreted as: abandoning oneself, and one is distraught. *Anhalonium* have a psychodynamic need to leave their 'self'; the more they stay in their body the more likely they are to feel burdened. The simillimum will not be *Anhalonium* unless the patient has abandoned 'being in their body' in preference for the experience of being merged with their ethereal body.

1. Denial: *Delusion* rubric: *immortality, of*: anh. [1] 1. *Delusion* rubric: *eternity*: *merged with present*: anh. [1] 1. *Delusion* rubric: *transparent*: *everything is*: *Anh. Delusion* rubric: *transparent*: *he is*: anh. *Delusion* rubric: *floating*: *air, in*: anh. *Delusion* rubric: *hearing*: *illusions of*: anh. *Delusion* rubric: *body*: *out of the body*: *Anh. Delusion* rubric: *visions, has*: *beautiful*: *kaleidoscopic changes; varied*: anh. *Delusion* rubric: *voices*: *hearing*: anh. *Delusion* rubric: *sounds*: *color; are like*: anh. [1] 1.

2. Forsaken: *Delusion* rubric: *standing; beside oneself*: anh. [1] 1. *Delusion* rubric: *separated*: *world; from the*: *he is separated*: *Anh.*

3. Causation: NONE.

4. Depression: *Delusion* rubric: *hindered; he is*: anh. *Delusion* rubric: *waiting*: *had to wait; he*: anh. [1] 1. [*Anhalonium* often feel depressed because they feel like they are bidding time 'on this worldly plane', waiting to die.]

5. Resignation: *Delusion* rubric: *body*: *immaterial, is*: anh. *Delusion* rubric: *body*: *out of the body*: Anh. *Delusion* rubric: *dead*: *he himself was*: anh. *Delusion* rubric: *emaciation; of*: Anh.

*   *Delusion*: *he answers to any delusion*: anh. aster.

Self deluding: This rubric is about self-imposed abandonment of the conscious self to *all* influences. This *Delusion* rubric indicates that the remedies listed are liable to be influenced or taken over by someone else, or desire another form.

Anhalonium: *Anhalonium* desire decomposition of their shape in the world so that they can become ethereal. *Anhalonium* like the sensation that they are *floating* without form; *transparent* and *immortal*. *Anhalonium* chose to be 'out of their body' so they can be merged with the spirits. *Anhalonium* have visions of spirits. *Anhalonium* have the *Mind* rubric: *clairvoyance* and the *Delusion* rubrics: *hearing illusions* and *seeing visions*. *Anhalonium* choose no form or body, they want to be *merged with eternity* so their psychic connectivity is able to hear and see and respond to all delusions.

Anhalonium want to abandon their body in preference for a connection to the ethereal energies of all other souls.

Asterias rubens is a homoeopathic remedy derived from Red Starfish. The theme within the sea remedies as a group is survival and protection, or predator versus victim. Sea creatures need constant protection from predators; they feel like they are being spied upon by predators and they only feel safe when they are alone and hiding in a safe hiding place [*home*]. Although this is the theme within the group of sea remedies as a whole, each remedy profile within that group will have a *peculiar* survival strategy.

The *Delusion* rubric: *he answers to any delusion* pertains to self-abandonment. *Asterias rubens* give themselves up to any outside influence in order to survive.

The Red Starfish is noted for its capacity to regenerate itself from its own discarded body parts. The Red Starfish reproduce asexually by fragmentation. Sea stars prey on clams and other mollusks. They are considered as a pest by fisherman who make a living from farming clams and mollusks. The fishermen used to kill the sea stars by chopping them up and throwing them back into the sea. This ultimately led to increased numbers until it was understood that a sea-star arm will regenerate into a new starfish, especially if a section of the central ring of the sea star is part of the chopped off arm. *Asterias rubens* are aware of predators. *Asterias rubens* have developed a unique survival strategy; they abandon themselves in order to survive. *Asterias rubens* are even influenced psychically by hearing voices. *Asterias rubens* have the *Delusion* rubric: *hearing voices and answers*. *Asterias rubens* have an interesting *Delusion* rubric: *conscious of suffering of women through the ages*. *Asterias rubens* are emotively and psychically attuned to misfortune and weariness. They have the *Delusion* rubric: *expecting bad news*. [1] 1. *Asterias rubens need* to feel invaded and penetrated in order to survive. *Asterias rubens* have the *Delusion* rubric: *own body has an offensive odor*. This *Delusion* rubric can indicate self-shame and self-disgust at being unclean (evil). This *Delusion* rubric can also indicate abandonment. *Asterias rubens* feel vulnerable to, and destabilized by, being taken over, not only by bad news but by their own body decaying. Believing that your body smells offensive is self-rejection. *Asterias rubens* have the *Mind* rubric: *confusion of mind, the muscles refuse to obey the will when the attention is turned away*.

They have been taken[48] over, they have lost control and answer to anyone's delusions. They have also been abandoned[49] by their own body which is *dirty* and smells offensive. The self-abandonment is psychic, emotional, mental, and physical.

Asterias rubens have the *Mind* rubric: *ailments from being abused and sexually raped.* [1] 2. [*Carc*]. *Asterias rubens* have the *Mind* rubrics: *ailments from bad news, emotional excitement, sensitive to moral impressions,* and *weakness of will. Asterias rubens* need to remain destructively exposed to all influences in order to survive. The simillimum will only be *Asterias rubens* if the patient deludes themselves that by remaining open to psychic influences that are stronger mentally and emotionally. The simillimum will only be *Asterias rubens* if the patient indicates that they need self-destruction and self-decay to feel 'attuned' to others. Within the alternative 'back to earth' movement there is the belief that if one doesn't wash it enhances the spiritual connection to the earth. I have only had one *Asterias rubens* patient. She was a young woman who believed that if she offered up her body to anyone within her 'spiritual group' she was able to be attuned psychically to all the suffering within the world. She also held the belief that she shouldn't wash. If she smelt it indicated that she must have had a negative emotion or thought. All negative thoughts needed to be cleansed by offering her soul to humanity. Purity of mind was confirmed by allowing herself to be overwhelmed [*weeping*] with all the suffering in the world. If she wasn't overwhelmed with everyone else's psychic energy and suffering she didn't believe that she was worthy. In her history she had been raped by her father when she was thirteen years old. She consulted me for a boil on her breast. *Asterias rubens* (30 one dose a day, for one week), cured the boil, but she stopped the remedy and did not make another appointment with me because she felt the remedy "made her less sensitive to other's energies". It was not until writing this section on *Asterias rubens* that I truly understood the self-denial within the belief that she needed to be conscious of all the suffering of others in the world.

The simillimum will only be *Asterias rubens* if the patient needs to abandon themselves in order to know the suffering of others.

1. Denial: *Delusion* rubric: *voices: hearing*: aster. *Delusion* rubric: *voices: hearing: answers; and*: aster. *Delusion* rubric: *suffering: women through the ages; conscious of*: aster. [1] 2. [lac-lup[50].]

2. Forsaken: *Delusion* rubric: *he answers to any delusion*: aster. *Delusion* rubric: *home: away from home; he is*: Aster. *Delusion* rubric: *strangers: surrounded by*: aster. *Delusion* rubric: *strangers: control of; under*: aster. *Delusion* rubric: *smell, of: own body has offensive odor*: aster. [1] 1. [This rubric is indicative of self-decay (the body has abandoned them) and also of self-disgust (they have abandoned themselves).]

3. Causation: *Delusion* rubric: *dirty: he is: inside and smells badly*: aster. [1] 1. *Delusion* rubric: *smell, of: own body has offensive odor*: aster. [1] 1. [This *Delusion* rubric can indicate self-disgust over being unclean (evil).]

4. Depression: *Delusion* rubric: *weep; he would*: aster. *Delusion* rubric: *news: expecting news: bad news*: aster. [1] 1.

5. Resignation: *Delusion* rubric: *smell, of: own body has offensive odor*: aster. [1] 1. *Delusion* rubric: *dirty: he is: inside and smells badly*: aster. [1] 1. [Both of these rubrics can indicate self-disgust towards one's decaying body, or they can be indicative of shame and disgust over being unclean (evil).]

-   *Delusions: robbed, is going to be*: bar-c. borx. caust. maias-l. rhus-g. sep.

Self-deluding: A patient will not say in a consultation "I am going to be robbed". What they will say is: *everyone has always taken everything that I own, it happens all the time. Everyone is copying what I do and what I have. As soon as I*

*get something, my friend wants it or my sister takes it. It has
even started to happen at work. The woman next to me, I am
sure she bought the same pen as my new pen that I bought
last week. Even my cleaner asked me last week if she could
have the shirt I was actually wearing. When I was finished with
it of course! Because she liked it!* Psychological delusions
concerning the loss of possessions is something which a lot of
patients experience.

> If a constitutional remedy profile has any *Delusion* rubrics pertaining to
> being forsaken, then all material possessions, or loved ones, or themselves,
> will be hyper-vigilantly guarded.

Baryta carbonica in particular hoard food because they
are fearful it will be taken away from them. *Baryta carbonica*
have the *Delusion* rubric: *is forsaken*, and the *Mind* rubric:
borrowing from everyone, desire to nibble, and *impelled to
touch everything. Causticum* hoard family memorabilia and are
particularly vigilant and possessive of any possession which
holds a history of their childhood. *Causticum* suffer from anxiety
over the safety of their family, and pets in particular, and are
hypersensitive to all loss. *Causticum* have the *Delusion* rubric:
about criminals, and the *Mind* rubric: *jealousy for an inanimate
object or an animal. Causticum* are particularly sensitive to
anyone copying any of their ideas. *Causticum* also have
the *Mind* rubric: *love for family,* and numerous *Mind* rubrics
of ailments from grief, especially concerning family. In *Rhus
glabra* the theme of abandonment is about being *deceived*
and *cheated, robbed, betrayed, attacked, tricked* and *stabbed
in the back.* The psychological 'delusions of persecution' are
disproportionately exaggerated within *Rhus glabra. Sepia* are
paranoid about financial loss. They have the *Delusion* rubric: *he
is poor* and *family will starve. Sepia* have the *Delusion* rubric:
he or she is neglected, and the *Mind* rubric: *neglected by one's
mother. Sepia* also have the *Delusion* rubric: *being alone in
a graveyard. Sepia* suffer from early pre-verbal[51] neglect and
abandonment, and it is these early psychosomatic memories of

neglect from the mother which fuels their exaggerated, hyper-vigilant fears about loss. *Sepia* also have the *Mind* rubric: *anxiety about household matters*. Their anxiety is centered around the primal centre of the home; hence the reason they are fearful of robbery and further loss.

Borax are fearful of their own 'ego' abandoning them. They have psychological delusions around *being robbed* of themselves – *Delusion* rubric: *is going to be robbed*. *Borax* have the *Mind* rubric: *ailments from being magnetized*.

Borax are fearful of being possessed and consumed in case they lose themselves.

Borax have the *Delusion* rubric: *possessed of a devil*. *Borax* have several *Mind* rubrics about fear of falling and fear of loss. *Borax* have the *Mind* rubric: *starting from unexpected news*. [1] 1. *Borax* also have the *Mind* rubrics: *clinging to persons or furniture*, and *child clings to mother as if frightened*. *Borax* as a homoeopathic remedy is recognized as being wonderfully effective for the highly anxious child who wakes up startled and who is terrified of being put back down to sleep. *Borax* as a constitutional remedy profile are unable to form psychological boundaries in order to feel secure within their own being. The *Mind* rubric: *ailments from being magnetized* means that *Borax* are under constant psychic threat. Their lack of psychic boundaries also means they are fragile in their own somatic form, which is why they are convinced they will *fall*. *Borax* live in a highly frightened state. They have only one Denial rubric of grandeur, the *Delusion* rubric: *has visions*. This *Delusion* rubric adds to their 'delusions of persecution'; it is not able to strengthen. The *visions Borax* have frighten them [*possessed of the devil*] rather than inspire them with hubristic visions [*has visions*].

The simillimum will only be *Borax* if the patient is consumed[52] with personal loss.

1. Denial: *Delusion* rubric: *visions, has*: borx. [This adds to their 'persecution complex'; it is not a 'delusion of grandeur'.]
2. Forsaken: *Delusion* rubric: *robbed, is going to be*: borx.
3. Causation: *Delusion* rubric: *devil*: *possessed of a devil*: *he is*: borx.
4. Depression: *Delusion* rubric: *fright*: *as if in a fright*: borx.
5. Resignation: *Delusion* rubric: *falling*: *bodies*: Borx. [2] 1.

   • *Delusions: annihilation; about to sink into*: calc. cann-i. carbn-h. *Carc.* moni.

Avoidance: Each constitutional remedy in this *Delusion* rubric has a vastly different profile.

The difference between *Calcarea carbonica* and *Cannabis indica* could not be more profound. The essence is that each constitutional remedy profile in this rubric disproportionately needs structure to avoid feeling unsure about themselves.

Calcarea carbonica are fearful of loss of structure [*annihilation*] when they become sick. *Calcarea carbonica* are the only remedy listed in the *Delusion* rubrics: *body being dashed to pieces*, and *brain was dissolving and she was going crazy*. *Cannabis indica* need inner security to allay their fears that their own body will abandon them. *Cannabis indica* are the only remedy listed in the *Delusion* rubric: *about to die, one will soon be dissected*. The only *Delusion* rubric attached to the remedy *Carboneum hydrogenisatum* is the above rubric: *about to sink into annihilation*. *Carboneum hydrogenisatum* is a homoeopathic remedy derived from Carbureted Hydrogen[53] (methane) and as such they are acutely aware of losing their own consciousness. *Carboneum hydrogenisatum* have the *Mind* rubrics: *deep coma, sudden unconsciousness* and *vanishing of thoughts*. *Carcinosin* are fearful that their own body will abandon them. *Carcinosin* are the only remedy listed in the *Delusion* rubrics: *hand does not belong to her*, and *feet do not belong to her*. *Monilia albicans* feel threatened because they are being *annihilated* from within their own body.

If a patient concentrates *obsessively* on the need for structure around health so they do not feel threatened (abandoned), the *Delusion* rubric: is *about to sink into annihilation*.

Monilia albicans is a homoeopathic remedy derived from the fungi known as monilia, (*Candida albicans*). *Candida albicans* is in gut flora, the many organisms which live in the human mouth, and gastrointestinal tract. Under normal circumstances, *Candida albicans* lives in 80% of the human population with no harmful effects, although overgrowth results in candidiasis. Normally, the bacteria and fungi are present in the digestive tract and vagina of healthy individuals; each holds each other in check. If the bacteria are killed off in an immune compromised patient, the fungi multiplies causing candidiasis (thrush) in the mouth, throat, vagina and gut. Candidiasis is often observed in immune-compromised individuals such as HIV-positive patients. Candidiasis, also known as 'thrush', is a common condition which is usually easily cured in people who are not immune-compromised. To infect host tissue, the yeast-like form of *Candida albicans* reacts to environmental cues and switches to invasive, multicellular filamentous forms.

The theme in the remedy profile of *Monilia albicans* is abandonment, and the attack is from inside the body as well as from the outside world. *Monilia albicans* are listed in the majority of the Forsaken rubrics.

Monilia albicans feel compromised about their own safety. They are obsessive about any real or perceived threats because they are being *annihilated* from inside their own body. The simillimum will only be *Monilia albicans* if the patient feels vulnerable to impending death.

1. Denial: *Delusion* rubric: *floating*: *air, in*: moni. [For *Monilia albicans,* this rubric is not necessarily a dissociative rubric. Because they feel so threatened and have the Resignation *Delusion* rubric: *body is thin*, this rubric is more indicative of *Monilia albicans* fading away rather than denying reality.]

2. Forsaken: *Delusion* rubric: *annihilation; about to sink into*: moni. *Delusion* rubric: *alone, being*: *world; alone in the*: moni. *Delusion* rubric: *animals*: *devoured by*: *being*: moni. *Delusion rubric*: *despised; is*: moni. *Delusion* rubric: *enemy*: *surrounded by enemies*: moni. *Delusion* rubric: *persecuted*: *he is persecuted*: moni. *Delusion* rubric: *separated*: *world*; *from the*: *he is separated*: moni. *Delusion* rubric: *pursued; he was*: moni. *Delusion* rubric: *danger, impression of*: moni.

3. Causation: *Delusion* rubric: *wrong*: *done wrong; he has*: *Moni.*

4. Depression: *Delusion* rubric: *stupid; one is*: moni. [1] 1.

5. Resignation: *Delusion* rubric: *thin*: *body is*: moni. [Candidiasis is often observed in immune-compromised individuals especially HIV-positive patients.]

- *Delusions: bed*: *sold his bed; someone has*: nux-v.[1] 1.
- *Delusions: bed*: *someone*: *gets into his bed and there is no more room*: nux-v.[1] 1.
- *Delusions: bed*: *someone*: *over the bed; someone is*: calc.[1] 1.
- *Delusions: bed*: *someone*: *under the bed; someone is*: am-m. ars. **BELL**. calc. canth. colch.

Avoidance: This rubric is useful when the patient feels threatened about losing their position in the world. One's bed is synonymous with the inner sanctum of one's home.

To feel threatened in one's bed indicates deep paranoia about loss of position.

For *Calcarea carbonica,* the underlying feeling is fear of poverty and loss of their home. For *Nux vomica,* it is indicative of a threat to their kingdom or inner sanctum.

Nux vomica: The underlying paranoia in *Nux vomica* relates to loss of status. The abandonment fear specific to *Nux vomica* is the threat of someone taking over their territory [*bed*]. *Nux vomica* have grand *illusions of fancy* and 'delusions of grandeur' all pertaining to the need to prove their wealth. *Nux vomica* have the *Delusion* rubric: *delusions of wealth and makes useless purchases.* [2] 1.

Nux vomica need to prove their status because they suffer from numerous 'persecution complexes': *insulted, laughed and mocked at, persecuted, pursued, teased, abandoned from his home* and loss of their *mother who is murdered.* They fear rejection and loss of societal status.

If there is a contradiction between Stage one, Denial ('delusions of grandeur') and Stage five, Resignation ('delusions of hypochondria'), the inconsistency indicates an instability in the psyche which will undermine confidence and mental and emotional stability. On the one hand *Nux vomica* have the *Delusion* rubric: *delusions of wealth and makes useless purchases*, and on the other hand they have the *Delusion* rubric: *he is poor. Nux vomica* have the *Mind* rubrics: *ailments from loss of position, increased ambition for fame*, and *increased ambition to make money. Nux vomica* have the *Mind* rubric: *anxiety, hypochondria, mania to read medical books.* If *Nux vomica* feel undermined and threatened internally over fears about being small and needing to project enlarged grandness, then this instability will lead to 'delusions of paranoia' and 'delusions of hypochondria'. *Nux vomica* have numerous *Mind* rubrics emphasizing their hyper-vigilant reactivity: *ailments from intolerance*, [1] 1., and *disposition to contradict. Nux vomica* have numerous *Delusion* rubrics which reflect paranoia: *seeing vermin crawl about, creeping worms, seeing strangers, pursued by enemies, pursued by animals*, and *sees dead people.*

Nux vomica have one *Delusion* rubric which specifically alludes to their need to protect themselves from all real or perceived threats to their well being: *Delusion* rubric: *he can live without heart.* [1] 1. *Nux vomica* abandon their emotive empathy in order to protect themselves from abandonment.

The simillimum will only be *Nux vomica* if the patient is paranoid about losing status.

1. Denial: *Delusion* rubric: *enlarged*: nux-v. [This rubric can often intensify illusionary fears. With *Nux vomica* it alludes to their delusional belief that they have a large territory over which they reign.]

    Versus

5. Resignation: *Delusion* rubric: *small*: *body is smaller*. nux-v.

1. Denial: *Delusion* rubric: *enlarged*: nux-v. *Delusion* rubric: *fancy, illusions of*: nux-v. *Delusion* rubric: *wealth, of*: *purchases; and make useless*: *Nux-v*. [2] 1. *Delusion* rubric: *stimulant; had taken a*: nux-v.

2. Forsaken: *Delusion* rubric: *bed*: *someone*: *gets into his bed and there is no more room*: nux-v.[1] 1. *Delusion* rubric: *criminals, about*: nux-v. *Delusion* rubric: *injury*: *about to receive injury; is*: nux-v. *Delusion* rubric: *insulted, he is*: nux-v. *Delusion* rubric: *laughed at and mocked at; being*: nux-v. *Delusion* rubric: *persecuted*: *he is persecuted*: nux-v. *Delusion* rubric: *people*: *beside him; people are*: nux-v. *Delusion* rubric: *people*: *pranks with him; people are*: **NUX-V**. *Delusion* rubric: *home*: *away from home; he is*: *Nux-v*. *Delusion* rubric: *murdered*: *mother had been murdered; her*. nux-v. [1] 1. *Delusion* rubric: *poor; he is*: nux-v.

3. Causation: *Delusion* rubric: *crime*: *committed a crime; he had*: nux-v.

4. Depression: *Delusion* rubric: *fail, everything will*: nux-v. *Delusion* rubric: *depressive*: nux-v. *Delusion* rubric: *unfair to him; that life is*: nux-v. *Delusion* rubric: *poor; he is*: nux-v.

5. Resignation: *Delusion* rubric: *die*: *about to die; one was*: nux-v. *Delusion* rubric: *poisoned*: *he*: *has been*: nux-v. *Delusion* rubric: *small*: *body is smaller*. nux-v. *Delusion* rubric: *fermenting*: *everything was fermenting*: nux-v. [1] 1.

    *   *Delusions*: *dreams*: *belong to another; dreams*: choc.[1] 1.

Self deluding: *Chocolate* abandon themselves and their dreams and their somatic hold on their body.

Chocolate have abandoned their body and have delusions that they are transformed into the body of animal. *Chocolate* suffer from 'delusions of zooanthropy'. (Zooanthropy is the delusion that you have assumed the form of an animal.) *Chocolate* also abandon themselves psychically. *Chocolate* suffer from 'nihilistic delusions'. 'Nihilistic delusion' is the delusion that everything, including the self, does not exist; a sense that reality and the somatic does not exist and that everything outside of the self is also unreal. A somatic delusion is a delusion concerning the body image or parts of the body. *Chocolate* also suffer from 'delusions of persecution' that society will abandon them. *Chocolate* have the *Delusion* rubrics: *he is persecuted*, *watched*, *alone* and *separated from the world*. *Chocolate* have the *Delusion* rubric: *others will observe her confusion*. *Chocolate* have the *Mind* rubric: *fear of her condition being observed*. *Chocolate* are unsure about their own sense of reality. *Chocolate* have the *Mind* rubric: *desire to fly*, [1] 1., and the *Mind* rubric: *desires to see great distances*. On the one hand, *Chocolate* have the *Mind* rubric: *attempts to escape from her family and children,* and on the other hand they have the *Mind* rubrics: *estranged from society,* and *estranged from his family*. The nihilistic self-denial within *Chocolate* causes them to abandon themselves and leave their family and society. *Chocolate* are the only remedy listed in the *Mind* rubric: *does not recognize his own face*, and the *Delusion* rubric: *his own face looks unfamiliar*. *Chocolate* will not literally say in a consultation, *I have turned into an animal or a hedgehog*. Nor will they say, *my dreams have been stolen*. They will say: *I am sick. I have nothing left. Do you know I can't even remember my dreams anymore. Everything has been taken away from me, even my looks. I can't even recognize who I am anymore. This cancer has made me feel like I want to be an Echidna*

(Australian native equivalent to the hedgehog) *who is able to quickly disappear from sight, or I want to transform myself into a bird which is able to fly away. I want to be above myself and look down on myself and see that my body has been transformed into some beautiful creature, like a cicada with beautiful wings, who is no longer sick and dying. I have decided to completely let myself go. I eat all of the food that is bad for me. I eat chocolate all day. I even go to bed not brushing my teeth because I want the taste of the chocolate to completely consume my sensations. I don't care anymore, I just want to be consumed by chocolate. Do you know Liz there is even a shop called Death by Chocolate?* Chocolate addiction can be viewed as nihilistic self-abandonment because the addiction causes the person to abandon all concern of the consequences to their body size from consuming large amounts of chocolate. Chocolate is often described by patients as 'comfort food' for feelings of hurt, rejection and abandonment. Chocolate is also something which is viewed as a replacement for not having a lover.

The simillimum will only be *Chocolate* if the patient shows evidence of self-rejection as well as having experienced real or perceived societal rejection.

1. Denial: *Delusion* rubric: *visions, has: simultaneous from above and below*: choc. [1] 1. *Delusion* rubric: *nursing; she is: animals or hairy babies*: choc. [1] 1. [This rubric can pertain to their vision of themselves as a mother to all creatures; this is a 'delusion of grandeur'.]

2. Forsaken: *Delusion* rubric: *dreams: belong to another; dreams*: choc. [1] 1. *Delusion* rubric: *alone, being: world; alone in the*: choc. *Delusion* rubric: *persecuted: he is persecuted*: choc. *Delusion* rubric: *separated: world; from the: he is separated*: choc. *Delusion* rubric: *watched, she is being*: choc. *Delusion* rubric: *dreams: stolen; dreams have been*: choc. [1] 1.

3. Causation: NONE.

4. Depression: *Delusion* rubric: *face: unfamiliar; his own face looks*: choc. [1] 1. [This rubric pertain to self-abandonment or loss of identity.]

5. Resignation: *Delusion* rubric: *hedgehog: she is a*: choc. [1] 1. *Delusion* rubric: *animals: she is an animal*: choc. *Delusion* rubric: *back: opens and wings are forming*: choc. [1] 1. *Delusion* rubric: *dead: he himself was*: choc. *Delusion* rubric: *wings: back were opening and wings were forming; as if*: choc. [1] 1. *Delusion* rubric: *blood: pouring out of mouth*: choc. [1] 1. *Delusion* rubric: *divided: four parts; into*: choc. [1] 1. *Delusion* rubric: *small: he is*: choc.

*   *Delusions: belong to her own family; she does not*: lac-lup. *Plat.*

Self deluding: This rubric is an excellent example of the importance of looking at why the psychological delusion or misrepresentation is of advantage to each individual remedy profile. On the one hand, *Platina* have the *Delusion* rubric: *she is not appreciated*, and on the other hand they have the *Delusion* rubric: *he is better than others*. *Platina* use their contemptuousness and their 'superiority complex' (*Delusion* rubric: *humility and lowness of others; while he is great*) to extricate *themselves* from the rest of humanity.

Platina need to believe they are superior to compensate for feeling *alone in the world*. In turn, their superiority is what isolates them. Consequently, the numerous rubrics pertaining to 'delusions of abandonment' are the undermining force which in turn fuels their need to maintain their numerous 'delusions of superiority'. *Platina* believe they are not being recognized for their *nobility*.

Platina feel that they are so superior that no one could possibly be worthy of them, but they deliberately separate themselves from the *lowliness of others* to prove to themselves how *great* they are.

They also maintain this distance between themselves

and others so they can reinforce their superiority. *Platina* maintain their *nobility* at a cost to themselves. In the process of constructing their 'delusions of superiority' *Platina* are overwhelmed by believing, and/or perceiving that they will be undermined. This is why they have numerous 'persecution complexes' and 'delusions of abandonment', and why they are fearful that *everyone is an enemy* about to *cut them in two* or *cut their throat*. *Platina* have eight *Mind* rubrics that allude to their desire to *kill their children* and *beloved husband*. The simillimum will not be *Platina* unless the homoeopath can perceive that the patient is torn between, on the one hand needing to remain separate from their family because it reinforces their 'delusions of superiority'. And on the other hand feeling distraught that they feel abandoned by their family.

1. Denial: *Delusion* rubric: *humility and lowness of others; while he is great*: plat. *Delusion* rubric: *noble, being*: plat.

2. Forsaken: *Delusion* rubric: *belong to her own family; she does not*: Plat. *Delusion* rubric: *alone, being: world; alone in the*: Plat. *Delusion* rubric: *appreciated, she is not*: plat. *Delusion* rubric: *family, does not belong to her own*: plat. [1] 1. *Delusion* rubric: *enemy: everyone is an*: plat. *Delusion* rubric: *family, does not belong to her own*: plat. [1] 1. *Delusion* rubric: *forsaken; is*: Plat. *Delusion* rubric: *place: no place in the world; she has*: Plat. *Delusion* rubric: *strange: land; as if in strange*: plat. *Delusion* rubric: *disgraced: she is*: plat. *Delusion* rubric: *disgraced: family or friends; he has disgraced his*: plat. *Delusion* rubric: *neglected: he or she is neglected*: plat. *Delusion* rubric: *devil: all persons are devils*: **PLAT**. *Delusion* rubric: *choked: he is about to be: night: waking on*: Plat.

3. Causation: *Delusion* rubric: *devil: possessed of a devil: he is*: plat.

4. Depression: *Delusion* rubric: *insane: become insane; one will*: plat.

5. Resignation: *Delusion* rubric: *body: cut though; he is: two; in:* plat.

• *Delusions: division between himself and others:* arge-pl. dream-p. falco-pe. hippoc-k. hydrog. nat-c. phasco-ci.

Self-deluding: A belief that there is a division between oneself and others can be allocated to the *Delusion* rubrics of hubristic 'delusions of superiority', or to the *Delusion* rubrics of being forsaken. The division is proof that one is either above everyone else, or that there is a division between oneself and society because one has been abandoned.

Hydrogenium: The division in *Hydrogenium* between themselves and others can be analyzed as an indication of their desire to live in a higher consciousness [*God*], or as evidence that they are unable to live connected to the world. Underpinning their delusional conflict about living in their higher consciousness is fear of being rejected by, and divorced from, society. *Hydrogenium* feel separated from others. *Hydrogenium* have the *Delusion* rubric: *he is separated from the world*. The separation conflict in *Hydrogenium* undermines their belief in their right to exist, and this is why *Hydrogenium* have numerous *Delusion* rubrics all pertaining to 'persecution complexes'. *Hydrogenium* have the *Delusion* rubric: *out of the body*. When they are sick, *Hydrogenium* will literally believe that the world will reject them because they are sick. *Hydrogenium* will also literally believe that their body (which is separate to themselves) has abandoned them.

The simillimum will only be *Hydrogenium* if the patient presents with delusional arrogance that they are greater than everyone else. Conversely, the simillimum will only be *Hydrogenium* if the patient presents with expectations of abandonment. *Hydrogenium* will often refuse treatment because they are so disconnected from their body that they cannot believe they are sick.

Hydrogenium need to continue to feel abandoned and

separated from their body and the world so that they can delude themselves that they will die and be merged with a *higher consciousness*. *Hydrogenium* are divided between their body and soul. *Hydrogenium* have the *Delusion* rubric: *body is separated from soul*. *Hydrogenium* will often refuse treatment because they desire death so they can merge into a unification with a higher consciousness.

Hydrogenium have only one *Delusion* rubric pertaining to 'delusions of original sin'. *Hydrogenium* have the *Delusion* rubric: *that she is frightening others*. This *Delusion* rubric reinforces their feeling of separation and division from society.

1. Denial: *Delusion* rubric: *consciousness: higher consciousness; unification with*: hydrog. [1] 1. *Delusion* rubric: *God: presence of God; he is in the*: hydrog: [1] 1. *Delusion* rubric: *beautiful: thinks look*: hydrog. *Delusion* rubric: *heaven, is in*: hydrog. *Delusion* rubric: *enlarged*: hydrog. *Delusion* rubric: *energy: air, moving around in the*: hydrog. [1] 1. *Delusion* rubric: *separated: body: soul; body is separated from*: Hydrog. [This rubric can pertain to 'delusions of superiority' that one's soul is not associated with one's body or it can pertain to abandonment.]

2. Forsaken: *Delusion* rubric: *division between himself and others*: hydrog. [This rubric can be allocated to Denial or Forsaken.] *Delusion* rubric: *people: pranks with him; people carry on all sorts of*: hydrog. *Delusion* rubric: *murdered: will be murdered; he: conspire to murder him; others*: hydrog. *Delusion* rubric: *persecuted: he is persecuted*: hydrog. *Delusion* rubric: *betrayed; that she is*: hydrog. *Delusion* rubric: *repudiated; he is: society; by*: hydrog. [1] 1. *Delusion* rubric: *separated: world; from the: he is separated*: **HYDROG**.

3. Causation: *Delusion* rubric: *frightening others; that she is*: hydrog. [1] 1.

4. Depression: *Delusion* rubric: *hell: in; is*: hydrog. *Delusion* rubric: *diminished: all is*: hydrog.

5. Resignation: *Delusion* rubric: *diminished*: *all is*: hydrog. [I have allocated this rubric to this section because *Hydrogenium* have the 'nihilistic delusion' that their somatic body does not exist.] *Delusion* rubric: *body*: *out of the body*: *Hydrog.*

• *Delusions*: *consciousness*: *belongs to another*. *Alum.* [2] 1.

Avoidance: A belief that one's consciousness belongs to another, on the one hand can allude to a refusal to take responsibility for one's actions or it can pertain to an inability to maintain control over one's consciousness in the face of stronger outside influences.

Alumina abandon themselves.

In *Alumina* there is confusion about who owns their identity. Their consciousness belongs either to God or to the devil or to someone else; but *Alumina* themselves struggle to feel like they have the right to *own* their own consciousness. Because *Alumina* struggle to have control over their own consciousness they can become victims of suicide. As soon as *Alumina* are exposed to the *sight of blood*, or see a *knife or gun*, they have a desire to suicide. Everything can possess *Alumina*, even a *knife*.

Alumina is a remedy profile of someone who has suppressed and abandoned their own hold on their consciousness. *Alumina* have psychological delusions of being possessed, *being double*, and of *their head belonging to another*. *Alumina* have the *Delusion* rubric: *she is someone else's identity*. *Alumina* are the only remedy listed in the *Mind* rubric: *courageous alternating with fear*. [2] 1. *Alumina* struggle to be confident enough that others will not take away their right to exist. *Alumina* have the *Mind* rubric: *fear that people behind him might hit him*. [1] 1.

Alumina have the *Delusion* rubric: *when he is speaking, someone is talking*. The psychosis in *Alumina* presents as fear that everyone will take their consciousness.

Psychoses are a mental derangement that develop from the conflict between the 'ego' and the external world. The organized *realistic* part of the psyche is the 'ego'. If a remedy profile has a weakened 'ego' then their psyche is under threat. The psyche is the personification of the soul, spirit, and mind. *Alumina* can be convinced that they have committed numerous crimes. *Alumina* have such a weakened 'ego' that they psychosomatically respond to all suggestions, even being *possessed by the devil*. There is a conflict between their hubristic belief that they are a *great person* and their numerous rubrics of being *possessed by the devil* for *crimes committed*.

The consequences of the confusion in *Alumina* means that they will continually feel like they need to change prescriptions and practitioners. *Alumina* have changing psychosomatic symptoms.

It is extremely difficult to convince *Alumina,* whose mind *always belongs to another,* that that they should not abandon the prescription because of a new somatic sensation that has enveloped their mind and body. The homoeopath should not respond to the continually changing and confusing psychosomatic symptoms when treating an *Alumina* patient, and should not prescribe according to the new presenting symptoms. The very nature of the remedy profile is one of confusing symptoms of psychosis or self-abandonment of the psyche, and as such the patient will always be possessed by new symptoms of derangement.

1. Denial: *Delusion* rubric: *great person, is a*: alum. *Delusion* rubric: *consciousness: outside of his body; his consciousness were*: alum. [1] 1. *Delusion* rubric: *seeing: cannot see; he; transfer himself into another, and only then he could see; he could*: alum. [1] 1. *Delusion* rubric: *possessed; being*: alum. *Delusion* rubric: *consciousness: belongs to another. Alum.* [2] 1. [This can be by God or the devil or by someone else.]

2. Forsaken: *Delusion* rubric: *consciousness: belongs to another. Alum.* [2] 1. [This rubric can be interpreted as self-abandonment or a 'delusion of grandeur'.] *Delusion* rubric:

friendless, he is: alum. *Delusion* rubric: *talking: someone is talking: he is speaking; when*: alum. *Delusion* rubric: *consciousness: outside of his body, his consciousness were*: alum. [1] 1. *Delusion* rubric: *identity; someone else, she is: Alum. Delusion* rubric: *seeing: cannot see; he; transfer himself into another, and only then he could see; he could*: alum. [1] 1. [These can be interpreted as rubrics of self-abandonment or rubrics of 'delusions of grandeur'.]

3. Causation: *Delusion* rubric: *criminal, he is a*: alum. *Delusion* rubric: *crime: committed a crime; he had*: alum. *Delusion* rubric: *devil: possessed of a devil*: alum. *Delusion* rubric: *wrong: done wrong; he has*: alum. *Delusion* rubric: *possessed; being*: alum.

4. Depression: *Delusion* rubric: *melancholy*: alum. *Delusion* rubric: *insane: become insane; one will*: alum. *Delusion* rubric: *suicide: impelled to commit: knife; on seeing a*: alum. [1] 1.

5. Resignation: *Delusion* rubrics: *die: about to die; one was*: alum. *Delusion* rubric: *disease: incurable disease; he has an*: alum. *Delusion* rubric: *enlarged: body is: parts of body*: alum. [This rubric can also be placed in 'hubristic denial'.] *Delusion* rubric: *head: belongs to another. Alum.*

- *Delusions: person: other person; she is some*: androc. cann-s. dream-p. gels. haliae-lc. ignis-alc. lac-c. *Lach.* mosch. olib-sac. oxal-a. phos. plb. puls. valer.

- *Delusions: identity: errors of personal identity*: aids. *Alum.* androc. anh. ant-c. bapt. cann-i. cann-s. cic. gard-j. kali-br. lac-c. lach. lil-t. mosch. myric. naja. ol-j. orig. petr. phos. plb. pyrog. pyrus. raja-s. stram. thuj. valer. **VERAT**.

- *Delusions: identity; someone else, she is: Alum.* cann-i. cann-s. gels. *Lach.* mosch. phos. plb. pyrog. *Valer.*

- *Delusions: head: separated from body; head is*: allox. alum. anac. ant-t. arg-n. bell. bufo cann-i. cocc. *Daph.* falco-pe. kali-bi. lac-lup. lyc. m-ambo. mez. nat-c. ol-eur. plut-n. **PSOR**. ther.

- *Delusions: separated: body: mind are separated; body and:* anac. arb-m. arge-pl. bit-ar. cann-i. corv-cor. cypra-eg. dioxi. dream-p. lac-lup. limest-b. loxo-recl. melal-alt. mucs-nas. musca-d. oncor-t. ozone. polys. sabad. suis-em. thuj.

- *Delusions: body: divided, is: Agath-a.* cann-i. choc. lil-t. olib-sac. *Petr.* sil. *Stram.*

- *Delusions: divided: two parts; into: Anac.* aq-mar. *Bapt.* bell. cann-i. cypra-eg. des-ac. fic-m. lil-t. neon. ol-eur. olib-sac. ozone. petr. positr. puls. *Ruta.* sal-fr. sil. stram. thuj.

- *Delusions: divided: two parts; into: real him, one is not the:* sal-fr. [1] 1.

- *Delusions: double; being:* alum. *Anac.* anh. ara-maca. *Bapt.* calc-p. cann-i. glon. haliae-lc. lach. lil-t. mosch. *Nux-m.* op. *Petr.* phos. psil. pyrog. rhus-t. sec. sil. *Stram.* thuj. valer.

- *Delusions: double: being; controls the other; one self: Cann-i.* [2] 1.

- *Delusions: double: existence; having a double:* ara-maca. cann-i. [1] 1.

Avoidance: The *Delusion* rubrics: *being double, having a double existence,* and *she is some other person*, are allocated in the Forsaken rubrics because they all reflect personality Dissociative Disorders and/or Multiple Personality Disorders. These psychological disorders all reflect abandonment of the 'ego'. This group of *Delusion* rubrics are not only applicable to complicated Dissociative Disorders; they can simply reflect intense self-doubt and/or self-denegation. The above group of rubrics can also be allocated to Depression because they also indicate depressive self-doubt. The above group of rubrics can also be allocated to Resignation in that they reflect abandonment of one's body.

Rajania subsamarata have only one *Delusion* rubric: *errors of personal identity*. *Rajania subsamarata* is a plant remedy which belongs to the Anacardiaceae family. *Rajania subsamarata* are able to lose their personal identity to connect psychically. *Anacardium* similarly have the *Mind* rubrics: *clairvoyant* and *clairaudient*. Julian, notes in his *Dictionary of Homeopathic Materia Medica*, that *Rajania subsamarata* is "Psychic with a loss of personality." *Rajania subsamarata* have the *Mind* rubrics: *religious affections, too occupied with religious songs,* and *sensitive to sacred music.* Similarly to *Anacardium* they are also listed in the *Mind* rubric: *rage*.

Salix-fragilis is a plant remedy derived from crack willow. Stirling proved *Salix-fragilis*. These notes are taken from Stirling's notes listed on Radar™: "The Anglo-Saxon wellig from which willow is derived means pliancy. Almost all varieties are used in basketry, being extremely pliable. Male and female catkins grow on separate trees. Even if planted upside down, it will 'take', as the branches can become roots, and the roots branches. The crack willow has an advantage by snapping off so easily, in that twigs and branches that are snapped off by the wind can float downstream and root themselves in the bank further down. They will continue to grow, even if split right down the middle, and sometimes other saplings will take root in the split." When transposed to a personality profile, the characteristics Stirling has identified in crack willow equate with a profile that is able to transpose, adapt, split themselves off, and bend to all powerful influences.

Salix-fragilis have numerous psychological 'delusions of persecution'. The personality profile is of someone who is able to deflect blame on to others.

Salix-fragilis are adaptive to the environment. They are influenced by whomever is the most powerful[54] – they can break off and shoot a new persona which is able to match any current situation. *Salix-fragilis* can also deny that their own disease belongs to them. *Salix-fragilis* have no *Delusion* rubrics in Resignation. *Salix-fragilis* will not acknowledge disease and/ or impending death.

Salix-fragilis display a capacity to abandon themselves, adapt personas, and deny their own body.

Salix-fragilis believe that they are a *great person;* consequently they will only 'sell themselves to the highest bidder[55]'. *Salix-fragilis* have the *Delusion* rubrics: *is an imposter* and *two different trains of thought influenced him at the same time.* *Salix-fragilis* will abandon themselves and allow others to abandon them as long as they continue to survive and grow and sprout[56] again at any costs. *Salix-fragilis* is a 'double agent' who trusts no one and who deceives everyone. *Salix-fragilis* is particularly applicable to the person who has separate lives. Every now and again, one hears of someone who has been living a double life, with two wives and children in two different cities – this is the profile of the constitutional remedy *Salix-fragilis*. *Salix-fragilis* have the *Mind* rubrics: *desire for change in life,* and *confusion of mind as to his sense of duality of identity.*

1. Denial: *Delusion* rubric: *great person, is a:* sal-fr. *Delusion* rubric: *disease: belong to her, her disease does not:* sal-fr. [1] 1. *Delusion* rubric: *thoughts: two different trains of thought influenced him at the same time:* sal-fr. *Delusion* rubric: *imposter, is an:* sal-fr. [1] 1. *Delusion* rubric: *influence; one is under a powerful:* Sal-fr. *Delusion* rubric: *possessed; being:* sal-fr. [The last four rubrics can pertain to God or the devil].

2. Forsaken: *Delusion* rubric: *divided: two parts; into:* sal-fr. *Delusion* rubric: *divided: two parts; into: real him, one is not the:* sal-fr. [1] 1. *Delusion* rubric: *persecuted: he is persecuted:* sal-fr. *Delusion* rubric: *separated: world; from the: he is separated:* sal-fr. *Delusion* rubric: *conspiracies: against him; there are conspiracies:* sal-fr. *Delusion* rubric: *confusion; others will observe her:* sal-fr. *Delusion* rubric: *misunderstood; she is:* sal-fr. *Delusion* rubric: *wrong: suffered wrong; he has:* sal-fr.

3. Causation: *Delusion* rubric: *thoughts*: *two different trains of thought influenced him at the same time*: sal-fr. *Delusion* rubric: *imposter, is an*: sal-fr. [1] 1. *Delusion* rubric: *influence; one is under a powerful*: Sal-fr. *Delusion* rubric: *possessed; being*: sal-fr. [The last four rubrics can pertain to God or the devil].

4. Depression: *Delusion* rubric: *beaten, he is being*: sal-fr. *Delusion* rubric: *succeed, he does everything wrong; he cannot*: sal-fr. *Delusion* rubric: *pressed down by a great force*: sal-fr. *Delusion* rubric: *wretched; she looks: looking in a mirror; when*: sal-fr.

5. Resignation: NONE.

- *Delusions: will power; as if loss of*: carb-v. chinin-s. nit-ac. pop.
- *Delusions: head: swaying: head was swaying: back and forth*: carb-v. zinc.
- *Delusions: oppressed; he was*: carb-v. positr.

Self-deluding: These rubrics should be used in case-repertorisation for patients who have abandoned themselves to a dominant power. That dominant power can be either the illusion of God or the devil or any stronger force within or outside of themselves. This rubric is particularly relevant to consider for the patient who finds themselves in an abusive relationship.

Carbo vegetabilis are the only remedy listed in both of the *Delusion* rubrics: *if he had postponed waking any longer he would faint*, and *he is awakening himself from a dream*. *Carbo vegetabilis* is a homoeopathic remedy which is used when a patient is in a state of collapse or near death from a grave illness. It has traditionally been viewed as a remedy which is able to loosen 'the grip of death' and revive an almost lifeless patient. *Carbo vegetabilis* have the *Mind* rubric: *accelerated respiration with coma*. *Carbo vegetabilis* as a homoeopathic is used for the patient who is extremely weak and exhausted. Their vitality is so diminished that their digestion is sluggish.

They experience constipation and excessive flatulence from such a disordered gut. Their gut expands [*large*] considerably with excess flatulence. Their circulation is notably cold and unresponsive, and their respiration is diminished and underperforming. Their lung capacity is critically diminished [*small*] so it is an excellent remedy for cyanosis, asthma and blue skin. *Carbo vegetabilis* as a homoeopathic is commonly used for a dying patient who is struggling to hold on to consciousness [*coma*]. *Carbo vegetabilis* as a constitutional remedy profile have the psychosomatic theme of not being able to keep a strong enough grip on their own consciousness and psyche.

Carbo vegetabilis do not necessarily abandon themselves; it is more the case that they struggle to hold on to their belief that they should continue to live.

Carbo vegetabilis have the *Mind* rubric: *yielding disposition.* [4] *Carbo vegetabilis* also have the *Mind* rubric: *weary of life.* [2] 1. *Carbo vegetabilis* lose their grip on their psyche because they are overwhelmed by *dark delusions* that they carry within themselves. They also loosen their grip on their psyche because they have numerous paranoid 'delusions of persecution'. *Carbo vegetabilis* have numerous *Delusion* rubrics of *people beside them, near their bed,* being surrounded by *criminals,* and of *walls falling* on them. *Carbo vegetabilis* have the *Mind* rubric: *desire to be flattered.* It is their desire to surrender themselves to the *will power* of others that weakens them. *Carbo vegetabilis* struggle to hold their own opinion. The *Delusion* rubric: *head was swaying back and forth,* can be interpreted literally. However, it is much more significant if it is interpreted psychosomatically. *Carbo vegetabilis* surrender their *head* (consciousness): psychically to the *ghosts,* emotionally to their *anxious delusions of the dark,* mentally to others who *possess* and *oppress* them, and physically to their *small or large body* which they can't control.

The simillimum will not be *Carbo vegetabilis* unless the patient feels like they are a victim to their own body sensations. The simillimum will not be *Carbo vegetabilis* unless the patient feels like they are a victim to someone who is stronger than they are.

1. Denial: *Delusion* rubric: *fancy, illusions of*: carb-v. *Delusion* rubric: *possessed; being*: carb-v. [This can pertain to possession by God, or the devil, or someone who is a stronger force.]

2. Forsaken: *Delusion* rubric: *oppressed; he were*: carb-v. *Delusion* rubric: *head: swaying: head was swaying: back and forth*: carb-v. *Delusion* rubric: *forsaken; is*: carb-v. *Delusion* rubric: *footsteps; hearing*: carb-v. *Delusion* rubric: *criminals, about*: carb-v. *Delusion* rubric: *people: beside him: people are*: carb-v. *Delusion* rubric: *bed: someone: comes near his bed; as if someone*: carb-v. [1] 1. *Delusion* rubric: *specters, ghosts, spirits: seeing*: carb-v.

3. Causation: *Delusion* rubric: *crime: committed a crime; he had*: carb-v. *Delusion* rubric: *possessed; being*: carb-v.

4. Depression: *Delusion* rubric: *anxious*: carb-v. *Delusion* rubric: *falling: walls*: carb-v. *Delusion* rubric: *dark: in the dark; delusions*: carb-v. [1] 1.

5. Resignation: *Delusion* rubric: *small: body is smaller*: carb-v. *Delusion* rubric: *large: parts of body seem too large*: carb-v.

    -   *Delusions: devil: persecuted by the devil; he is; crimes he had never done; for*: zinc.[1] 1.
    -   *Delusions: accused, she is*: laur, zinc.

Self-deluding: These rubrics should be used in case-repertorisation for patients who deny any wrong doing and who believe they are being wrongly accused by others in their life.

Laurocerasus and *Zincum* are under the *Delusion* rubric: *she is accused*, yet each react profoundly differently to acknowledging personal fault. *Laurocerasus* have no *Delusion* rubrics pertaining to acknowledgment of personal blame or acknowledgement of sin. *Zincum* have the *Delusion* rubrics: *he committed a crime* and *had done some evil.* Regardless of their avoidance which they transfer on to the devil who has possessed them, *Zincum* are aware of personal blame. *Laurocerasus* react with anger when accused because they have no acknowledgement of self-blame. *Laurocerasus* have the *Mind* rubric: *anger when misunderstood. Laurocerasus* carry within their somatic memory the nature of the substance from which the homoeopathic remedy is derived. *Laurocerasus* is derived from the plant *Prunus laurocerasus* which contains cyanogenic glycosides. Cyanogenic glycosides contain the element nitrogen in the form of hydrocyanic acid which is one of the most toxic of all plant compounds.

All homoeopathic substances derived from any substance which contains poison will have several persecutory fears within their psyche.

Laurocerasus have the *Delusion* rubric: *she is criticized.* When compiling the *Delusion* rubrics in case-taking we have to use a psychotherapeutic model which allows us to probe why the patient has chosen to concoct a complicated system of excuses to justify their emotional stance. *Laurocerasus* have numerous *Delusion* rubrics pertaining to persecution and annihilation because the homoeopathic remedy is derived from a poisonous substance.

Laurocerasus as a homoeopathic remedy is often used for sudden loss of memory and speech especially with the onset of vertigo. *Laurocerasus* have the *Mind* rubric: *forgetful on motion.* [1] 1. *Laurocerasus* also have the *Mind* rubrics: *confusion of mind, aphasia, unconsciousness and semi-consciousness,* and *sudden and periodical weakness of memory. Laurocerasus* have the *Delusion* rubrics: *everything turned in a circle,* and *everything turned round and round.* [1] 1. It is a mistake to assume that this rubric only reiterates the inherent tendency to vertigo within the homoeopathic remedy of *Laurocerasus*. The remedy profile of *Laurocerasus* have the ability to turn the truth around and around until they can create their own version of reality which they prefer. *Laurocerasus* avoid reality by creating a complex set of avoidance techniques, the most profound being a dream-like, cheerfulness. The 'hubristic denial' and avoidance that *Laurocerasus* have is reflected in the *Mind* rubric: *cheerful,* and *Dream* rubrics: *dreams of high places,* and *dreams unremembered*. *Laurocerasus* will often refuse to mention or acknowledge their illness in consultation after consultation. *Laurocerasus* have the *Mind* rubrics: *unfeeling,* and *indifference with sleepiness*. *Laurocerasus* avoid feeling. This is the significance of the psychotherapeutic meaning of the *Delusion* rubric: *he was stunned*. [1] 1.

The simillimum will only be *Laurocerasus* if the patient is in total denial about the seriousness of their illness.

Laurocerasus have the *Mind* rubric: *loathing of life*. In a repertory if the only *Mind* rubric mentioned is *cheerfulness,* then the homoeopathic student can be left with a limited understanding of the contradictory states within a psychological profile. *Laurocerasus* have the *Mind* rubrics: *loathing of life,* and *cheerful*. All mental and emotional states which contradict each other will show up in the *Delusion* rubrics especially if the rubric only lists one remedy. The *Delusion* rubric: *he was stunned* is reflective of the mental and emotional dissociation within the psychological profile of *Laurocerasus*. *Laurocerasus* prefer to keep their consciousness buried in their unconscious. *Laurocerasus* as a homoeopathic remedy is also used for paralysis, especially of the respiratory system. The simillimum will only be *Laurocerasus* if the patient needs to stay in a depressive unresponsive state [*stunned*]. *Laurocerasus* will never acknowledge self-blame.

Laurocerasus prefer to remain unresponsive to protect themselves from others criticism and persecution. The simillimum will only be *Laurocerasus* if the patient prefers to remain in lachrymose despondency.

1. Denial: *Delusion* rubric: *fancy, illusions of: Laur. Delusion* rubric: *enlarged*: laur. [This rubric can pertain to grandeur or persecutory fears.]

2. Forsaken: *Delusion* rubric: *accused, she is*: laur. *Delusion* rubric: *criticized, she is*: laur. *Delusion* rubric: *fire: visions of*: laur. *Delusion* rubric: *man: old men: seeing: beards and distorted faces; seeing old men with long*: laur. [1] 1. *Delusion* rubric: *dead: persons, sees*: laur.

3. Causation: NONE.

4. Depression: *Delusion* rubric: *stunned; he was*: laur. [1] 1.

5. Resignation: *Delusion* rubric: *sick: being*: laur. *Delusion* rubric: *turn: everything turned: round and round*: laur. [1] 1.

Zincum transfer their illusions and psychological 'delusions of original sin' on to the devil within who has possessed them. *Zincum* have the *Delusion* rubrics: *devil is after her,* and *sees devil. Zincum* have the *Delusion* rubric: *voices from within him are speaking abusive and filthy language.* [2] 1. 'Transference neuroses' are a conflict between the realistic part of the psyche, or 'ego', and the 'id' which is unconscious, socially unrestrained and selfish. *Zincum* have the *Mind* rubric: *malicious desire to play dirty tricks on others or their teachers. Zincum* have an unrestrained malicious streak. *Zincum* also have the *Mind* rubric: *violent delirium is restrained and calmed with great difficulty.* [1] 1. *Zincum* suppress their conscious psyche. They have the *Mind* rubric: *frequent spells of unconsciousness.*

Transference is characterized by unconscious, self-deluding denial which allows for the redirection of feelings on to another person. 'Transference neuroses' can be found in the *Delusion* rubrics of 'hubristic denial' in which the patient transfers 'cause and effect' on to God. These are the *Delusion* rubrics: *in communication with God.* 'Transference neuroses' are also found in the *Delusion* rubrics of sin in which the patient transfers 'cause and effect' on to the devil. These are the *Delusion* rubrics: *in communication with the devil*. *Zincum* distance themselves from their own guilt and transfer blame on to the devil. The 'devil' is synonymous with whatever part of themselves they believe to be evil or controlled by evil forces. A neurosis is a disorder of the behavioral system which shows an inability to have a rational or realistic objective view of one's life.

Zincum spend their lives in a constant 'flight or fight' state. They are in 'flight' from their unconscious demons which are aligned to the devil or the 'id'. They 'fight' with their rational psyche or 'ego' which can inadvertently reveal them to the outer world. *Zincum* need to suppress and fight their own psyche. *Zincum* are highly neurotic and highly anxious that they will be 'found out'.

This heightened state of arousal means that *Zincum* suffers from an exhausted nervous system. Their inner conflict means that *Zincum* will present with very suppressed or compromised immune systems. Boger notes, in *Synoptic Key to Materia Medica*, Radar™, that *Zincum* are: "fagged, enervated or depressed; can't throw things off; develop exanthema[57]. Increasing weakness. Descending paralysis. Easily startled, excited or intoxicated."

Zincum have the *Mind* rubric: *tormenting everyone with his complaints*. [3] 3. *Zincum* as a homoeopathic remedy is used for psychological delusions arising from loss and grief. *Zincum* are neurotically obsessed with their own emotional processing, they can't let anything go. *Zincum* have the *Mind* rubric: *delusions from grief*. [2] 1., and the *Delusion* rubric: *delusions from grief and anger*. [2] 2. *Zincum* abandon themselves and subject themselves to undermining neurotic annihilation of their 'ego'. *Zincum* have the *Mind* rubric: *calmly thinks of the presentiment of death*. [1] 1. All neuroses are self-destructive and by their very nature have their origin in inner conflict. *Zincum* have the *Mind* rubrics: *discontented with himself, sensation of being good for nothing,* and *contentment alternating with sadness.* [1] 1. When *Zincum* are sick they exaggerate [*enlarged*] their illness. They neurotically exaggerate their inability to deal with being sick [*body is small*] and they are neurotically obsessed with the fact that others have caused their illness. When *Zincum* are sick they exaggerate all their 'delusions of persecution'. The 'never-well-since-event' or causation in any *Zincum* case will always have its origins in 'delusions of abandonment'. *Zincum* in *particular* have real and perceived psychological persecution delusions of being abandoned because they are bad.

Zincum are listed in the hubristic *Delusion* rubric: *he is counting his money.* Financial success is extremely important to all adults who have been orphaned or abandoned as children because wealth is synonymous with importance. *Zincum* have the *Delusion* rubric: *seeing thieves. Zincum* are obsessively neurotic about protecting their possessions and their health.

Zincum are neurotically possessive of everything they think can be taken away from them.

Zincum have the *Delusion* rubric: *deprived of sleep. Zincum* also have the *Mind* rubrics: *ailments from alcohol, ailments from bad news, ailments from emotions, ailments from grief* and *confusion after wine. Zincum* are easily overwhelmed and persecuted by everything.

1. Denial: *Delusion* rubric: *fancy, illusions of:* zinc. *Delusion* rubric: *money: counting money; he is:* zinc. *Delusion* rubric: *enlarged:* zinc. *Delusion* rubric: *voices: hearing:* Zinc. [This rubric can indicate 'delusions of hubristic denial' or 'delusions of persecution'.]

2. Forsaken: *Delusion* rubric: *devil: persecuted by the devil; he is; crimes he had never done; for:* zinc.[1] 1. *Delusion* rubric: *accused, she is:* zinc. *Delusion* rubric: *arrested, is about to be:* Zinc. *Delusion* rubric: *devil: after her; is:* Zinc. *Delusion* rubric: *murdered: will be murdered; he:* zinc. *Delusion* rubric: *persecuted: he is persecuted:* Zinc.

Delusion rubric: *poisoned: he has been*: zinc. *Delusion* rubric: *pursued; he was: enemies, by*: zinc. *Delusion* rubric: *pursued; he was: police, by*: zinc. *Delusion* rubric: *specters, ghosts, spirits: seeing*: zinc. *Delusion* rubric: *court; called before: menopause; during*: zinc. [1] 1. *Delusion* rubric: *voices: hearing: Zinc*. [This rubric can indicate 'delusions of persecution' or 'delusions of hubristic denial'.]

3. Causation: *Delusion* rubric: *crime: committed a crime; he had*: zinc. *Delusion* rubric: *evil: done some evil; had*: zinc.

4. Depression: *Delusion* rubric: *grief: anger; delusions from grief and: Zinc*. [2] 2. *Delusion* rubric: *fright: as if in a fright*: zinc.

5. Resignation: *Delusion* rubric: *die: about to die; one was*: zinc. *Delusion* rubric: *small: body is smaller*. zinc.

Causation

"I have caused my disease."

"This is my fault."

"I must have done something wrong to deserve this."

"I have been bad."

"I have sinned."

I have allocated all the *Delusion* rubrics which pertain to psychological 'delusions of original sin' or self-blame into Causation. If the trauma inside your patient starts with them feeling guilty and unrealistically responsible for their illness then the simillimum is listed in the all the *Delusion* rubrics: *he is sinful, he has committed a crime* or *he has done wrong*, and is allocated to the section Causation.

Kübler-Ross identified bargaining as the third stage. Bargaining is when a patient believes that if they are, for example, being good with their diet by juice fasting, or if they are meditating, they can do a deal with God and be cured.

Underlying the patient's active processing of bargaining is their underlying delusional belief that they have been bad, and that is what fuels their desire to now be good. I have identified Causation as the third stage. This is characterized by the patient blaming themselves for their loss of good health. A patient often blames their loss of good health on themselves by assuming they were bad, most commonly relating it to a time when they were not living their life in harmony.

A *Delusion* rubric is used when there is an assumption or perception which is a misrepresentation of reality.

The various 'New-Age' philosophies of 'you are what you think', and 'you are your disease', have their basis in the concepts of punishment for being bad.

I have sadly to say that I have never treated a patient with a permanent illness, whether it be life threatening or not, who has not become a victim to the delusional belief that their disease is a punishment. More often than not they have voluntarily taken on this belief in the guise of a 'New-Age' philosophy so they can find an explanation of the cause of their disease.

Since the emergence of 'New-Age' ideology we have developed a delusional belief that we are entitled to good health if we have been living a mindful life. This incorrect assumption of entitlement of good health fuels all the delusional conspiracy theories which have sprung up in the alternative health industry.

In the majority of the cases in my *Case Companion* to *Homoeopathic Psychiatry*, the relevance of each of the *Delusion* rubrics in Causation will throw light on the underlying guilt and the overwhelming effect that the concept of 'original sin' and the expulsion of Adam[58] and Eve has had on our psyche. 'Original sin' or the belief in good and evil[59] holds a powerful position in the Jewish, Islamic and Christian religions as well as in 'New-Age' philosophies that influence the alternative health industry. The absorption of good and evil by our modern-day psyche has affected our understanding of the reason for disease. I have added the psychological 'delusions of original sin' to the stages of refusing to acknowledge illness because in each case presented in my *Case Companion* to *Homoeopathic Psychiatry* the patient believes deep within their own self that they deserve the disease or emotional pain they are currently suffering. The psychological process of bargaining or of trying to be good is masking the underlying delusional belief in punishment for being bad.

I have found in my practice that every patient who presents with any serious disease, whether it be emotional, mental, or physical always presents with the *Delusion* rubrics of abandonment and the underlying guilt of being cast out of Paradise because they are evil. Each case presented also resonates with the patient's delusional expectation that if they are in communication with God or a 'higher being' or their 'inner spiritual spirit' they should be able to cure their disease.

If they can't cure their disease then they believe that their disease is a result of God's judgment or karma for the sins they have committed.

Adam and Eve don't just appear in Genesis and the Quran; they are the underlying psychological theme in all 'New-Age' books which have influenced the modern-day view we have of disease. Adam and Eve are expelled from Paradise, forsaken, abandoned, separated from God, and they lose their immortality. The assumption of the concept of 'original sin' and the attributing of personal blame will, in my experience, always present itself when a patient faces the loss of their health, regardless of whether it is fatal or non-fatal. The psychotherapeutic formation of the development of the five psychological steps: denial, forsaken, causation, depression and resignation which the patient will move through as they struggle to acknowledge and accept their illness is reminiscent of the steps Adam and Eve undertook in their story when they had to acknowledge their sin, subsequent abandonment and ultimate loss of immortality. The story of Adam and Eve is also the basis of an enormous number of the *Delusion* rubrics in the *Mind* section in our repertory and I have categorized them accordingly. If the trauma inside your patient starts with them feeling guilty and responsible for being sick then the simillimum is listed in the *Delusion* rubrics: *he is sinful* and *he has committed a crime.*

Invariably, in all the consultations I have had with patients facing a fatal illness, they will bring the conversation around to the subject of *why me*? I have found it is not helpful, or useful, to offer any explanations of the potential cause of their illness.

It is impossible to know the cause of many diseases, and even if, there is a logical explanation, as is the case with exposure to asbestos, for example, the patient will still want to find their own reason for why *they* got asbestosis and not their friend who was standing next to them when they were exposed. The patient wants and needs to arrive at what they themselves believe to be the cause. Even if there has been an established genetic link, as is the case with cancer of the bowel, for example. The patient still wants to find their own reason for why *they* got bowel cancer. If the homoeopath interferes with this crucial process by reiterating the genetic link, then the homoeopath will not get to find out the information they need to be able to pick the *peculiarities specific* to that patient and not to the disease.

It is also not appropriate to offer any homoeopathic explanations of miasms to a patient who is trying to find the cause of their illness. I have as a teacher watched students and qualified homoeopaths do this in consultations. If you offer homoeopathic miasmic philosophy to the patient they will not offer you *their* explanation; *their* explanation is a gem which will indicate the simillimum. What the patient offers as their explanation will, of course, indicate the simillimum in the case.

When a patient is faced with failure in their life, whether it is fiscal failure, failure in their marriage, or whether it is failure of their health they will consistently relate the cause back to a period of time in their life when they felt that they were not living in harmony with themselves. Typically the patient will relay the following explanations of the cause of their illness: *I was chasing the mighty dollar. – I was not in touch with my true self. – I was always living the high life. – There was a time when I was pushing too many drugs. – I knew I had been drinking way too much, for too long. – I knew this would happen because I have had very negative thoughts. – I have been working too hard and well, it has to catch up with you doesn't it?* None, or all, of these sorts of explanations might, or might not, have contributed to a patient's illness. So far, in this process, there is nothing in the above possible explanations of the cause for their illness which is indicative of the patient having any psychological delusions. The above causes that patients have come up with are in proportion to the situation, and in proportion to their feelings of having no control. Because your patient is facing a loss of control over their health, and potentially their life, they will seek to regain control by finding the cause of their illness; this is a normal response. It is also a normal appropriate response for a patient to blame themselves for their current illness if, for some time, they have been drinking, or smoking, or taking too many drugs.

A *Delusion* rubric can only be used in the case if you can see a conflicting struggle which is *self-punishing* in your patient's psyche.

If your patient says to you with the intensity of the 'eye of the storm', that they know *why* they are ill, and they reveal their sins, and conclude that their illness is their *just desert*, then this is indicative of the psychological delusions of punishment.

In psychiatry, self-inflicted exile or self-imposed punishment is a consequence or end result of a 'persecution complex[60]'. In homoeopathy 'delusions of self-persecution' are repertorised by using the *Delusion* rubrics pertaining to sins. The word devil or sinful is no longer in common usage. In the *Delusion* rubrics the use of the word devil should not be interpreted literally. The devil in the *Delusion* rubric: *he is possessed of a devil*, does not refer to the personification of the devil, Satan. The *Delusion* rubric: *he is possessed of a devil* can refer to the wicked or bad side of one's nature which has led one astray. The *Delusion* rubric: *he is possessed of a devil* can also refer to predictions of impending damnation or doom. The person possessed by the devil can also refer to someone who is luckless or wretched. Nowadays it is rare for a patient to refer to their 'devil' within, or the 'devil' who is the tempter of mankind. If a patient refers to the 'dark-side of their nature' who tempts them to do 'bad things', this should be repertorised as the *Delusion* rubric: *he is possessed of a devil*. Similarly, a patient will rarely use the word sinful. If a patient believes they have been 'bad', this should be repertorised as the *Delusion* rubric: *he is possessed of a devil*, or *he has committed a crime*.

If your patient believes that they truly *deserve* their illness and this is why they are sick then this is representative of the *Delusion* rubrics of having *sinned* and *committed a crime*. If your patient believes in a system of just punishment for their sins, this is an indication of disproportionate retribution. If their reactions to their feelings of being bad are disproportionately an *over-reaction* and misrepresentation of reality then it is important to consider the *Delusion* rubrics pertaining to *wrongs committed*. These rubrics are also important to consider for patients who believe that the reason they are sick is because they are essentially bad people [*evil*]. These are the *Delusion* rubrics of being *in communication with the devil* or *being the devil*, or *being evil*. This group of rubrics is crucial to case-taking for patients who believe that in some way *they* are the cause of their illness or misfortune. Self-persecution is commonly referred to as psychological 'delusions of original sin'.

Psychological delusions of guilt are fueled by a *disproportionate* reaction to crimes most commonly committed in childhood. These crimes are often held as deep dark secrets which, because they are suppressed for so long in the emotional memory of a child, become blown out of proportion to their seriousness. Psychological 'delusions of original sin' are easily accessed by the patient; the memories of wrongs committed sit in our subconscious and conscious mind. As soon as the homoeopath asks a patient why they think they are sick, the patient will be drawn into confessing their 'original sin'. Firstly, the patient will be drawn to confessing sins because their childhood guilt will have kept the memories alive, and secondly because the desire to find the reason they are sick will compel them to confess all their deeply held secrets, even if the secrets are self-condemning. All the remedies listed in *Delusion* rubrics: *evil*, *being the devil*, *being a criminal* and *having done wrongs*, know in their subconscious and conscious mind that they have committed crimes. The essence of avoidance and self-deluding is that it is a psychological technique which allows the patient to over-react to their sins. The disproportionate reaction is either used to their advantage or used as self-destructive, self-punishing condemnation. The next questions to ask the patient which will reveal the simillimum are: "what happens when they feel accused and what happens if they feel they have done something wrong"?

The homoeopath needs to understand how each constitutional remedy reacts or tries to avoid acknowledging perceived or real psychological delusions of fault. Each remedy will present with a specific and *peculiar* interpretation which will reveal the simillimum.

Self-destructive depression and predictions of failure underpin and also cover up the psychological delusions of self-blame and psychological 'delusions of original sin'. Self-destructive depression and predictions of failure advantageously protect the patient from having to acknowledge sins committed, or alliances made with the 'evil-side' of themselves. Self-destructive behavior and self-blame will be maintained and nurtured because they help protect the patient from their innermost dark secrets about themselves.

Delusion Rubrics in Causation

In this section I analyze and explain the meaning of each individual *Delusion* rubric. I offer previously unexplored explanations of the psychological delusional state inherent in each *Delusion* rubric. Furthermore, I explain their psychotherapeutic meaning and application by analyzing how each remedy listed under the rubric heading has utilized the delusional stance to its advantage. The reasons why each constitutional remedy is listed under a rubric will often be vastly different. Understanding the need for the psychological delusions within each of the constitutional remedy profiles will aid in remedy recognition.

Each selection of *Delusion* rubrics discussed are shaded. Analyses of the remedy profiles follow each sub-section. The psychological development of *Delusion* rubrics for each constitutional remedy profile is analyzed according to either **avoidance** or **self-deluding** need.

- *Delusions: God: he is God, then he is the devil:* **STRAM**. [3] 1.
- *Delusions: God: vengeance; he is the object of God's:* **KALI-BR**. [3] 1. [This rubric can be an admission of guilt or an indication of 'delusions of persecution'.]
- *Delusions: devil:* anac. *Bell.* cupr. hyos. *Plat.*
- *Delusions: devil: connected to devil, he is arrogant towards those who strive to purity, light and love:* ozone. [1] 1.
- *Delusions: devil: he is a devil:* **ANAC**. camph. cann-i. *Hyos.* kali-br. pegan-ha. positr. stram.

- *Delusions*: *devil*: *possessed of a devil*: aluni. lyss. mand.

- *Delusions*: *devil*: *possessed of a devil; he is*: borx. cann-i. *Hyos*. plat. positr. stram.

- *Delusions*: *devil*: *sits in his neck, devil*: Anac. [1] 1.

- *Delusions*: *devil*: *sits in his neck, devil; prompting to offensive things*: anac. [1] 1.

- *Delusions*: *devil*: *speaking in one ear, prompting to murder; angel in the other ear, prompting to acts of benevolence; and an*: Anac. [2] 1.

- *Delusions*: *evil*: *done some evil; had*: cycl. lat-h. zinc.

- *Delusions*: *executioner; visions of an*: stram. [1] 1.

- *Delusions*: *influence*: *one is under a powerful*: ambr. brass-n-o. carc. cere-b. dream-p. foll. *Hyos*. irid-met. kali-br. *Lach*. ozone. positr. psil. *Sal-fr*. *Stram*. thuj. verat. [This rubric can pertain to God or the devil.]

- *Delusions*: *possessed, being*: alum. *Anac*. bell. canth. carb-v. helo-s. hydrog. *Hyos*. lach. lyss. **MANC**. mand. op. orot-ac. plat. positr. psil. sal-fr. sil. stram. *Sulph*. verat.

- *Delusions*: *possessed; being: evil forces; by*: ignis-alc. manc.

- *Delusions*: *visions, has; horrible*: absin. ambr. atro. **BELL**. calc-sil. **CALC**. camph. carb-an. carb-v. **CAUST**. hep. ign. indol. **KALI-BR**. lac-c. lyc. merc. nicot. **NUX-V**. op. phos. positr. **PULS**. rad-br. rhod. samb. sil. **STRAM**. sulph. tarent.

- *Delusions*: *devil*: *squeezed dry in the devil's fist; she is*: positr. [1] 1.

- *Delusion*: *God*: *God's works are ill made and ill done*: positr. [1] 1.

- *Delusions*: *evil*: *he is evil and does not care*: positr. [1] 1.

- *Delusions*: *devil, sees*: absin. ambr. *Anac*. ars. *Bell*. cann-i. cupr. dulc. *Hell*. *Hyos*. ignis-alc. *Kali-br*. kali-c. lach. *Manc*. nat-c. *Op*. orig. *Plat*. *Puls*. stram. sulph. *Zinc*.

- *Delusions*: *devil*: *taken by the devil; he will be*: bell. manc. *Puls*.

- *Delusions*: *stabbed*: *person who passed on the street; he had stabbed a*: Bell. [2] 1.

- *Delusions*: *murdering; he is*: *husband and child; she is about to murder her*: kali-br. [1] 1.

- *Delusions: murdering; he is: struck friends who came to help him: Stram.* [2] 1.
- *Delusions: evil: happened to him; feeling as though some evil had:* lach. meny.

Avoidance: The *Delusion* rubrics of being evil and in communication with the devil apply to the constitutional remedies which are haunted by deep dark secrets about their 'past sins' or they experience guilt over their desire to align themselves to 'the dark-side' of their nature.

Each constitutional remedy listed over-react to their evilness. Their guilt is a psychological delusion which is either a misinterpretation or exaggeration of how bad they are.

Or alternatively, an avoidance of acknowledging, or taking responsibility for their sins by blaming them on the power of the 'de√il' who has led them astray. In homoeopathic case analysis it is important to understand why each constitutional remedy will choose to hold on to their guilt.

Guilt over sins committed is always a psychological avoidance technique which is maintained because it is advantageous to the patient.

A lot of the remedies listed are also capable of acts of cruelty. This is why they over-react to their evilness, and why they lay the blame for their evilness at the feet of the devil rather than acknowledge that it is their own instinctual impulse. The psychological delusion of avoidance implies that all the constitutional remedy profiles are aware in their conscious or subconscious mind of the 'dark-side' of their personality which haunts them. We should not assume that modern-day patients do not identify with the devil as a real person.

When faced with fatal illness and impending death the psychological 'delusions of original sin' and the power of God to save them and the devil as the person who has led them astray from good health are as real today as they were in medieval times. Death elicits myths.

Anacardium have intense fear of their own hate and 'devil-like' rage which flares[61] intensely if they are contradicted or criticized. *Anacardium* have the *Delusion* rubric: *surrounded by enemies*. This delusional paranoiac feeling of being surrounded by enemies leaves them open to being hypersensitive about all real, or perceived criticisms. *Anacardium* consequently over-react when they are criticized. This is why *Anacardium* are listed so prominently in the rubrics for the devil in one ear, and the angel in the other. *Anacardium* have the *Mind* rubric: *antagonism with self*. *Anacardium* avoid facing their fear of being criticized and avoid feeling vulnerable to their own lack of self-confidence by relying on their 'divine' (whether it be devil or angel) auditory intervention.

Anacardium spend an enormous amount of time berating themselves for their 'devil-like' rage and hate, which they try to make up for by over-compensating with 'god-like' generosity.

Guilt over their reactivity keeps them separate from the world – *Delusion* rubric: *separated from the world*. Separating themselves from the world allows them protection from being criticized and contradicted. As there is no peace from their internalized dilemma of the *devil speaking in one ear, prompting to murder; and angel in the other ear, prompting to acts of benevolence, Anacardium* solve the debate by avoiding the world. This avoidance then becomes a self-fulfilling prophecy for *Anacardium* as they then believe they have been abandoned (forsaken) because they are evil. The simillimum will only be *Anacardium* if the patient periodically needs to avoid people, especially proceeding any kind of dispute. If the simillimum is *Anacardium* the homoeopath must perceive that the patient has approached their illness with the same internalized separation. The simillimum will not be *Anacardium* unless the patient indicates that they want to hide their illness.

Their self-destructive behavior is separating themselves from the world and remaining in self-inflicted exile. *Anacardium* are difficult to treat when they are sick because they do not want to talk about their illness or acknowledge they are sick. This is avoidance. Illness exposes them to criticism and illness is proof of their 'dark-side' [*devil*]. Disease and illness is also viewed by *Anacardium* as proof of their failure to succeed.

Their dark secret or innermost fear is that they will not be recognized. *Anacardium* have the *Delusion* rubric: *seeing everybody's face in the mirror except his own.* [1] 1. *Anacardium* fear everyone else will be reflected in the mirror and not them. When they are sick *Anacardium* become *religious*. It is a mistake to assume the *Delusion* rubric: *religious* applies to institutionalized religious practices. *Anacardium* will align themselves with various 'New-Age' ideologies, firstly so they can assure themselves that they are 'seeking a cure', and secondly because they need to believe they are spiritual [*angel*]. *Anacardium* will not present as an evil person, they will see themselves as righteously 'good'. *Anacardium* prefer to hide (deny) their 'devil-side' from themselves and others; it is only if they are criticized that one sees the *devil* in *Anacardium*.

The simillimum will only be *Anacardium* if the patient believes that they can cure themselves by being good.

Anacardium have the *Delusion* rubric: *body is separated from soul*. The simillimum will only be *Anacardium* if the patient believes that it is their body which is sick not their 'true self' [*soul*]. The homoeopath must be able to detect that the patient is 'split' or in denial about the bad [*devil*] part of them which is sick.

The simillimum will not be *Anacardium* unless the patient shows signs of denial, as well as signs of exaggerated self-blame ('delusions of original sin'). The simillimum will only be *Anacardium* if the homoeopath can perceive that the patient believes that they and the homoeopath *will not succeed* in making them well. *Anacardium* have the *Delusion* rubrics: *he is worthless*, and *he does everything wrong, he cannot succeed*. On one hand, *Anacardium* are in denial about their illness and on the other hand they are fatalistic, they believe they are already *in their grave.*

1. Denial: *Delusion* rubric: *religious*: Anac. *Delusion* rubric: *separated*: *body*: *soul; body is separated from*: Anac.

2. Forsaken: *Delusion* rubric: *outcast; she were an*: anac. *Delusion* rubric: *enemy*: *surrounded by enemies*: Anac. *Delusion* rubric: *separated*: *world; from the*: *he is separated*: Anac.

3. Causation: *Delusion* rubric: *devil*: *he is a devil*: **ANAC**. *Delusion* rubric: *superhuman*: *is*: *control; is under superhuman*: anac. [In *Anacardium* this rubric can pertain to the devil or God.]

4. Depression: *Delusion* rubric: *anxious*: Anac. *Delusion* rubric: *succeed, he does everything wrong; he cannot*: Anac. *Delusion* rubric: *worthless; he is*: anac.

5. Resignation: *Delusion* rubric: *grave, he is in his*: anac. *Delusion* rubric: *separated*: *body*: *soul; body is separated from*: Anac.

Belladonna: In all the rubrics pertaining to sin, *Belladonna* are only listed in two *Delusion* rubrics: *devil,* and *he had stabbed a person who passed on the street. Belladonna* are listed in more of the rubrics pertaining to fear and terror of being taken by the devil and seeing horrible visions of spirits. *Belladonna* have numerous *Delusion* rubrics: *hears dead people's voices, sees horrible visions, sees people as animals, sees the devil, will be taken by the devil, will be murdered,* and conversely *beautiful, things look beautiful. Belladonna* are highly impressionable and reactive; they see the world as a horrible, threatening place and conversely as a beautiful place. Psychological illusions of the world as beautiful can be a smoke screen shielding violent reactivity and rage; this is an avoidance technique. *Belladonna* are listed in numerous *Mind* rubrics for rage and violent desires to kill, and conversely numerous *Mind* rubrics for sensitivity.

Belladonna have intense fear of the devil and intense fear that they *are* the devil.

Belladonna are listed under the *Delusion* rubric: *violent,* and the *Delusion* rubric: *after vexation.* It is their violent, reactive rage which confirms their view that they *are* the devil. *Belladonna* are then overcome with 'god-like' remorse – *Delusion* rubric: *religious.* If you apply the five psychological processes to the rubric-repertorisation of the remedy *Belladonna,* your understanding of their hubristic 'delusions of grandeur' will be greatly deepened. If *Belladonna* externalize their devil it allows them to delude themselves about their own violent reactivity.

Belladonna are one of only two remedies listed in the *Delusion* rubric: *she has her own little world. Belladonna* need to believe they are a great person to shield their fears that they *are* the devil. *Belladonna* also need to believe they are a great person to allay fears of being taken over by the devil. Their violent reactivity is a well constructed technique which gives them protection from being taken over by the devil inside of themselves.

Belladonna are similar to *Anacardium* in that they are difficult to treat when they are sick; with *Belladonna* however, their anger about being sick is directed towards the practitioner rather than internalized, which is what *Anacardium* tend to do. *Belladonna* use their violent reactivity to protect themselves when they are vulnerable. When *Belladonna* are sick they feel extremely vulnerable to attack – *Delusion* rubric: *about to receive injury. Belladonna* get swamped by depressive fears that their illness will consume them – *Delusion* rubrics: *body will putrefy,* and the *devil will take them. Belladonna* can view the homoeopath as the devil and the homoeopathic medicine as a poison which is going to cause them *injury* – *Delusion* rubrics: *sees devil,* and *possessed.*

The simillimum will only be *Belladonna* if the homoeopath can perceive an equal psychological split between acknowledging blame for sins (rage) and feeling like a persecuted victim of the world. The simillimum will only be *Belladonna* if the homoeopath can also perceive that the patient deals with their fear of the world and themselves, by creating an imaginary world in which everything is *beautiful* and everyone is their *friend*.

1. Denial: *Delusion* rubric: *religious*: bell. *Delusion* rubric: *great person, is a*: bell. *Delusion* rubric: *well, he is*: bell. *Delusion* rubric: *beautiful: things look*: bell. *Delusion* rubric: *friend: surrounded by friends; being*: bell. *Delusion* rubric: *magician, is a*: bell. [1] 1. *Delusion* rubric: *wealth, of*: bell.

2. Forsaken: *Delusion* rubric: *home: away from home; he is*: bell. *Delusion* rubric: *injury: about to receive injury; is*: bell. *Delusion* rubric: *devil: taken by the devil; he will* be: bell. *Delusion* rubric: *caught; he will be*: bell. *Delusion* rubric: *gallows with fear; vision of*. *Bell*. [2] 1.

3. Causation: *Delusion* rubric: *devil*: *Bell*. *Delusion* rubric: *stabbed*: *person who passed on the street; he had stabbed a*: *Bell*. [2] 1. *Delusion* rubric: *gallows with fear; vision of*. *Bell*. [2] 1. [This rubric can also pertain to an admission of guilt.]

4. Depression: *Delusion* rubric: *doomed, being*: bell.

5. Resignation: *Delusion* rubric: *body: putrefy, will*: bell. *Delusion* rubric: *sick; being*: bell.

Hyoscyamus can be extremely sweet and loving one minute, and extremely violent and malicious the next. Their affection is a calculated, manipulative technique to ensure they are in total control of everyone's love. *Hyoscyamus* are hyper-vigilant to any perceived loss of love. *Hyoscyamus* have the *Mind* rubrics: *delirium from jealousy,* and *animus possession*. *Hyoscyamus* are the only remedy listed in the *Delusion* rubric: *going to be married,* and the only remedy listed in the *Delusion* rubric: *being sold*. *Hyoscyamus* obsessively desire marriage or union with another and fear being sold or abandoned by another. *Hyoscyamus* when they are sick feel trapped and tied to the practitioner, as well as suspicious and untrusting of the practitioner and the medication – *Delusion* rubrics: *about to be poisoned*. On the one hand they feel like they will lose themselves to their illness, and on the other hand they are convinced they are well and do not need you. *Hyoscyamus* have the *Delusion* rubrics: *he has suffered wrong,* as well as *he has done wrong,* and the *Delusion* rubrics: *will be murdered,* and *has to murder someone. Hyoscyamus* blame their sins on the devil, who is possessing them. *Hyoscyamus* have the *Delusion* rubric: *being in debate. Hyoscyamus* will avoid all acknowledgment of sins inflicted on others and avoid acknowledgment of any illness because illness is viewed as acknowledging fault. *Hyoscyamus* will only acknowledge their illness through endless lamentations of righteous jealous rage about others' wellbeing.

If you ask *Hyoscyamus* what it means to be sick, they will answer that it means they need you and because of that they hate you; this is why *Hyoscyamus* need the hubristic illusion that they are well.

The simillimum will not be *Hyoscyamus* unless the patient indicates that they feel trapped [*possessed*] and bound by their disease. *Hyoscyamus* have the *Delusion* rubric: *hand bound by chains*. [1] 1. *Hyoscyamus* have exaggerated reactions to being controlled [*married*].

1. Denial: *Delusion* rubric: *religious*: Hyos. *Delusion* rubric: *visions, has fantastic*: hyos. *Delusion* rubric: *well, he is*: hyos.

2. Forsaken: *Delusion* rubric: *poisoned*: *he*: *about to be poisoned; he is*: Hyos. *Delusion* rubric: *friend*: *affection of; has lost the*: hyos. *Delusion* rubric: *home*: *away from home; he is*: Hyos.

3. Causation: *Delusion* rubric: *devil*: hyos. *Delusion* rubric: *devil*: *he is a devil*: Hyos. *Delusion* rubric: *devil*: *possessed of a* devil: *he is*: Hyos. *Delusion* rubric: *possessed; being*: Hyos. *Delusion* rubric: *criminal, he is a*: hyos. *Delusion* rubric: *murdering; he is*: *has to murder someone; he*: hyos.

Delusion rubric: *offended people; he has*: **HYOS**.

4. Depression: *Delusion* rubric: *collect senses; unable to*: hyos. *Delusion* rubric: *insane: become insane; one will*: hyos. *Delusion* rubric: *hand: bound: chains; with*: hyos. [1] 1. *Delusion* rubric: *sinking; to be: floor; through the*: hyos. [This rubric should not be interpreted literally, it pertains to sinking depression.]

5. Resignation: *Delusion* rubric: *weight: no weight; has*: hyos. [This rubric should not be interpreted literally, it pertains to hypochondriacal fears of the loss of one's health.]

Kali bromatum are prone to paranoid delusions about being the victim of God's vengeance. *Kali bromatum* have the *Delusion* rubric: *is forsaken by God*. [1] 1. *Kali bromatum* exaggerate God's vengeance; they are helplessly resigned to their fate – *Delusion* rubric: *destruction of all near her impending*. [2] 1. *Kali bromatum* have an internal conflicting discord about accepting their own mortality. Death is the ultimate failure in life. *Kali bromatum* misinterpret and misrepresent failure. *Kali bromatum* is a crucial remedy to consider when a patient who is critically ill cannot abide or accept that they could possibly die. They suffer intensely from embarrassment about any loss or failure, whether it is business failure, declining health, or relationship failure. They avoid their fears of failure by projecting all their failure on to the wrath of God. They also exaggerate the power and potency of the devil's influence. This allows them to avoid acknowledging their part in the failure, while simultaneously exaggerating their part in the 'original sin' by believing they are inherently evil. *Kali bromatum* have the *Delusion* rubrics: *he is a devil,* and *he is the object of God's vengeance.*

Kali bromatum are convinced that their disease is God's punishment because they are the devil.

It is important to realize that no one is going to come into your consulting room and say that they are the devil, or that their disease is evidence of God's vengeance. *Kali bromatum* have the *Delusion* rubrics: *melancholy,* and *he would go out of his mind. Kali bromatum* will present in your clinic and tell you: *my illness is causing me unbearable suffering, everyone can see I am sick; it is proof to the world that I have something truly wrong with myself. My illness has been caused by pressure in the world to always succeed and be good. It is being good and others' goodness which has caused this illness.* Psychotherapeutic understanding of the avoidance techniques within this statement is crucial to finding the simillimum in this case.

The pressure to be good is their allegiance to God; and God has deceived them. Their illness is an indicator of impending doom and proof of God's punishment. Illness is proof of their allegiance to the devil. *Kali bromatum* will never acknowledge that they are solely to blame – they are under the influence of a *superhuman* force.

Kali bromatum align themselves with their murderous rage [*devil*] and wring their hands because they fear God's vengeance. *Kali bromatum* have the *Mind* rubric: *desire to kill loved ones. Kali bromatum* are vulnerable to believing that God and/or the devil has instructed them to murder. Believing one is controlled by someone else can be a pretentious and dangerous psychological 'delusion of grandeur' which allows for the redirection of responsibility on to another person. *Kali bromatum* have 'transference neuroses'. *Kali bromatum* transfer blame on to either God or the devil.

The simillimum will not be Kali bromatum unless the patient transfers blame on to everyone else other than themselves.

1. Denial: *Delusion* rubric: *religious*: *Kali-br. Delusion* rubric: *influence; one is under a powerful*: kali-br. *Delusion* rubric: *superhuman; is*: *control; is under superhuman*: kali-br. [These last two rubrics can be interpreted as God or the devil.]

2. Forsaken: *Delusion* rubric: *forsaken: is: God; by:* kali-br.
   [1] 1. *Delusion* rubric: *God: vengeance; he is the object of
   God's:* **KALI-BR**. *Delusion* rubric: *life threatened; life is:*
   kali-br. [1] 1. [This rubric can pertain to persecution or can
   be an indication of hypochondria and fear of ill health.]

3. Causation: *Delusion* rubric: *devil, he is a devil:* kali-br.
   Delusion rubric: *murdering; he is: husband and child;
   she is about to murder her.* kali-br. [1] 1. *Delusion* rubric:
   superhuman; is: control; is under superhuman: kali-br.
   [This rubric can be interpreted as God or the devil.]

4. Depression: *Delusion* rubric: *melancholy:* **KALI-BR**.
   Delusion rubric: *painful, with sadness:* kali-br. [1] 1.
   Delusion rubric: *mind: out of his mind; he would go: Kali-br.*
   Delusion rubric: *doomed, being: Kali-br.*

5. Resignation: *Delusion* rubric: *emptiness; of: around and
   under one on standing; emptiness:* kali-br. [1] 1. *Delusion*
   rubric: *life: threatened; life is:* kali-br. [1] 1. *Delusion* rubric:
   destruction of all near her; impending: Kali-br. [2] 1. [These
   last three rubrics can be allocated into Resignation,
   indicating predications of ill health and/or death. Or it can
   be allocated into Depression indicating predications of
   doom.]

Mancinella fear they will be taken by the devil. *Mancinella*
are tormented[62] by obsessive thoughts. *Mancinella* have the
Mind rubric: *tormenting thoughts* and *persistent thoughts of
evil. Mancinella* fear being consumed by the devil from inside
and from outside of themselves.

Mancinella fear the devil will possess them and they will become the
devil. Their sin is that they have let themselves be possessed by the devil.
Mancinella fear their cancer taking them over, rather than believing *they*
have created the cancer. *Mancinella* succumb to disease.

If they have Chronic Fatigue Syndrome, they are *consumed*
with Chronic Fatigue Syndrome. If they have a simple cold

or a seasonal bout of influenza they are *consumed* with the influenza which is *invading* and taking over every cell in their body.

Each patient reacts in an individual, *peculiar* way which is determined by their psychological delusions. The psychological delusions are reflected in the *Delusion* rubrics and this is why understanding homoeopathic psychiatry is essential.

Mancinella will say in a consultation: *I have never been well since I got Ross River Fever; I can feel the poison of this virus still inside of me; it is penetrating every muscle of my whole being. I can't even walk or lift my head off the pillow. Every time I lift my head I feel like I am floating and my head is swimming. I feel like I just want to leave my body, float off and go somewhere else.* [*Delusion* rubrics: *floating in air,* and *swimming in the air.*] *I have been singled out, of all my friends, it is only me who was bitten by the mosquitoes in Queensland and who got this virus.* [*Delusion* rubrics: *he was pursued,* and *he is persecuted.*] Their sin is that they have let themselves be possessed by their illness. When they are possessed by the illness they will succumb and loose all rational thought; *become insane.*

The simillimum will only be *Mancinella* if the patient indicates that they (personally), have nothing to do with being responsible for their illness.

1. Denial: *Delusion* rubric: *floating: air; in:* manc. [*Mancinella* disassociate from themselves when they are sick.] *Delusion* rubric: *voices; hearing:* manc. [This rubric can pertain to auditory illusions of persecution or illusions of grandeur.]

2. Forsaken: *Delusion* rubric: *pursued; he was:* manc.

3. Causation: *Delusion* rubric: *possessed; being:* **MANC**. *Delusion* rubric: *possessed; being: evil forces; by:* manc.

4. Depression: *Delusion* rubric: *insane: become insane; one will:* **MANC**.

5. Resignation: *Delusion* rubric: *light*: *is light; he*: manc. [This rubric reinforces physical vulnerability.]

Positronium: One of the themes of *Positronium* is not caring and being uncaring. *Positronium* have a conflicting debate between matter and anti-matter; between substance and lack of substance; between structure and destruction. *Positronium* embrace the destruction of disease.

The theme of self-abandonment is reinforced in the *Delusion* rubric: *he is evil and doesn't care*. *Positronium* are unique in their indifference and lack of inner conflict over guilt for crimes or wrongs committed.

Positronium have a self-fulfilling prophecy of creating structure, and then allowing themselves and the structure to be decimated. *Positronium* have the *Delusion* rubrics: *she cannot bend, body will turn to stone,* and *hypnotized*. On one hand they are hard and will not be influenced by anyone, and on the other hand they allow themselves to be hypnotized. *Positronium* also have the *Mind* rubric: *desires activity alternating with lassitude*. On the one hand, *Positronium* hang on to their structure; *Delusion* rubric: *a stone statue,* and on the other hand they let it go; *body torn to pieces. Positronium* have the *Delusion* rubric: *final acceptance of being slaughtered like something innocent.* [1] 1. They also have the *Delusion* rubric: *God's works are ill made and ill done. Positronium* are disturbingly fatalistic when sick. In fact, there is a relishing of destruction and embracing of death's final decay of matter. *Positronium* enjoy their allegiance to the devil and illness and decay because it proves God is powerless. *Positronium* will enjoy being sick and they will enjoy seeing that their friends and family are terrified and confronted with their illness and decay. *Positronium* enjoy the self-abandonment of illness. *Positronium* have the *Delusion* rubric: *squeezed dry in the devil's fist; she is*: positr. [1] 1.

The self-abandoning depression in *Positronium* is particularly notable; but what is *peculiar* and *specific* to *Positronium* is *that they do not care about the evil inside of them.*

Usually, the psychological 'delusions of original sin' play a significant role in the remedy profiles and the case analysis because the patient is so overcome with guilt and the need for redemption that they create an inner conflict which is the precipitating cause of inner conflict in existing, or future ill health. *Positronium* are fatalistically self-destructive and feel they deserve death. *Positronium* is a remedy derived from positronium which is a short-lived atomic system formed of an electron and a positron before they interact to annihilate each other. *Positronium* are significantly not overcome with guilt and self-redemption; they embrace death with final *acceptance*. Significantly, *Positronium* believe themselves to be *innocent and sacrificed*; they have not absorbed any residual guilt or self-conflict over their acknowledgment that they are evil. *Positronium* have the *Mind* rubric: *alcoholism, drinking to see what oblivion is like*. [1] 1. *Positronium* also have the *Mind* rubrics: *lack of reaction to danger* and *desires death*. It is noteworthy that the final stage of Acceptance in the model by Kübler-Ross does not imply that the patient should feel they are *sacrificing* their life. Acceptance in the model by Kübler-Ross is a peaceful coming to terms with the finality of death. The *final acceptance of being slaughtered* in *Positronium* is noteworthy as a psychological delusion which highlights a disproportionate need to desire decay and death. *Positronium* have the *Delusion* rubric: *locked away within herself*. [1] 1.

The simillimum will only be *Positronium* if the patient is decidedly fatalistic. However, the simillimum will only be *Positronium* if their fatalism is glorified [*blessed*].

1. Denial: Delusion rubric: *blessed state; she is in a*: positr. [1] 1. Delusion rubric: *gifts; she is showered with*: positr. [1] 1. Delusion rubric: *value, she is*: positr. [1] 1. *Delusion rubric*: *beautiful*: positr. *Delusion* rubric: *sacrificed*: *acceptance of being slaughtered like something innocent; final*: positr. [1] 1. [This rubric can be perceived as an indication of glorified martyrdom or finality.]

2. Forsaken: Delusion rubric: *friendless, he is*: positr. Delusion rubric: *appreciated, she is not*: positr.

3. Causation: *Delusion* rubric: *evil*: *he is evil and does not care*: positr. [1] 1. *Delusion* rubric: *God*: *God's works are ill made and ill done*: positr. [1] 1. *Delusion* rubric: *devil*: *squeezed dry in the devil's fist; she is*: positr. [1] 1.

4. Depression: *Delusion* rubric: *crushed*: *she is*: positr. *Delusion* rubric: *locked away within herself*. posit.[1] 1.

5. Resignation: *Delusion* rubric: *disease*: *incurable disease; he has an*: positr. *Delusion* rubric: *sacrificed*: *acceptance of being slaughtered like something innocent; final*: positr. [1] 1. *Delusion* rubric: *decayed, tarnished and impure; everything is*: positr. [1] 1. *Delusion* rubric: *diminished*: *shrunken, parts are*: positr.

Stramonium have good reason to fear their own reactive tendencies towards violent rage because they know that they can *easily* be possessed by the devil. *Stramonium* are listed in numerous *Delusion* rubrics pertaining to communication with God because God protects them from themselves. *Stramonium* are listed in the *Delusion* rubrics: *in communication with God*, *is a great person*, and *she is the Virgin Mary*. *Stramonium* are the only remedy listed in the *Delusion* rubric: *she is beautiful and wants to be beautiful*, and the only remedy in the *Delusion* rubric: *poses as a statue to be admired*. Their religiosity and pretentious 'delusions of grandeur' are needed to protect themselves from becoming the 'devil', which they know is inside them.

The irony for *Stramonium*, which is why they are listed in the *Delusion* rubric: *he is God then the devil*, is that they are fearful of becoming the victim of their own violence.

Stramonium know that they are divided into two parts, possessed by the devil and God. They have fears and psychological delusions of being abandoned. *Stramonium* are the only remedy listed in the *Delusion* rubric: *being alone in the wilderness*. *Stramonium* will present with a split psychotic personality when they are sick. On the one hand, they will become extremely religious and spiritual and believe that God will save them from their illness – *Delusion* rubric: *he had power over all disease*. On the other hand, they will be crippled with fear because they believe that their illness is proof that the devil already possesses them and they are abandoned to the wilderness – *Delusion* rubric: *he has every disease,* and the *Delusion* rubric: *he is in his grave*. *Stramonium* are the only remedy listed in the *Delusion* rubric: *he had power over all disease*, and the *Delusion* rubric: *being inconsolable*. Both sides will try to avoid acknowledging that the other side exists – *Delusion* rubric: *divided, cut in two parts*. Their split personality means *Stramonium* will deny that they are sick. The simillimum will not be *Stramonium* unless the patient has evidence of a delusional belief that they have control over all illness at the same time as having delusional fears they are already *in their grave*.

1. Denial: *Delusion* rubric: *God: communication with God; he is in*: stram. *Delusion* rubric: *power; disease; he had power over all*: stram. [1] 1. *Delusion* rubric: *pure; she is*: stram. *Delusion* rubric: *beautiful: she is beautiful and wants to be*: stram. [1] 1. *Delusion* rubric: *divine, being*: stram. *Delusion* rubric: *delightful: she is or wants to be delightful*: stram. [1] 1.

2. Forsaken: *Delusion* rubric: *wilderness; being in*: stram. [1] 1. *Delusion* rubric: *murdered: will be murdered; he*: Stram.

3. Causation: *Delusion* rubric: *devil: he is a devil*: stram. *Delusion* rubric: *God: he is God, then he is the devil*: **STRAM**. [3] 1. *Delusion* rubric: *executioner; visions of an*: stram. [1] 1. *Delusion* rubric: *murdering; he is: struck friends who came to help him*: Stram. [2] 1.

4. Depression: *Delusion* rubric: *doomed, being*: stram.

Delusion rubric: *joy: nothing could give her any joy*: stram.
. [1] 1.

5.   Resignation: *Delusion* rubric: *die: about to die; one was*:
     stram. *Delusion* rubric: *grave, he is in his*: stram. *Delusion*
     rubric: *divided: two parts; into*: stram. *Delusion* rubric: *body*:
     cut through; he is: two; in: stram. *Delusion* rubric: *body*:
     scattered about; body was: stram.

Zincum are significantly the only remedy listed in the
Delusion rubric: *persecuted for crimes by the devil, for crimes*
he had never done. Although *Zincum* are listed in the *Delusion*
rubric: *he had committed a crime*, as well as the rubric: *had done*
some evil, *Zincum* have a classic passive-aggressive struggle
within themselves to acknowledge, or take responsibility for,
sins committed. (The passive-aggressive personality disorder
refers to people who express their aggression in a passive,
often undermining, way towards themselves and others. It can
manifest as obstructionist, learned helplessness, ineffectual
procrastination, passive resentment or defensiveness.) *Zincum*
have psychological 'delusions of persecution', and their modus
operandi for avoidance is defensive as well as unrequited
blaming of others. Even when extremely angry, [*Mind* rubric: *so*
angry they could have stabbed anyone] *Zincum* will internalize
their rage. *Zincum* are the only remedy listed in the *Delusion*
rubric: *hearing abusive and filthy language and voices from*
within him.

The attack is from inside and outside of themselves, which is why *Zincum*
have such a compromised nervous system.

Zincum literally undermined their immune system to the
point where they can not tolerate foods. *Zincum* are listed in
the *Mind* rubric: *anxiety of conscience as if guilty of a crime*.
Zincum when sick will always accuse others of causing their
illness as well as accusing themselves. *Zincum* precariously
balance everything in their life, especially their fragile hold over
their health.

Their passive-aggressive procrastination and avoidance will often mean that they do nothing about their illnesses until it is too late and the disease has rendered them helpless – *Delusion* rubric: *one was about to die*. *Zincum* are listed in the *Delusion* rubrics pertaining to 'hubristic denial', *illusions of fancy*, and *hearing voices*. With *Zincum* it could be said that "hearing voices" could be their own inner rage. It could also be said that the *Delusion* rubric: *illusions of fancy* is a 'delusion of grandeur' which aids their ability to deny alleged sins.

The simillimum will not be *Zincum* unless the patient shows signs of a struggle to acknowledge that they could have contributed to their illness in any way. On the one hand they have contributed to their disease and on the other hand they are the *persecuted* victim of the disease.

1. Denial: *Delusion* rubric: *fancy, illusions of*: zinc. *Delusion* rubric: *voices: hearing*: Zinc. [This rubric can pertain to persecutory illusions or hubristic illusions.]

2. Forsaken: *Delusion* rubric: *devil*: *persecuted by the devil*; *he is*: *crimes he had never done; for*: zinc. [1] 1. *Delusion* rubric: *persecuted*: *he is persecuted*: *Zinc*.

3. Causation: *Delusion* rubric: *evil*: *done some evil; had*: zinc. *Delusion* rubric: *crime*: *committed a crime; he had*: zinc.

4. Depression: *Delusion* rubric: *grief*: *anger; delusion from grief and*: Zinc. *Delusion* rubric: *fright*: *as if in a fright*: zinc.

5. Resignation: *Delusion* rubric: *die*: *about to die; one was*: zinc.

   • *Delusions*: *crime*: *committed a crime; he had*: agath-a. alum-sil. alum. am-c. anac. ars. carb-an. carb-v. caust. chel. chinin-s. cina. cocc. conch. cycl. dig. hell. *Ign*. *Kali-bi*. kali-br. lac-h. lach. med. merc. nux-v. petr-ra. plb. puls. rheum. rhus-t. ruta. sabad. staph. *Verat*. zinc-o. zinc.

   • *Delusions*: *crime*: *about to commit a*: *Kali-bi*. kali-br. *Lach*. thea.

   • *Delusions*: *criminal, he is a*: agath-a. alum. am-c. ars. carb-v. caust. cina cob. coff. crot-c. cycl. dig. ferr. graph. hyos. *Ign*. m-arct.

Merc. nat-c. nux-v. op. phos. puls. ruta. sabad. sarr. sil. stront-c. sulph. thuj. verat.

- *Delusions: criminal, he is a; others know it; and:* calc-br. cob.

- *Delusions: murdered: had murdered someone; he:* ars. phos.

- *Delusions: neglected: duty; he has neglected his:* arizon-l. *Ars.* aur-m-n. aur-s. **AUR.** crot-c. cur. cycl. dream-p. falco-pe. hell. hyos. ign. kali-br. kola. lac-e. *Lyc.* melal-alt. myos-a. naja. nat-ar. petr-ra. ptel. puls. staph. ulm-c.

- *Delusions: wrong: done wrong: he has:* agath-a. aids. alum. *Ars.* aur-ar. *Aur-m-n.* aur-s. *Aur.* cina. cob. cocc. con. crot-c. cycl. dig. digin. ferr. germ-met. granit-m. *Hell.* hyos. *Ign.* lac-h. *Lach. Lil-t.* lyc. merc. *Moni.* myric. naja. nat-ar. *Nux-m.* oncor-t. op. positr. puls. ruta. sarr. sil. sulph. thuj. verat.

- *Delusions: offended people; he has:* aids. ap-g. **ARS.** cere-b. **HYOS.** nit-ac.

- *Delusions: sinned: one has; day of grace; sinned away his:* ars. aur. kali-p. plb. podo. psor. puls. stram. sulph.

- *Delusions: sinned: one has; unpardonable sin; he had committed the:* aur. chel. hell. med.

- *Delusions: vow: breaking her vow: she is:* ign.[1] 1.

- *Delusions: voices: hearing; commit crime; voice commands him to:* lach.[1] 1.

- *Delusions: wrong: doing something wrong; he is:* germ-met. hell.

- *Delusions: reproach; he has neglected his duty and deserves: Aur.* germ-met.

- *Delusions: disgraced, she is:* caust. kali-s. mag-s. nat-s. nux-v. plat. rob. sarr. sec. staph. sulph.

- *Delusions: doomed, being: expiate her sins and those of her family; to: Lil-t.* [2] 1.

- *Delusions: family, does not belong to her own: get along with her; cannot:* lil-t. [1] 1.

Avoidance: These *Delusion* rubrics are used in the case analysis if the patient shows signs of over-reacting to guilt for their real or perceived sins. The psychotherapeutic need behind the perception that one *is a criminal*, is a guilt ridden need to atone for sins so one's sense of self-worth can be restored.

The question which will reveal the simillimum is: do you feel you have done something wrong to contribute to your illness?

This question could be rejected by many homoeopaths as a leading question. I ask leading questions because they elicit leading answers which point me in the direction of the simillimum.

Arsenicum album have the *Delusion* rubric: *everything one is touching is contaminated.* All their underlying obsessive fears about health and disease have their foundations in a guilty conscience. The internal anguish in *Arsenicum album* is profound. *Arsenicum album* have the *Delusion* rubric: *he will never be happy in his own house.*

Arsenicum album believe they have failed in providing for their friends and family – *neglected his duty.*

Arsenicum album have the *Delusion* rubric: *he has done wrong.* Feelings of failure in business and in their marriage underpin their psychological delusion of *crimes committed.* *Arsenicum album* are very hypercritical of themselves; they have 'sinned away their day of grace'. Their way of making amends is to be responsible and conservatively reliable. *Arsenicum album* have the *Delusion* rubric: *they are pursing ordinary business,* and the *Delusion* rubric: *he is engaged in some ordinary occupation.* Both of these rubrics in *Arsenicum album* pertain to 'delusions of grandeur' because it reinforces their belief that they are dependable. *Arsenicum album* need to see themselves as *ordinary* so as to alleviate internal anguish over feelings of having *neglected their duty. Arsenicum album* have the *Delusion* rubric: *the family will starve.*

The simillimum will only be *Arsenicum album* if there is evidence in the patient's life that they have sacrificed what they want to do for a conservative occupation.

Whilst exacting order, *Arsenicum album* can become censorious. *Arsenicum album* have numerous *Delusion* rubrics all pertaining to psychological 'delusions of persecutions'. They fear that everyone is able to perceive that they have sinned – *policeman coming into the house.* Their carefulness in creating order in their lives leads them to be harsh and exacting. This in turn fuels their psychological delusions of guilt for their wrongs. *Arsenicum album* are then hypercritical of themselves as well as others. I have an *Arsenicum album* patient who, as he is ageing, has embraced alternative health practices. Not only is he obsessively convinced about its curative qualities for himself, all of his work colleagues and his partner have to be convinced as well. *Arsenicum album* are obsessively worried about potential decay of their body as they age, which is why it is a remedy which is graded so highly in all the *Mind* rubrics pertaining to anxiety about health. *Arsenicum album* have eighty-five *Anxiety Mind* rubrics, eighteen *Anguish Mind* rubrics, one hundred and twenty-three *Fear Mind* rubrics and forty-nine *Restlessness Mind* rubrics as well as numerous other *Mind* rubrics emphasizing internal anguish over their health. *Arsenicum album* have the *Mind* rubrics: *doubtful of recovery, doubtful of recovery, thinks the medicine is useless,* and *doubtful of salvation.* The simillimum will only be *Arsenicum album* if the patient questions whether the medicine will work on them. *Arsenicum album* have numerous psychological 'delusions of hypochondria'. Underlying their *despair of recovery* is the perception that they are *doomed. Arsenicum album* have twenty *Suicide Mind* rubrics as well as the *Delusion* rubrics: *impelled to commit suicide,* and *wants to hang himself.* [2] 1. *Arsenicum album* have the *Delusion* rubric: *has a body threefold.* This rubric in *Arsenicum album* pertains to 'delusions of grandeur' because it reinforces their belief that they are strong [*threefold*] and obsessively healthy. There is a symbiosis between the 'delusions of grandeur' and the 'delusions of hypochondria' in *Arsenicum album*. *Arsenicum album* need to believe that they are strong and healthy to be able to overcome their self-damnation. The simillimum will only be *Arsenicum album* if the patient needs to obsessively prove their worth by being exceedingly strong [*threefold*] and physically well. *Arsenicum album* have a contradiction between Stage one and Stage five in the rubric-repertorisation. They need to be *well* to avoid fears that their body will *putrefy*. All inconsistencies in the rubric-repertorisation indicate internal anguish and conflict which is either present in existing disease states or will proceed to future pathology. The simillimum will only be *Arsenicum album* if the patient does not feel they are worthy of recovery. *Arsenicum album* will maintain psychological 'delusions of deprivation' because they reinforce underlying exaggerated perceptions of having *sinned*. Suffering redeems *Arsenicum album* of exaggerated feelings of having *neglected their duty*.

The homoeopath working with an *Arsenicum album* patient needs to be alerted to the need to reinforce in them that they are *worthy* of life. Because of their exaggerated perceptions of having neglected their duty *Arsenicum album* have a propensity to believe they are *lost for salvation*. The numerous psychological 'delusions of original sin' in *Arsenicum album* prevent them from feeling worthy of not only the homoeopathic treatment but they can also feel unworthy of all enjoyment in life.

1. Denial: *Delusion* rubric: *well, he is*: ars. *Delusion* rubric: *business: ordinary, they are pursing*: ars. [This rubric in *Arsenicum album* pertains to 'delusions of grandeur' because it reinforces their belief that they are reliable [*ordinary*] and stable.] *Delusion* rubric: *body: threefold, has a*: ars. [1] 2. [petr.] [This rubric in *Arsenicum album* pertains to 'delusions of grandeur' because it reinforces their belief that they are strong [*threefold*] and healthy.] *Delusion* rubric: *house: people; house is full of*: ars. [This rubric in *Arsenicum album* pertains to 'delusions of

grandeur' because it reinforces their belief that they are more important if they have a large family.]

2. Forsaken: *Delusion* rubric: *friend: affection of; has lost the*: ars. *Delusion* rubric: *lost; she is*: ars. *Delusion* rubric: *lost; she is*: *salvation for*: ars. *Delusion* rubric: *conspiracies*: *against him; there are conspiracies*: ars. *Delusion* rubric: *thieves: seeing: listens under the bed*: ars. [1] 1. *Delusion* rubric: *policeman: coming into house; he sees a policeman*: ars. *Delusion* rubric: *starve: family will*: ars.

3. Causation: *Delusion* rubric: *crime: committed a crime; he had*: ars. *Delusion* rubric: *offended people; he has*: **ARS**. *Delusion* rubric: *wrong: done wrong; he has*: Ars. *Delusion* rubric: *neglected: duty; he has neglected his*: Ars. *Delusion* rubric: *sinned; one has: day of grace; sinned away his*: ars.

4. Depression: *Delusion* rubric: *hang himself, wants to*: Ars. [2] 1. *Delusion* rubric: *suicide; impelled to commit*: ars. *Delusion* rubric: *doomed, being*: ars.

5. Resignation: *Delusion* rubric: *die: time has come to*: ars. *Delusion* rubric: *sick: being*: Ars. *Delusion* rubric: *body: putrefy, will*: Ars. *Delusion* rubric: *contaminated: everything one is touching is contaminated*: ars.

Aurum metallicum suffer an intensely over-exaggerated, guilty conscience and depressive remorse for perceived wrongs and neglected duty because they have a higher sense of purpose and far grander visions of hubristic perfection than anyone else. *Aurum metallicum* have the *Mind* rubrics: *censorious*, and *contemptuous of oneself*. *Aurum metallicum* have the *Delusion* rubrics: *he is worthless, he has neglected his duty and deserves reproach*, and *she is lost for salvation*. *Aurum metallicum* also have the *Delusion* rubric: *religious*. It is this higher purpose to which they aspire.

Aurum metallicum have such high expectations of themselves that their goals become self-fulfilling prophecies of doom as they can never be pure enough or good enough to meet them. They are doomed to be overcome with fits of censorious anger which they direct mainly towards themselves.

Aurum metallicum avoid doing wrong by being pure and religious. When sick they will present with intensely depressing self-blame and 'fundamentalist' dictatorial health regimes which cause them extreme pain and suffering and do more harm than good because the intent behind the regimes is one of self-punishment. For example, *Aurum metallicum* can juice fast and become sick because the intent behind their regime is self-punishment. As a homoeopath it is important to identify 'delusions of grandeur' and 'delusions of self-deserving persecution' in our patients and inside ourselves, so that we do not become victim to either by colluding with our patients' psychological delusions. The simillimum will only be *Aurum metallicum* if the patient has evidence of self-punishment which is justified by hubristic perfectionism. *Aurum metallicum* will punish and berate themselves for being sick and needing to come to the health practitioner in the first instance.

1. Denial: *Delusion* rubric: *religious*: aur.
2. Forsaken: *Delusion* rubric: *forsaken; is*: Aur. *Delusion* rubric: *lost: she is: salvation: for.* Aur.
3. Causation: *Delusion* rubric: *neglected: duty; he has neglected his*: **AUR.** *Delusion* rubric: *neglected: friends, his*: Aur. [2] 1.
4. Depression: *Delusion* rubric: *fail, everything will*: Aur. *Delusion* rubric: *doomed, being*: aur. *Delusion* rubric: *depressive*: Aur. *Delusion* rubric: *melancholy*: Aur. *Delusion* rubric: *emptiness; of: internal*: aur. [1] 1. [This rubric can pertain to depression or physical decay.]
5. Resignation: *Delusion* rubric: *hollow: body is hollow; whole*: aur. *Delusion* rubric: *emptiness; of: internal*: aur. [1] 1.

Aurum muriaticum natronatum have prophecies of doom. *Aurum muriaticum natronatum* have the *Delusion* rubrics: *he does everything wrong, he cannot succeed,* and *unfit for the world.* When *Aurum muriaticum natronatum* become sick it will only ever be up to them (never the practitioner), to prove their worth by becoming well. Feelings of failure sit underneath the psychological 'delusions of self-deserving punishment' for crimes committed. *Aurum muriaticum natronatum* are self-destructively condemning of themselves. *Aurum metallicum* similarly have high expectations of themselves, however, in contrast, they believe that if they can be pure enough, or good enough God will redeem them – *Delusion* rubric: *religious*. *Aurum muriaticum natronatum* on the other hand have no listings in the *Delusion* rubrics pertaining to 'delusions of grandeur'. All of the ten *Delusion* rubrics for *Aurum muriaticum natronatum* resonate with feelings of abandonment, self-deserving punishment and self-blame. No one, not God nor their inner 'spirit guide' is going to save them; including the homoeopathic practitioner.

The simillimum will only be *Aurum muriaticum natronatum* if the patient is fatalistic.

Aurum muriaticum natronatum brood internally because they are not able to meet their ambition to achieve more worldly goals of excellence. *Aurum muriaticum natronatum* have the *Mind* rubrics: *increased ambition, anger about his mistakes, antagonism with herself,* and *ailments from unusual responsibility.* [1] 1. *Aurum muriaticum natronatum* have an interesting inner guilt which undermines their confidence and which fuels all the *Delusion* rubrics of having done wrong – *Mind* rubric: *love with the wrong person. Aurum muriaticum natronatum* believe that they have married the wrong person; it is this which fuels their inner antagonism.

1. Denial: NONE.
2. Forsaken: *Delusion* rubric: *forsaken; is: Aur-m-n. Delusion*

rubric: *friend: affection of; he has lost the*: aur-m-n. *Delusion* rubric: *dead: mother is, his*: aur-m-n. [This rubric pertains to fear of abandonment.]

3. Causation: *Delusion* rubric: *wrong: done wrong; he has: Aur-m-n. Delusion* rubric: *unfit: world; he is unfit for the*: aur-m-n.

4. Depression: *Delusion* rubric: *succeed, he does everything wrong; he cannot: Aur-m-n. Delusion* rubric: *unfit: world; he is unfit for the*: aur-m-n.

5. Resignation: *Delusion* rubric: *unfit: world; he is unfit for the*: aur-m-n. [This rubric pertains to admission of sins, or feelings of depressive unworthiness. In relation to *Aurum muriaticum natronatum* I have also allocate this rubric into Resignation because when sick they feel their illness makes them unworthy [*unfit*].

Causticum have a significant amount of rubrics which all pertain to 'delusions of persecution'.

They are listed in numerous *Delusion* rubrics to do with horrible visions of specters and ghosts. *Causticum* are listed in so many because they have a guilty conscience. *Causticum* over-react to and over-emphasize, the importance of their own dictates of moral and political conscience[63].

In their own eyes they have fallen, and have failed to meet their own expectation of *illusions of fancy* – *Delusion* rubric: *he is falling*. The *Delusion* rubric: *illusions of fancy,* alludes to a psychological 'delusion of idealism'. A patient who is suffering *illusions of fancy* is someone who has grand visions of persona. Their expectations of what they can achieve, or what they *have* achieved, or who they are in the world, are over-exaggerated. *Causticum* feel overly responsible for their crimes; they have no psychological 'delusions of abandonment' which they can project on to others. All their *Delusion* rubrics in Forsaken pertain to persecutory complexes and not to 'delusions of abandonment'. *Delusion* rubrics pertaining to feeling personally abandoned allocate blame for misfortune on to others. Although *Causticum* might have the *Delusion* rubric: *he is unfortunate*, their suffering comes from deep internal questioning and self-blame because they feel *they* are responsible – *Delusion* rubric: *disgraced*.

Causticum feel they have personally wronged, even if there is only *one* wrong in the world which they have not been able to personally correct.

Feelings of failure sit underneath the psychological delusions of self-deserving punishment for crimes committed. The homoeopath has to be careful not to reinforce self-blame and self-punishment during the patient's treatment. *Causticum* need to have it re-enforced constantly that they are not responsible for the psychological welfare of others. *Causticum* will sink into self-deprivation in their lives because they feel solely responsible for their sins, and the sins of the whole world. (The most common form this self-deprecation takes is one of self-imposed poverty. As long as there is poverty in the world, *Causticum* will deprive themselves of material wealth.)

Their anxious forebodings and sensitivities to loss and grief, their own and others, often means that when they are sick they will forgo treatment because they believe that they must have done a great wrong – *Delusion* rubric: *he is a criminal*. *Causticum* have the *Mind* rubrics: *defiant*, and *refusing treatment in spite of being very sick*. Over-exaggerated guilt will keep them trapped in self-punishing situations. *Causticum* find it hard not to trap themselves in 'causes', which they become embroiled in because they need to fight for the 'under-dog'. The Materia medica *Causticum* profile the homoeopath is familiar with is reflected in the *Mind* rubrics: *exhilaration about politics, revolutionist,* and *inclined to discuss political disputes*. [1] 1. *Causticum* have the *Mind* rubric: *love for animals. Causticum* are well known for their ideological revolutionary zeal, especially in pursuit of protecting animal rights.

What is not commonly noted is that *Causticum* are listed in twenty-eight *Ailments from cares and worry Mind* rubrics, forty-six *Anxiety Mind* rubrics, two hundred and sixty-four *Fear Mind* rubrics, and thirty-three *Weeping Mind* rubrics. This degree of intense internal anguish is precipitated by 'delusions of original sin'.

Self-destructive predictions of feeling *disgraced* are psychological delusions which reinforce self-blame. The simillimum will not be *Causticum* unless the patient feels *personally* responsible for alleviating the suffering in the world. *Causticum* have so many *Delusion* rubrics pertaining to 'delusions of persecution' because they feel undermined and haunted by all the ills of the world.

When *Causticum* are sick they often feel like they are unable to enact change. They have the *Delusion* rubric: *there is an empty space between the brain and skull*. This rubric indicates that the patient feels that the thoughts in their brain are not able to connect – there is an *empty space* in their brain which is making it hard to think. This rubric should not be taken literally – rather it indicates fears of *falling* and fear of failure to enact changes in their lives and in the lives of others. *Causticum* have seventeen *Mind* rubrics for concentration being difficult.

The simillimum will only be *Causticum* if the patient feels disappointed [*disgraced*] with themselves as well as with the world. When *Causticum* are sick they feel so *disgraced* with themselves that they are unable to enact change to make themselves well.

1. Denial: *Delusion* rubric: *fancy, illusions of*: caust.
2. Forsaken: *Delusion* rubric: *robbed, is going to be*: caust. *Delusion* rubric: *insects, sees*: caust. *Delusion* rubric: *dead: persons, sees*: caust. *Delusion* rubric: *visions, has*: *horrible*: Caust. *Delusion* rubric: *absurd, ludicrous: figures are present*: caust. *Delusion* rubric: *faces, sees: diabolical faces crowd upon him*: caust. *Delusion* rubric: *images, phantoms; sees: closing eyes, on*: Caust.

3. Causation: *Delusion* rubric: *criminal, he is a*: caust. *Delusion* rubric: *disgraced: she is*: caust.

4. Depression: *Delusion* rubric: *falling: he is*: caust. *Delusion* rubric: *unfortunate: he is*: caust. *Delusion* rubric: *space: between brain and skull; there is empty space*: caust. [1] 1. [This rubric can pertain to feelings of failure and depression.]

5. Resignation: *Delusion* rubric: *sick: being*: caust. *Delusion* rubric: *die: about to die; one was*: caust. *Delusion* rubric: *space: between brain and skull; there is empty space*: caust. [1] 1.

Cyclamen are so distraught with fear at the thought of having to face their real or perceived sins that they are paralyzed. Similarly to *Causticum* they feel overly responsible for their crimes. In their own eyes they have failed to meet their own expectation of *illusions of fancy* – *Delusion* rubric: *illusions of fancy.* Their expectations of what they should have achieved are over-exaggerated. Exaggerated perceptions of guilt perpetuate 'persecution complexes'. *Cyclamen* have numerous persecution rubrics as well as the *Delusion* rubric: *as if two persons lay in the bed, the body of the other person overlapping hers.* [1] 1. This rubric should not be interpreted literally rather it is reflective of how hard it is for *Cyclamen* to feel deserving of their right to their own space [*bed*].

Cyclamen feel undeserving. When *Cyclamen* are sick they believe their illness is deserved.

Cyclamen will not want to talk[64] or confront their real or perceived 'delusions of original sin'. They will do nothing to seek treatment or help. *Cyclamen* stay at home by themselves and isolate themselves from society. *Cyclamen* have the *Mind* rubrics: *taciturn, aversion to company desire for solitude, aversion to going out,* and *brooding over imaginary grief. Cyclamen* use their emotionally paralyzed state as a self-fulfilling prophecy to reinforce their punishment. *Cyclamen* have the *Delusion* rubric: *he is on the ridge of a descending mountain.* [1] 1. *Causticum* punish themselves by perpetuating and intensifying internal anxiety and anguish. *Cyclamen* punish themselves by inflicting pain. The simillimum will not be *Cyclamen* unless the patient is self-punishing in order to absolve themselves of 'delusions of original sin'. *Cyclamen* will continually put themselves in precarious situations, stranded on the ridge of descending mountains. Self-destructive behavior and self-blame will be maintained and nurtured because they help protect the *Cyclamen* patient from their innermost dark secrets about themselves. The simillimum will only be *Cyclamen* if the patient appears to be stuck [*paralyzed*] in their feelings of guilt. *Cyclamen* have the *Mind* rubric: *anorexia nervosa*. There are sixty-three other remedies listed in that particular *Mind* rubric. *Cyclamen* are specifically listed because they enjoy losing their senses. *Cyclamen* like starving themselves so they can lose conscious awareness. *Cyclamen* have the *Delusion* rubric: *deprived of his senses.* [1] 1. *Cyclamen* like losing all connection to their own psyche. *Cyclamen* have the *Mind* rubric: *unconsciousness, mental insensibility*. The simillimum will only be *Cyclamen* if the patient wants to numb all senses and stay alone in isolation from themselves and from the world.

The homoeopath working with a *Cyclamen* patient needs to do a lot of counselling around helping them forgive themselves for real or perceived sins committed. The homoeopath working with a *Cyclamen* patient also needs to be alerted to the self-destructive need they have to position themselves on the *ridge of a descending mountain*. *Cyclamen* place themselves in self-destructive situations.

1. Denial: *Delusion* rubric: *fancy, illusions of*: cycl.
2. Forsaken: *Delusion* rubric: *forsaken; is*: Cycl. *Delusion* rubric: *alone, being: world; alone in the*: cycl. *Delusion* rubric: *animals: large animal is running over her whole body*: cycl. [1] 1. *Delusion* rubric: *animals: surrounded by*

ugly animals: cycl. *Delusion* rubric: *bed*: *two persons in bed with her*: cycl. [1] 2. [petr.] *Delusion* rubric: *persecuted*: *he is persecuted*: *Cycl. Delusion* rubric: *persecuted*: *he is persecuted*: *everyone; by*: *Cycl. Delusion* rubric: *pursued*: *he was*: *enemies, by*: cycl.

3. Causation: *Delusion* rubric: *crime: committed a crime; he had*: cycl. *Delusion* rubric: *neglected*: *duty; he has neglected his*: cycl. *Delusion* rubric: *evil*: *done some evil; had*: cycl.

4. Depression: *Delusion* rubric: *paralyzed; he is*: cycl. *Delusion* rubric: *insane*: *become insane; one will*: cycl. *Delusion* rubric: *doomed, being*: cycl. *Delusion* rubric: *troubles: great troubles had just come over him*: cycl. [1] 1. *Delusion* rubric: *brain*: *wobble; brain seems to*: *to and fro*: cycl. [1] 2. [spira.] [This rubric should not be interpreted literally. *Cyclamen* feel continually disempowered and unable to control their thinking processes enough to enact positive change.]

5. Resignation: *Delusion* rubric: *paralyzed; he is*: cycl. *Delusion* rubric: *senses*: *deprived of his senses*: cycl. [1] 1. [These rubrics can pertain to depression or physical deprivation.] *Delusion* rubric: *mountain; he is on the ridge of a*: *descending*: cycl. [1] 1. [This rubric can also be allocated in Depression. In Resignation it pertains self-destructive tendencies in *Cyclamen*.]

Ignatia believe they are unable to be saved when they become sick with any illness, regardless of whether it is a minor ailment or a serious ailment. *Ignatia* are the only remedy listed in the *Delusion* rubric: *she is lost, everything is lost*, and the *Delusion* rubric: *cries and rages, being doomed, soul cannot be saved*. *Ignatia* are listed as a grading of two in all the *Delusion* rubrics for wrongs and crimes committed, and have the *Mind* rubric: *ailments from shame*. The underlying dilemma is that *Ignatia* are crippled with shame that they are sick. Illness is hysterically viewed as proof of their crimes. Other than the

Delusion rubrics: *hearing voices,* and *illusions of fancy, Ignatia* is not listed in any other rubrics of 'hubristic denial'. In relation to *Ignatia, fanciful illusions* only exasperate the anxiety. *Ignatia* are hysterically[65] crippled in the face of illness – *Delusion* rubric: *cannot walk.* The advantage of understanding the five psychological steps a patient will move through when they are sick is that they help to identify the rubrics which are relevant to the case-repertorisation.

Ignatia are easily identifiable because they believe they have no hope of being saved; this in itself is a clear indication of the *Delusion* rubrics pertaining to assumption of sin – *Delusion* rubric: *cries and rages, being doomed, soul cannot be saved.*

The simillimum will only be *Ignatia* if the hysteria and collapse is across all levels – emotionally, mentally, and physically. *Ignatia* are crippled and broken by all tragedy. Hysterical anguish over having *neglected their duty* will be a keynote mental and emotional characteristic which will accompany all physical collapse. The 'never-well-since-event' in an *Ignatia* case will always center around the perception that they have broken a promise [*vow*].

1. Denial: *Delusion* rubric: *fancy, illusions of*: **IGN.** [It is debatable in relation to *Ignatia* whether this rubric adds to 'delusions of grandeur' or 'delusions of hypochondria'.]

2. Forsaken: *Delusion* rubric: *deceived, being*: *Ign. Delusion* rubric: *lost; she is: everything is lost*: ign. [1] 1. *Delusion* rubric: *unfair to him; that life is*: ign. *Delusion* rubric: *laughed at and mocked at; being*: ign. *Delusion* rubric: *trapped; he is*: ign. [This rubric can be allocated into 'delusions of persecution' or 'delusions of impending doom'.]

3. Causation: *Delusion* rubric: *criminal, he is a*: *Ign. Delusion* rubric: *crime: committed a crime; he had*: *Ign. Delusion* rubric: *neglected: duty; he has neglected his*: ign. *Delusion* rubric: *vow: breaking her vow; she is*: ign. [1] 1.

4. Depression: *Delusion* rubric: *anxious*: ign. *Delusion* rubric:

trapped; he is: ign. *Delusion* rubric: *ruined*: *is ruined; he*:
IGN. *Delusion* rubric: *doomed, being*: *soul cannot be
saved*: *cries and rages*: *Ign*. [2] 1. *Delusion* rubric: *sinking;
to be*: *Ign*. *Delusion* rubric: *emptiness; of*: *Ign*.

5. Resignation: *Delusion* rubric: *walking*: *cannot walk, he*:
    Ign. *Delusion* rubric: *legs*: *belong to her; her legs don't*: ign.
    Delusion rubric: *body*: *brittle is*: ign.

Lachesis: Although *Lachesis* feel overwhelmed by guilt for
their anger and jealousy they are equally torn between feeling
wronged and acknowledging their wrongs. *Lachesis* have the
Delusion rubric: *he has suffered wrong,* and the *Delusion* rubric:
feeling as though some evil had happened to him, as well as the
Delusion rubric: *he has done wrong,* and the *Delusion* rubric:
he has to murder someone. As with *Hyoscyamus, Lachesis* can
dramatically switch from guilt and shame about their illness to
raging accusation and jealousy of others' health. *Lachesis* live
up to our expectations of a remedy derived from a snake[66] and
they are expert at all avoidance techniques.

Lachesis have numerous *Delusion* rubrics pertaining to 'delusions of
persecution' so they can delude themselves that they have been wronged
more than they have wronged anyone else. *Lachesis* also absolve
themselves of all sins by choosing to believe they are influenced by a
higher power. *Lachesis* can dramatically switch from guilt and shame to
accusatory rage for being threatened or persecuted.

Lachesis will over-exaggerate disease and predictions of
destruction from disease, but they have strong 'delusions of
grandeur' and righteousness so the blame will not become
self-deprecating like the other remedies discussed in this
chapter. When *Lachesis* are sick, the blame is not directed at
themselves; *Lachesis* will not remain in a state of self-blame
and shame for too long. The simillimum will only be *Lachesis* if
the patient in the very next sentence after acknowledging guilt,
accuses others of persecution.

1. Denial: *Delusion* rubric: *charmed and cannot break the spell*: Lach [2]1. *Delusion* rubric: *great person, is a*: Lach. *Delusion* rubric: *proud*: lach.

2. Forsaken: *Delusion* rubric: *friendless, he is*: lach. *Delusion* rubric: *lost; she is*: *salvation; for. predestination, from*: Lach [2]1. *Delusion* rubric: *hated; by others*: lach. *Delusion* rubric: *criticized, she is*: lach. *Delusion* rubric: *conspiracies*: *against him; there are conspiracies*: lach. *Delusion* rubric: *wrong*: *suffered wrong; he has*: lach. *Delusion* rubric: *poisoned*: *medicine; being poisoned by*: lach.

3. Causation: *Delusion* rubric: *crime*: *committed a crime; he had*: lach. *Delusion* rubric: *wrong*: *done wrong; he has*: Lach.

4. Depression: *Delusion* rubric: *doomed, being*: lach.

5. Resignation: *Delusion* rubric: *die*: *about to die; one was*: Lach. *Delusion* rubric: *die*: *about to die; one was*: *exhaustion; she would die from*: lach. [1] 1. *Delusion* rubric: *disease*: *incurable disease; he has an*: Lach. *Delusion* rubric: *body*: *disintegrating*: Lach.

Lilium tigrinum have the *Mind* rubric: *too occupied with religion, conflict between religious ideals and sexuality at night*. [2] 1. *Lilium tigrinum* demonstrate remorse for their sexual perversities. They have other remorseful *Mind* rubrics: *anxiety about salvation, fear moral obliquity alternating with sexual excitement*, and *lasciviousness alternating with remorse*. *Lilium tigrinum* also have the *Mind* rubric: *rage alternating with remorse*. [1] 1. All these *Mind* rubrics demonstrate remorse which is reminiscent of the confessional box. *Lilium tigrinum* will also behave remorsefully when sick, they promise to be good and pure.

If a patient presents in the first consult after they have found out they have a severe illness, and they are full of promises that they will redeem themselves by *abstaining from all fun,* then this is a clear pointer towards the remedy *Lilium tigrinum*.

Lilium tigrinum have a struggle between religion and sexual desires. Although *Lilium tigrinum* have several *Delusion* rubrics indicating internal conflict they have no *Delusion* rubrics specifically mentioning sexual and religious conflict. All the rubrics mentioning sexual and religious conflict are *Mind* rubrics. Internal struggles between religion and sexuality perpetuate abuse. *Lilium tigrinum* have the *Mind* rubrics: *rage from suppressed sexual desire* and *wild feeling in head from suppression of sexual desire.* [1] 2.

All suppression causes internal discord and instability. *Lilium tigrinum* have the *Delusion* rubrics: *being double, errors of personal identity, one will become insane,* and *body is divided. Lilium tigrinum* have the *Mind* rubrics: *mutilating his body, desire to pull her own hair,* and *tormenting himself.*

Lilium tigrinum have the *Delusion* rubric: *one will become insane unless she got out of her body.* [1] 1. *Lilium tigrinum* have the *Delusion* rubric: *as if he could fly.* All the *Delusion* rubrics: *flying, in the air,* and *floating,* indicate 'Dissociative Disorders'. 'Dissociation' is a normal response to the trauma of illness. If the patient dissociates, it allows themselves space to distance themselves from the feelings which are overwhelming them. *Lilium tigrinum* have the ability to split (dissociate) from their self and their body and allow one part of themselves to indulge in sexual desire. *Lilium tigrinum* have the *Mind* rubric: *confusion of mind, muscles refuse to obey the will when the attention is turned away.*

Lilium tigrinum behave remorsefully and suppress their sexuality and mutilate their body to redeem their sins.

Lilium tigrinum have only one significant 'delusion of grandeur' – *everything is depending on them.* This 'delusion of grandeur' elevates *Lilium tigrinum* into a position of importance which allows them to feel entitled to adoration as well as sexual adoration.

'Delusions of grandeur' combined with a dissociative split, and sexual *lasciviousness* combined with *religious remorsefulness,* perpetuate self-abuse and abuse of others.

Lilium tigrinum is a remedy derived from the Tiger Lily. The theme of the *Liliales* is adoration and praise for their perfection. Their self-punishment is also disproportionate for guilt over abandonment of their family. The 'hubristic denial' for *Lilium tigrinum* refers to their belief that everyone is depending on them. Their failure and sin, which has become a psychological delusion, is that they have abandoned their family – *Delusion* rubric: *cannot get along with her family, does not belong to her own family.* [1] 1. They then feel guilt for their family – *Delusion* rubric: *doomed to expiate her sins and those of her family.* The self-fulfilling prophecy for the *Liliales* family, which predisposes *Lilium tigrinum* to this psychological delusion, is that they feel so entitled to adoration and praise that it has removed them from their family. Their lofty position predisposes them to also feeling *forsaken with no one to care for them.*

1. Denial: *Delusion* rubric: *depending on him; everything is*: lil-t. *Delusion* rubric: *flying: could fly; as if he*: lil-t. [This rubric should not be interpreted literally. This rubric pertains to Dissociative Disorders.]

2. Forsaken: *Delusion* rubric: *forsaken; is*: lil-t. *Delusion* rubric: *forsaken; is*: *care for her; no one would*: lil-t. *Delusion* rubric: *family, does not belong to her own*: *get along with her; cannot*: lil-t. [1] 1. *Delusion* rubric: *poisoned*: *he*: *has been*: lil-t.

3. Causation: *Delusion* rubric: *wrong: done wrong; he has*: Lil-t. *Delusion* rubric: *doomed, being*: *expiate her sins and those of her family; to*: Lil-t. [2] 1. *Delusion* rubric: *family, does not belong to her own*: *get along with her; cannot*: lil-t. [1] 1. [This rubric is an admission of guilt and an admission of abandonment.]

4. Depression: *Delusion* rubric: *insane*: *become insane; one*

will: *unless she got out of her body*: lil-t. [1] 1. *Delusion* rubric: *insane*: *become insane; one will*: lil-t. *Delusion* rubric: *doomed, being*: Lil-t. *Delusion* rubric: *double*: *being*: lil-t. *Delusion* rubric: *identity*: *errors of personal identity*: lil-t. *Delusion* rubric: *unreal*: *everything seems unreal*: lil-t.

5. Resignation: *Delusion* rubric: *die*: *about to die; one was*: lil-t. *Delusion* rubric: *divided*: *two parts; into*: lil-t. *Delusion* rubric: *disease*: *incurable disease; he has an*: Lil-t. *Delusion* rubric: *body*: *divided, is*: lil-t. *Delusion* rubric: *insane*: *become insane; one will*: *unless she got out of her body*: lil-t. [1] 1. [This rubric can pertain to internal anxiety or fears of disease.]

Mercurius are undermined by any possibility that they will be exposed as a criminal even though they are listed in the *Delusion* rubric: *he is a criminal*. They will want to kill anyone who has criticized them – *Mind* rubric: *desire to kill the person who contradicts them*. Their persecution complex is also fueled by delusions that they are being attacked – *Delusion* rubric: *surrounded by enemies*. The colloquial saying 'the best defense is attack', is a good example of the avoidance techniques of *Mercurius*. *Mercurius* is the only remedy listed in the *Delusion* rubric: *take people by the nose*. This is a wonderful rubric which reflects the mercurial ability, and need, to coerce and delude. *Mercurius* are the only remedy listed in the *Delusion* rubric: *body is made of sweets*. *Mercurius* have an obsessive need to 'charm their way into your good book'. In the process of charming you, they need to present themselves as pure and untouchable. *Mercurius* have the *Delusion* rubrics: *religious* and *fancy illusions*, in the rubrics of 'hubristic denial'. If *Mercurius* are humiliated and exposed as being a criminal they can be very dominating and, conversely, self-destructive in their attempt to protect their inherent instability. Their intuitive ability to protect/hide their instability reflects the reactive and unstable nature of the metal mercury. The reason I identify

Mercurius as being inherently self-destructive is that as soon as any fault is exposed they have to fight and charm. When they fight to defend their 'ego' it consequently exposes them to the world; the more exposed their weaknesses are, the more they disintegrate. *Mercurius* enact the same self-destructive, self-fulfilling prophecy in their homoeopathic health treatment. As soon as the homoeopath gets them healthy in the homoeopathic treatment process, they immediately need to self-destruct by consuming excessive amounts of alcohol or drugs.

If they allow you, the practitioner, any control over, or effectiveness in, making them well through your treatment, it is viewed as an humiliation because it is proof that they were sick in the first place. *Mercurius* cannot allow themselves to be put in a vulnerable position. This is a classic psychological avoidance technique. Self-destructive behavior and self-blame will be maintained and nurtured because they help protect *Mercurius* from their innermost dark secrets about themselves.

The conflict between their 'hubristic denial' rubrics: *religious* and *body made of sweets*, and their presumptions of disease rubrics: *sick* and *about to die*, places *Mercurius* in an unstable and untenable position; the only possible outcome is failure. The simillimum will only be *Mercurius* if the patient believes they are being tormented without acknowledging to themselves the true cause. *Mercurius* have the opposing *Delusion* rubric: *is in hell* – which pertains to acknowledgment of sins committed – and the *Delusion* rubric: *suffers in hell, without being able to explain why* – which is a retraction of acknowledged sins or blame.

Mercurius will only be the simillimum if the patient retracts acknowledgment of blame.

1. Denial: *Delusion* rubric: *religious*: merc. *Delusion* rubric: *body: sweets, is made of:* merc. [1] 1.

2. Forsaken: *Delusion* rubric: *home: away from home; he is*: merc.

3. Causation: *Delusion* rubric: *criminal, he is a: Merc. Delusion*

rubric: *hell*: *in; is*: merc. OPPOSING *Delusion* rubric: *hell*: *torments of hell without being able to explain; suffers the*: *Merc.*

4. Depression: *Delusion* rubric: *fail, everything will*: merc. *Delusion* rubric: *hell: torments of hell without being able to explain; suffers the*: *Merc.* [This rubric acknowledges feelings of suffering but does not acknowledge self-blame.] *Delusion* rubric: *hell*: *in; is*: merc.

5. Resignation: *Delusion* rubric: *die: about to die; one was*: merc. *Delusion* rubric: *sick: being*: merc.

Natrum carbonicum sink into the belief that there is a division between themselves and others which can never be repaired. They will never become well, they are going to be sick forever, and the treatment will never succeed. It is important that one is aware of the crippling desperation and self-inflicted punishment *Natrum carbonicum* suffer. *Natrum carbonicum* are so self-punishing that they believe they are not worth saving. *Natrum carbonicum* are weighted heavily in all the rubric categories pertaining to persecution and failure. Their treatment process will be slow; this is consistent with the carbonicum element. With the salt element added to the carbonicum, their internal questioning will cause *Natrum carbonicum* to continually be confronted with their self-worth. *Natrum carbonicum* believe nothing they do will be right [*he is doing nothing right*].

Natrum carbonicum have the *Mind* rubric: *never succeeds,* and the *Delusion* rubric: *he cannot succeed, he does everything wrong. Natrum carbonicum* will continually question whether they (as a patient) are doing the right thing and whether the remedy is right.

Natrum carbonicum have the *Mind* rubric: *desire for company,* and the *Mind* rubric: *aversion to company yet fear of being alone* [3]. Their self-inflicted exile [*division between himself and others*] is maintained to avoid further abandonment and/or persecution. *Natrum carbonicum* have the *Mind* rubric: *suspicious, fear of company* and the *Delusion* rubric: *sees devils*. If the homoeopath understands this psychological process they will be better able to show patience when *Natrum carbonicum* are suspicious about the treatment.

Natrum carbonicum have an interesting *Delusion* rubric – *of a wedding.* The one delusional desire *Natrum carbonicum* have in this world is to be wedded, if they give up this journey their heart will literally break. Every single time *Natrum carbonicum* take the remedy they will feel emotionally closer to others' feelings, and their own. *Natrum carbonicum* have the *Mind* rubric: *inconsolable, continuous weeping from consolation.* [1] 1. The consequence of feeling more connected to others is that emotional fears of being abandoned and persecuted will confront *Natrum carbonicum*. The homoeopath treating a *Natrum carbonicum* must predict that they have created a division between themselves and others for a particular reason. The gulf between others and *Natrum carbonicum* are self-imposed to avoid feeling close. *Natrum carbonicum* have the *Delusion* rubric: *body has become heavy and thick.* The psychosomatic meaning of the *Delusion* rubric: *body has become heavy and thick* is that they will never be moved, or penetrated, or touched by others. *Natrum carbonicum* not only separate themselves, they separate their body from their lovers as well. It is this separation and *division between themselves and others* which perpetuates their obsession with bonding [*wedding*]. *Natrum carbonicum* have several *Dream* rubrics: *amorous,* and *amorous with erections,* and *amorous with pollutions.* *Natrum carbonicum* struggle to feel confident enough in real life to connect with others; all their amorous desires are played out in their dreams. *Natrum carbonicum* have the *Mind* rubrics: *estranged from his family, estranged from friends and relatives,* and *estranged from her husband.* *Natrum carbonicum* have the *Dream* rubrics: *wedding,* and *wedding with two women.* The simillimum will only be *Natrum carbonicum* if the patient struggles with being able to emotionally bond and sexually connect to others. *Natrum carbonicum* struggle to bond emotionally in relationships because they are convinced the other person will deceive them. Sankaran, in *The Soul of Remedies*, writes that in a proving of *Natrum carbonicum* it was noted that they had "a desire to be at their mother's breast". *Natrum carbonicum* have no rubrics confirming this symptom. I have had however, two cases of *Natrum carbonicum* where the male patients were more comfortable having a sexual relationship with their mother because they were frightened that any other woman, other than their mother, would deceive them.

The questions which will reveal the simillimum are: what happens when they feel accused, and what happens if they feel they have done something wrong? Underlying their fears is their self-inflicted exile which is maintained because of the belief that they have committed serious crimes.

Natrum carbonicum believe that they are being isolated from others because they have been 'bad'.

Natrum carbonicum have several *Dream* rubrics which all indicate that they ruminate about remorseful acts – *Dreams: remorse, events of previous evening, events long forgotten*, and *conversations of the previous day*. The 'never-well-since-event' in *Natrum carbonicum* will have its origins in an event in which the patient believes they have *committed a crime* against their family. *Natrum carbonicum* have the *Delusion* rubric: *head is separated from body*. This rubric reinforces that they cannot not always trust themselves. Depressive feelings of past and future failure underpin their psychological delusions of self-deserving banishment.

Natrum carbonicum have the *Delusion* rubric: *he is on a journey,* and *illusions of fancy. Natrum carbonicum* will not arrive at a consultation and literally say they are on a journey, therefore it is important to consider the psychotherapeutic meaning of this *Delusion* rubric. *Natrum carbonicum* need to believe they are on a spiritual quest. *Natrum carbonicum* have the *Mind* rubrics: *benevolence,* and *dignified.* If one is inspired by a mission which is greater than oneself, it is possible to overcome and deny all one's underlying fears of persecution for sins committed. Their benevolent sacrifice of themselves is needed to alleviate fears of persecution. Benevolence is a position of superiority which the *Natrum carbonicum* use to deny their weaknesses. *Natrum carbonicum* have the *Mind* rubric: *cheerful but fearful.* [1] 1. In our repertories it can become extremely confusing if on the one hand a remedy profile has the *Mind* rubric: *benevolence* and the *Mind* rubric: *avarice.* All *Mind* rubrics of superiority protect underlying fears of persecution because they have been so greedy.

1. Denial: *Delusion* rubric: *fancy, illusions of:* nat-c. *Delusion* rubric: *wedding, of a:* nat-c. [*Natrum carbonicum* delude themselves they are wedded.] *Delusion* rubric: *journey; he is on:* nat-c. *Delusion* rubric: *enlarged:* nat-c. [This rubric in *Natrum carbonicum* can pertain to exaggerated status or exaggerated persecutory fears.]

2. Forsaken: *Delusion* rubric: *forsaken; is:* nat-c. *Delusion* rubric: *division between himself and others:* nat-c. *Delusion* rubric: *persecuted: he is persecuted:* nat-c. *Delusion* rubric: *soldiers; surrounded by:* nat-c. [1] 1. *Delusion* rubric: *images, phantoms; sees: frightful:* nat-c. *Delusion* rubric: *thieves: seeing:* nat-c. *Delusion* rubric: *dead: persons, sees:* nat-c. *Delusion* rubric: *devil: sees:* nat-c. *Delusion* rubric: *pursued; he was: enemies, by:* nat-c. *Delusion* rubric: *criminals, about:* nat-c. *Delusion* rubric: *dead: persons, sees:* nat-c.

3. Causation: *Delusion* rubric: *criminal, he is a:* nat-c.

4. Depression: *Delusion* rubric: *right: doing nothing right; he is:* nat-c. *Delusion* rubric: *succeed, he does everything wrong; he cannot:* nat-c. *Delusion* rubric: *heavy; is:* nat-c.

Delusion rubric: *head*: *separated from body; head is*: nat-c.
[This rubric indicates that *Natrum carbonicum* cannot trust
that their head will know what is good for their body.]

5. Resignation: *Delusion* rubric: *sick, being*: nat-c. *Delusion*
    rubric: *body*: *thick, is*: nat-c. [1] 1. *Delusion* rubric: *heart*:
    disease; having an: Nat-c. *Delusion* rubric: *heavy; is*:
    nat-c. [This rubric can pertain to heaviness in the body or
    in the mind.] *Delusion* rubric: *body*: *heavy and thick; body
    has become*: nat-c. [1] 2. [positr] *Delusion* rubric: *head*:
    separated from body; head is: nat-c.

Nux moschata are listed in only one of the *Delusion*
rubrics pertaining to acknowledging sin: *he has done wrong.*

The *peculiar* psychological differences amongst remedies as they struggle
to acknowledge illness, or allocate blame for illness, hold the essence of
the simillimum. *Nux moschata* will argue with you that they are not really
sick – only *one* part of them is sick.

This is reflective of their psychotic ability to differentiate and
split from themselves. The *Delusion* rubric: *being double, his
real conscious self seemed to be watching his other self playing*,
is indicative of a psychotic ability to split off from acknowledging
what the 'other' self is doing. A *Nux moschata* patient suffering
with lung cancer will say in a consultation: *not all of me is sick.
It is only my lungs which have a tumor. Really, I know I might
have smoked all my life, but really it is not all my doing, my
wife has to acknowledge she has smoked our whole married
life.* The ability to find the simillimum in this case is based on
exacting listening, and understanding the true psychiatric
meaning of the *Delusion* rubrics. Because *Nux moschata* is
a remedy derived from nutmeg it has been allocated to the
group of remedies known as the 'hallucinogenic remedies'.
Homoeopaths have presumed that the *Delusion* rubrics: *body
is enlarged, expansion of space*, and *he is three people* have
reflected Dissociative Disorders normally associated with the

remedies which are derived from hallucinogenic substances. The *Delusion* rubrics: *body is enlarged, expansion of space,* and *he is three people* are all reflective of 'selective consciousness' and 'selective conscientiousness'. *Nux moschata* are the only remedy listed in the *Delusion* rubric: *being double; his real conscious self seemed to be watching his other self playing.*

Nux moschata will never acknowledge that *they* have contributed to their predicament; the 'other' is responsible.

The consequence of having a limited understanding of the *Delusion* rubrics has meant that students of homoeopathy, as well as qualified homoeopaths, expect a patient to literally say in a consultation that their *conscious self seems to be watching his other self.* It will not happen as literally as that: a *Nux moschata* patient will say in a consultation, *I am not totally sick, it is only my lungs which have a tumor. I don't have cancer.* This is an avoidance of body-ownership which is exquisitely exclusive and *peculiar* to *Nux moschata.*

Nux moschata will also apply the same deflective ability to the assumption of guilt. *Nux moschata* will concentrate on *minor* details of their health rather than acknowledge what they have done *overall* to contribute to ill health. *Nux moschata* have the *Delusion* rubric: *about pins.* [3] 2. *Nux moschata* will never acknowledge *personal* wrong doing; it will always be the 'other' who has *done wrong. Nux moschata* have a contradiction between the *Delusion* rubrics: *body is enlarged* and *parts are shrunken.* They also have a contradiction between the *Delusion* rubrics: *he has done wrong* and *watching his other real conscious part playing.* If there are contradictions within the rubrics attached to a remedy then those contradictions have to be reflected in the patient's behavior. The simillimum will only be *Nux moschata* if the patient is struggling to take personal responsibility for their health. *Nux moschata* have the *Mind* rubric: *facility for arguing. Nux moschata,* although acknowledging they might have done wrong, blame their illness on the 'other' *sleepy* or *intoxicated* part of themselves which can't be held responsible.

1. Denial: *Delusion* rubric: *three persons, he is*: *Nux-m*.
   Delusion rubric: *fancy, illusions of*: nux-m. *Delusion* rubric:
   enlarged: nux-m. *Delusion* rubric: *enlarged*: *body is*: *parts
   of body*: nux-m. *Delusion* rubric: *space*: *expansion of*:
   nux-m. *Delusion* rubric: *objects; about*: *large*: nux-m. [This
   rubric can pertain to illusions of grandeur or perceptions of
   persecution.]

2. Forsaken: *Delusion* rubric: *execute him; people want to*:
   nux-m. *Delusion* rubric: *images, phantoms; sees*: *dwells
   upon*: nux-m. [1] 3. [arn. nux-m. sil.] *Delusion* rubric: *pins;
   about*: **NUX-M**. [3] 2. [*Sil*.] *Delusion* rubric: *talking*: *someone
   is talking*: *he is speaking; when*: nux-m.

3. Causation: *Delusion* rubric: *wrong*: *done wrong; he has*:
   nux-m. OPPOSING *Delusion* rubric: *double*: *being*:
   *watching his other self playing; his real conscious self
   seemed to be*: nux-m. [1] 1. [This rubric indicates an ability
   to avoid ownership of 'the other' in wrong doing.]

4. Depression: *Delusion* rubric: *existence*: *surroundings did
   not exist*: nux-m. *Delusion* rubric: *sleepy; he is*: nux-m.
   Delusion rubric: *intoxicated*: *is; he*: nux-m. [These rubrics
   reflect unconsciousness.]

5. Resignation: *Delusion* rubric: *sick*: *being*: nux-m. *Delusion*
   rubric: *diminished*: *shrunken, parts are*: nux-m.

Silicea doubt their integrity. *Silicea* have the *Delusion*
rubrics: *illusions of fancy,* and *he is on a journey*. Both are
Delusion rubrics of idealism which *Silicea* strive to live up to.
Silicea need their meticulous conscientiousness because it
is their *only* salvation from their psychological delusions that
they have done something wrong. The internal questioning
and agonizing about wrong doing is reflected in the *Delusion*
rubric: *divided, left side did not belong to her,* in which *Silicea*
are the only remedy listed, and in the *Mind* rubrics: *anxiety
of conscience* and *always washing her hands. Silicea* avoid

becoming 'criminals' by being *obsessively perfect* – *Silicea* have the *Delusion* rubric: *sees needles* – the attention to detail[67] is obsessively maintained to avoid future wrong doing.

> It is crucial to ask a patient in a consultation: *What do you think about yourself being sick?* The answer to that question highlights *peculiarities* which indicate the simillimum. *Silicea* will answer the question by referring to their perceived failure *to be perfect.*

The psychotherapeutic interpretation of the *Delusion* rubric: *divided, left side did not belong to her,* reveals an internal somatic dilemma where the patient feels like they do not have total control over the two sides of themselves. *Silicea* are never quite sure that the left side of them is as perfect as the right side. *Silicea dwell* upon persecutions – *dwells upon seeing images and phantoms.*

> *Silicea* dwell upon everything which they have done wrong in *minute* detail.

Silicea will say: *I must have done something wrong to be sick and now I need to be extra careful with everything that I do; this will ensure I do not get sick again. I will watch every single thing I eat and I will not do anything to upset myself.* Internal doubt [*will become insane*] and predictions of failure [*everything will fail*] underpin their perceptions of wrong doing. *Silicea* will be particularly obsessive in order to avoid having to face their fear of failure. *Silicea* have the *Delusion* rubric: *about pins. Silicea* chose to concentrate on all the *minor* details of everything they, or someone else has done wrong rather than allow themselves to be inspired by the greater overall view or overall improvement in their health. The simillimum will only be *Silicea* if the patient has to continually concentrate on the minor ailments, (such as a small blemish on their face), which have not been 'cured' in the homoeopathic treatment rather than the overall cure of a major disease.

1. Denial: *Delusion* rubric: *fancy, illusions of:* sil. *Delusion* rubric: *journey; he is on a:* sil.

2. Forsaken: *Delusion* rubric: *persecuted*: *he is persecuted*: sil. *Delusion* rubric: *images, phantoms; sees*: *dwells upon*: sil. [1] 3. [arn. nux-m. sil.] *Delusion* rubric: *injury*: *about to receive injury; is*: sil. *Delusion* rubric: *needles; sees*: *Sil.* [2] 2. [merc.] *Delusion* rubric: *pins; about*: *Sil.* [2] 2. [**NUX-M**.] *Delusion* rubric: *pursued; he was*: sil.

3. Causation: *Delusion* rubric: *wrong*: *done wrong; he has*: sil. *Delusion* rubric: *criminal, he is a*: sil.

4. Depression: *Delusion* rubric: *insane*: *become insane; one will*: sil. *Delusion* rubric: *fail, everything will*: sil.

5. Resignation: *Delusion* rubric: *body*: *divided, is*: sil. *Delusion* rubric: *divided*: *two parts; left side did not belong to her; and*: sil. [1] 1. *Delusion* rubric: *die*: *about to die; one was*: sil.

Veratrum album: Identifying the psychological processes and the psychodynamic avoidances and self-delusions which come into play in each constitutional remedy not only explains the remedy and expands our knowledge – it is necessary for identifying the simillimum. When a patient is sick they are in conflict; when someone is in conflict they self-delude or avoid reality. When a patient is sick they will move through the five psychological processes as they struggle to acknowledge or accept their illness.

Identifying the prominence of one remedy in a particular psychological process will indicate the simillimum. *Veratrum album* are religiously and self-righteously consumed with their guilt.

Veratrum album feature prominently in all the *Delusion* rubrics of grandeur to do with being one with God. The *Delusion* rubric: *he is in heaven talking to God*, and *she is the virgin Mary*, and *he is a prince*, indicates the elevated status that *Veratrum album* have for themselves. From such a lofty height, *Veratrum album* fall a long way when they acknowledge sin. *Veratrum album* have the *Delusion* rubric: *must keep a vow.* The *Veratrum album* (case) in my *Case Companion* to *Homoeopathic Psychiatry* highlights the intensity of the guilt they feel for having committed a sin; the patient in that case did not feel she was worthy of treatment for her cancer because she had fallen so far in the eyes of God.

Veratrum album have numerous rubrics which all indicate hubristic 'delusions of grandeur'. Their religious fanaticism is a 'hubristic denial' and arrogance which allows them to feel pure and purified in the eyes of God.

- *Delusion* rubric: *Christ, himself to be*: **VERAT.**
- *Delusion* rubric: *God*: *communication with God; he is in*: verat.
- *Delusion* rubric: *God*: *messenger from God; he is a:* verat. [1] 1.
- *Delusion* rubric: *great person, is a*: *Verat.*
- *Delusion* rubric: *heaven, is in*: *Verat.*
- *Delusion* rubric: *heaven, is in: talking with God*: *Verat.*[2] 1.
- *Delusion* rubric: *Mary; Virgin: she is*: verat.
- *Delusion* rubric: *prince; he is a: verat.* [1] 1.
- *Delusion* rubric: *power: all powerful; she is*: verat.
- *Delusion* rubric: *religious*: *Verat.*
- *Delusion* rubric: *rank; he is a person of*: verat.

The *Veratrum album* (case) in my *Case Companion* to *Homoeopathic Psychiatry* highlights the consequences of being unable to accept her illness. *Veratrum album* have the *Delusion* rubrics: *has a cancer,* and *will be murdered. Veratrum album* have the *Delusion* rubrics: *proud,* and *must keep a vow.*

The hardest issue to tackle in a *Veratrum album* case is their belief in righteous self-punishment. Self-destructive behavior and self-blame is justified because it is God's punishment.

If one is punished for sins committed then one is worthy

cf being let into heaven. Punishment is redemption and purification. *Veratrum album* believe that they deserve to be *doomed* forever for the *crimes they have committed. Veratrum album* have the *Delusion* rubric: *compelled to suicide,* and the *Mind* rubric: *suicidal disposition from religious despair. Veratrum album* have religious convictions of martyrdom. *Veratrum album* have the *Mind* rubric: *religious psychotic preaching.*

There is hubris in the way *Veratrum album* embrace punishment.

All perceived faults cause them to flee into religious fanaticism so they can purify themselves; this is 'hubristic denial' and avoidance. *Veratrum album* have the *Delusion* rubric: *he is deaf and dumb, and has the disease cancer.* [1] 1. The simillimum will only be *Veratrum album* if the patient has a very low opinion of themselves when they are sick.

Veratrum album believes illness is proof of having been evil.

Underlying righteousness is fear of God's vengeance. The simillimum will only be *Veratrum album* if the patient believes that they deserve to be punished by being sick and that the punishment (sickness) will purify their soul.

1. Denial: *Delusion* rubric: *distinguished; he is*: verat. *Delusion* rubric: *Christ, himself to be*: **VERAT**. *Delusion* rubric: *heaven, is in: talking with God*: Verat.[2] 1.

2. Forsaken: *Delusion* rubric: *home: away from home; he is*: verat.

3. Causation: *Delusion* rubric: *criminal, he is a*: verat.

4. Depression: *Delusion* rubric: *doomed, being*: Verat.

5. Resignation: *Delusion* rubric: *disease: deaf, dumb and has cancer; he is*: verat. [1] 1.

   • *Delusions: lost: she is: salvation; for*: ars. Aur. hell. hura. plb.

   • *Delusions: lost: she is: salvation; for; predestination, from*: Lach. [2] 1.

Avoidance: Underneath the belief that one's soul is beyond salvation will be an intensely exaggerated overwhelming fear or guilt about one's 'original sin'. *Aurum metallicum* have the *Delusion* rubric: *he has neglected his duty. Arsenicum album, Helleborus, Lachesis,* and *Plumbum* all have the *Delusion* rubrics: *he had committed a crime. Arsenicum album* and *Plumbum* are also listed in the *Delusion*: rubric: *one has sinned away his day of grace. Arsenicum album, Helleborus,* and *Lachesis* are all listed in the *Delusion* rubric: *he has done wrong. Hura* are listed in the *Delusion* rubric: *his friends have lost all confidence in him*; this is their 'original sin'.

Hura believe their soul is beyond salvation because they feel intensely exaggerated guilt over having abandoned their friends. *Hura* have the *Mind* rubrics: *anxiety about salvation, religious despair of salvation, reproaching oneself, despair of recovery, biting nails, hands,* and *himself*. All of these reflect their inner turmoil and anguish about salvation.

Hura are however, disturbingly and disproportionately reconciled to their fate and their inability to be saved.

The last psychological stage in the *Delusion* rubrics repertorisation is Resignation. *Hura* are not listed in the *any Delusion* rubrics of *exaggerated* predictions of decay. The homoeopath needs to understand the complexities of the remedies, and *which* constitutional remedies allow anxiety and fear and predictions of death to overwhelm them and which remedy profiles do not, and *why. Hura* also have no *Mind* rubrics: *fear of disease* or *fear of death*, or *anxiety about health*. They have the Mind rubrics: *despair of recovery, despair of religious salvation,* and *aggravated thinking of his complaints. Hura* have dreams of crimes and death. *Hura* have the *Mind* rubrics: *thoughts of death,* and *desires death, fear of misfortune,* and the *Delusion* rubric: *he is unfortunate,* but they have no *Mind* rubrics or *Delusion* rubrics pertaining to hypochondria. If a remedy profile have no fear of illness or death then it is disproportionate to expected normality. *Hura* have the *Mind* rubric: *moaning with pain*. This rubric is indicative of being passively reconciled to one's pain. *Hura* are also disproportionately reconciled to their fate of being an *outcast*. *Hura* dissociate themselves from their misfortune. *Hura* have the dissociative *Delusion* rubric: *floating in air*.

If a remedy profile has no *Mind* or *Delusion* rubrics pertaining to fear of death, then it indicates something extremely unusual and psychologically disturbing.

Hura have 'depersonalization disorder'. 'Depersonalization disorder' is an ability to inappropriately distance oneself emotionally from one's pain and from the pain inflicted on oneself from the outer world. It is these periods of detachment which allow *Hura* distance from feeling *appropriate* fear of illness or death. If your patient is frightened about being sick then the simillimum is *not Hura*. Conversely, if your patient is in conflict and self-denial about their psychological 'delusions of original sin', the simillimum is not *Hura*. *Hura* feel deserving of their banishment from salvation. *Hura* have the *Delusion* rubric: *on falling asleep he or she is hanging three feet from the ground.* [1] 1. This rubric either reinforces their dissociative tendencies or else it reinforces suicidal doom.

Hura is listed in Boericke as being a good remedy for the skin complaints of leprosy. Sankaran also allocates *Hura* to the leprosy miasm. Sankaran notes in *The Soul of Remedies,* that *Hura* is "longing to be part of normal society, to be among his friends, and the feeling of hopelessness of coming out of this destructive process that is leprosy." The feeling of hopelessness in *Hura* is reinforced because they passively dissociate themselves from acknowledging the pain inflicted on them by society. Sankaran notes in *The Soul of Remedies* that "the main feeling in the leprosy miasm is that even with intense, rapid, hectic activity to come out of this destructive process (leprosy), there is little hope." There is *no* struggle within *Hura*. *Hura* are passively resigned about their *despair of recovery* and *loss of salvation*. Their 'depersonalization disorder' gives them an ability to distance themselves emotionally from their pain and from the pain inflicted on them from the outer world. *Hura* are passively resigned to their separation from society.

The simillimum will only be *Hura* if the patient feels deserving of their illness and death, and separation from society because of their illness.

1. Denial: *Delusion* rubric: *floating: air, in*: hura.
2. Forsaken: *Delusion* rubric: *forsaken; is*: hura. *Delusion* rubric: *outcast; she were an*: hura. *Delusion* rubric: *repudiated; he is: relatives; by his*: hura. *Delusion* rubric: *alone, being: world; alone in the*: hura. *Delusion* rubric: *despised; is*: hura. *Delusion* rubric: *dead: persons, sees*: hura. *Delusion* rubric: *friend: lose a friend; she is about to*: hura. [1] 1. *Delusion* rubric: *confidence in him; his friends have lost all*: hura.
3. Causation: *Delusion* rubric: *lost: she is: salvation; for.* hura. *Delusion* rubric: *confidence in him; his friends have lost all*: hura. *Delusion* rubric: *repudiated; he is: relatives; by his*: hura. [These last two rubrics can also be allocated into 'delusions of abandonment' or 'delusions of persecution'.]
4. Depression: *Delusion* rubric: *unfortunate, he is*: hura. *Delusion* rubric: *hanging; is: he or she was hanging: three feet from the ground: asleep; on falling*: hura. [1] 1. [This rubric pertains to feeling dissociation, or abandonment, or depressive suicidal thoughts.]
5. Resignation: NONE.
   - *Delusions: hell: going to hell because he had committed a unpardonable crime*: med.[1] 1.
   - *Delusions: hell: in; is*: camph. cann-i. germ-met. haliae-lc. hydrog. ignis-alc. lyss. merc. orig-v. *Orig.*
   - *Delusions: lost; she is: salvation; for. sexual desire; with violent*: orig. [1] 1.

Self-Deluding: The list of *Delusion* rubrics above all resonate with the theme of 'fire and brimstone' (God's punishment) and of being cast into the fires of hell and damnation as a result of having been bad. Self-deluding means that the remedy will hide their sins from themselves so they do not have to change their behavior. Self-deluding can also mean that if they do not acknowledge sins committed, they cannot understand why they are being punished in hell.

Lyssinum is a homoeopathic remedy derived from the saliva of a dog suffering with rabies. *Lyssinum* have the *Mind* rubric: *desire to cut, mutilate or slit others*. *Lyssinum* have the *Delusion* rubric: *is in hell*.

Lyssinum are *in hell* but in their mind *they* are not responsible for getting themselves there. *Lyssinum* have the *Delusion* rubric: *he could do nothing*. The simillimum will not be *Lyssinum* if the patient indicates that *they* are responsible for their predicament.

Lyssinum have the *Delusion* rubric: *momentary loss of consciousness*. The simillimum will not be *Lyssinum* if the patient acknowledges blame. *Lyssinum* helplessly negate responsibility and attribute their desire to attack others to being possessed by the devil.

Lyssinum does not acknowledge inner fault for being sick. The blame for their illness is viciously reflected outwards with the same intensity of a dog with rabies.

The *Delusion* rubric: *torments of hell without being able to explain,* indicates self-deluding denial of any blame. *Lyssinum* will never acknowledge in a consultation that the reason they have, for example, a fatty liver is that they have been overindulging in too much alcohol and rich food. I have never treated *Lyssinum* when they are seriously or fatally ill, so I am not sure of the intensity of their self-deluding, but I imagine they would be equally intense, if not more so, when they have to change even one small part of their health regime by avoiding alcohol, for example. *Lyssinum,* even though they have the *Mind* rubric: *desire to attack others,* take no responsibility for being in hell. This is self-deluding behavior. Similarly, *Lyssinum* feel *they* have suffered wrong. *Lyssinum* have the *Delusion* rubric: *he has suffered wrong. Lyssinum* have the *Delusion* rubric: *being possessed,* and *possessed by the devil.*

Lyssinum have the *Delusion* rubric: *great person,* and the *Delusion* rubric: *he had received joyful intelligence.* [1] 1. Psychological 'delusions of superiority' will mean that the *Lyssinum* patient will have a tendency to deflect responsibility. *Lyssinum* have the *Delusion* rubric: *two different thoughts influenced him at the same time.* [1] 2. *Lyssinum* also have the *Delusion* rubrics: *expecting joyful news,* and *expecting unpleasant news.* The simillimum will not be *Lyssinum* unless the patient demonstrates delusional denial over their health.

Lyssinum have the *Delusion* rubric: *she could not hold her head straight, something was drawing her around in a circle.* [1] 1. This rubric should not be taken literally, rather it indicates abdication of responsibility.

Lyssinum refuse to acknowledge they are responsible for holding their own head straight, nor are they responsible for moving in a circle. *Lyssinum* refuse to acknowledge they are responsible for any health predicament in which they find themselves. The *unpleasant news* the homoeopath delivers to the *Lyssinum* patient is not their fault.

1. Denial: *Delusion* rubric: *great person, is a:* lyss. *Delusion* rubric: *news: expecting news: joyful news:* lyss. [1] 2. [valer.] *Delusion* rubric: *intelligence: joyful intelligence; he had received:* lyss. [1] 1.

2. Forsaken: *Delusion* rubric: *forsaken; is:* lyss. *Delusion* rubric: *attacked; being:* lyss. *Delusion* rubric: *criticized, she is:* lyss. *Delusion* rubric: *deceived; being:* lyss. *Delusion* rubric: *injury: being injured; is:* lyss. *Delusion* rubric: *insulted, he is:* lyss. *Delusion* rubric: *laughed at and mocked at; being:* lyss. *Delusion* rubric: *wrong: suffered wrong; he*

has: *Lyss*. *Delusion* rubric: *tormented; he is*: lyss.

3. Causation: *Delusion* rubric: *hell*: *in*; *is*: lyss. OPPOSING *Delusion* rubric: *hell*: *torments of hell without being able to explain; suffers the*: lyss. *Delusion* rubric: *devil*; *possessed of a devil*: lyss. *Delusion* rubric: *possessed; being*: lyss. *Delusion* rubric: *dogs*: *he is dog*: *growls and barks*: lyss.

4. Depression: *Delusion* rubric: *tormented; he is*: lyss. *Delusion* rubric: *nothing*: *do nothing; he could*: lyss. [1] 1. *Delusion* rubric: *news*: *expecting news*: *unpleasant news*: lyss. *Delusi on* rubric: *falling*: *he is*: lyss. *Delusion* rubric: *sinking*: *to be*: lyss.

5. Resignation: *Delusion* rubric: *consciousness*: *lose consciousness; he would*: *momentarily; he had lost consciousness*: lyss. [1] 1. *Delusion* rubric: *die*: *about to die; one was*: lyss. *Delusion* rubric: *swallow, cannot*: lyss. [1] 1. *Delusion* rubric: *mouth*: *cannot open mouth, lower jaw stiff and painful*: lyss. [1] 1.

Medorrhinum[68] struggle intensely with inner questioning and doubt about their motives because they appear, even to themselves, to be extremely unstable. The contrasting themes within their nature mean that they are extremely reactive and go into flight from themselves, as well as over-react and go into flight from all other constraints or social expectations. *Medorrhinum* have the *Mind* rubric: *aversion to responsibility*, and the *Mind* rubric: *restlessness, must constantly move, goes from one room to the next*. Their reactivity is evident in the *Mind* rubric: *has to restrain himself in order not to curse*.

Medorrhinum condemn themselves and throw themselves into the fires of hell, especially with *despair from the smallest criticism.*

Medorrhinum have numerous *Delusion* rubrics pertaining to paranoia: *hearing voices behind him, someone whispering behind him*, and *sees faces looking from behind bed and furniture*. In my *Case Companion* to *Homoeopathic Psychiatry*, the *Medorrhinum* (case) highlights the seriousness with which they take their *unpardonable crimes*. *Medorrhinum* will be tormented by their sins, which is why *Medorrhinum* are the only remedy listed in the *Delusion* rubric: *she must do something to rid her mind of the torture*.

When sick, *Medorrhinum* are totally sure that they deserve to die.

Medorrhinum have the *Delusion* rubric: *time has come to die*. When *Medorrhinum* have even the smallest of health problems, like acne or a boil, they will seriously evaluate whether they should continue to live and whether they are worthy of your attention and care. Self-deluding is evident in the way *Medorrhinum* abandon themselves and avoid all responsibility even for living and preserving their life – *Delusion* rubric: *life was unreal*. *Medorrhinum* will choose to condemn themselves to die rather than take responsibility for getting themselves out of the hell and torment they are in. Their passive-aggressive ineffectualness becomes a procrastination and crippling undermining of their own self-confidence. This is self-deluding behavior which they continue because it helps them avoid responsibility.

It is important to identify the psychological steps a patient will move through as they struggle to acknowledge or resign themselves to illness.

Medorrhinum religiously and righteously condemn themselves for their perceived sins; this is why they have the *Delusion* rubric: *going to hell because he had committed an unpardonable crime*.

Medorrhinum have strong, self-defeating, psychological 'delusions of persecution' which will need to be acknowledged when you are treating them, as they desire death so they can avoid the responsibilities involved in living.

A neurosis indicates an inability to have a rational or realistic objective view of one's life. *Medorrhinum* have no personal 'delusions of grandeur'; all their power is transferred outwards on to their 'spiritual guides' who stand beside them *caressing their head. Medorrhinum* struggle to separate their psyche from the influences of others. This instability perpetuates their numerous 'persecution complexes'. 'Transference neuroses' are a conflict between the 'ego' and the 'id'. The realistic 'ego' in *Medorrhinum* is undermined. The unconscious and unfettered 'id' in *Medorrhinum* is suppressed by their disproportionate 'delusions of impending doom'. *Medorrhinum* have the *Delusion* rubrics: *being doomed*, and *something dreadful has happened*. [1] 1. The 'id' is unconscious and is not restricted by social conventionality. The 'id' is unrestrained, selfish self-gratification. *Medorrhinum,* for all their supposed social unconventionality, restrain their own 'id', *cut their own legs off,* and surrender personal power into persecutory paranoia because of their exaggerated 'delusions of original sin'. The 'never-well-since-event' or causation in a *Medorrhinum* case will always come from an over-exaggerated reaction to an *unpardonable crime*.

1. Denial: *Delusion* rubric: *religious*: med. *Delusion* rubric: *caressed on head by someone*: *Med*. [2] 1. *Delusion* rubric: *hand*: *smoothing her; felt a hand*: med. [1] 1. *Delusion* rubric: *women*: *bedside; by*: med. [1] 1. *Delusion* rubric: *hearing: illusions, of*: med. [This rubric can allude to hubristic illusions or to 'delusions of persecution'.]

2. Forsaken: *Delusion* rubric: *persecuted*: *he is persecuted*: med. *Delusion* rubric: *people*: *beside him; people are*: *Med*. *Delusion* rubric: *people; behind him; someone is*: *Med*. *Delusion* rubric: *faces, sees: looking from behind bed and furniture*: med. [1] 1. *Delusion* rubric: *faces, sees: wherever he turns his eyes, or looking out from corners*: med. *Delusion* rubric: *people*: *behind him; someone is*: *whispering*: med. [1] 1.

3. Causation: *Delusion* rubric: *hell*: *going to hell because he had committed a unpardonable crime*: med.[1] 1. *Delusion* rubric: *crime*: *committed a crime; he had*: med.

4. Depression: *Delusion* rubric: *doomed, being*: med. *Delusion* rubric: *anxious*: med. *Delusion* rubric: *insane*:

become insane; one will: med. *Delusion* rubric: *trembling*: *he was trembling*: *without trembling; but*: med. *Delusion* rubric: *torture*: *rid her mind of the torture; she must do something to*: med. [1] 1. *Delusion* rubric: *intoxicated: is; he*: med. [This rubric pertains to unconsciousness.] *Delusion* rubric: *happened; something has*: *dreadful has happened; something*: med. [1] 1. *Delusion* rubric: *unreal*: *life was unreal*: med. *Delusion* rubric: *business*: *accomplished; business could never be*: med. [1] 1.

5. Resignation: *Delusion* rubric: *die*: *time has come to*: med.

Origanum majorana believe they are deserving of punishment because they are sexually perverse. *Origanum majorana* have the *Delusion* rubric: *is despised with violent sexual desire,* and the *Delusion* rubric: *she is lost for salvation with violent sexual desire* [1] 1. *Origanum majorana* desire punishment. *Origanum majorana* have the *Delusion* rubric: *being in the chains of hell*. Below I have listed all the *Delusion* rubrics for *Origanum majorana.*

Origanum majorana have no *Delusion* rubrics pertaining to psychological 'delusions of grandeur'. Because there are no rubrics of 'hubristic denial', the self-condemnation is more profound than in other remedies.

All the remedies listed in this section know in their conscious and subconscious mind that they have committed crimes or that they are 'bad'. The essence of avoidance which sits in the conscious and subconscious mind is a psychological technique which allows the patient to either over-react to their sins or to use their over-reaction to their advantage.

Origanum majorana have strong, self-defeating psychological 'delusions of persecution'. These will need to be acknowledged when you are treating them as, in my experience, they desire death.

Origanum majorana have the *Mind* rubrics: *desires death, suicidal disposition, hysterical insanity, suicidal disposition throwing himself from a height,* and *suicidal disposition with violent sexual desire.* [1] 1. Self-destructive behavior, self-blame, and self-abuse will be maintained and nurtured because they reinforce their innermost dark secrets about themselves.

The simillimum will only be *Origanum majorana* if the patient enjoys being abused either by themselves or others.

- *Delusion* rubric: *despised; is*: Orig.
- *Delusion* rubric: *despised; is*: *sexual desire; with violent*: orig. [1] 1.
- *Delusion* rubric: *devil*: *after her. is; sexual desire; with violent*: orig.
- *Delusion* rubric: *devil*: *sees*: orig.
- *Delusion* rubric: *hell*: *chains of; in*: Orig. [2] 1.
- *Delusion* rubric: *hell*: *chains of; in; sexual desire; with violent*: orig. [1] 1.
- *Delusion* rubric: *hell*: *in; is*: Orig.
- *Delusion* rubric: *identity*: *errors of personal identity*: orig.
- *Delusion* rubric: *insane*: *he is insane*: orig.
- *Delusion* rubric: *lost; she is*: *salvation; for. despised in erotomania; and*: orig. [1] 1.
- *Delusion* rubric: *lost; she is*: *salvation; for. sexual desire; with violent*: orig. [1] 1.

1. Denial: NONE.
2. Forsaken: *Delusion* rubric: *despised; is*: Orig.
3. Causation: *Delusion* rubric: *lost; she is*: *salvation; for. sexual desire; with violent*: orig. [1] 1. *Delusion* rubric: *hell*: *chains of; in*: Orig. [2] 1.
4. Depression: *Delusion* rubric: *insane*: *he is insane*: orig.
5. Resignation: NONE.

- *Delusions*: *looked down upon; she is*: Lac-c. lac-lup. pin-con.

- *Delusions: confusion; others will observe her.* Calc. choc. limest-b. sal-fr.
- *Delusions: body: ugly; body looks:* bar-c. brass-n-o. bry. bufo. *Cham.* cina cygn-be. falco-pe. haliae-lc. loxo-recl. melal-alt. *Nux-v.* ol-eur. positr. pycnop-sa. *Thuj.* tub.
- *Delusions: dirty, he is:* aster. cygn-be. hydrog. *Lac-c.* limest-b. lycps-v. nat-p. neon. olib-sac. plut-n. positr. rhus-t. sanguis-s. *Syph.* thuj.

Self Deluding: The *Delusion* rubrics: *she is looked down upon, others will observe her confusion, body looks ugly*, or *he is dirty*, are all reflective of paranoid inner questioning and doubt about one's motives. The remedies listed in the rubrics above all have, in one way or another, an exaggerated over-reaction to their internal crisis of conscience which is disproportionate to their sins. These rubrics can all also be analyzed in 'delusions of persecution'. All these remedies are sure that someone is able to perceive their faults. This is a self-deluding exaggeration of their inner assumption of guilt.

One of the most notable dilemmas that patients face in acknowledging their illness or disease is what other people will say about them. Fear of exposure is a strong underlying indication of either a guilty conscience, or an exaggerated conscientiousness evident in psychological delusions of self-blame; this is the basis of the *Delusion* rubrics of sin.

One of the most pressing concerns people have over needing to change their diet when they find out they have an allergy to gluten, wheat, or fructose, for example, is what work colleagues, friends, and family will say about them being different and needing to eat different food. It is important in case-taking to consider the above group of rubrics whenever a patient is upset about how they are going to survive in society when others find out they are sick.

When something as simple as their diet being different, or something as profound as the 'world' finding out they have cancer, can make them feel fearful of being exposed to ridicule and blame, it is indicative of inner psychological delusions of guilt for unspecified sins.

Illness can be viewed as proof of inner fault. I have noticed that self-blame for illness has become more prevalent in society since the emergence of the 'New-Age' philosophies that attribute the cause of illness to the patient's negative emotions or thoughts. Since the emergence of 'New-Age' philosophies, my patients who have cancer have been exposed to an extra stress on top of what they are already having to deal with. I am frequently being told by patients, that friends, and family, and work colleagues, look down upon them and think lesser of them because *they* have caused their cancer. The first time that this became prevalent in my health practice was in the late eighties. My patient relayed how she felt about this rejection: *It is bad enough that I have cancer, but the worst part is that all my friends and family think that I am bad inside. I am bad inside because I have not been able to cure myself of this cancer. They are all angry with me because they don't think I have tried hard enough to live. I know I am very negative inside, and this cancer is proof of that.* My patient had bowel cancer, by the time it was diagnosed it had already spread into her liver. Both her parents had died of bowel cancer. The patient who 'takes on' this view of themselves feels that everyone is looking at them, thinking that they are in some way, 'negative'. The pain of the rejection from family and friends was more distressing for this patient than her distress about dying. The *Delusion* rubrics which should be used in the rubric-repertorisation are – *she is looked down upon, others will observe her confusion, body looks ugly*, or *he is dirty*.

We are all in some way, to a lesser or greater degree, 'negative'. Illness uncovers our negativities; whether our negativities are the direct 'cause' of disease is a contentious issue. The role of the homoeopath is to find the simillimum which is able to contain within its profile similarities to the patient's profile. This section, which contains all the *Delusion* rubrics of sin, is critical to understanding constitutional homoeopathy. Each constitutional remedy will absorb their sins, or absolve themselves of sin, in unique and individual ways.

Calcarea carbonica suffer from paranoid fears of being *watched by someone behind* them because they are fearful of having not been 'good'. *Calcarea carbonica* misinterpret their own perceived illusions of having sinned. *Calcarea carbonica* have intense religious affections. *Calcarea carbonica* have the *Mind* rubric: *religious affections, wants to read the bible all day.*

Calcarea carbonica is a very important remedy profile to consider if the patient has an over-exaggerated conscientiousness about having been the cause of their illness because they have not been 'good'.

Calcarea carbonica feel that they have been 'bad', and that *someone has seen them* being 'bad', and this is why they are being punished. On one hand, *Calcarea carbonica* have friends around them to make them feel secure, and on the other hand the friends observing them are part of an unfounded guilty conscience. *Calcarea carbonica* have the *Delusion* rubric: *others will observe her confusion*, and are the only remedy listed in the *Delusion* rubric: *someone is over the bed*. *Calcarea carbonica* over-react to their fears of being abandoned and left alone and *away from their home*[69]. *Calcarea carbonica* equate abandonment with punishment for having been 'bad'. *Calcarea carbonica* fear *sinking into annihilation* and this is why they need their *religious affections* and their connection to God to save them. *Calcarea carbonica* live in a *fantasy world of imaginary friends* because they need reassurance that they are being protected. Furthermore, to help them feel secure, *Calcarea carbonica* live in a fantasy world of *wealth* where they are not abandoned without money. All of the *Delusion* rubrics of being *watched* or someone *standing over the bed* can indicate paranoia or exaggerated 'delusions of abandonment'. The *peculiarity* specific to *Calcarea carbonica* is that they equate illness with proof of having been 'bad' and this is why they are so obsessive about their religious affections. Since the emergence of all the 'New-Age' philosophies that attribute the cause of illness to the patient's negative emotional or mental thinking all my *Calcarea carbonica* patients have suffered from the perception that they must be guilty. *Calcarea carbonica* need support from *people beside them* otherwise they feel distraught – *Delusion* rubric: *body dashed to pieces*. The simillimum will only be *Calcarea carbonica* if the patient is extremely anxious that their illness will mean they will be rejected by society.

Calcarea carbonica need to be well to assure themselves that they are good people.

1. Denial: *Delusion* rubric: *wealth, of*: calc. *Delusion* rubric: *friend: fantasy world of imaginary friends; lives in a*: calc. [1] 1. *Delusion* rubric: *people: beside him; people are*: calc. [This rubric can indicate illusions of God standing next to you, or it can indicate paranoia.]

2. Forsaken: *Delusion* rubric: *bed: someone: over the bed; someone is*: calc. [1] 1. *Delusion* rubric: *home: away from home; he is*: calc. *Delusion* rubric: *watched, she is being*: Calc. *Delusion* rubric: *people; behind him; someone is*: calc. *Delusion* rubric: *people: beside him; people are*: calc. *Delusion* rubric: *criticized, she is*: calc.

3. Causation: *Delusion* rubric: *confusion; others will observe her. Calc. Delusion* rubric: *bed: someone: over the bed; someone is*: calc. [1] 1. *Delusion* rubric: *watched, she is being*: Calc. *Delusion* rubric: *people; behind him; someone is*: calc. *Delusion* rubric: *people: beside him; people are*: calc. [These rubrics can indicate exaggerated guilt or 'delusions of persecution'.]

4. Depression: *Delusion* rubric: *anxious*: calc. *Delusion* rubric:

ruined: *is ruined; he*: calc. *Delusion* rubric: *insane*: *become insane; one will*: *Calc.*

5. Resignation: *Delusion* rubric: *annihilation; about to sink into*: calc. *Delusion* rubric: *disease: incurable disease; he has an*: calc. *Delusion* rubric: *die: about to die; one was*: calc. *Delusion* rubric: *sick: being*: **CALC**. *Delusion* rubric: *body: dashed to pieces, being*: calc. [1] 1.

Lac caninum: Sankaran, in *The Soul of Remedies,* states: "Lac caninum is a sycotic remedy. It is prepared from the milk of the dog (bitch). This remedy has in it the nature of the dog, an animal that has been totally controlled and civilized so that it has to suppress its basic animal nature and can only express its controlled, civilized side. It is dependent on its master for food and so it is out to please him. Its survival depends upon keeping its master happy by its performance, its affection, etc. It has to perform or it won't be wanted anymore and its master will kick it out. This need to please is the animal side of Lac caninum, but the dog knows that no matter how much it tries to please, it will never be equal to the human. It feels inferior, knows that it is at the bottom of the hierarchy." *Lac caninum* have been noted for the rubrics which emphasize their self-contempt. The *Delusion* rubric: *she is looked down upon,* as well as the rubrics listed below, all resonate with self-loathing flagellation, reminiscent of the lowly dog laying themselves at their master's feet ready to be kicked. *Lac caninum* have endless *Mind* rubrics: *loathing oneself, contemptuous of self,* and *doubtful of recovery,* which resonate with the image of a downtrodden dog. As soon as there is conflict inside a remedy, there will be *Delusion* rubrics which mirror the perversity of self-deprecating inner conflict. Sankaran says, "The dog knows that no matter how much it tries to please, it will never be equal to the human." *Lac caninum* compensate for their feelings of servitude by dissociating from reality. *Lac caninum* have the *Delusion* rubrics: *has beautiful visions, as if exalted,* and *floating in air like a spirit.* Because

Lac caninum have psychological 'delusions of grandeur' and dissociative denial they will, when sick, deny the process of their illness by somatically *floating off into the air like a spirit.* The *Delusion* rubric: *crazy if she could not get out of her body,* indicates a need to dissociate from their body.

> If you expect *Lac caninum* to present in a consultation as a downtrodden, self-loathing, pitiful creature who believes themselves to be a *loathsome, horrible mass of disease*, then you will not recognize the simillimum. I cannot stress strongly enough the need to know and understand the psychological process that a patient will progress through as they struggle to accept or resign themselves to their illness. In their first consultation, a seriously sick *Lac caninum* will present in an *exalted* state of 'hubristic denial'.

When *Lac caninum* start to come to terms with being sick, their first defense will be that you have insulted them; this defense mechanism is associated with psychological 'delusions of abandonment'. They will then blame themselves and tell you with exaggerated intensity that they are dirty and diseased. The next phase is depressive feelings of worthlessness. Finally, they will move into the psychological delusions of being a *loathsome mass of disease*. Below are the five stages of psychological processing that *Lac caninum* will move through as they struggle to acknowledge their illness. Feelings of worthlessness and self-loathing underpin the psychological 'delusions of original sin'. The *Delusion* rubric: *looked down upon*, reiterates the self-deprecating self-punishment that resonates in all of the rubrics attached to *Lac caninum*.

1. Denial: *Delusion* rubric: *exalted; as if*: lac-c. *Delusion* rubric: *floating; air, in; spirit; like a*: lac-c. *Delusion* rubric: *visions, has; beautiful*: lac-c.

2. Forsaken: *Delusion* rubric: *insulted, he is*: lac-c. *Delusion* rubric: *looked down upon; she is*: Lac-c. [This rubric can indicate persecutory paranoia or self-loathing.] *Delusion* rubric: *despised; is*: lac-c.

3. Causation: *Delusion* rubric: *dirty; he is*: Lac-c. *Delusion* rubric: *looked down upon; she is*: Lac-c. *Delusion* rubric: *prostitute, is a*: lac-c.

4. Depression: *Delusion* rubric: *worthless; he is*: lac-c. *Delusion* rubric: *body: out of the body; crazy if she could not get out of her body; she would become*: lac-c. [1] 1. *Delusion* rubric: *insane: become insane; one will; sitting still and thinking; when*: lac-c.[1]1.

5. Resignation: *Delusion* rubric: *disease: loathsome, horrible mass of disease; he was a*: lac-c.

   • Delusions: devil: sees: bed; sees devils about his: op. [1] 1.

   • Delusions: criminal: he is a: executed, to be: **OP**. [3] 1.

   • Delusions: wrong: done wrong; he has: punished; and is about to be: op. [1] 1.

Opium: Although *Opium* are listed in the *Delusion* rubric: *he has done wrong*, it is the above *Delusion* rubric: *he is a criminal to be executed*, which is most *peculiar* and *specific* to *Opium*. *Opium* do not want to remain in a conscious mind state. *Opium* is a remedy derived from the opium poppy. In addition to alleviating pain, the psychological effects of opium, the drug, convey a sense of peace and contentment and 'emotional distance' from cares and worries. *Opium* have the *Mind* rubric: *indifference to joy and the suffering of others,* and the *Mind* rubric: *content, forgets all his ailments and pains.* *Opium* need to maintain delusional denial, illusions of beauty, and the psychological delusion that they are in a *euphoric* state because they don't want to care. *Opium* are overwhelmed by feeling. *Opium* have the *Mind* rubrics: *ailments from joy,* and *ailments from grief.* The history of the use of the opium poppy as a narcotic which allows the user to elevate themselves above the worldly pain of their everyday worries and grief of living is well documented. *Opium* choose to delude themselves that they are beautiful to avoid the harshness of the world. The simillimum will not be *Opium* unless the patient feels guilty because they don't care. The simillimum will only be *Opium* if the patient tells you that they deserve their disease because they have never cared about anyone else's suffering.

The intensity of the 'persecution complex' in *Opium* is so self-condemning they believe they should be *executed*. The simillimum will only be *Opium* if the patient tells you that they have always lived to enjoy life and now they deserve their punishment (disease).

1. Denial: *Delusion* rubric: *beautiful*: op. *Delusion* rubric: *heaven, is in*: op. *Delusion* rubric: *visions, has beautiful*: OP. *Delusion* rubric: *superhuman; is control*: *is under superhuman*: op. [This rubric can be aligned to God or the devil.] *Delusion* rubric: *pleasing delusions*: op. *Delusion* rubric: *visions, has*: *fantastic*: op. *Delusion* rubric: *well, he is*: op. *Delusion* rubric: *enlarged*: *tall; he is very*: op. *Delusion* rubric: *enlarged*: *body is*: op. *Delusion* rubric: *flying*: op. *Delusion* rubric: *laughter, with*: op.

2. Forsaken: *Delusion* rubric: *execute him; people want to*: OP. *Delusion* rubric: *poisoned: he, has been*: op. *Delusion* rubric: *home: away from home; he is*: Op. *Delusion* rubric: *injury: about to receive injury; is*: Op. *Delusion* rubric: *journey; he is on a*: op. *Delusion* rubric: *stabbed; someone threatened to stab him; as if*: op. [1] 1. *Delusion* rubric: *murdered: will be murdered; he*: Op. *Delusion* rubric: *house: own house; not being in one's*: Op. *Delusion* rubric: *visions, has*: *horrible*: op.

3. Causation: *Delusion* rubric: *criminal; he is a*: *executed, to be*: OP. [3] 1. *Delusion* rubric: *wrong: done wrong; he has*: *punished; and is about to be*: op. [1] 1. *Delusion* rubric: *devil*: *sees*: *bed; sees devils about his*: op. [1] 1. [This rubric can pertain to admission of guilt or persecution.] *Delusion* rubric: *criminal, he is a*: op. *Delusion* rubric: *wrong: done wrong; he has*: op. *Delusion* rubric: *possessed; being*: op. *Delusion* rubric: *superhuman; is control*: *is under*

superhuman: op. [These last two rubrics can be alignment to God or the devil.]

4. Depression: *Delusion* rubric: *doomed, being*: op. *Delusion* rubric: *drugged; as if*: op.

5. Resignation: *Delusion* rubric: *weight: no weight; has*: op. *Delusion* rubric: *body: lighter than air; body is*: Op. *Delusion* rubric: *brain: smoke on brain*: op. [1] 1. *Delusion* rubric: *dying: he is*: op.

Depression

"I will never become well."

"I will never succeed."

"I will always fail."

"This is my fate."

I have allocated all the *Delusion* rubrics which pertain to psychological 'delusions of impending doom' into Depression. If the trauma inside your patient starts with them feeling hopeless doom about being sick or them feeling like they will never succeed in becoming well in life, then the simillimum is listed in the *Delusion* rubrics: *failure* and *he will not succeed* and is allocated to the section Depression.

Kübler-Ross identified depression as the fourth stage. When someone finds out that they have a serious illness it is normal for them to find their thoughts sinking into depressive fear. The rubrics used in the rubric-repertorisation that would match these *very normal imaginations* are the *Mind* rubrics: *fear of disease* or *fear of death*, and *anxiety about health*. Furthermore, it is normal for a patient to feel depressed during or after an illness, and continue to feel depressed even when they have been given a good prognosis. When a patient is confronted with mortality for the first time, they can feel so anxious about their lack of control over life and death that they lose all confidence in themselves for years following the disease. It is incorrect to presume that a patient will become 'a positive person' after a good prognosis. It is normal for a patient to become a more positive person after a good prognosis but it is also normal for a patient to become pessimistic, and fatalistic after a good prognosis. When a patient is confronted with mortality for the first time they are also confronted with the reality that they are not perfect; their body has failed them. Homoeopaths should not underestimate the impact this can have on a patient. Every day all health practitioners confront the reality of disease and death. The majority of my patients are experiencing for the first time their body having failed them. It is a shock which reverberates within their psyche for years afterwards. The shock is so profound that I often need to explain to patients that they are suffering from post-traumatic stress disorder. The way I explain this to patients is to use the analogy that until they became sick, or before they experienced loss in their lives, they believed that life was a wonderful fairy story in which everything turned out right in the end, and good always triumphed over bad. Now their belief in fairy castles and good triumphing over bad is shattered. Without fail when I use this analogy, patients confirm that I am correct and that it is not fair because they believed if they were good then this would not have happened to them; bad things only happen to bad people. I collect children's fairy stories from all around the world. In all fairy stories, regardless of the country of origin, the moral of the story is that if one's deeds are motivated by greed or evilness then the outcome will be bad. If one is motivated by good then they will be rewarded with three wishes and their Prince Charming and a wonderful castle. Fairy stories and cultural mythology form the moral guidance which is instilled in us by our parents from a very young age.

The belief that good deeds are rewarded is also the moral premise of all Eastern and Western religious ideologies and all 'New-Age' philosophies. The dismay which preempts a patient sinking into feelings of pessimistic hopelessness when they find out they are sick dates back to the beliefs that were instilled in them through the fairy stories of their childhood. Patients who experience illness or loss for the first time in their life are angry that their belief in life being a fairy story is incorrect. Disease and death is not the ending for 'a good person' in a fairy story.

The *Mind* rubrics applicable in the rubric-repertorisation are: *hypochondriasis, hysteria, thoughts of death, depressive mania, sadness, discouraged, doubtful of recovery, dwells on disappointments, exaggerating symptoms, fear something bad will happen, fear of suffering, forebodings, horrible things affect her, impatience about trifling things, inconsolable, lack of initiative, mental insecurity, introspection, irritability, irresolution about trifles, desire to kill, lamenting, laughing with weeping, sardonic laughing, loathing of life or work, weakness of memory, making mistakes with speech or time, moaning about complaints, morose, easily offended, pities herself, pessimistic, postponing everything, prostration of mind, quarrelsome, rage, religious affections, remorse, reproaching himself, resignation, sadness, sighing, thoughtless staring, suicidal, taciturn, thinking of his complaints, feels unfortunate, weeping, weary of life,* and finally, *everything seems wrong.* The reason I have listed so many of the relevant *Mind* rubrics is to emphasize that illness can make one feel several, or all, of the above emotions.

A *Delusion* rubric is used only when there is an assumption or perception which is disproportionate to reality. If the shock of becoming ill for the first time has a *permanent* pessimistic influence on your patient even after they have a good prognosis then the simillimum is listed in the *Delusion* rubrics of Depression.

If the trauma inside your patient starts with them feeling *intense* hopeless doom about being sick, and/or always being sick, or feeling that they *will never succeed* in becoming well, then the simillimum is listed in the *Delusion* rubrics of Depression. These are the *Delusion* rubrics: *he cannot succeed, everything will fail, he does everything wrong, he is trapped, he is ruined, he will become insane,* and *being doomed,* to list just a few. Psychological 'delusions of impending doom' are disproportionate assumptions about future failure.

The need to believe that one is unfortunate in life is usually based on exaggerated psychological delusions of being evil, wrong, or bad. This is the reason that Causation, or 'delusions of original sin', precedes Depression in the five stage psychological model. If a patient needs to hang on to the belief that they are unfortunate, then they need to deflect responsibility for their situation from themselves. Commonly, patients will blame their unfortunate circumstances on past life laws of karma, fate, or God who is testing their faith, or God who is punishing them for past sins. These varying ideologies are covered in the *Delusion* rubrics of Depression because underpinning their assumption that they deserve punishment is the need to believe that they are *doomed* and are *unfortunate*. (Aside from believing that one is ill-fated, the other reason why a person may not be able to achieve 'self-actualization' is that realistically they do not have the capacity to solve their problems. This is not necessarily delusional and is covered in all the *Mind* rubrics of Depression).

In this chapter, I specifically concentrate on the remedy profiles for which a delusional belief in failure, or a need to believe one will always fail, is an all consuming problem which causes future pathology. The *Delusion* rubrics of Depression resonate with disturbance because the remedy profiles in this group wish to maintain their depression and their belief that they will *always* fail and they will *never* succeed.

The delusional belief in failure is self-destructive. To an outsider, or to the homoeopath observing the patient suffering 'delusions of impending doom', it is not always reflective of reality. A patient can maintain a perception of themselves as a failure whereas in reality they are very successful. The *peculiar* reason why a patient continues to need to believe they will not succeed will always indicate the simillimum.

The purpose in understanding the five stage psychological analysis of the *Delusion* rubrics is to highlight the specific *peculiarities* of a remedy profile. The constitutional remedy profiles which are profoundly consumed by 'delusions of impending doom' have no 'delusions of grandeur' or denial processes which are able to create a 'hubristic illusion' of success. The patient who has no delusional belief in cure or no 'hubristic denial' process in place within their psyche will be more likely to sabotage their success and their medical or homoeopathic treatment.

Delusion Rubrics in Depression

In this section I analyze and explain the meaning of each individual *Delusion* rubric. I offer previously unexplored explanations of the psychological delusional state inherent in each *Delusion* rubric. Furthermore, I explain their psychotherapeutic meaning and application by analyzing how each remedy listed under the rubric heading has utilized the delusional stance to its advantage. The reasons why each constitutional remedy is listed under a rubric will often be vastly different. Understanding the need for the psychological delusions within each of the constitutional remedy profiles will aid in remedy recognition.

Each selection of *Delusion* rubrics discussed are shaded. Analyses of the remedy profiles follow each sub-section. The psychological development of *Delusion* rubrics for each constitutional remedy profile is analyzed according to either **avoidance** or **self-deluding** need.

- *Delusions: worthless; he is*: adam. agn. anac. aur. falco-pe. lac-c. lac-h. nat-ar. positr. thuj.
- *Delusions: succeed, he does everything wrong; he cannot*: adam. Anac. Arg-n. arn. Aur-m-n. Aur. bamb-a. bapt. Bar-c. gels. germ-met. lyc. melal-alt. naja. nat-c. nat-m. ozone. petr-ra. phos. sal-fr. sulph.
- *Delusions: fail, everything will*: act-sp. aq-mar. Arg-n. Aur-m-n. Aur. bamb-a. carc. chir-fl. cob-n. conch. cygn-be. kola. lac-c. lac-e. merc. nux-v. psor. sil.
- *Delusions: right; doing nothing right; he is*: anac. arg-n. Aur. germ-met. nat-c. plac-s.

- *Delusions: wrong; everything goes wrong*: androc. bac. bamb-a. calc. coloc. falco-pe. hep. kali-br. naja. nux-v. phys. plac-s.
- *Delusions: wrong; suffered wrong; he has*: adam. bac. bar-c. carc. chin. cygn-be. **HYOS**. lach. *Lyss*. naja. petr-ra. positr. sal-fr. ulm-c.
- *Delusions: unfortunate, he is*: bry. caust. *Chin*. cub. dream-p. graph. hura. ip. lyc. petr-ra. sep. *Staph*. verat.
- *Delusions: work: accomplish her work; she cannot*: bry. limen-b-c.
- *Delusions: poor; he is*: bamb-a. bell. bry. calc-f. coli. gink-b. hep. mez. nux-v. psor. sal-fr. *Sep*. stram. valer.
- *Delusions: ruined: is ruined; he*: calc. **IGN**. verat.
- *Delusions: misfortune: approaching: as if some misfortune were*: brass-n-o. cupr. *Verat*.
- *Delusions: misfortune: inconsolable over imagined misfortune*: calc-s. *Verat*.
- *Delusions: misfortune*: calc-s. [1] 1.
- *Delusions: happened; something has*: calc. nux-v. *Staph*. sulph.
- *Delusions: happened; something has; dreadful has happened; something*: med. [1] 1.
- *Delusions: destruction of all near her; impending*: Kali-br. [2] 1.
- *Delusions: depressive*: ambr. *Aur*. **KALI-BR**. murx. nux-v. plat.
- *Delusions: clouds; black cloud enveloped her; a heavy*: Adam. arg-n. Cimic. dendr-pol. galla-q-r. irid-met. *Lac-c*. melal-alt. plut-n. puls. sal-fr.
- *Delusions: doomed, being*: acon. ars. aur. bell. cycl. hell. hyos. *Ign*. Kali-br. Kali-p. lach. *Lil-t*. lyc. med. meli. nat-m. op. *Plat*. psor. puls. stram. sulph. *Verat*.
- *Delusions: melancholy*: alum. *Aur*. **KALI-BR**. murx. nux-v. plat.
- *Delusions: wretched; she looks*: cygn-be. **NAT-M**.

Avoidance: Delusional belief in poverty or ruin or impending misfortune is very often disproportionate to reality.

A patient may need to believe they are unfortunate because they do not want to succeed. These group of *Delusion* rubrics are particularly applicable to patients who believe that they will never recover from an illness.

These group of *Delusion* rubrics are also applicable to patients who believe that they will never have enough material possessions to prove that they are successful. Believing that one has failed in life reinforces and perpetuates depression. Believing everything will always fail is an excuse for avoiding the fact that if one tried to succeed, one might fail. Believing that a homoeopathic treatment or any other health treatment will never be successful is far easier than believing in cure. If a patient believes that they might be cured, they have to confront whether they believe *they are worthy of cure*. Believing in failure is easier than believing in self-worth.

Why a patient will choose to fail rather than succeed is *peculiar* to their constitutional remedy profile.

Bryonia have disproportionate psychological 'delusions of failure'. Although *Bryonia* have the *Delusion* rubric: *illusions of fancy*, they have so many *Delusion* rubrics pertaining to *seeing frightful images, seeing dead persons* and *strangers* that *illusions of fancy* pertains more to illusions of terror about being away from home, than hubristic illusions of grandeur. As a homoeopathic remedy, *Bryonia* is commonly used for children suffering from homesickness. As a constitutional remedy profile, *Bryonia* have a recurring need to find security both within and outside of themselves. *Bryonia* have an obsessive compulsive need to work hard in order to create security. *Bryonia* have the *Delusion* rubrics: *is doing business, occupied about business,* and *is working hard*. *Bryonia* have psychological 'delusions of deprivation[70]' from feeling abandoned. *Bryonia* have the *Delusion* rubrics: *he is poor, unfortunate,* and *she cannot accomplish her work*. *Bryonia* do not have any psychological 'delusions of hubristic grandeur' which are *personally* attributed to themselves. Their *fancy illusions* pertain to their idealized need to see themselves as wealthy and secure. Sankaran, in *The Soul of Remedies,* notes: "One may also compare *Bryonia* with *Veratrum album*, but *Veratrum* is concerned more with the loss of position than with the loss of money. So egotism, extravagance and show become the theme in *Veratrum*, but are not so much seen in *Bryonia*." *Veratrum album* are listed in the *Delusion* rubric: *he is away from home* along with *Bryonia*. *Veratrum album* have numerous hubristic 'delusions of grandeur' that they are *a distinguished person* who *is a messenger from God*. *Bryonia* are concerned with creating the *illusion* of wealth outside of themselves so that they can feel secure. *Veratrum album* are concerned with creating illusions of *personal* grandeur. *Bryonia* have the *Mind* rubrics: *full of desires, more than she needs, fear of poverty,* and *fear of being sold*. The 'never-well-since-event' or causation in any *Bryonia* case will always be 'delusions of deprivation'. *Bryonia* have the *Mind* rubric: *desires to go out and when there, desires to go home*.

Bryonia also have the *Delusion* rubric: *floating in air.* This is a *Delusion* rubric which I have previously allocated to Denial because it pertains to deluded feelings of being above the mundane. In relation to *Bryonia,* this is not a rubric emphasizing 'hubristic denial'; it instead pertains to *Bryonia* being disconnected from their own ability to achieve success. *Bryonia* have the *Delusion* rubric: *occupied about business*: *Bry*. [2] 2. [op.] I have discussed this rubric in relation to *Opium* as a 'delusion of grandeur' because *Opium* feel empowered doing business – with *Bryonia* it pertains to drudgery. *Bryonia* are consumed with work because they have psychological 'delusions of failure'. *Bryonia* have the *Delusion* rubrics: *he is poor,* and *she cannot accomplish her work*. *Bryonia* have the *Mind* rubrics: *full of desires for unattainable things*, *thoughts of persistent desires,* and *ungrateful from avarice* (greed).

Bryonia maintain their feelings of *being unfortunate* because they are *never* satisfied that they have been able to meet their own idealistic level of achievement. The *Delusion* rubric: *illusions of fancy,* can pertain to unattainable illusions. They never think they have done enough work.

They never think they have enough material possessions, and they always think they will be poor. *Bryonia* have the *Mind* rubrics: *feels unfortunate, fear of poverty,* and *capriciousness, when offered, rejecting things for which he has been longing.* *Bryonia* have psychological delusions of perpetual dissatisfaction which they maintain because they are not satisfied with their own achievements.

They have the *Mind* rubric: *despair of recovery.* When *Bryonia* are sick they are convinced they will not recover. *Bryonia* have the *Delusion* rubric: *body looks ugly.* Just as *Bryonia* are never satisfied with their material possessions, they transfer the same avaricious desires on to their body; *Bryonia* desire the unattainable body because their *body is ugly.* My aim in the *Rubric-categories* is to highlight the self-destructive perspectives within the *Delusion* rubrics. *Bryonia* obsessively seek security in money and business, and in their home. What has not been previously understood about *Bryonia* is that regardless of how much money they obtain, they always feel *poor* and *unfortunate* because they scorn themselves. *Bryonia* have the *Mind* rubric: *ailments from being scorned,* and the *Mind* rubrics: *discontented with everything,* and *discontented with himself.*

Bryonia have the *Delusion* rubrics: *head was going around in a circle* and *when standing surroundings whirled around.* [1] 1. *Bryonia* are not able to stand still for long enough to appreciate their achievements.

Bryonia work at such a feverish pace that they are exhausted [*faint*]. *Bryonia* need to work until they exhaust themselves because they believe they will never become accomplished. Their self-doubt keeps them in a perpetual trap of feeling like a failure. Their unsatisfied greed also keeps them in a perpetual trap of feeling like a failure.

1. Denial: NONE. [*Delusion* rubric: *fancy, illusions of*: bry.]

2. Forsaken: *Delusion* rubric: *home: away from home; he is: must get there*: **BRY**. *Delusion* rubric: *home: away from home; he is*: **BRY**. *Delusion* rubric: *strange: land; as if in a strange*: bry. *Delusion* rubric: *strangers: control of; under*: bry. *Delusion* rubric: *soldiers: seeing*: bry. *Delusion* rubric: *figures: seeing figures*: bry. *Delusion* rubric: *beaten, he is being*: bry. *Delusion* rubric: *injury: being injured; is*: bry. *Delusion* rubric: *pursued; he was*: bry. *Delusion* rubric: *dead: persons, sees*: bry. *Delusion* rubric: *strangers: friends appears as strangers*: bry. *Delusion* rubric: *images, phantoms; sees: frightful*: bry.

3. Causation: *Delusion* rubric: *work: accomplish her work; she cannot*: bry. [This rubric can pertain to an admission of guilt as well as an expression of failure.] *Delusion* rubric: *drunk: been drunk; he had: night; before*: bry. [1] 1. [This rubric emphasizes their guilt over not being sober at work the next morning.]

4. Depression: *Delusion* rubric: *unfortunate, he is being*: bry. *Delusion* rubric: *work: accomplish her work; she cannot*: bry. *Delusion* rubric: *poor; he is*: bry. *Delusion* rubric: *business: doing business; is*: Bry. *Delusion* rubric: *business: occupied about business*: Bry. [2] 2. *Delusion* rubric: *work: hard; is working*: bry. *Delusion* rubric: *smoke; of*: Bry. *Delusion* rubric: *bed: sinking: she is sinking: down deep in bed*: bry. [This rubric should not be taken literally. The psychodynamic interpretation is that the patient feels like they are swallowed up by depression and cannot get out of bed.] *Delusion* rubric: *floating: air, in*: bry. [In relation to *Bryonia* this rubric reinforces their belief that they cannot accomplish anything.]

5. Resignation: *Delusion* rubric: *body: ugly; body looks*: bry. *Delusion* rubric: *faint; he would*: bry.

Calcarea sulphuricum is a remédy profile which is renowned for predictions of *misfortune*. *Calcarea sulphuricum* are particularly noted for their anger at being overlooked. Sankaran, in *The Soul of Remedies,* writes: "Calcium sulphate is commonly known as gypsum and is most familiar to us as plaster of Paris, from which are made the plaster casts used to immobilize a fractured limb, to help healing by providing stability. In addition to a need for stability of Calcarea, Sulphur introduces an element of ego and appreciation to the salt. Hence the main feeling of Calcarea sulphurica is that he is not appreciated at the place of security, for example by his parents. Thus the Calcarea sulphurica person is constantly trying to do things that will gain him appreciation. There is a constant feeling of not being appreciated or valued, of being put down and suppressed at the place of security." *Calcarea sulphuricum* have the *Mind* rubrics: *lamenting because he is not appreciated* [1] 1., and *hatred of persons who do not agree with him* [1] 1. *Calcarea sulphuricum* have the *Mind* rubrics: *inclination to sit and meditate over imaginary misfortune*, and *quarrelsome from jealousy*. Sankaran, in *The Soul of Remedies,* writes: "He is perhaps the second or third child in the family who has not yet learned to struggle on his own, he cannot be independent but his parents praise other children more than him. So he laments passionately so that they realize how he feels."

Calcarea sulphuricum not only ruminate over *perceived misfortune*, they also have delusional expectations and *visions of misfortune*.

Calcarea sulphuricum have numerous 'delusions of persecution' which are projected on to *frightful images and phantoms. Calcarea sulphuricum* have *visions* which confirm their *imagined misfortune. Calcarea sulphuricum* will over-exaggerate and disproportionately imagine that they are being overlooked and persecuted.

The need to continue to *imagine misfortune* and be persecuted by *frightful images* is maintained and negatively nurtured by *Calcarea sulphuricum* because they wish to avoid the fact that they have no faith in their own abilities.

Calcarea sulphuricum doubt their capacity to succeed and rather than confront their fear of having failed in the past, or the possibility of failing in the future they transfer blame for their lack of achievement on to others. *Calcarea sulphuricum* have the *Mind* rubrics: *self-depreciation, want of self-confidence, cowardice,* and *dullness.* [3]. *Calcarea sulphuricum* will choose to sabotage rather than admit they lack the confidence to succeed. My aim in writing the *Rubric-categories* is to highlight the psychodynamic crisis within each constitutional remedy profile. *Calcarea sulphuricum* will also choose to sabotage homoeopathic treatment rather than admit that they lack the belief they can become healthy. The homoeopath needs to actively support the growth of self-belief while they are treating the *Calcarea sulphuricum* patient.

1. Denial: NONE.
2. Forsaken: *Delusion* rubric: *visions; has: Calc-s.* [In relation to *Calcarea sulphuricum* this rubric pertains to 'delusions of persecution' and not hubristic visions.] *Delusion* rubric: *images, phantoms; sees: frightful:* calc-s. *Delusion* rubric: *images, phantoms; sees:* calc-s. *Delusion* rubric: *images, phantoms; sees: frightful: night: sleep; while trying to:* calc-s. *Delusion* rubric: *images, phantoms; sees: frightful: night: sleep: going to; on:* calc-s.
3. Causation: NONE.
4. Depression: *Delusion* rubric: *misfortune: inconsolable over imagined misfortune:* calc-s. [1] 2. *Delusion* rubric: *misfortune:* calc-s. [1] 1.
5. Resignation: NONE.

Murex as a homoeopathic remedy is often applicable for a female patient who has extreme anxiety and distress before her menses. *Murex* is a homoeopathic remedy derived from

the shellfish, Murex brandaris. Similarly to *Sepia*, the uses
and themes of all the sea remedies are often ideal remedies
for depression with climatic disorders. *Murex* have the *Mind*
rubrics: *desire to weep all the time*, and *sadness aversion to
company and desire for solitude*. *Murex* sink into psychological
delusions of melancholia and depressive hypochondria. If
a patient is able to transfer blame for their depression on to
sins they have committed then there is some evidence of self-
assessment in their persona.

The simillimum will not be *Murex* unless the patient is so depressed that
are unable to assess their life. *Murex* have no sense that anything can
possibly change in their lives.

If a patient looks back on their life and believes they are
able to find where they went wrong then there is evidence
that the patient feels empowered enough to enact change.
If a patient is able to transfer blame for their depression
on to others for forsaking them, then there is at least some
evidence within the personality profile of some degree of belief
in oneself. *Murex* have no rubrics in the Denial, Forsaken or
Causation stages of the rubric-repertorisation. The reason the
psychological delusional stance of depression is maintained by
Murex is that they lack 'delusions of grandeur' in their psyche.
Consequently, without any egotistical delusions to uphold them
they are unable to avoid sinking into depression. *Murex* the
homoeopathic remedy is derived from Murex brandaris which is
a shellfish which has been noted to cause paralytic poisoning.

If a homoeopathic remedy is derived from a substance which causes
paralysis then within the psyche of the remedy profile there has to be the
same paralysis across all levels of the persona – emotionally, mentally,
and physically.

Murex alternate between feeling highly sexed and
depressed. *Murex,* in contrast to the remedy profile of *Sepia,*
are noted for their strong sexual desire. *Murex* and *Platina*
are the only remedies in the *Mind* rubric: *women who become*

lascivious at every touch. [2] 2. *Murex* also have the *Mind* rubric: *satyriasis* (excessive sexual desire in males) – therefore it cannot be assumed that it is predominantly a female remedy.

The simillimum will only be *Murex* if there is evidence that sexual excitement is the *only* thing that is able to lift the patient out of depression.

1. Denial: NONE.

2. Forsaken: NONE.

3. Causation: NONE.

4. Depression: *Delusion* rubric: *depressive*: murx. *Delusion* rubric: *melancholy*: murx.

5. Resignation: *Delusion* rubric: *sick*: *being*: murx.

- *Delusions: insane; become insane; one will*: *Acon*. act-sp. agar. ail. alum. ambr. aq-mar. arg-n. ars. asar. brom. *Calc*. **CANN-I**. cann-s. cann-xyz. cham. *Chel*. chlor. **CIMIC**. colch. cupr. cycl. cypra-eg. *Eup-per*. falco-pe. gels. glon. ham. hydrog. hyos. *Ign*. iod. iris-t. kali-bi. kali-br. kali-p. lac-c. *Lac-e*. lam. lil-t. limen-b-c. maias-l. **MANC**. med. merc. nat-m. nat-s. nitro-o. nux-v. pall. phys. plat. psor. sil. streptoc. sulph. *Syph*. tanac. tarent. vario.

- *Delusions: insane; he is insane*: *Cimic*. falco-pe. germ-met. *Kali-br*. maias-l. ol-j. orig. pall. phys. sanic. spong. sulph. *Thuj*.

- *Delusions: insane; people think her or him being insane*: aids. **CALC**. germ-met. hydrog. sal-fr.

- *Delusions: mind; out of his mind; he would go*: ambr. calc. cot. eup-per. ham. *Kali-br*. *Lac-c*. nit-ac. ol-j. paraf. petr. visc.

- *Delusions: brain: dissolving and she were going crazy; brain were*: calc.[1] 1.

- *Delusions: confusion; others will observe her*. *Calc*. choc. limest-b. sal-fr.

Avoidance: A patient will maintain psychological delusions of insanity so they can avoid the struggle involved in trying to succeed.

Chelidonium are noted for their exaggerated personal blame and shame. *Chelidonium* have the *Mind* rubric: *fear that she has ruined her health*, as well as the *Delusion* rubric: *he has ruined his health*.

The importance of understanding that *Chelidonium* is weighted so heavily with rubrics pertaining to Causation, Depression, and Resignation is that it is not possible the simillimum will be *Chelidonium* if the patient does not have intense predictions of self-ruin. *Chelidonium* feel solely responsible for the welfare of their health. *Chelidonium* are noted for exaggerated personal blame for indulgences.

Chelidonium as a homoeopathic remedy is strongly recommended for the patient suffering from liver toxicity as a result of excessive alcohol use. *Chelidonium* have the *Mind* rubrics: *stupor in jaundice*, and *unconsciousness in jaundice* [3] 1. *Chelidonium* have the *Mind* rubric: *violence*. [3] 3. Their violence is directed inwards in the form of self-punishing indulgences which damage their health. All the *Mind* rubrics and *Delusion* rubrics which emphasize their ruined health indicate that the ruin is violently self-inflicted punishment for sins committed. *Chelidonium* have the *Mind* rubrics: *reproaching oneself*, and *remorse*. *Chelidonium* have the *Delusion* rubric: *he had committed the unpardonable sin*. With no psychological 'delusions of grandeur' *Chelidonium* are left with intensely disproportionate anxiety and despair of salvation for their health and soul. *Chelidonium* feel solely responsible for the welfare of their soul.

The simillimum will only be *Chelidonium* if the patient shows signs of shame. *Chelidonium* have the *Mind* rubric: *fear of her condition being observed.*

The *Delusion* rubrics: *I am dying, sick, I have ruined my health,* and *I have an incurable disease*, are all examples of exaggerated predictions of decay which are predominately in *Chelidonium* because they have no *Delusion* rubrics in Denial to be able to elevate them out of their obsessive psychological 'delusions of hypochondria'.

The simillimum will only be *Chelidonium* if the patient is filled with obsessive fears about their health.

Chelidonium have no psychological delusions of pretentiousness to use as tools of self-denial. *Chelidonium* have the *Mind* rubric: *discontented with surroundings*. *Chelidonium* have the *Delusion* rubric: *one will become insane*. *Chelidonium* have the *Mind* rubrics: *causeless moroseness, feeling helplessness*, and *feels unfortunate*.

The simillimum will only be *Chelidonium* if the patient is filled with psychological delusions of depressive doom.

Vermeulen, notes in *Prisma,* that *Chelidonium*, "never wastes time with analyzing emotions". And that they are "not overtaken by their emotions". *Chelidonium* do not want to allow themselves to get in touch with their emotions because it overwhelms them with confusion. *Chelidonium* have the *Mind* rubric: *causeless feeling as though she must shriek* [1] 1. *Chelidonium* also have the *Mind* rubric: *weeping when carried*. [1] 1. *Chelidonium* do not want to allow themselves to get in touch with their emotions because it overwhelms them with self-hate. *Chelidonium* are deeply affected if they are emotionally supported [*carried*] by others.

Chelidonium have intense self-hate and self-blame for sins committed. *Chelidonium* have no *Delusion* rubrics in Denial which allow themselves to feel self-love. *Lycopodium* are often compared to *Chelidonium*. *Lycopodium* in comparison have 'delusions of grandeur' – they believe they *are a great person*.

Lycopodium suffer with underlying fears of failure but their capacity to rely on their delusional hope [*childish fantasies*] elevates them into delusional positivity and self-love. The simillimum will not be *Chelidonium* if the patient shows signs of self-love. Furthermore, the simillimum will not be *Chelidonium* if the patient shows signs of being willing to allow themselves to be emotionally supported.

Chelidonium have the *Delusion* rubric: *everything turned in a circle*. It is a mistake to interpret this rubric literally because in relation to *Chelidonium* it reemphasizes the degree to which they feel defeated by life.

Chelidonium are unable 'to think their way out' of dilemmas in life.

Vermeulen quotes Grandgeorge in *Prisma* as noting, "They make an effort to avoid speculation or abstraction, and never try to understand the situation they face, since they see this as a waste of time. In short, they remain in the material world and only with great difficulty can they rise to a more elevated perspective, to an outlook of a spiritual nature." *Chelidonium* have no 'delusions of grandeur' which elevate them into a position of spiritual hope, therefore they are unable to have speculation or abstraction or a 'spiritual outlook'. *Chelidonium* have the *Delusion* rubric: *she cannot think*. The simillimum will only be *Chelidonium* if the patient is filled with confusion.

Chelidonium have the *Mind* rubrics: *religious affections too occupied with religion, fear about his social position, despair, religious despair of salvation*, and *fear, insanity with restlessness and heat* [3] 1. *Chelidonium* need religion to protect them from their own insanity.

Chelidonium have the *Delusion* rubric: *is falling forward*. The simillimum will only be *Chelidonium* if the patient is filled with despair. *Chelidonium* have the *Delusion* rubric: *being a soldier at night*. This rubric should not be interpreted literally. This rubric indicates a hyper-vigilant need to guard oneself from potential attack. *Chelidonium* often appear 'in control'. It is a mistake to interpret this external appearance of control as mental and emotional rationality, rather it is an external defense to protect *Chelidonium* from their own fears of insanity and societal exposure. The simillimum will only be *Chelidonium* if the patient has exaggerated fears about their sanity.

1. Denial: NONE.

2. Forsaken: *Delusion* rubric: *soldiers: being a soldier.*

night: chel. [1] 1. [This rubric pertains to 'delusions of persecution'].

3. Causation: *Delusion* rubric: *sinned; one has*: *unpardonable sin; he had committed the*: chel. *Delusion* rubric: *crime*: *committed a crime; he had*: chel.

4. Depression: *Delusion* rubric: *insane*: *become insane; one will*: *Chel*. *Delusion* rubric: *think*: *cannot think; she*: *Chel*. *Delusion* rubric: *skull diminished*: chel. *Delusion* rubric: *turn*: *everything turned*: *circle; in a*: chel. *Delusion* rubric: *turn*: *everything turned*: *sitting up; on*: chel. [1] 1. *Delusion* rubric: *falling*: *forward*: *is falling forward; she*: chel. [It is a mistake to interpret these last three rubrics literally. These *Delusion* rubric emphasize the tendency *Chelidonium* have of never being able to achieve anything.]

5. Resignation: *Delusion* rubric: *health, he has ruined his*: chel. *Delusion* rubric: *sick: being*: chel. *Delusion* rubric: *die*: *about to die; one was*: *Chel*. *Delusion* rubric: *disease*: *incurable disease; he has an*: chel. *Delusion* rubric: *skull diminished*: chel. [This rubric can pertain to an inability to think or it can pertain to physical deficiency].

Natrum sulphuricum is a homoeopathic remedy which is commonly used for mental confusion arising from physical injuries to the head. *Natrum sulphuricum* have the *Mind* rubrics: *confusion of mind after injury to the head* [3], and *mental symptoms from injuries to the head.* [2] 1. Within the profile of *Natrum sulphuricum* is evidence of a desire to remain unconscious. *Natrum sulphuricum* wish to obliterate their psyche. *Natrum sulphuricum* as a constitutional remedy profile is traditionally thought of as a strong suicide remedy. *Natrum sulphuricum* are the only remedy in the two *Mind* rubrics: *loathing life, must restrain herself to prevent doing injury*, and *suicidal thoughts, must restrain himself because of his duties to his family.* [3]. 1. *Natrum sulphuricum* feel overwhelmed by the seriousness of responsibility. *Natrum sulphuricum* have the

Mind rubrics: *too much sense of duty, never succeeds,* and *taking responsibility too seriously.* *Natrum sulphuricum* choose to maintain the belief that they cannot cope [*insane*] to avoid the fact that too much responsibility can make them feel like they will not *succeed* [*disgraced*]. The *Mind* profile of *Natrum sulphuricum* is abandonment of life [*suicide*] and abandonment of all belief in the self.

The psychodynamic theme in the *Delusion* rubrics attached to *Natrum sulphuricum* is unconscious self-effacement. *Natrum sulphuricum* have a delusional need to deface [*disgrace*] themselves – they unconsciously sabotage everything they attempt. *Natrum sulphuricum* is a remedy profile for a patient who displays passive-aggressive behavior.

Natrum sulphuricum have the *Mind* rubric: *strongly attached to others,* and conversely they have the *Mind* rubrics: *aversion to his wife.* *Natrum sulphuricum* will sabotage their relationships (including their relationship with the homoeopath) because they are frightened of becoming dependent. Passive-aggressive behavior is passive, sometimes obstructionist resistance to following through with expectations in interpersonal relationships. It can manifest itself as learned helplessness, or deliberate failure to accomplish requested tasks for which one is responsible. The passive-aggressive person 'defends himself' from others by retaliating with passivity and unconscious sabotage. Passive-aggressive behavior can manifest as a destructive need to deliberately sabotage relationships by withholding intimacy. What underpins passive-aggressive behavior is a deep feeling of rage (in the unconscious mind) which is transferred on to anyone upon whom one becomes dependent. The 'never-well-since-event' in all *Natrum sulphuricum* cases will arise from abandonment in childhood. For many constitutional remedy profiles, abandonment is part of their 'never-well-since-event'. The *specific* and *peculiar* interpretation (aphorism 153) of a particular trauma by an individual patient is the inner disturbance which is the core of our case-taking. This disturbance is always reflective of what is *unusual* or disturbing to the homoeopath's inner sensibilities. *Natrum sulphuricum peculiarly* interpret abandonment shamefully. *Natrum sulphuricum* have delusional feelings of shame [*disgraced*] over being abandoned. Understanding this helps explain why *Natrum sulphuricum* need to withhold intimacy. Intimacy is disproportionately associated with feeling abandoned; acknowledgment of abandonment is associated with acknowledgment of shame. Feeling disgraced in turn is proof of never succeeding in life. Never succeeding is continually reinforced because whenever they take on responsibility they are overcome with the pressure of the responsibility and subsequently collapse.

1. Denial: NONE.
2. Forsaken: *Delusion* rubric: *disgraced*: *she is*: nat-s[71]. [This rubric can pertain to abandonment or admission of guilt.]
3. Causation: *Delusion* rubric: *disgraced*: *she is*: nat-s.
4. Depression: *Delusion* rubric: *insane: become insane; one will*: nat-s[72].
5. Resignation: NONE.

- *Delusions*: *paralyzed; he is*: agar. cist. con. cycl. falco-pe. hippoc-k. sacch-l. sang. syph.
- *Delusions*: *prisoner; she is a*: falco-pe. germ-met. haliae-lc. *Moni.* olib-sac. positr.
- *Delusions*: *trapped; he is*: cygn-be. dendr-pol. falco-pe. haliae-lc. hippoc-k. ign. lac-e. lath. limest-b. naja. ol-eur. oncor-t. positr. sal-fr. stry. *Tub.*

Self-deluding: It is a mistake to interpret these rubrics literally.

The psychodynamic need behind the delusional belief that one is trapped is maintained by the patient because it is an excuse which justifies non-action.

Passive-aggressive patterning or learned helplessness allows the patient to delude themselves about the need to break free and succeed in life. When I was studying psychotherapy, there was a cartoon drawing of a bird in a cage on the wall in our study room. Even though the cage door was open the bird stayed in the cage. The patient who stays trapped needs to believe they are trapped so they can avoid their fear of failure; this is learned passivity. Furthermore, the patient who stays trapped needs to believe they are trapped so they can transfer punishment on to the person who they believe is holding them prisoner; this is learned aggressive transference. Learned passivity and learned aggressive transference are the psychological patterns evident in passive-aggressive behavior.

Cistus canadensis are listed in only one *Delusion* rubric: *he is paralyzed*. Passive-aggressive behavior is characterized by obstructionist resistance to demands. Deliberate resistance can occur within the work place by repeated failure to accomplish tasks, or it can occur within relationships by withholding intimacy. Learned helplessness is needed by the patient because it helps them to defend themselves against their own fears that they might not succeed. Their behavior results in increased anger being directed towards them because of their lack of involvement. The anger directed towards them reinforces their need to maintain 'control' and defend themselves by not responding to others' demands. This in turn sparks off another round of procrastinating behavior. The bird who stays in the cage after the door has been opened can stay there because it is too frightened to fly free, or it can stay there because it believes that it is resisting demands put upon it to be free. The symptom which confirms a passive-aggressive psychological patterning is a *strong resistance to feeling*. The bird did not want to be disturbed in its cage and similarly the passive-aggressive patient does not want to feel any emotion. The sabotage within the behavior of the passive-aggressive patient is unconscious. The passive-aggressive patient *wants* *and needs to remain calm* and *tranquil*. Sabotage is a classic characteristic of withholding intimacy or emotional involvement. More significantly, the passive-aggressive patient does not want to tap into their unconscious. If the passive-aggressive patient is confronted with their behavioral patterns they deflect responsibility for their behavior and become extremely angry with the person who they believe has trapped them in the cage. Their own anger in turn disturbs them as the force of the emotion starts to tap into their unconscious. In the unconscious mind of *Cistus canadensis* is the psychodynamic crisis which holds the secret of their 'never-well-since-event'.

The remedy profile of *Cistus canadensis* contains a strong resistance to feeling, a strong desire to remain calm, and a strong reaction to feeling their own anger. If a patient does not want to learn how to use their anger positively to motivate themselves out of whatever stasis they are encapsulated in, then they remain stuck [*paralyzed*].

The irony is that the patient then spends their time being angry at how stuck they are rather than redirecting their anger into self-motivation. This behavior is exemplified in the *Mind* rubric: *anger feels as if paralyzed*. This is the psychological pattern evident within the remedy profile of *Cistus canadensis*.

When *Cistus canadensis* are sick they remain in stasis and hold on to their illness.

Cistus canadensis is a homoeopathic remedy which is used for patients suffering from swollen glands associated with influenza, malignant tumors, or sepsis. The stasis [*paralyzed*] evident in stagnant swollen glands is also evident within the constitutional remedy profile. When *Cistus canadensis* are sick they psychologically need to maintain the delusional belief that they are unable to become well; this is the psychodynamic meaning of the *Delusion* rubric: *he is paralyzed*.

- *Mind: anger: paralyzed; feels as if: Cist.*
- *Mind: ailments from: anger: cist.*

- *Mind*: *ailments from*: *emotions*: cist.
- *Mind*: *ailments from*: *excitement*: *emotional*: *Cist*.
- *Mind*: *tranquility*: cist.
- *Mind*: *mood*: *agreeable*: cist.

1. Denial: NONE.
2. Forsaken: *Delusion* rubric: *paralyzed; he is*: cist. [This rubric can pertain to 'delusions of persecution' – the passive-aggressive patient blames their entrapment upon others].
3. Causation: NONE.
4. Depression: *Delusion* rubric: *paralyzed; he is*: cist.
5. Resignation: *Delusion* rubric: *paralyzed; he is*: cist. [When sick *Cistus canadensis* need to maintain the delusional belief that they will remain sick [*paralyzed*].]

Lac-equinum is a homoeopathic remedy derived from horses' (mares') milk. Within the tethered psyche of the domesticated horse is conflict between their desire to run free and their desire to *connect* to man. The psyche of the horse wants to remain free, they do not want to be tamed by man, they only want to have a working relationship with man. The horse needs to maintain their free spirit.

Lac-equinum are deeply depressed patients who *trap themselves* in depression because like the horse they have allowed themselves to be tamed and trapped, and domesticated.

Lac-equinum patients *trap* themselves in depression because they believe they have failed. The Achilles-Heel that traps them is their self-destructive need to stay in servitude because they need to prove their worthiness.

The psychological system of allocating rubrics into the five stages highlights what is *peculiar* to each remedy. The reason *Lac-equinum* judge themselves and life so harshly is that they have no hubristic 'delusions of grandeur'.

Lac-equinum have the *Delusion* rubric: *losing control over one's organization*, and the *Mind* rubric: *ailments from poor job performance*. [1] 1. *Lac-equinum* have the *Delusion* rubric: *neglected his duty*. It is their 'delusions of original sin' that they have let their boss (owner) down, or that their *organization* will fail, which traps them into feelings of depressive failure.

Lac-equinum have the delusional need to stay trapped because they believe life is hard and will always remain hard [*life is hardship*]. They have the *Mind* rubrics: *anxiety for his family's safety,* and *attempts to escape from her family and children*. *Lac-equinum* have the *Dream* rubrics: *escaping,* and *danger from escaping*. *Lac-equinum* are trapped between caring for their family, and needing to escape from their family. They dream of escaping and they dream of the dangers of escaping.

The 'never-well-since-event' or psychodynamic crisis within *Lac-equinum* is formulated in their psyche at a moment when they feel like they have not fulfilled their duty, specifically towards *family* or *friends*.

Lac-equinum have the *Mind* rubric: *ailments from discord between family members*. [2] 1. *Lac-equinum* disproportionately judge their performance at work, in relationships and life in general. It is this delusional judgment of their worthiness that entraps *Lac-equinum* in servitude. *Lac-equinum* have the *Mind* rubric: *suicidal thoughts*. A *Delusion* rubric is attached to a remedy profile if within the persona of the remedy profile there is evidence of a psychological pattern which traps the patient in self-destructive behavior. *Lac-equinum* are *trapped* in their own depression because they believe they will *always* fail [*everything will fail*]. *Lac-equinum* have the *Mind* rubric: *suffocative breathing from anxiety*. [1] 1. When *Lac-equinum* are sick they sink into a depressive anxiety which has such a tight grip on their psyche that they believe there is no hope of cure [*sinking in quicksand*]. The homoeopath treating *Lac-equinum* needs to instill hope into their patient. *Lac-equinum* remain in *suffocating* servitude because they have no *Delusion* rubrics allocated into Denial. *Lac-equinum* have no *Delusion* rubrics allocated into psychological 'delusions of grandeur' which would enable them to have a grandeur vision of themselves.

Lac-equinum have the following *Dream* rubrics.

* *Dreams: animals: restrained by collar.* lac-e. [1] 1.
* *Dreams: betrayed, having been:* lac-e.
* *Dreams: escaping: Lac-e.*
* *Dreams: escaping: danger; from:* lac-e.
* *Dreams: helping people:* lac-e.
* *Dreams: friends:* lac-e.

1. Denial: NONE.

2. Forsaken: *Delusion* rubric: *stalked; he is being:* lac-e. [1] 1. *Delusion* rubric: *house: surrounded; house is:* lac-e. *Delusion* rubric: *insulted, he is: Lac-e.*

3. Causation: *Delusion* rubric: *neglected: duty; he has neglected his:* lac-e.

4. Depression: *Delusion* rubric: *trapped; he is:* lac-e. *Delusion* rubric: *fail, everything will:* lac-e. *Delusion* rubric: *hard; everything is:* lac-e. *Delusion* rubric: *hardship; life is:* lac-e. [1] 1. *Delusion* rubric: *hindered; he is: Lac-e. Delusion* rubric: *insane: become insane; one will: Lac-e. Delusion* rubric: *sinking; to be:* lac-e. *Delusion* rubric: *sinking; to be: quicksand; in:* lac-e. [1] 1. *Delusion* rubric: *control; out of: organization; losing control over one's:* lac-e.

5. Resignation: *Delusion* rubric: *sinking; to be: quicksand; in:* lac-e. [1] 1. [When *Lac-equinum* are sick, they sink into deep hopelessness. It is hard for the homoeopath to loosen its grip.] *Delusion* rubric: *noise: exaggerated, loud; seems:* lac-e. [1] 1. [When *Lac-equinum* are sick they are aggravated by all noise.]

- *Delusions: ground: coming up to meet him; ground were:* bell. calc. cann-xyz. pic-ac. sil.
- *Delusions: ground; gave way beneath his feet:* arg-n. con. cypra-eg. digin. *Kali-br.* sulph. tep. visc.

Self-deluding: It is a mistake to interpret these rubrics literally. The psychodynamic belief behind the perception that the ground beneath your feet will give way is reflective of deep emotional insecurity about one's existence.

Digitalinum is an active principle (glucoside) of *Digitalis*. Allen states in *Encyclopedia of Materia Medica*: "*Digitalinum* acts with great energy on the heart, throwing it into violent and disorderly contractions, which quickly end in a cessation of movement. The frequency of the contractions is not increased, but is progressively diminished, and the functions of the heart are abolished very early, voluntary power surviving the death of the organ." *Digitalis* in comparison to *Digitalinum* are able to live in a semi-conscious state which affords them a sense of hope. *Digitalis* escape into *illusions of fancy* which create an imaginary world in which they have assured confidence over life. Although *Digitalis* struggle to get over the sense that they have failed and that it is their fault, in comparison to *Digitalinum* they have the *illusion* of hope. *Digitalinum,* similarly to *Digitalis,* have psychological 'delusions of original sin' that they have caused their own demise. *Digitalinum* have the *Delusion* rubric: *he has done wrong.*

In comparison to *Digitalis, Digitalinum* have *no* 'delusions of grandeur' which are able to lift them out of their *morose unconsciousness. Digitalinum* have the *Mind* rubrics: *fear of misfortune, stupefaction, morose, indifference,* and *unconsciousness. Digitalinum* will be the applicable simillimum in a case in which the patient is assured of guilt and assured of death.

1. Denial: NONE.
2. Forsaken: *Delusion* rubric: *ground: gave way beneath his*

feet: digin. [This rubric can pertain to self-abandonment of the body].

3. Causation: *Delusion* rubric: *wrong: done wrong; he has*: digin.

4. Depression: *Delusion* rubric: *ground: gave way beneath his feet*: digin.

5. Resignation: *Delusion* rubric: *ground: gave way beneath his feet*: digin. [This rubric can pertain to self-abandonment of the body].

* *Delusions*: *love is impossible*: dioxi. hippoc-k.

* *Delusions*: *bad: triumphs over good because good is not good enough*: dioxi. [1]1.

* *Delusions*: *seeing: river of tar*: dioxi. [1]1.

Self-deluding: The psychodynamic need behind the delusional belief that love is impossible is maintained by the patient because it is an excuse which re-enforces failure.

Dioxin is a homoeopathic remedy derived from a dioxin. Dioxin belongs to a large group of chemicals that are created as a byproduct during the manufacturing or burning of organic chemicals and plastics that contain chlorine. The most toxic of these chemicals is 2,3,7,8-tetrachlorodibenzo-p-dioxin or TCDD. On the internet there are numerous scientific papers proving and disproving possible carcinogenic effects of dioxin. The homoeopathic proving of Dioxin (the substance) has had debilitating and destructive effects on the provers' psyches, so it is safe to assume that arguments warning of its carcinogenic effects are more than likely true. *Dioxin* (the homoeopathic remedy) is an extremely relevant remedy to consider for extreme depression and debility.

Robbins writes in *Evolving homeopathy, Towards a developmental Approach to Homeopathy,* EH., Radar™: "This new remedy was introduced to me by a local, self-taught homoeopath, Mathew Lines, who claimed that it could cure depression and chronic fatigue, especially in cases caused by chemical exposure. He had been using it himself for some time. Mathew was involved in an earlier proving of DNA and in exchange for some potencies of DNA he swapped me a bottle of Dioxin 30c. Soon after this, a colleague of mine who is sensitive to remedies undertook a blind, proving of this remedy on herself. Her main finding was that this remedy would be useful for people overloaded by toxicity from any source. Quite a useful attribute I thought. Another colleague, Linda Grierson, became enthusiastic about this remedy and offered to supervise a full proving of it. This she did most effectively. Several potencies of the remedy were purchased from Helios Pharmacy in England and a proving was conducted in September and October 2000. All provers were blind to the remedy (being proved) and had a homeopathic supervisor."

The following list of mental and emotional responses to the proving of *Dioxin* were taken by Robbins from the provers' notes.

- Depression and despair.
- Negative.
- No interest in communication with people.
- Lethargic.
- Total isolation.
- I didn't set up energy so that I would connect with others.
- Melancholy, lack focus, purpose.
- Not much inspiration.
- I feel exhausted, old, stiff and fat and totally uninspired.
- Didn't feel much joy and happiness in situations that he normally would.
- Mentally and emotionally drained.
- Low energy, achy muscles, fatigued.

- I have to work so hard.
- Deep sadness, disappointment.
- I am never good enough.
- Tears.
- Deep feeling of being alone, lost in this feeling, nothing penetrates this mood, not friends, children, partner, music.
- No connection between mind and feelings.
- Not in touch with mental facilities.
- Devoid of light/love.
- Insidious, kept in emotional realm where it is dense and dark and I am alone.
- Exhausted with my deep dark depths.
- Immediate lifting of chronic depressed state.
- Unable to change mood.
- Strong line of negativity.
- I don't want this.
- Opposite of creativity.
- No thought, more feeling of lethargy.
- Withdrawn into self.
- Distinct negativity pertaining to self.
- I am no good.

The *Dioxin* patient will have *no* sense of hope. *Dioxin* have no *Delusion* rubrics pertaining to psychological 'delusions of grandeur'. The overwhelming number of *Delusion* rubrics are all allocated in Depression.

Dioxin is a chemical which has been detected in breast milk. Every person has supposedly been exposed to the dangerous chemical Dioxin in one form or another. *Dioxin,* along with *Carcinosin,* have the *Delusion* rubric: *has no defense protection. Dioxin* also have the *Mind* rubric: *sensitive to psychic environment.*

Dioxin have the *Delusion* rubric: *seeing a river of tar.* This rubric should not be interpreted literally. The psychodynamic implications of *seeing a river of tar* are that all forward movement is impeded. The desolation and hopeless despair in *Dioxin* is soul destroying.

Dioxin have the *Mind* rubrics: *fear of embracing life,* and *fear of asking for what I want.* [1]1. *Dioxin* do not even feel able to have control over their own body – they have the *Delusion* rubric: *limbs have their own brain.* [1] 1. *Dioxin* is destructive on all levels – the patient's emotional will to live is destroyed, their mental capacity to feel empowered is non-existent, and their physical control is defenseless to attack from within and from outside.

The simillimum will not be *Dioxin* if the homoeopath can detect emotional hope, or positive thoughts, or physical wellness. *Dioxin* believe that wellness is not achievable. *Dioxin* have the *Delusion* rubric: *bad triumphs over good because good is not good enough.* The simillimum will not be *Dioxin* unless the patient believes that there is no point in becoming well because good health will change nothing in their life; they will remain depressed.

1. Denial: NONE.

2. Forsaken: *Delusion* rubric: *separated: world: from the: he is separated:* dioxi.

3. Causation: *Delusion* rubric: *place: wrong place; he was in the:* dioxi. [This rubric is an admission of failure by default. The expression, 'he was in wrong place at the wrong time' can apply to this rubric.]

4. Depression: *Delusion* rubric: *love is impossible:* dioxi. *Delusion* rubric: *bad: triumphs over good because good is not good enough:* dioxi. [1]1. *Delusion* rubric: *seeing: river of tar:* dioxi. [1]1. *Delusion* rubric: *help: wanted; is not:* dioxi. [1]1.

5. Resignation: *Delusion* rubric: *protection, defense; has no:* dioxi. [1] 2. [carc.] *Delusion* rubric: *separated: body: mind are separated; body and:* dioxi. *Delusion* rubric: *limbs: brain; have own:* dioxi. [1]1.

Resignation

"I am dying."

"I am sure I have cancer."

"I am sure I have a terrible disease."

"I am too weak to survive this world."

I have allocated all the *Delusion* rubrics which pertain to psychological 'delusions of hypochondria' into Resignation. If the patient's trauma starts with hypochondria or delusional doom about being sick, or you feel that your patient is exaggerating their weakness or sickness then the simillimum is listed in the *Delusion* rubrics: *death*, and *disease* and is allocated to the section Resignation.

When someone finds out that they have a serious illness it is normal for them to find their thoughts alternating between believing they will be cured, and the very next minute morbidly dwelling on imagining their death. The rubrics used in the rubric–repertorisation that would match these *very normal imaginations* are the *Mind* rubrics: *fear of disease* or *fear of death*, and *anxiety about health*. It is neither exceptional nor unusual to find that a patient will develop irrational, paranoiac fears about their health or their family's health after they have experienced for the first time a friend or family member dying of cancer. If these fears are present and predominant for an appropriate amount of time then this is not exceptional or *unusual*. For example, in this last year in my practice I have consulted with a significant number of patients who have had bowel cancer. Because my mother died of bowel cancer, it would not be unusual for me to become anxious about developing bowel cancer. This is a normal, expected anxiety which will, every three or four years, remind me that I must go to the doctor for a colonoscopy to check for bowel cancer. It is not in the fore front of my mind daily, nor do I suffer any obsessive fears about bowel cancer. However, I do expect to feel anxious when I have a colonoscopy and I also expect my mind will travel off into the imaginary fears of 'what if'? These imaginary fears are not *unusual* or significantly disproportionate. All patients are likely to experience the same imaginary fears when they are having medical check-ups. It is only significant in case analysis if the fears take precedence and become a 'never-well-since-event', leading to crippling anxiety about health.

The fifth stage in Doctor Elisabeth Kübler-Ross's model is acceptance. Acceptance is a *realistic* acknowledgment of mortality. Coming to terms with impending death can be a painful, long and confronting process and peaceful acceptance only comes after: denial, anger, bargaining, and depression. Illness is loss of personal control and freedom. Illness which is potentially life-threatening is loss of our life and loss of our future experiences, loss of our future with our loved ones and loss of everything which we know and depend on. I have chosen the word 'resignation' as the fifth stage in my model because the *Delusion* rubrics pertaining to death, and disease resonate with *exaggerated* internal self-damnation. Doctor Elisabeth Kübler-Ross's fifth stage of acceptance assumes that the patient has arrived at a place inside of themselves which has allowed them to finally be able to peacefully consent to receiving their death. When one has to resign oneself to a situation, it implies that even if one is able to *reconcile* themselves to the situation they find themselves in, they are not in peace. Resignation is an uncomplaining *endurance* or *exaggerated* resignation of the situation rather than a consenting peaceful acceptance of death. If the patient sinks into overblown or *exaggerated* resignation of disease and death then the homeopath should be alerted to a disproportionate *need* within the patient to resign themselves to illness.

The theme of the *Delusion* rubrics in this group include the psychological 'delusions of hypochondria'. Hypochondria is a morbid, unfounded anxiety about one's health. The theme of hypochondria within the *Delusion* rubrics in this group pertain to psychological delusions of *exaggerated* fragility and weakness and *disproportionate* predictions of disease and death.

The mental and emotional trauma of acknowledging the lack of control we have over disease and death can easily become a paranoiac misrepresentation of reality. Hypochondria is an obsessive-compulsive need to become so morbidly anxious about one's health that one's perception is no longer correct, and fears of possible diseases are blown out of proportion.

If there is no indication that the patient has an invested interest in maintaining their 'delusions of hypochondria', and that the patient is realistically assessing the gravity of their illness, then the rubrics are simply the *Mind* rubrics: *fear of disease* or *fear of death*, and *anxiety about health*.

If there are contradictions and inconsistencies in the rubric-repertorisation pertaining to a remedy profile then there is inner conflict which is indicative of the psychological pathology of conflict between acknowledging disease and reconciliation and resignation. The self-denial is evident in the inconsistencies between the rubrics pertaining to 'delusions of grandeur' or denial, and the rubrics pertaining to disease and death or resignation. In particular, if there are inconsistencies between Stage one and Stage five, then this is evidence of self-denial and suppression and internal discord in the acknowledgment process. This internal discord will either accelerate present pathology or precede future pathology, especially exaggerated hypochondria.

If it is advantageous for your patient for them to believe they are weak and fragile then it is essential that a *Delusion* rubric is used in the case analysis. Furthermore, if it is advantageous for your patient to believe they are sick and dying then it is also essential that a *Delusion* rubric is used in the case analysis. The *Delusion* rubrics: *I am dying, sick, I am dead, I have an incurable disease, diminished, disintegrating, cut through, emaciated,* are all examples of *exaggerated* predictions of decay.

The other reason a *Delusion* rubric is used is if there are signs of avoidance. Avoidance of reality enables the person to justify their misrepresentation of reality and this is a psychological delusional stance. In this section I want to emphasize that if the patient is presenting with an energy which is predominantly weighted in the rubrics pertaining to 'delusions of hypochondria', then the homoeopath needs to understand why it is advantageous to the patient to have over-exaggerated predications of illness and fragility and over-blown predictions of death. The homoeopath also has to understand the complexities of the remedies, and *which* constitutional remedies allow anxiety and fear and predictions of death to overwhelm one, and *why*.

One reason the psychological delusional stance is maintained by the patient is because it is advantageous to them to delude themselves of reality; this is the case in the example of *Pulsatilla* below. *Pulsatilla* have the *Delusion* rubric: *he is well,* versus the *Delusion* rubric: *one was about to die.* Preceding the rubrics pertaining to illness and death are the section of rubrics pertaining to depression and failure. It is advantageous to *Pulsatilla* to remain dependant to protect themselves from internal anxiety which can become cripplingly out of proportion. If *Pulsatilla* concentrates on over-exaggerating their illness, then they feel justified in remaining dependant. It is emotionally advantageous to *Pulsatilla* to maintain their position as it allows them to remain fragile and needy. *Pulsatilla* know they need to seek continual reassurance and protection.

1. Denial: *Delusion* rubric: *well, he is*: puls.
2. Forsaken: *Delusion* rubric: *alone, being*: *world; alone in the*: *Puls.*
3. Causation: *Delusion* rubric: *sinned; one has*: puls.

4. Depression: *Delusion* rubric: *anxious*: *Puls.*

5. Resignation: *Delusion* rubric: *sick: being*: **PULS**. *Delusion* rubric: *die*: *about to die*; *one was*: puls.

The other reason the psychological delusional stance is maintained by the patient is that they have none, or not enough, of the 'delusions of grandeur' in their psyche to enable them to avoid anxiety and the psychological 'delusions of hypochondria'.

This is the case in the example of *Aconite* below. *Aconite* are predominantly weighted in the rubrics pertaining to 'delusions of hypochondria', and predictions of death. The homoeopath needs to understand why *Aconite* maintain delusional predictions of death. *Aconite* is also weighted significantly in numerous *Mind* rubrics: *fear of death*, *anxiety about health*, *ailments from fear, fright,* and *grief*. One reason the psychological delusional stance is maintained by the patient is because it is advantageous to them to delude themselves of reality. The other reason is that they have none of the 'delusions of grandeur' which strengthen their psyche to avoid anxiety and hypochondria. This is the case for *Aconite*. *Aconite* will only be the simillimum for the patient who is extremely unsure and uncertain of themselves. Hypochondriac psychoses are a conflict between the sense of one's self or the strength of 'ego'[73] and the external world. The *Delusion* rubrics: *I am dying*, *sick*, *I am dead*, *I have an incurable disease*, are all examples of *exaggerated* predictions of decay which emphasize the threat the world poses to the weakened self-esteem in *Aconite*.

1. Denial: *Delusion* rubric: *fancy, illusions of*: *Acon.* [This is significantly the only *Delusion* rubric from the rubrics pertaining to 'delusions of grandeur'. Because *Aconite* are listed in numerous other *Delusion* rubrics: *seeing specters, ghosts, spirits,* and the *Delusion* rubric: *hearing voices,* and the *Delusion* rubric: *sees images and phantoms*, the relevance and strength of this rubric is undermined and diminished. The *Delusion* rubrics: *seeing specters, ghosts,*

spirits, and the *Delusion* rubric: *hearing voices,* and the *Delusion* rubric: *sees images and phantoms,* pertain to 'persecutory fears' which undermine *Aconite. Aconite* have no significant 'delusions of grandeur' which psychologically protect them from their overwhelming fears and *illusions* of death.]

2. Forsaken: *Delusion* rubric: *home: away from home; he is*: acon.

3. Causation: *Delusion* rubric: *jostling against everyone she meets*: acon. [1] 1.

4. Depression: *Delusion* rubric: *anxious*: *Acon. Delusion* rubric: *doomed, being*: acon. *Delusion* rubric: *insane: become insane; one will*: *Acon.*

5. Resignation: *Delusion* rubric: *body: deformed, some part is*: acon. *Delusion* rubric: *die: about to die*; *one was*: **ACON**.

The essential relevance of the above process is that it allows one to understand that an *Aconite* patient will not present with psychological 'delusions of grandeur'. As a direct psychological consequence of that lack, an *Aconite* patient will be overcome with all the psychological 'delusions of hypochondria'.

In this section it is important to note the inconsistencies between Stage one and Stage five. It is important to understand why the avoidance or self-denial is maintained. The preoccupation with hypochondriacally orientated delusions will either be advantageously needed, as it is with *Pulsatilla,* or it will be as a result of deficiencies, as is the case with *Aconite.*

Another example is the remedy profile of *Chelidonium.* The *Delusion* rubrics: *I am dying, sick, I have ruined my health,* and *I have an incurable disease,* are all examples of exaggerated predictions of decay which predominate in *Chelidonium* because they have no *Delusion* rubrics in Denial to be able to elevate them out of their obsessive psychological 'delusions of hypochondria'. The simillimum will only be *Chelidonium* if the patient is filled with obsessive fears about their health. *Chelidonium* is weighted so heavily with rubrics pertaining to

Causation, Depression, and Resignation that it is not possible the simillimum will be *Chelidonium* if the patient does not have intense, restless anxiety of conscience. *Chelidonium* is noted for exaggerated personal blame. The simillimum will only be *Chelidonium* if the patient is filled with psychological delusions of depressive doom. With no psychological 'delusions of grandeur' *Chelidonium* are left with intensely disproportionate anxiety and despair of salvation for their health and soul.

1. Denial: NONE.

2. Forsaken: *Delusion* rubric: *criminals, about*: Chel. *Delusion* rubric: *soldiers: being a soldier: night*: chel. [1] 1. [These rubrics pertain to 'delusions of persecution'.]

3. Causation: *Delusion* rubric: *sinned; one has: unpardonable sin; he had committed the*: chel. *Delusion* rubric: *crime: committed a crime; he had*: chel.

4. Depression: *Delusion* rubric: *insane: become insane; one will*: Chel. *Delusion* rubric: *think: cannot think; she*: Chel. *Delusion* rubric: *skull diminished*: chel. *Delusion* rubric: *turn: everything turned: circle; in a*: chel. *Delusion* rubric: *turn: everything turned: sitting up; on*: chel. [1] 1. *Delusion* rubric: *falling: forward: is falling forward; she*: chel. [It is a mistake to interpret these last three rubrics literally. These *Delusion* rubrics emphasize, and pertain to, the tendency of *Chelidonium* to never being able to achieve anything.]

5. Resignation: *Delusion* rubric: *health, he has ruined his*: chel. *Delusion* rubric: *sick: being*: chel. *Delusion* rubric: *die: about to die; one was*: Chel. *Delusion* rubric: *disease: incurable disease; he has an*: chel.

The importance of the five psychological processes is that it allows the homoeopath to understand the varying layers attached to the simillimum and match those to the constitutional remedy profile, and the patient, and to the behavior of the patient when they are sick.

Delusion Rubrics in Resignation

In this section I analyze and explain the meaning of each individual *Delusion* rubric. I offer previously unexplored explanations of the psychological delusional state inherent in each *Delusion* rubric. Furthermore, I explain their psychotherapeutic meaning and application by analyzing how each remedy listed under the rubric heading has utilized the delusional stance to its advantage. The reasons why each constitutional remedy is listed under a rubric will often be vastly different. Understanding the need for the psychological delusions within each of the constitutional remedy profiles will aid in remedy recognition.

Each selection of *Delusion* rubrics discussed are shaded. Analyses of the remedy profiles follow each sub-section. The psychological development of *Delusion* rubrics for each constitutional remedy profile is analyzed according to either **avoidance** or **self-deluding** need.

- *Delusions: dying, he is*: acon. ant-t. apis cact. cann-i. chlf. *Lac-lup.* morph. nux-v. op. podo. pot-e. rhus-t. stram. ther. thyr. vesp. xan.
- *Delusions: die: about to die; one was*: **ACON.** agn. alum. am-c. ant-t. *Arg-n.* arn. ars. asaf. asar. bar-c. bar-m. bell. cact. calc. cann-i. caps. caust. cench. *Chel. Croc.* cupr. gels. glon. graph. hell. iris-t. kali-c. lac-d. *Lach.* lil-t. lyc. lyss. mag-p. magn-gr. med. meli. merc. mur-ac. *Nit-ac.* nux-v. petr. phos. *Plat. Podo.* positr. psor. puls. pyrus raph. rhus-t. ruta sil. stram. sulph. tab. thea. *Thuj.* v-a-b. verat. *Xan.* zinc.
- *Delusions: die: about to die; one was: exhaustion; she would die from*: lach. [1] 1.

- *Delusions: die: about to die; one was; lie down and die; she must:* kali-c. [1] 1.
- *Delusions: die: time has come to:* ars. bell. dendr-pol. lach. med. sabad. thuj.
- *Delusions: die: rather die than live; one would:* xan. [1] 1.
- *Delusions: disease: every disease; he has: Aur-m.* stram.
- *Delusions: disease: incurable disease; he has an:* acon. adam. alum. *Arg-n.* arn. cact. calc-sil. calc. chel. *Ign.* lac-c. *Lach. Lil-t.* macro. mag-c. nit-ac. petr-ra. phos. plb. podo. positr. *Sabad. Stann. Syph.*
- *Delusions: health, he has ruined his:* bamb-a. chel.
- *Delusions: ideas: rush of ideas prevented him from completing his work:* stann. [1] 1.
- *Delusions: cancer, has a:* carc. sabad. verat.
- *Delusions: dead; he himself was:* agn. anac. anh. apis ars. camph. cann-i. choc. cypra-eg. graph. *Lach.* mosch. oena. *Op.* phos. plat. raph. sil. stram.
- *Delusions: mutilated bodies; sees:* ant-c. arn. con. mag-m. maias-l. marb-w. merc. *Nux-v.* sep.
- *Delusions: grave, he is in his:* anac. *Gels.* lepi. stram.

Self-deluding: The *Delusion* rubrics: *I am dying, sick, I am dead*, and *I have an incurable disease*, are all examples of exaggerated predictions of decay which are maintained because it is psychologically advantageous.

The homoeopath looking at a case analysis has to be able to understand why it is advantageous for the patient to maintain the obsessive psychological 'delusions of hypochondria'. Alternatively, the homoeopath needs to understand what the patient is *lacking* which will cause them to be swamped with obsessive fears about their health, and predictions of death.

Aconite are predominantly weighted in the rubrics pertaining to 'delusions of hypochondria', and predictions of death. The homoeopath needs to understand *why Aconite* are *so* vulnerable to predictions of death every time they become ill. *Aconite* as a homoeopathic remedy is frequently used for the patient who, after shock, feels convinced that they are going to die. *Aconite* have the *Mind* rubrics: *fear of death, anxiety about health, ailments from fear, fright,* and *grief. Aconite* is a homoeopathic remedy used for permanent anxiety after shock. *Aconite* have the *Mind* rubric: *timidity after fright.* [2] 1. *Aconite* as a homoeopathic remedy is often used for intense attacks of diarrhoea when the patient becomes convinced that they are going to die. *Aconite* have the *Delusion* rubric: *thoughts come from the stomach.* [1] 1. *Aconite* have the *Mind* rubric: *anguish before stool,* and *anguish during peritonitis.* [3] 1. and the *Mind* rubric: *anguish driving from place to place with restlessness. Aconite* overreact to all illness, especially stomach problems, and are convinced they are going to die.

Aconite will easily be overcome with anxiety because their high expectations of self predispose them to predictions of doom. A patient suffering *illusions of fancy* has grand visions of persona: their expectations of what they *should* achieve are exaggerated. *Aconite* have not lived up to their own expectations of success. As a constitutional remedy, *Aconite* will only be the simillimum for the patient who is extremely unsure and uncertain of themselves because they have previously failed in their life. Insecurity as a result of not having met their own expectations of perfection is the predetermining personality trait which predisposes *Aconite* to exaggerated fears of death with every health complaint, regardless of its severity.

The simillimum will not be *Aconite* unless the patient is able to display evidence of perfectionism. *Aconite* have the *Mind* rubrics: *increased ambition, audacity* and *boaster.* Their need to maintain control predisposes them to extreme shock if they have not managed to achieve perfect predictability [*illusions of fancy*]. It is fair to say that every person, to one degree or another, likes to be in control. The 'never-well-since-event' in an *Aconite* case will not only involve an accident or intense shock. The simillimum will only be *Aconite* if the patient feels that they made a fool of themselves at the time of the accident.

Aconite have numerous Resignation rubrics which all pertain to them looking foolish – some part is *deformed*, their *head is large*, or their *body is small*. The simillimum will not be *Aconite* unless the patient reveals they are vulnerable to unpredictability. *Aconite* as a constitutional remedy profile will have within their persona a *strong* need for known predictable stability across all levels – emotionally, mentally, and physically.

Aconite have only one *Delusion* rubric: *jostling against everyone she meets*, which can be allocated to the Causation rubrics or acknowledgments of personal blame or sins. This rubric can be analyzed in two ways. On the one hand, it can be seen that *Aconite* are always in such a highly anxious state that they irritate others. The other interpretation of this rubric, which is more relevant to *Aconite,* is that they lack strength and self-esteem. They are so unsure of themselves that they will always be the cause of, or the recipient of, contradictions and *jostling*. This integral lack of societal self-confidence predisposes *Aconite* to anxiety. The idealistic fanciful illusions of *Aconite* predispose them to becoming anxious because they can't hope to fulfill their own high expectations of themselves. *Aconite* have the *Mind* rubric: *tormenting himself.* [2] 8.

1. Denial: *Delusion* rubric: *fancy, illusions of*: Acon.

2. Forsaken*: Delusion* rubric: *home: away from home; he is*: acon. *Delusion* rubric: *assembled things, swarms, crowds etc.*: acon. *Delusion* rubric: *images, phantoms*: sees: acon. *Delusion* rubric: *figures: seeing figures*: acon. *Delusion* rubric: *voices: hearing*: acon. [These last two rubrics can pertain to 'God by one's side'; however, in relation to *Aconite* they pertain to persecutory fear.]

3. Causation: *Delusion* rubric: *jostling against everyone she meets*: acon. [1] 1.

4. Depression: *Delusion* rubric: *anxious*: Acon. *Delusion* rubric: *doomed, being*: acon. *Delusion* rubric: *insane: become insane; one will*: Acon. *Delusion* rubric: *weeping; with*: acon.

5. Resignation: *Delusion* rubric: *die: about to die; one was*: **ACON**. *Delusion* rubric: *body: deformed, some part is*: acon. *Delusion* rubric: *dying: he is*: acon. *Delusion* rubric: *small: body is smaller*. acon. *Delusion* rubric: *swollen, is*: acon. *Delusion* rubric: *head: large: too large; seems*: acon. *Delusion* rubric: *large: parts of body seem too large*: acon. *Delusion* rubric: *thoughts: stomach; come from*: acon. [1] 1.

Gelsemium are listed in numerous *Delusion* rubrics pertaining to 'delusions of hypochondria' – *he is in his grave, about to die, he has been poisoned,* and *his heart stops beating when sitting.* Gelsemium are also listed in numerous *Mind* rubrics: *ailments from anticipation, ailments from death of loved ones, fear of death, forebodings,* and *anxiety with fear.* Sankaran notes in *The Soul of Remedies,* "So the main feeling in *Gelsemium* is: 'I have to keep my control when going through ordeals. I have to be able to withstand very difficult, trying situations, I have to be able to withstand shock and bad news without losing my control'. So they keep courage when facing ordeals, and are not shaken up even by frightening situations. This courageous *Gelsemium* is exactly the opposite of the picture we read in the books, of the coward who is unable to face any unexpected event." *Gelsemium* is a homoeopathic remedy derived from a plant containing poisonous properties. Vermeulen notes in *Prisma,* "Many members of the Loganiaceae are extremely poisonous, causing death by convulsions. Poisonous properties are largely due to indole alkaloids such as those found in *Strychnos, Gelsemium* and *Mostuea.* Due to its very rapid effects, the species Gelsemium elegans is used in China as a criminal poison. Glycosides in the form of pseudo-indicans are also present, as loganin in *Strychnos,* and the related substance aucubin in *Buddleja.* The alkaloids in *Gelsemium* have the following activities: convulsant, hypotensive, cardiodepressant, and, chiefly, CNS (Central Nervous System) depressant. All parts of G. sempervirens are toxic, including the flower and nectar. The plant can cause skin allergies and it is possible that the plant toxins can be absorbed through the skin, especially if there are cuts. The primary toxic compounds are gelsemine and gelseminine, which act as motor nerve depressants. Symptoms of toxicity in humans include difficulty in use of voluntary muscles, muscle rigidity and weakness, dizziness, loss of speech, dry mouth, visual disturbances, trembling of extremities, profuse sweating, respiratory depression, and convulsions. Cattle, sheep, goats, horses and swine have been poisoned by feeding on the plants. Symptoms in animals include muscular weakness; convulsive movements of head, front legs and sometimes hind legs; slow respiration; decreased temperature; excessive perspiration; death due to respiratory failure."

The alkaloids in *Gelsemium* act as a CNS depressant. Similarly, *Gelsemium* (the constitutional remedy profile) force themselves into a paralytic immobilized state, reminiscent of the nature and action of the poison. This suppression of their emotive and somatic responses to perceived danger allows them to shut down all feelings and responses to fear. *Gelsemium* have the *Mind* rubric: *fear of losing self-control*. *Gelsemium* allow themselves to move into a catatonic state of immobilized paralysis [*emptiness*] because their *enlarged* imagination is likely to overwhelm them with crippling fears. *Gelsemium* as a homoeopathic remedy is frequently used for the patient who is overcome with crippling stage fright. *Gelsemium* have the *Mind* rubrics: *cowardice, anticipation, stage fright in singers and speakers,* and *timidity about appearing in public.* [4] 31.

The homoeopath should not expect to find *Gelsemium* in a frantic [*delirious*] and worried state about their impending fears of disease and death; rather they are calmly controlled. However, it is a mistake for Sankaran to interpret this calm control as a "courageous *Gelsemium*". *Gelsemium* have several *Mind* rubrics which all indicate that they are mentally and emotionally 'shut down'.

Gelsemium have the *Mind* rubrics: *answering in monosyllables, unable to answer when emotionally hurt, confusion of mind, muscles refuses to obey the will when attention is turned away,* and *confusion of mind, as to his identity, sense of duality. Gelsemium* somatically suppress feeling; this is not courage, it is suppression. *Gelsemium* shut down their exaggerated responses to fear. The suppressive [*emptiness*] in *Gelsemium* makes the patient appear as if they are mentally and emotionally unconscious of all of their feelings. The homoeopath should not presume that *Gelsemium* will appear *hysterically delirious.* The CNS suppression inherent in its origins allows them to suppress their mental and emotional responses to trauma.

Gelsemium have no *Delusion* rubrics of self-blame for real or supposed sins. The relevance of this fact is crucial. If a constitutional remedy has psychological 'delusions of original sin' which they need to flagellate themselves for, or hide from, it creates within their psyche an internal dialogue of self-blame. *Gelsemium* have no self-blame.

The simillimum will not be *Gelsemium* if the patient is filled with guilt.

1. Denial: *Delusion* rubric: *enlarged*: *Gels. Delusion* rubric: *large*: *everything looks larger. Gels.* [These rubrics, when analyzed along with the overwhelming number of exaggerated *Delusion* rubrics of predictions of death, have to be interpreted as a psychological delusion of hypochondriac foreboding, and not as a psychological 'delusion of grandeur' which increases their confidence[74]. For *Gelsemium* the *Delusion* rubric: *enlarged*, and *everything looks larger* reinforce their exaggerated fears and forebodings.]

2. Forsaken: *Delusion* rubric: *snakes*: *in and around her.* gels. *Delusion* rubric: *poisoned*: *he: has been*: gels.

3. Causation: NONE.

4. Depression: *Delusion* rubric: *succeed, he does everything*

wrong; he cannot: gels. *Delusion* rubric: *insane: become insane; one will*: gels. *Delusion* rubric: *falling: height; from a*: gels. *Delusion* rubric: *emptiness; of*. Gels. *Delusion* rubric: *identity: someone else, she is*: gels. *Delusion* rubric: *person: other person; she is some*: gels.

5. Resignation: *Delusion* rubric: *die: about to die; one was*: gels. *Delusion* rubric: *grave, he is in his*: Gels. *Delusion* rubric: *delirious: become delirious; he would*: gels. [1] 1. *Delusion* rubric: *body: lighter than air; body is: hysteria; in*: gels. [1] 1. *Delusion* rubric: *heart: stops beating when sitting*: gels.

Kali carbonicum are noted for internal antagonism and conflicting behavior; on the one hand needing company, and on the other hand rejecting company. This is reflected in the *Mind* rubrics: *antagonism with self, desire for company yet treats those who approach outrageously*, and the *Mind* rubric: *quarrelsome with her family*. Conversely, they also have the *Mind* rubrics: *love for family*, and the *Mind* rubric: *loyal*. [3] 3. The *Mind* rubrics: *love for family,* and *quarrelsome with family*, highlight a self-conflicting dynamic within the remedy profile which reflects internal confusion.

My aim in understanding the delusional states in the five stages of illness and death is to shed light on psychological inconsistencies within the remedy profile. If, in a repertory, the homoeopath only notes particular rubrics for *Kali carbonicum,* like the *Mind* rubric: *antagonism with self*, and the *Mind* rubric: *quarrelsome with family,* then the student homoeopath can be left with an incorrect understanding of the remedy profile of *Kali carbonicum. Kali carbonicum* were always noted, when I was a student, as the 'demanding' patient who would be most likely to complain; conversely, they are also noted as loyal patients. Sankaran notes, in *The Soul of Remedies*, that the sycotic theme of *Kali carbonicum* is seen in the feeling: "I am too weak to support myself and need the company of family". *Kali carbonicum* are noted for their lack of self-confidence. This is reflected in the *Mind* rubrics: *want of self-confidence*, and *full of inexpressible desires*. The abandonment within *Kali carbonicum* is self-abandonment which is covered up, and supported by a need for social conservatism. *Kali carbonicum* are noted for the *Mind* rubrics: *conformism*, [3] 3., *dress conservative*, [1] 1., *dogmatic*, and *too much sense of duty*. *Kali carbonicum* need a secure 'nine to five' job or a conservative stable profession to strengthen their self-confidence. *Kali carbonicum* lack the self-confidence which fuels a person's ability to propel themselves into financial risk-taking. *Kali carbonicum* needs the homoeopath who is treating them, yet they continually complain. *Kali carbonicum* needs family, yet they also reject them. *Kali carbonicum* are *full of inexpressible desires* which they don't have enough confidence or emotional strength to express. *Kali carbonicum* need financial predictability, yet they become overwhelmed by pressure [*duty*] and expectations. *Kali carbonicum* are noted for the *Mind* rubric: *too much sense of duty*.

If *Kali carbonicum desires company, yet treats those who approach him outrageously* then it equates to self-sabotage. If in the case analysis the patient is *not* noted for 'shooting themselves in the foot', especially in the area of family and intimate relationships, then the simillimum will *not* be *Kali carbonicum*.

For internal confusion and self-sabotage to be significant (in the case) there must be evidence that they are have become the precursor for deeper destructive pathology. If the rubric-repertorisation (of the five stages) reveals that a remedy profile is weighted with *Delusion* rubrics of abandonment, then the homoeopath has to expect the patient to display self-deserting unassertiveness.

Furthermore, if the rubric-repertorisation (of the five stages) reveals that a remedy profile is weighted with *Delusion* rubrics relating to hypochondria, then the homoeopath has to expect the patient to display internal self-deserting self-destructive anguish. *Kali carbonicum* have the *Delusion* rubric: *about to die, she must lie down and die.* [1] 1. *Kali carbonicum* feel abandoned and will abandon themselves.

Kali carbonicum are one of three remedies listed in the *Delusion* rubric: *seeing mask*. I have listed this rubric in the *Delusion* rubrics pertaining to abandonment. A mask is traditionally associated with the image of someone hiding behind a mask. Seeing a mask on others is, on the other hand, reflective of the ability to discern another's falsity. The conflict within *Kali carbonicum* stems from the fact that the abandonment is viewed as coming from within and outside of themselves; this fuels their lack of self-confidence. *Kali carbonicum* will literally abandon their own thoughts and psyche and project their need for security outwards to family and the world. *Kali carbonicum* only feel confident if they are hiding behind the mask of either their family, or their conservative job, or their health practitioner. Furthermore, *Kali carbonicum* continually question the mask they present to the world, as well as the mask the world presents to them. The psychodynamic need to self-examine comes from the lack of psychological 'delusions of grandeur' which strengthen egotism. Their only Denial rubric: *illusions of fancy*, predisposes *Kali carbonicum* to illusions of fanciful idealism which they cannot achieve.

The homoeopath needs to continually alert *Kali carbonicum* to the downfalls of maintaining hubristic idealism. Their idealism predisposes them to continual perceptions of failure. Furthermore, their illusions of fanciful idealism preempt their continual need to re-examine all of their decisions. *Kali carbonicum* continually need to re-examine everyone else as well as themselves; it is this characteristic which sheds light on the psychological inconsistencies within the remedy profile. *Kali carbonicum* struggle to trust their own perceptions. If in the case analysis the patient is *not* noted for 'shooting themselves in the foot' in the area of trust then the simillimum will not be *Kali carbonicum*.

Kali carbonicum maintain their 'delusions of hypochondria' because it reinforces their need for the homoeopathic practitioner. The simillimum will only be *Kali carbonicum* if the patient indicates that they *need* illness even though they are obsessed and terrified of illness and death. *Kali carbonicum* have the *Mind* rubrics: *hypochondriacal anxiety,* and *fear of impending disease.* [3]. *Kali carbonicum* have a passive/ aggressive relationship with the world and with their own health.

Kali carbonicum maintain their 'delusions of hypochondria' because it allows them to avoid examining their own self-deserting abandonment.

If the patient presents with conflicting behavioral patterning within their personality profile, then they will always have *Delusion* rubrics within the case analysis, which will explain their *peculiar* internal anguish and self-destruction. *Kali carbonicum* are aware of their own internal *abyss,* which always threatens their security. *Kali carbonicum* have the *Delusion* rubrics: *to be sinking,* and *their whole body is hollow.* The consequence of always *turning around and finding nothing but emptiness* is that *Kali carbonicum* feel that even their own thoughts have abandoned them. Self-questioning is what fuels their need to rely on the homoeopathic practitioner; conversely their self-questioning also fuels their disbelief in their cure.

The psychological delusion which preempts the self-abandonment and anxiety in *Kali carbonicum* is self-doubt. *Kali carbonicum* have the *Delusion* rubrics: *thoughts had vanished,* and *abyss behind him.*

Kali carbonicum are noted for anxiety, but the anxiety which is *peculiar* to *Kali carbonicum* is their ability to abandon all confidence *in themselves.* *Kali carbonicum* will only be the simillimum if the patient has no faith or hope in themselves being cured.

Furthermore, *Kali carbonicum* will only be the simillimum if the patient has no faith in being able to cure themselves. *Kali carbonicum* need to maintain their belief that they will always be sick because to abandon psychological delusions of impending death would require them to come to terms with how alone [*emptiness*] and abandoned they feel [*abyss behind them*].

The homoeopath working with a *Kali carbonicum* patient needs to slowly reinforce and encourage self-confidence; only then will they become well across all levels.

1. Denial: *Delusion* rubric: *fancy, illusions of*: kali-c. *Delusion* rubric: *visions, has*: kali-c. [These rubrics, when analyzed along with the overwhelming number of exaggerated *Delusion* rubrics of predictions of death, and the numerous abandonment rubrics pertaining to forebodings and exaggerated ailments from fear have to be interpreted as psychological delusions of hypochondriac foreboding, not as psychological 'delusions of grandeur' which increase egotism. *Kali carbonicum* have numerous persecutory rubrics of seeing images and phantoms, *Delusion* rubric: *sees dead persons, sees devil*, and *sees faces, vermin, pigeons flying around the room, sees creeping worms*, and is the only remedy listed in the *Delusion* rubric: *seeing figures of old repulsive persons*. [2] 1.]

2. Forsaken: *Delusion rubric: abyss: behind him*: Kali-c. [2] 1. *Delusion* rubric: *emptiness; of: behind one on turning around; emptiness*: kali-c. [1] 1. *Delusion* rubric: *murdered: will be murdered; he*: kali-c. *Delusion* rubric: *poisoned: he, has been*: kali-c. *Delusion* rubric: *mask: seeing*: kali-c. *Delusion* rubric: *hollow: body is hollow; whole*: Kali-c. [This last rubric pertains to self-deserting abandonment as well as indicating physical weakness.]

3. Causation: NONE [*Kali carbonicum* have the *Delusion* rubric: *sees devil*, but they have no psychological delusions of *personal* guilt.]

4. Depression: *Delusion* rubric: *sinking; to be*: kali-c. [This rubric should not be interpreted literally. This rubric reflect

feelings of impending doom.] *Delusion* rubric: *thoughts*: *vanish*: *had vanished; thoughts*: kali-c. [This rubric reflects self-doubt.]

5. Resignation: *Delusion* rubric: *die*: *about to die; one was; lie down and die; she must*: kali-c. [1] 1. *Delusion* rubric: *sick, being*: *Kali-c. Delusion* rubric: *hollow*: *body is hollow; whole*: *Kali-c.* [This last rubric indicates feelings of exaggerated physical weakness.] *Delusion* rubric: *faint; he would*: kali-c. *Delusion* rubric: *die*: *about to die; one was*: kali-c.

Lilium tigrinum have exaggerated pretensions about their self-importance. This is reflected in the *Delusion* rubric: *everything is depending on him.* The theme of the Liliales is adoration of self-perfectionism. On the one hand *Lilium tigrinum* fee' as if they are so important that everything depends on them, and on the other hand they feel that everything is depending *on them,* and that no one is able to care *for them. Lilium tigrinum* have the *Delusion* rubric: *is forsaken, no one to care for her. Lilium tigrinum* maintain the feeling that no one can possibly take care of them to reinforce delusional self-importance. *Lilium tigrinum* have the *Mind* rubric: *taking responsibility too seriously. Lilium tigrinum* maintain their grandiose belief in their high position to deny fears of insanity. *Lilium tigrinum* have the *Delusion* rubrics: *one will become insane,* and *if he did not hold himself he would become insane. Lilium tigrinum* also maintain their grandiose belief in their high position to deny their sins. *Lilium tigrinum* have the *Delusion* rubric: *being doomed to expiate her sins and those of her family.* [2] 1.

'Hubristic denial' for *Lilium tigrinum* refers to their belief that everyone is depending on them. Their failure and sin, which is a psychological delusion, is that they have abandoned their family – *Delusion* rubric: *cannot get along with her family, does not belong to her own family.* [1] 1. Their internal conflict stems from the feeling or belief that they are entitled to adoration and praise. This feeling or belief removes them from their family. If a patient has 'delusions of grandeur', their denial is maintained to avoid acknowledging reality.

If there are inconsistencies between Stage one and Stage five, then that is evidence of self-denial and suppression which will either accelerate present pathology or precede future pathology. On the one hand *Lilium tigrinum* believe *everything is depending on them,* and on the other hand *they are going to go insane unless they can get out of their body.* If a patient has an urgent need to prove themselves, they are more likely to push their body to extreme levels of exhaustion. Continual exhaustion is the precursor of hypochondria.

Lilium tigrinum leave themselves open to internal instability [*insanity*] because they invest so much of their psyche in delusional denial. This internal conflict will accelerate collapse and disease because *Lilium tigrinum* will exhaust their energy in the attempt to live up to their own expectations of importance.

Lilium tigrinum are in continual exaggerated fear of disease and dying because they have exhausted themselves as a result of their internal battle to control their sexual lasciviousness. All suppression which is based on needing to deny part of ourselves will eventuate in mental and emotional instability [*insanity*] or self-destruction.

Lilium tigrinum have the *Mind* rubrics: *mutilating his body, desire to pull her own hair, tormenting himself,* and the *Mind* rubric: *wild feeling in head from suppression of sexual desire.* [1] 2. [med.] *Lilium tigrinum* have numerous *Mind* rubrics pertaining to their *conflict between religious ideals and sexuality* which I have discussed further in Causation. *Lilium tigrinum* struggle between religion and sexual desires. Their inner guilt and turmoil is reflected in the *Delusion* rubrics: *divided into two parts,* and *body is divided.*

Conflict and suppression will always be the precursor to the development of destructive pathology.

1.   Denial: *Delusion* rubric: *depending on him; everything is*: lil-t. [1] 2. [lac-lup]

2. Forsaken: *Delusion* rubric: *forsaken; is: care for her; no one would*: lil-t. *Delusion* rubric: *forsaken; is*: lil-t. *Delusion* rubric: *poisoned: he: has been*: lil-t.

3. Causation: *Delusion* rubric: *wrong: done wrong; he has*: *Lil-t.* *Delusion* rubric: *doomed, being: expiate her sins and those of her family; to*: *Lil-t.* [2] 1. *Delusion* rubric: *family, does not belong to her own: get along with her; cannot*: lil-t. [1] 1.

4. Depression: *Delusion* rubric: *insane: become insane; one will*: lil-t. *Delusion* rubric: *doomed, being*: *Lil-t.* *Delusion* rubric: *insane: become insane; one will: hold himself; if he did not*: lil-t. [1] 1. *Delusion* rubric: *insane: become insane; one will: unless she got out of her body*: lil-t. [1] 1. *Delusion* rubric: *divided: two parts; into*: lil-t.

5. Resignation: *Delusion* rubric: *die: about to die; one was*: lil-t. *Delusion* rubric: *disease: incurable disease; he has an*; *Lil-t.* *Delusion* rubric: *insane: become insane; one will: unless she got out of her body*: lil-t. [1] 1. *Delusion* rubric: *body: divided, is*: lil-t. *Delusion* rubric: *divided: two parts; into*: lil-t.

Podophyllum have an intensely *disproportionate* amount of *Delusion* rubrics relating to illness and death. *Podophyllum* have the *Delusion* rubrics: *about to die, he is dying, he has an incurable disease*, as well as, *he will die of heart or liver failure*. *Podophyllum* also have the *Mind* rubric: *anxiety about one's health*.

Podophyllum have extreme psychological 'delusions of hypochondria'.

Podophyllum as a homoeopathic remedy is often used for rectal incontinence associated with the condition Irritable Bowel Syndrome, or gastroenteritis, where similarly, the patient feels powerless to stop bowel evacuations.

As a constitutional remedy, the profile of *Podophyllum* has the same theme of not being able to 'hold on' to themselves. *Podophyllum* are sure they are going to die.

The simillimum will not be *Podophyllum* unless the patient indicates that they have persecutory fears. *Podophyllum* is derived from a poisonous plant. If ingested in large amounts along with alcohol, poisoning symptoms may occur, typically, headaches, gastroenteritis and collapse.

If a homeopathic remedy is derived from any poisonous substance, within the psyche of the homoeopathic profile there is always an element of collapse and/or self-destruction.

Podophyllum is applicable to the patient who is easily overwhelmed with illness. *Podophyllum* have the *Delusion* rubric: *body is smaller*. This rubric should not be interpreted literally. Rather it is indicative of how powerless *Podophyllum* feel. I have only used *Podophyllum* once, constitutionally, and it was for a woman who was 'spiritually attached' to her gastric disturbances. Every time she was overcome by an explosive bowel motion she felt depressed and thought she was going to die. However, every time I tried to encourage diet changes she subconsciously sabotaged my efforts. Eventually, after a few months of persisting with my prescription of *Podophyllum* she revealed to me that she felt that her extreme sensitivity to food proved she was highly attuned to the universe; this is a 'delusion of grandeur' or 'spiritual ego'. When her diarrhoea stopped she felt like everyone else who *had gross insensitive bodies and lacked spiritual sensitivity*. Cure in this case came when the patient was able to realize that she could maintain her *heightened spiritual sensitivity* without needing to have it validated by extreme food sensitivities.

In 'New-Age' groups I have noticed a common myth that 'sensitivity' to the environment or to particular foods is proof of 'spiritual sensitivity' or 'spiritual awareness'.

None of the dietary changes I had tried to enforce were effective. The action of simillimum exposed her delusional denial, she was subsequently able to release her attachment to maintaining her psychological delusion, and her diarrhoea stopped. The first action of the simillimum will expose or heighten psychological denial. The importance of understanding the psychological delusional stages will alert the homoeopath to predominant delusional states. Each remedy profile has a predominance in one area, whether it be 'delusions of grandeur', 'delusions of abandonment', 'delusions of original sin', 'delusions of impending doom' or 'delusions of hypochondria'. I have discussed each remedy profile in the five stages according to the predominant delusional themes within the profile. Cure from the action of the simillimum will first expose psychological denial. *Podophyllum* have an intensely *disproportionate* amount of *Delusion* rubrics relating to 'delusions of hypochondria'. *Podophyllum* will maintain their 'delusions of hypochondria' for a specific reason. Furthermore, if there are inconsistencies between Stage one and Stage five, then there is evidence of self-denial and suppression which will either accelerate present pathology or precede future pathology.

Podophyllum have the *Delusion* rubric: *he is well* and the contradictory *Delusion* rubric: *he is going to be sick*. Inconsistencies within the remedy profile should alert the homoeopath to the patient's need of self-destructive psychological patterning to maintain their delusional perceptions. The collapse within *Podophyllum* is immediate. *Podophyllum* presume that they will always become unwell; they do not believe they can sustain well-being. *Podophyllum* need to suppress their physical well-being to support their 'delusions of grandeur' of being united with a *higher consciousness*.

It is this degree of suppression which leaves them vulnerable to persecutory fears and 'delusions of hypochondria'. *Podophyllum* maintains the perception they are *smaller* to avoid being persecuted. In the psyche of all the remedy profiles which are derived from poisons is a somatic hypersensitivity to perceived annihilation. Ironically, remaining in a *small* state leaves *Podophyllum* exposed to annihilation.

Podophyllum will only be the simillimum if the patient is mentally and emotionally attached to remaining vulnerable.

Podophyllum have the *Mind* rubric: *desire to be magnetized,* and the *Delusion* rubric: *unification with higher consciousness.* The simillimum will not be *Podophyllum* unless the patient indicates that their sensitivity is a result of their heightened spiritual connection to a higher consciousness. *Podophyllum,* along with *Hydrogen,* choose to live in the presence of a higher consciousness. *Hydrogenium* experience a psychological delusional conflict between their higher consciousness and their existence in the world. *Podophyllum* on the other hand, as a result of their heightened consciousness, suffer from exaggerated awareness of their vulnerability. The simillimum will not be *Podophyllum* unless the patient indicates that they are extremely vulnerable to all outside influences across all levels – emotionally, mentally, and physically.

1. Denial: *Delusion* rubric: *well, he is*: podo.
    Versus
5. *Delusion* rubric: *sick: going to be sick; he is*: podo.

1. Denial: *Delusion* rubric: *well, he is*: podo. *Delusion* rubric: *consciousness: higher consciousness; unification with*: podo. [1] 2. [hydrog.]
2. Forsaken: *Delusion* rubric: *criticized, she is*: podo. *Delusion* rubric: *assaulted, is going to be*: podo. *Delusion* rubric: *persecuted: he is persecuted*: podo. *Delusion* rubric: *place: strange place; he was in a*: podo.
3. Causation: *Delusion* rubric: *sinned; one has: day of grace; sinned away his*: podo.
4. Depression: *Delusion* rubric: *sick: going to be sick; he is*: podo. *Delusion* rubric: *unreal: everything seems unreal*: podo.
5. Resignation: *Delusion* rubric: *die: about to die; one was*: Podo. *Delusion* rubric: *dying: he is*: podo. *Delusion* rubric:

disease: *incurable disease; he has an*: podo. *Delusion* rubric: *liver disease; that he will have*: podo. [1] 1. *Delusion* rubric: *sick*: *being*: podo. *Delusion* rubric: *heart*: *disease*: *going to have a heart disease and die; is*: podo. *Delusion* rubric: *sick*: *going to be sick; he is*: podo. *Delusion* rubric: *small*: *body is smaller*: podo.

Sabadilla are listed in numerous rubrics pertaining to extreme hypochondria. *Sabadilla* have only one 'delusion of grandeur', the *Delusion* rubric: *illusions of fancy*. The essence of understanding the psychological profile within the five stages is that it will always highlight *peculiarities,* or *strange* and *rare* aspects of each remedy profile.

Sabadilla have numerous *Delusion* rubrics pertaining to 'delusions of hypochondria' and not enough 'delusions of grandeur' which can boost their stature. It is debatable whether in the case of *Sabadilla* the fanciful idealism inherent in the *Delusion* rubric: *illusions of fancy*, is a psychological 'delusion of fancy' or the precursor of their overwhelming illusions of illness and disease. If the latter is correct, which I suspect is the case, then it indicates that *Sabadilla* do not have the 'ego' strength to be able to resist their delusional hypochondria.

Sabadilla have several physical, psychosomatic and imaginary [*illusions of fancy*] illnesses. Their obsessive, neurotic hypochondria, illusions and imaginations are turned inwards against themselves. They have numerous *Delusion* rubrics which all center around self-repulsion.

Sabadilla the homoeopathic remedy is derived from seeds of the South American lily (*Schoenocaulan officinale*). The seeds of the Sabadilla are used as an insecticide. The seed dust is the least toxic and is used as a botanical insecticide against armyworms, harlequin bugs, stink bugs, cucumber beetles, leafhoppers, and blister beetles. It is considered among the least toxic of botanical insecticides and breaks down rapidly in sunlight. Although Sabadilla is classified as slightly toxic, it is toxic to honey bees. Sabadilla dust causes irritation to eyes and produces sneezing if inhaled. The purified alkaloid is very toxic. It is a severe skin irritant and even small amounts cause headaches, nausea, and vomiting. Large doses can cause convulsions, respiratory failure and cardiac arrest. *Sabadilla* (the homoeopathic remedy) is commonly used for hay fever, sneezing, throat irritation, headaches and skin irritation. *Sabadilla* is also used for nausea and diarrhoea. If a homoeopathic remedy is derived from a poisonous substance, then within the profile of the remedy there will always be evidence of self-destruction and fear of annihilation (persecution).

Within *Sabadilla,* obsessive self-destruction stimulates psychological illusions of their body devouring itself from the inside out. *Sabadilla* have the *Delusion* rubric: *his stomach is devoured. Sabadilla* have several physiological imaginings: *imagining they are pregnant, filled with flatus,* and illusions they *are pregnant.*

'Phantom pregnancy' is the appearance of clinical, and/or sub-clinical, signs and symptoms associated with a pregnancy, when the patient is not pregnant. Psychodynamic theories attribute the 'phantom pregnancy' to a somatic manifestation of internal mental and emotional conflict. Either the patient has an intense desire to become pregnant, or an intense fear of becoming pregnant. *Sabadilla* have a psychosomatic desire to be pregnant.

Sabadilla need to be taken over by something inside of themselves or by someone outside of themselves. *Sabadilla* have no strength of 'mind over body'.

Sabadilla have the *Mind* rubrics: *persistent thoughts of mind and body separated, feigning to be sick, wakes his wife and child talking anxiously about his hypochondriasis,* and *runs recklessly about and jumps out of bed, wants to destroy himself but lacks the courage.* The *Delusion* rubric: *the house is coming down on her,* should not be taken literally, rather it is indicative of fear of annihilation ('delusions of persecution'). *Sabadilla* have a psychosomatic desire to imagine themselves sick, deformed, and dying of cancer. The simillimum will only be *Sabadilla* if the patient indicates that they are unable to resist their imaginings that their body is diseased from the inside out.

The rubric-list below lists the numerous body delusions of *Sabadilla*.

* *Delusions: diminished, all is*: sabad.
* *Delusions: separated: body, mind are separated: body and*: sabad.
* *Delusions: thoughts: outside of body; thoughts are*: sabad. [1] 1.
* *Delusions: die: time has come to*: sabad.
* *Delusions: cancer, has a*: sabad.
* *Delusions: disease: incurable disease; he has an*: Sabad.
* *Delusions: disease: throat disease, which ends fatal; has*: **SABAD**.
* *Delusions: emaciation; of*: sabad.
* *Delusions: poisoned: he, has been*: sabad.
* *Delusions: sick: being*: Sabad.
* *Delusions: withering, body is*: sabad.
* *Delusions: faint; he would*: sabad.
* *Delusions: brain: round and round; brain seemed to go*: sabad. [1] 1.
* *Delusions: body: shrunken, like the dead; body is*: Sabad. [2] 1.
* *Delusions: diminished: shrunken, parts are*: Sabad.
* *Delusions: disease: throat disease, which ends fatal; has*: **SABAD**. [3] 1.
* *Delusions: enlarged: scrotum is swollen*: sabad. [1] 1.

- *Delusions*: *falling*: *hold on to something; she would fall if she did not*: sabad. [1] 1.
- *Delusions*: *small*: *body is smaller*: sabad.
- *Delusions*: *pregnant, she is*: Sabad.
- *Delusions*: *pregnant, she is*: *distension of abdomen from flatus; with*: **SABAD**.
- *Delusions*: *body*: *deformed, some part is*: **SABAD**.
- *Delusions*: *abdomen*: *fallen in; abdomen is*: **SABAD**. [3] 1.
- *Delusions*: *stomach*: *devoured; his stomach is*: **SABAD**. [3] 1.
- *Delusions*: *stomach*: *ulcer in stomach; has corrosion of an*: sabad.

1. Denial: [*Delusion* rubric: *fancy, illusions of*: Sabad.] NONE.

2. Forsaken: *Delusion* rubric: *poisoned*: *he, has been*: sabad. *Delusion* rubric: *house*: *house coming down on her; house is*: sabad. [1] 1. [This rubric can pertain to 'delusions of persecution' or 'delusions of impending doom'.]

3. Causation: *Delusion* rubric: *crime*: *committed a crime; he had*: sabad. *Delusion* rubric: *criminal, he is a*: sabad.

4. Depression: *Delusion* rubric: *thoughts*: *outside of body; thoughts are*: sabad. [1] 1. *Delusion* rubric: *diminished, all is*: sabad. *Delusion* rubric: *separated*: *body, mind are separated*: *body and*: sabad. *Delusion* rubric: *house*: *house coming down on her; house is*: sabad. [1] 1. *Delusion* rubric: *house*: *falling on her; as if houses were*: sabad. [1] 1. *Delusion* rubric: *dull*: *liquor; from taking*: sabad. [1] 1. [This rubric should not be interpreted literally. It indicates unconsciousness.]

5. Resignation: *Delusion* rubric: *die*: *time has come to*: sabad. *Delusion* rubric: *cancer, has a*: sabad. *Delusion* rubric: *body*: *deformed, some part is*: **SABAD**. *Delusion* rubric: *disease*: *incurable disease; he has an*: Sabad. *Delusion*

rubric: *disease: throat disease, which ends fatal; has*: **SABAD**. *Delusion* rubric: *emaciation; of*: sabad. *Delusion* rubric: *sick: being*: *Sabad*. *Delusion* rubric: *withering, body is*: sabad. *Delusion* rubric: *faint; he would*: sabad.

Stannum is a homoeopathic remedy derived from tin. The theme within the metal remedies is mental stimulation. *Stannum* have abundant ideas, but they are not able to control their ideas.

The mental debility is marked in *Stannum*. *Stannum* feel unable to complete anything in their life. *Stannum* are overwhelmed by their own mental stimulation. Their ideas cause disintegration.

Stannum have many *illusions* of *fancy* but they lack the ability to be able to sustain their energy. *Stannum* have the *Mind* rubrics: *undertaking many things, persevering in nothing*, and *ailments from writing*. [1] 3. *Stannum* have several *Mind* rubrics which all confirm instability – *fear of spending money in order not to be short of it in the future* [1] 3., *praying timidly* [1] 1., *begging in sleep* [1] 1., *jumps out of bed from fear* [1] 3., *weeping feels like crying all the time but it makes her worse*. [1] 1. *Stannum* lack stamina; not only do they struggle with the practicalities of living, they are overwhelmed by their own feelings and thoughts. The simillimum will only be *Stannum* if the patient shows evidence of not being able to enact change in their lives. *Stannum* have the *Delusion* rubrics: *objects too far off, distances are enlarged* and *rush of ideas prevented him from completing his work*. *Stannum* are overwhelmed by everything in their lives, everything is too hard to achieve and everything is unattainable. The simillimum will only be *Stannum* if the patient has totally fallen [*fainted*] into their resigned predictions of illness and impending death. *Stannum* have no *Delusion* rubrics allocated to Forsaken or Causation. The simillimum will not be *Stannum* if the patient presents with psychological delusions of being abandoned or psychological delusions of exaggerated guilt.

Stannum fully embrace predictions of decline, they do not transfer their abandonment of health on to others.

1. Denial: *Delusion* rubric: *fancy, illusions of:* stann.
2. Forsaken: NONE.
3. Causation: NONE.
4. Depression: *Delusion* rubric: *objects; about: far off; too:* stann. *Delusion* rubric: *emptiness; of:* stann. *Delusion* rubric: *enlarged: distances are:* stann. [These rubrics should not taken literally. They allude to everything being unattainable.] *Delusion* rubric: *visions of fire.* [This rubric should not be taken literally. Patients who are overwhelmed with *visions of fire* suffer from predictions of impending doom.] *Delusion* rubric: *afternoon, it is always:* stann. [1] 2. [This rubric should not be interpreted literally. *Stannum* are physically exhausted by the afternoon. This rubric indicates a foreboding of exhaustion.]
5. Resignation: *Delusion* rubric: *disease: incurable disease; he has an*; Stann. *Delusion* rubric: *ideas: rush of ideas prevented him from completing his work:* stann. [1] 1. [This rubric confirms physical decline from mental excitement. Therefore it should be allocated to Resignation.] *Delusion* rubric: *faint; he would:* stann.

Xanthoxylum desert their own body [*floating in air*] and their own body deserts them; they would rather die than live. *Xanthoxylum* have numerous depression rubrics which perpetuate predictions of decline. *Xanthoxylum* literally feel like they fall to pieces and sink into their bed.

The simillimum will be only *Xanthoxylum* if the patient fully embraces predictions of decline. *Xanthoxylum* want to die because they do not have enough mental and emotional energy to desire life.

Xanthoxylum (the homoeopathic remedy) is derived from the Prickly Ash tree (*Zanthoxylum americanum*). If the fruit of the plant is rubbed on the skin (especially on the lips and face) it has a numbing effect. The pulverized root and bark chewed has been used as a cure for toothache. The fruits are considered more active than the bark, they are also antispasmodic, carminative, and excellent for rheumatic pain. *Xanthoxylum* as a homoeopathic remedy is commonly used for neuralgic pain, spinal disorders, nerve numbness and headaches, especially associated with dysmenorrhea. Boericke notes that the remedy is for mental depression.

Xanthoxylum (constitutionally) carry within their psyche a numbing unresponsiveness to life. *Xanthoxylum* would rather sink into decline and die, than make the choice to live.

Xanthoxylum are the only remedy listed in two *Delusion* rubrics: *floor was soft like walking on wool,* and *while walking, the ground is soft like wool. Xanthoxylum* feel thwarted in life, they feel like they are unable to make a mark in the world [*like walking on wool*]. The simillimum will be only *Xanthoxylum* if the patient displays evidence of extreme depressive weakness across all levels – emotionally, mentally, and physically.

1. Denial: *Delusion* rubric: *floating: air, in*: xan. [This rubric indicates a 'Dissociative Disorder'.] *Delusion* rubric: *floating: air, in: sitting; when*: xan. [1] 1.

2. Forsaken: NONE.

3. Causation: NONE.

4. Depression: *Delusion* rubric: *bewildered; he is*: xan. [1] 1. *Delusion* rubric: *die: rather die than live; one would*: xan. [1] 1. *Delusion* rubric: *bed: sinking: she is sinking; down deep in bed*: xan. *Delusion* rubric: *decline; is going into a: Xan.* [2] 1. *Delusion* rubric: *walking: wool on walking; floor was soft like*: xan. [This rubric indicates that the patient feels unable 'to make their mark in life'.] *Delusion* rubric: *falling: forward: is falling forward; she*: xan. [This rubric should not be interpreted literally, it pertains to predictions of failure.]

5. Resignation: *Delusion* rubric: *die*: *about to die*; *one was*:
    Xan. *Delusion* rubric: *die*: *rather die than live; one would*:
    xan. [1] 1. *Delusion* rubric: *dying*: *he is*: xan. *Delusion* rubric:
    head: *divided; is*; xan. *Delusion* rubric: *body*: *pieces*: *falling
    to pieces; body is*: xan. *Delusion* rubric: *body*: *lighter than
    air; body is*: xan. *Delusion* rubric: *enlarged*: *body is*: xan.

    • *Delusions: sick, being*: ambr. arg-n. *Ars*. asar. bar-c. bell. *Calc*.
      caust. cham. chel. cic. *Colch*. graph. hell. *Iod*. *Kali-c*. lac-c. laur.
      led. *Lyc*. merc. mosch. murx. naja. nat-c. nat-m. nit-ac. nux-m.
      Nux-v. petr. phos. podo. psor. *Puls*. *Sabad*. sel. sep. spig. spong.
      Staph. stram. tarax. *Tarent*. valer. verat.

Self deluding: The exaggerated belief that one is sick can be
maintained and nurtured for varying reasons. The homoeopath
looking at a case analysis has to be able to understand why
it is advantageous for the patient to maintain the belief that
they will always be sick. One reason that the psychological
delusional stance is maintained by the patient is that they lack
the 'delusions of grandeur' in their psyche which would enable
them to avoid anxiety and hypochondria. Secondly, if there are
inconsistencies between Stage one and Stage five then there
will always be evidence of internal discord which will either
accelerate the present pathology of hypochondria or precede
future obsessive health anxieties.

Colchicum have numerous persecutory *Delusion* rubrics:
sees insects, sees mice, sees rats, and *someone under the
bed*. Given that they have so many persecutory fears it is
questionable whether their *illusions of fancy* and their *illusions
of hearing* indicate hubristic visions or paranoiac illusions.
Colchicum have no *Delusion* rubrics pertaining to personal
blame.

Their internal distress is not coming from within. *Colchicum* have several
Mind rubrics which indicate that they are overwhelmed by others who are
upsetting their equilibrium. *Colchicum* are a very sensitive remedy profile.

Colchicum have the *Mind* rubrics: *ailments from the rudeness of others, insanity from intolerable pain*, and *fear of being touched*. Because *Colchicum* are lacking in psychological 'delusions of grandeur' they are easily dismissive of themselves and consequently they are also easily overwhelmed by others. *Colchicum* have the *Mind* rubrics: *indifference, does not complain unless questioned, says nothing of his condition* [1] 1., and *indifference, aversion to answer, says nothing when questioned.* [2] 1. *Colchicum* as a homoeopathic remedy is commonly used for the treatment of gout; it is especially applicable to the patient who is so overwhelmed by the pain they cannot move. *Colchicum* (the homoeopathic remedy) is derived from *Colchicum autumnale* which is highly toxic and fatal. The symptoms of poisoning have been compared to arsenic because the victim experiences paralysis of all organs.

Within the psyche of all homoeopathic remedies which are derived from poisonous or toxic substances is fear of annihilation, and powerlessness in the face of illness. *Colchicum* are overwhelmed by outside influences. *Colchicum* sees attacks coming from all directions. The simillimum will only be *Colchicum* if the patient shows signs (across all levels) of paralytic helplessness in the face of presenting health conditions.

1. Denial: NONE. [*Delusion* rubric: *fancy, illusions of*: colch. *Delusion* rubric: *hearing: illusions of*: colch. Both of these rubrics are more likely to reflect persecutory visions than 'hubristic illusions' of grandeur.]

2. Forsaken: *Delusion* rubric: *bed: someone under the bed; someone is*: colch. *Delusion* rubric: *insects, sees*: colch. *Delusion* rubric: *rats, sees*: colch. *Delusion* rubric: *mice: sees*: colch.

3. Causation: NONE.

4. Depression: *Delusion* rubric: *insane*: become insane; one will: colch.

5. Resignation: *Delusion* rubric: *sick: being*: Colch.

Iodum have inconsistencies between Stage one and Stage five which is evidence of internal discord; that discord accelerates the externalized destructive pathology that is associated with *Iodum*.

1. Denial: *Delusion* rubric: *well, he is*: *Iod*.

   Versus

5. Resignation: *Delusion* rubric: *sick*: *being*: *Iod*.

Iodum have the psychological delusion that they are a *great person*. The value of understanding the five stages within the rubric-repertorisation is that it will immediately highlight *peculiar* weaknesses. *Iodum* are overwhelmed by their fear of falling sick.

Iodum have the *Mind* rubrics: *disgust oneself, must check twice or more*, and *says he is well when very sick* – all of these rubrics indicate obsessive unstableness. *Iodum* fear that they will become insane. If such stark inconsistencies exist between Stage one and Stage five, it immediately highlights instability in the remedy profile. Psychological discord in their psyche between grandeur and failure [*insanity*] means that *Iodum* cannot afford to rest or sit still within themselves. *Iodum* are noted for frightful thoughts when they are forced to sit still. *Iodum* have the *Delusion* rubric: *one will become insane*, and the *Mind* rubric: *fear of insanity he must always move if he wants to repose* (rest). [1] 2. [ars.]. *Iodum* have no *Delusion* rubrics for self-blame. *Iodum* have five *Mind* rubrics relating to an impulsive need to kill, especially an *irresistible impulse and desire to kill a woman*. [2] 1. Noted within the typical psychotic persona are the classic fears of society; those fears justify their need to protect themselves by impulsive desires to kill.

Iodum have the *Mind* rubric: *aversion to being approached by people*, and *morbid impulse to do violence*. *Iodum* will only be the simillimum if the patient forcefully denies that they are sick. *Iodum* will only be the simillimum if the patient forcefully denies that they are sick, and if they have no guilt over any aspect of their life. The psychotic personality type denies guilt for sins committed and always needs to pretend that they are perfect [*says he is well when very sick*].

Iodum have the *Delusion* rubric: *is a great person*. If there is an inconsistency between Stage one and Stage five there has to be evidence of destructive psychotic behavior which will always be the precursor to physical illness.

1. Denial: *Delusion* rubric: *fancy, illusions of*: iod. *Delusion* rubric: *great person, is a*: iod. *Delusion* rubric: *well, he is*: Iod.

2. Forsaken: *Delusion* rubric: *dead persons, sees*: iod. *Delusion* rubric: *iodine; illusions of fumes of*: iod. [1] 1. [The homoeopath should not assume that this rubric is literally reflective of the substance from which the homoeopathic remedy is derived. It is a persecutory *Delusion* rubric.]

3. Causation: NONE.

4. Depression: *Delusion* rubric: *insane: become insane; one will*: iod.

5. Resignation: *Delusion* rubric: *sick: being*: Iod. *Delusion* rubric: *falling; walking; when if she walks*: iod. [1] 2. [calc]. [This rubric implies physical weakness.]

Tarentula hispanica[75] is a homoeopathic remedy derived from the spider *Lycosa tarantula*. Although *Tarentula hispanica* have the *Delusion* rubrics: *illusions of fancy,* and *religious* listed in Denial, they have *so many Delusion* rubrics of being attacked and persecuted that their presentation is overwhelmingly one of fear of being persecuted. The *Delusion* rubrics *religious, illusions of fancy,* and *visions* are rubrics which pertain more to superstitious self-protection than to self-empowerment or 'delusions of grandeur' rubrics. Their continual insecurity about their safety predisposes *Tarentula hispanica* to exhaustion and illness.

Tarentula hispanica present in a highly anxious state when they are sick. They are convinced that they will be rejected[76] [*persecuted*] by society when they are sick. The *Delusion* rubrics: *legs cut off* and *body is smaller* should be taken literally; they are a true representation of the somatic dilemma of powerless that overwhelms *Tarentula hispanica.*

Ironically, *Tarentula hispanica* have the *Mind* rubric: *feigning fainting* [1] 1., and *feigning to be sick.* [2]. My aim in presenting the five psychological stages is to highlight inconsistencies which could explain and highlight *peculiarities* within each remedy profile. All psychological delusions are maintained because they serve a purpose. The *Lycosa tarantula* spider does not spin a web as a snare but as a subterfuge to hide behind as it waits for prey to walk past its burrow. The first symptom reported after being bitten is a state of depression and lethargy which the sufferer will usually only come out of if they are roused by music and dance. The Materia medica presentations of *Tarentula hispanica* often concentrate on their erratic, high energy behavior and their need for, and love of music and dancing. If the homoeopath is looking for *Tarentula hispanica* to present with this picture then they will miss the predominant picture of *Tarentula hispanica.*

When sick, *Tarentula hispanica* are more likely to present with depressive psychological 'delusions of persecution' and an overwhelming fear of people.

The confusing dilemma inherent in all psychological delusional states is *why* a patient would maintain the delusional perception.

Tarentula hispanica have no *Delusion* rubrics of self-blame, therefore the simillimum will not be *Tarentula hispanica* if the patient looks internally into their own consciousness for their contribution to their predicament. *Tarentula hispanica* project all of their 'persecution complexes' outwards on to others. *Tarentula hispanica* feign sickness and maintain their psychological 'delusions of hypochondria' because it allows them to project all blame outwards on to others who have persecuted them.

The homoeopath working with a *Tarentula hispanica* patient should be alerted to the fact that they do not *want* to become well. *Tarentula hispanica* choose to maintain their 'delusions of hypochondria' because it allows them to remain hidden from self-responsibility.

The one Denial rubric which is indicative of the dissociative avoidance inherent within *Tarentula hispanica* is the *Delusion* rubric: *floating in air*. Within the psyche of all the homoeopathic remedies derived from poisonous substances or poisonous venom is fear of annihilation. This is also true for *Tarentula hispanica*. What is also inherent within the psyche is the same escape hatch that is inherent within the cure of poisoning from the *Lycosa tarantula* spider. I stated above that the first symptom reported after being bitten is a state of depression and lethargy which the sufferer will usually only come out of if they are roused by music and dance. *Tarentula hispanica* similarly disassociate by *floating into air*. I have come to understand this through working psychotherapeutically with *Tarentula hispanica* patients.

Tarentula hispanica feign illness and *feign fainting* and *need* sickness because it helps them hysterically rouse themselves out of crippling persecutory depression. *Tarentula hispanica* will only be the simillimum if there is evidence that the patient hysterically [*insanity*] enjoys reverting to sickness and ill health.

The trap the homoeopath can fall into when treating *Tarentula hispanica* is to presume that they have the wrong remedy because the patient has *feigned sickness*. Illness allows *Tarentula hispanica* to elevate their mood [*floating into air*] when they fear annihilation. Within *Tarentula hispanica* is a symbiosis between psychological 'delusions of persecution', 'delusions of hypochondria', and 'delusions of grandeur'.

1. Denial: *Delusion* rubric: *religious*: tarent. *Delusion* rubric: *fancy, illusions of*. Tarent. *Delusion* rubric: *visions, has*:

tarent. *Delusion* rubric: *floating air, in*: *Tarent.*

2. Forsaken: *Delusion* rubric: *assaulted, is going to be*: tarent. *Delusion* rubric: *figures: seeing figures*: tarent. *Delusion* rubric: *fall; something would*: *him; on:* tarent. [1] 2. *Delusion* rubric: *insulted, he is*: tarent. *Delusion* rubric: *persecuted: he is persecuted*: tarent. *Delusion* rubric: *visions, has: horrible*: tarent. *Delusion* rubric: *unseen things; delusions of*: tarent. [1] 1. *Delusion* rubric: *faces, sees: diabolical faces crowd up on him*: tarent. *Delusion* rubric: *voices: hearing*: tarent.

3. Causation: NONE.

4. Depression: *Delusion* rubric: *insane: become insane; one is*: tarent.

5. Resignation: *Delusion* rubric: *sick; being*: *Tarent.* *Delusion* rubric: *legs: cut off; legs are*: tarent. *Delusion* rubric: *small: body is smaller*: tarent.

- *Delusions: body: continuity of body would be dissolved*: thuj.[1] 1.
- *Delusions: body: pieces: coming in pieces; body is in danger of*: thuj. [1] 1.
- *Delusions: dissolving, she is*: aids. neon. olib-sac.
- *Delusions: body: absent; is*: cocain. germ-met. ozone.
- *Delusions: diminished; all is*: cann-i. cinnm. grat. hydrog. irid-met. lac-c. sabad. sulph.
- *Delusions: body: diminished; is*: agar. falco-pe.
- *Delusions: body: delicate, is*: *Thuj.* [2] 1.
- *Delusions: body, disintegrating*: *Lach.* marb-w.
- *Delusions: legs: glass; were made of*: *Thuj.* [2] 1.
- *Delusions: body: brittle, is*: falco-pe. gard-j. ign. lac-leo. nux-v. sars. seq-s. stram. *Thuj.*
- *Delusions: existence: longer; she cannot exist any*: thuj. [1] 1.
- *Delusions: emaciation; of*: *Anh.* nat-m. sabad. sulph. thuj.
- *Delusions: body: thin; is*: limest-b. thuj.

- *Delusions: light[77]: is light; he:* agar. agath-a. ara-maca. *Asar.* bit-ar. camph. cann-i. chin. chir-fl. coca-c. *Coff. Croc.* dendr-pol. dig. eup-pur. falco-pe. gels. hippoc-k. ignis-alc. lac-c. lac-leo. lac-lup. lach. lact-v. lact. manc. mez. mim-p. musca-d. neon. op. ozone. petr-ra. phos. pieri-b. *Plut-n.* puls. rhus-g. *Stict.* stram. tep. thuj. valer. zinc.

- *Delusions: emptiness[78]; of:* am-c. *Calad.* cann-i. **COCC.** Gels. germ-met. *Ign.* irid-met. *Kali-c. Kola.* lac-loxod-a. *Mur-ac.* oena. ol-eur. *Olnd.* ozone. petr-ra. *Plat.* plut-n. **PULS.** sars. **SEP.** stann. stry. *Sulph. Zing.*

- *Delusions: hollow: body is hollow; whole:* aur. *Kali-c.* oncor-t. pall.

- *Delusions: body: lighter than air[79]; body is:* asar. galla-q-r. ignis-alc. irid-met. lac-loxod-a. lac-lup. lach. limest-b. olib-sac. *Op.* psil. sanguis-s. thuj. visc. xan.

- *Delusions: weight: no weight; has:* cann-i. hyos. op.

Self-deluding: These *Delusion* rubrics indicate that each remedy profile suffers from the delusional belief that they are fragile.

The *Delusion* rubrics: *body diminished, body absent,* and *body brittle,* are examples of exaggerated predictions of decay which emphasize the threat that the world poses. The homoeopath needs to understand what the patient is lacking which causes them to believe that they will no longer be able to exist because they are too *hollow, thin, weak* or *delicate.*

Cocainum have the sensation of feeling absent from the world. The *Delusion* rubric: *body is absent,* indicates exaggerated self-abandonment. The Denial rubric for *Cocainum* – *floating in the air,* also indicates a desire to abandon reality.

The *Delusion* rubrics for *Cocainum* all indicate a self-protective pathology which is advantageously maintained to protect the patient from the harshness of reality.

The reason I have chosen to discuss the remedy profile of

Cocainum in the rubrics pertaining to 'delusions of hypochondria' is that it is not uncommon for a patient who is suffering from a potentially life threatening disease to present in a *Cocainum* state.

When someone finds out that they have a serious illness, it is normal for them to feel that their body has abandoned them [*body is absent*]. It is also normal to want to abandon reality and pretend that they are not sick – "this is not happening to me". When someone finds out that they have a serious illness, it is normal for them to find their thoughts alternating between believing they will be cured, and the very next minute morbidly dwelling on imagining their death.

Cocainum alternate between imagining cure, and persecutory anger; in both states their aim is to avoid the reality of being sick.

It has been reported to me by my patients that the effect of consuming cocaine (the drug from which the homoeopathic remedy is derived) is that they feel socially confident and self-important. *Cocainum* have the *Mind* rubric: *sensation as if he could do great deeds.* [2] 3. *Cocainum,* when faced with illness, abandon reality by *floating off* into fanciful illusions of grandiose cure. They also abandon their body or feel that their body has deserted [*absent*] them. *Cocainum* fixate on feeling undeservedly abandoned by others or feel undeservedly *persecuted* by their disease. The *Delusion* rubrics pertaining to disease resonate with *exaggerated* illusions of body decay. *Cocainum* have all the classic body illusions of being covered in worms and bugs. These are common hypochondriacal pathological fears which predominate in patients who feel attacked from inside and from outside of themselves by illness.

The simillimum will only be *Cocainum* if the patient is not willing to acknowledge personal guilt. The simillimum will not be *Cocainum* if the patient is depressed. *Cocainum* alternate between delusions of cure, and persecutory fears of attack from inside and from outside.

Cocainum maintain the psychological delusion that their *body is absent* because they prefer to either live in illusionary hope or persecutory anger.

I have observed in cocaine users that they present with either exaggerated perceptions of personal grandeur or persecutory fear or anger. The simillimum will only be *Cocainum* if the patient shows signs of wanting to avoid 'inhabiting their body'.

1. Denial: *Delusion* rubric: *visions, has*: cocain. *Delusion* rubric: *hearing: illusions of*: cocain. *Delusion* rubric: *floating: air, in*: cocain. [These all indicate 'Dissociative Disorders'.]

2. Forsaken: *Delusion* rubric: *abused, being*: cocain. *Delusion* rubric: *criticized, she is*: cocain. *Delusion* rubric: *persecuted*: he is persecuted: *Cocain*. *Delusion* rubric: *pursued; he was*: *enemies, by*: *Cocain*. *Delusion* rubric: *worms: covered with; he is*: cocain. [1] 1. *Delusion* rubric: *worms*: *Cocain*. [2] 1. *Delusion* rubric: *bugs; sees*: *Cocain*. [2] 1. *Delusion* rubric: *images, phantoms; sees*: *frightful*: cocain.

3. Causation: NONE.

4. Depression: NONE.

5. Resignation: *Delusion* rubric: *body: absent; is*: cocain.

Crocus is a homoeopathic remedy derived from the *Crocus sativus* herb which is the source of the dye and spice saffron. Vermeulen, in *Prisma,* draws a resemblance between the effects of opium and crocus – "In *small* quantities both exhilarate the mind, raise the passions, and invigorate the body; in *large* doses intoxication, languor, and stupor succeed this". *Crocus* and *Opium* share the *Mind* rubrics: *indifference to joy of others, ailments from excessive joy*, and *indifference to everything*. The profound difference is that *Crocus* have no *Delusion* rubrics pertaining to Causation or perceived sins. *Opium* have notable 'delusions of original sin'. (This aspect of the remedy profile of *Opium* is discussed in the chapter on Causation.) *Crocus* differs profoundly from *Opium* in that they have numerous *Mind* rubrics of religiosity, as well as the *Delusion* rubric: *religious*. *Crocus* feels remorseful shame, and anxiety of conscience, as distinct from guilt and self-blame. The aim of their remorse is to purify the soul, as distinct from *Opium* who need to annul their sins. The distinctive *Mind* rubrics (indicating anxiety of conscience) which differentiate between the two remedies are the *Mind* rubrics: *anger alternating with repentance, anxiety of conscience* and *anger followed by remorse.* [1] 1. *Crocus* repents quickly, whereas *Opium* have numerous 'delusions of grandeur' which allow them to avoid their multitude of sins. This distinction is significant.

Crocus diminish themselves because it reinforces their religious piety. *Crocus* will present in an exaggeratedly *small* and unworthy state when they are sick.

In the Denial chapter I comment on the fact that *Opium* are often attracted to Tibetan Buddhism. The same can be said for *Crocus*. 'Delusional piety', and the resonance of the saffron robes of a pious monk repenting for their anger and rage is the picture I associate with *Crocus*.

Peculiar to *Crocus* are the *Delusion* rubrics: *she is pregnant* and *animals in abdomen*. Both of these rubrics are associated with 'delusions of hypochondria'. False pregnancy (pseudocyesis, or what is most commonly termed 'phantom pregnancy' in humans) is the appearance of clinical and or sub-clinical signs and symptoms associated with a pregnancy, when the patient is not pregnant. An intense desire to become pregnant, and/or an intense fear of becoming pregnant, can create internal delusional conflict states. *Crocus* have an internal conflict of 'delusional piety'. It is wrong to think that the *Delusion* rubrics: *she is pregnant* and *animals in abdomen* should only be used in case analysis for the patient with pseudocyesis. The *Mind* rubric: *anger followed by remorse,* and *rage followed by remorse,* and the *Delusion* rubric: *religious,* all indicate exaggerated 'delusional piety' and purity.

A need to remain *pure* and pious in the mind creates a conflicting need to remain *pure* and pious in the body. The *Delusion* rubric: *body is smaller* is applicable to *Crocus* because they have an intense fear of becoming pregnant. *Crocus* have religious purity.

They are a pure monk or nun in saffron robes; this is why they need to appear in a small diminished state, *unfit for business* and unworthy of any life other than a religious life. *Crocus* have the *Mind* rubric: *religious affections, too occupied with religion,* and *religious affections, want of religious feeling.* 'Delusional piety' will create internal conflict and remorse. *Crocus* need to maintain the delusional perception that their body is small and light to avoid their fear of being pregnant. *Crocus* also maintain the perception that their *body is smaller* and they are *light* so they can reinforce their religious piety. *Crocus* have a symbiotic relationship between their 'delusions of grandeur' and their 'delusions of hypochondria'.

The simillimum will only be *Crocus* if the patient desires religious purity and shows evidence of needing to maintain the perception that they are small. Patients who believe that they are more 'spiritual' when they are small and light are vulnerable to developing anorexia. I have previously prescribed *Crocus* to a patient suffering from anorexia who was starting to lose her cognitive processing. *Crocus* have the *Delusion* rubric: *thoughts would suddenly vanish.* Within 'New-Age' spiritualism there is a perception that if one is *small and light* then one is more pious and 'spiritual'.

1. Denial: *Delusion* rubric: *fancy, illusions of:* croc. *Delusion* rubric: *religious:* croc. *Delusion* rubric: *music: thinks he hears:* croc.

2. Forsaken: *Delusion* rubric: *poisoned: he has been:* croc. *Delusion* rubric: *fire: visions of:* croc. *Delusion* rubric: *specters, ghosts, spirits: seeing:* Croc.

3. Causation: NONE.

4. Depression: *Delusion* rubric: *business: unfit for, he is:* Croc. [2] 1. *Delusion* rubric: *intoxicated: is; he:* croc. *Delusion* rubric: *thoughts: vanish: would suddenly vanish; as if thoughts:* croc.

5. Resignation: *Delusion* rubric: *small*: *body is smaller*: croc. *Delusion* rubric: *light*: *is light; he*: *Croc*. *Delusion* rubric: *animals*: *abdomen, are in*: *Croc*. *Delusion* rubric: *die*: *about to die; one was*: *Croc*. *Delusion* rubric: *pregnant, she is*: *Croc*.

Opium need to maintain the illusions and psychological delusions that they are in a beautiful heaven because it helps them avoid realism. *Opium* do not want to remain in a conscious mind state in which they allow themselves to acknowledge their real feelings. *Opium* do not want to acknowledge illness, especially an illness which is potentially life threatening. *Opium* is an extremely interesting constitutional remedy to consider for the psychological delusions that can overwhelm a patient when they are faced with predictions of death. It is not unusual that a patient, when presented with a diagnosis of a life threatening illness, will move into an *Opium* remedy profile. The homoeopathic remedy *Opium* is derived from the opium poppy. Morphine is the principal alkaloid of opium and is used most commonly for cancer sufferers. Morphine is the opiate analgesic which alters the central nervous system's perceptions of pain and emotional responses to pain. Morphine also produces changes in mood, including euphoria and drowsiness and mental cloudiness. The history of the opium poppy as a narcotic which allows the user to elevate themselves above the worldly pain of their everyday worries and grief of living is well documented. Ironically, this exalted euphoric state is similarly experienced when someone is faced with death.

It is not unusual for patients with cancer to present in a heightened state of meditative euphoria in which they are appreciating every leaf on the trees and reveling in every experience of living.

In the Tibetan tradition, meditation practice is most commonly obscured by two obstacles. One obstacle to meditation is dullness, the grossest form of which is falling asleep while mediating, while its most subtle form is allowing your mind to stay in a pleasant feeling of relaxation. The other obstacle to meditation is allowing your mind to be distracted by continual busy thoughts. The busyness can also manifest as euphoric meditative experiences which divert your mind from mindfulness. Both states of mind, sleepiness or dullness, and busyness or heightened euphoria, are an avoidance of conscious feeling or 'mindful awareness'. *Opium* similarly alternate between two states of mind: either a sleepy, pleasant nothingness or an excited, euphoric mental *agility*. Commonly, the majority of cancer sufferers delve into meditation as part of the experience of having cancer and dying from cancer. Quite often the patient will describe the experience of meditation as "euphoric". The patient will report that the experience of having cancer has heightened their perception of life and that everything is now much more meaningful and rich. In fact, when they become well or move into remission they often reminisce about the heightened experience that they had when they were sick. The underlying fear which they are often trying desperately to avoid acknowledging is the fear that they are dying.

Opium are fearful of death. This fear can become a delusional state in which *Opium* become paranoid and obsessive about the doctors and the medical system wanting to poison them with radiotherapy and chemotherapy drugs. *Opium* have the *Delusion* rubric: *he is poisoned* and *about to receive injury*. *Opium* are fearful of acknowledging all mindful reality.

Opium are listed in all the *Mind* rubrics: *ailments from fright, grief, homelessness, reprimands, mental shock* and even *sudden joy*. *Opium* have the *Mind* rubric: *indifference to joy and the suffering of others*. *Opium* also have the *Mind* rubrics: *ailments from joy* and *ailments from grief*. Their 'delusions of grandeur' and their belief that they are beautiful allows *Opium* to escape into a state which is *lighter than air*. *Opium* have the *Mind* rubric: *blissful feeling* and the *Delusion* rubric: *body is lighter than air. Opium* do not want to *feel. Opium* avoid conscious feeling or 'mindful awareness'.

Opium choose to delude themselves that they are *beautiful* and in *heaven* to avoid the harshness of the world. On the one hand they have psychological delusions that they are *well*, and on the other hand they have psychological delusions that they are *dying*.

A dying patient often feels that their heightened perceptions have created a blissful, God-like beauty which has penetrated their whole being. Dying patients often tell me that they think they emanate euphoria physically which assures them and their loved ones that they are cured. I have also noted that my patients' family and friends view their loved one as beautiful and blissful and God-like in their dying and death. I, on the other hand, see a body racked by pain and starvation. There is a contradiction between Denial and Resignation in *Opium. Opium* have the *Mind* rubric: *fear of death* and *desires death. Opium* have the *Mind* rubric: *contempt of death.* [2] 1. and the *Delusion* rubric: *he is dying*, and *he is well,* and *beautiful.* Inconsistencies within the remedy profile are always indicative of delusional conflict and destructive pathology.

The simillimum will only be *Opium* if the patient has a strong need to abandon their body so they can pretend they are merged with 'a higher energy'.

Vermeulen says in *Prisma* that *Opium* "withdraw into an inner world". My aim is to explain the psychological patterning of each remedy profile so that the homoeopath is able to match the concept of "withdrawal" to a patient's behavior. *Opium* will not acknowledge that they are sick.

The *Opium* patient will deny they are dying; in fact they will embrace meditation and having cancer because it has embellished them with experiences of heightened euphoria about living [*is under superhuman control*].

It will not be until death threatens that the homoeopath will see the converse profile of *Opium. Opium* have the *Delusion* rubric: *being double, there is another self and he is not sure which will conquer the other.* [1] 1. It is not until death threatens that *Opium* are forced into the position that they have to face reality. It is only then that the homoeopath will see the persecutory delusions [*poisoned*] and withdrawn, depressive, impending *doom* that *Opium* are renowned for.

Inconsistencies:

1. Denial: *Delusion* rubric: *well, he is*: op.

    Versus

5. Resignation: *Delusion* rubric: *dying*: *he is*: op.

Opium need to maintain their illusions and psychological delusions of being in a beautiful heaven because they have intense 'persecution complexes' and numerous psychological 'delusions of original sin' which are discussed in further detail in the chapter on Causation.

1. Denial: *Delusion* rubric: *beautiful*: op. *Delusion* rubric: *heaven, is in*: op. *Delusion* rubric: *visions, has beautiful*: **OP**. *Delusion* rubric: *superhuman; is control*: *is under superhuman*: op. *Delusion* rubric: *laughter, with*: op. *Delusion* rubric: *pleasing delusions*: op. *Delusion* rubric: *visions, has*: *fantastic*: op. *Delusion* rubric: *well, he is*: op. *Delusion* rubric: *body*: *lighter than air; body is*: *Op*. [This rubric can be allocated to Denial or Resignation. *Opium* use the perception that they are light to avoid bonding with the 'heaviness' of the world. Alternatively, this rubric can indicate physical weakness.]

2. Forsaken: *Delusion* rubric: *execute him; people want to*: **OP**. *Delusion* rubric: *poisoned: he, has been*: op. *Delusion* rubric: *home*: *away from home; he is*: *Op*. *Delusion* rubric: *injury*: *about to receive injury; is*: *Op*. *Delusion* rubric: *accidents*: *sees accidents*: op. *Delusion* rubric: *skeletons, sees*: op. *Delusion* rubric: *scorpions, sees*: **OP**. [3] 1. *Delusion* rubric: *rats, sees*: op. *Delusion* rubric: *snakes*: *in and around her*: op. *Delusion* rubric: *visions, has*: *horrible*:

op. *Delusion* rubric: *visions, has: monsters, of:* op. *Delusion* rubric: *soldiers: seeing:* op. *Delusion* rubric: *disorder; objects appear in:* op. [1] 2. [glon]

3. Causation: *Delusion* rubric: *criminal; he is a: executed, to be:* **OP.** [3] 1. *Delusion* rubric: *visions, has: horrible:* op. *Delusion* rubric: *wrong: done wrong; he has:* op. *Delusion* rubric: *possessed; being:* op. *Delusion* rubric: *superhuman; is control: is under superhuman:* op. *Delusion* rubric: *wrong: done wrong; he has: punished; and is about to be:* op. [1] 1. *Delusion* rubric: *criminal, he is a:* op.

4. Depression: *Delusion* rubric: *doomed, being:* op. *Delusion* rubric: *drugged; as if:* op.

5. Resignation: *Delusion* rubric: *body: lighter than air; body is:* Op. *Delusion* rubric: *weight: no weight; has:* op. *Delusion* rubric: *brain: smoke on brain:* op. [1] 1. *Delusion* rubric: *dying: he is:* op. *Delusion* rubric: *enlarged: body is:* op. *Delusion* rubric: *visions, has: coma vigil; in:* Op. [2] 1.

Ozonum fluctuate between the contradictory states of powerful grandeur and failure. The pathology inherent in the contrast between euphoria and emptiness is in the nature of the substance that the homoeopathic remedy is derived from.

Vermeulen, in his *Synoptic Materia medica 2,* writes the following: "The ozone layer, protecting life against harmful solar radiation, is located at a height of 20-50 kilometres above the earth's surface. Ozone produced in the lower atmosphere by industry and car exhaust is a pollutant. It damages crops and may be linked to breathing disorders. Destruction of the ozone layer would result in higher levels of ultraviolet radiation reaching the Earth's surface, which would in turn result in an increased incidence of skin cancer among persons exposed to sunlight. Ozone and water vapor in the atmosphere absorb solar radiation, and the heating and expansion of air that results are the major determinants of the oscillations in the atmosphere.

Thinning of the ozone layer contributes to the greenhouse effect, a global warming trend caused by rising levels of atmospheric carbon dioxide." These two opposing states are present within the remedy profile of *Ozonum*: they sit above it all secure in the atmosphere, but underneath the *euphoria* of the atmospheric layer is a layer of self-destruction. If there are contradictions and inconsistencies in the rubric-repertorisation then there is inner conflict which can be self-destructive as well as destructive to others. *Ozonum* have the *Mind* rubrics: *despair alternating with euphoria,* and *abusive, wishes others harm. Ozonum* are the only remedy listed in both rubrics. *Ozonum* will only be the simillimum if the patient shows internal self-destruction, as well as psychotic, destructive behavior towards others. *Ozonum* have the *Mind* rubrics: *indifference with a feeling of superiority,* and *indifference to the welfare of others. Ozonum* are once again the only remedy listed in both rubrics. *Ozonum* lack a *'heart'* for themselves as well as for others.

Ozonum are destructive. The self-destruction within *Ozonum* reflects the consequences of our modern day excesses on the ozone layer. *Ozonum* literally feel *choked* and abandoned by themselves. *Ozonum* have numerous *Delusion* rubrics all confirming that not only are they forsaken by society, but their body, heart, and mind will also abandon them. The simillimum will only be *Ozonum* if the patient is unable to recognize that their own excesses have caused them internal injury across all levels – emotionally, mentally and physically. *Ozonum* refuse to take responsibility for their internal abandonment [*emptiness*].

Ozonum can't afford to acknowledge their vulnerability because it would require them to give up their 'delusions of grandeur' that they are *powerful.* Generally speaking, the human race cannot acknowledge that we need to give up our excesses of living to protect our vulnerable ozone layer. The simillimum will only be *Ozonum* if the patient shows signs of psychotic behavior [*heart is absent*]. *Ozonum* are indifferent to their own *abyss* and indifferent to others. *Ozonum* are *connected to the devil and is arrogant towards those who strive for purity, light and love.* [1] 1.

1. Denial: *Delusion* rubric: *influence; one is under a powerful*: ozone. *Delusion* rubric: *floating*: *air, in*: ozone.

2. Forsaken: *Delusion* rubric: *forsaken; is*: ozone. *Delusion* rubric: *deceived; being*: ozone. *Delusion* rubric: *torture*: *tortured; he is*: ozone. [1] 1.

3. Causation: *Delusion* rubric: *devil*: *connected to devil, he is arrogant towards those who strive to purity, light and love*: ozone. [1] 1. *Delusion* rubric: *influence; one is under a powerful*: ozone. *Delusion* rubric: *heart*: *absent; is*: ozone. [1] 1. [This rubric can be allocated to Causation or Resignation. In Causation it pertains to alignment with the 'devil'. In Resignation it reflects self-abandonment.]

4. Depression: *Delusion* rubric: *road is long*: ozone. [1] 1. *Delusion* rubric: *succeed, he does everything wrong; he cannot*: ozone. *Delusion* rubric: *work*: *too much work; he has*: ozone. [1] 1. *Delusion* rubric: *abyss*: ozone. [1] 1. *Delusion* rubric: *snow blankets, sees black*: ozone. [1] 1. *Delusion* rubric: *emptiness; of*: ozone. [This rubric pertains to feelings of mental and emotional emptiness or, in Resignation, it pertains to abandonment and physical weakness.]

5. Resignation: *Delusion* rubric: *body*: *absent; is*: ozone. *Delusion* rubric: *emptiness; of*: ozone. *Delusion* rubric: *choked*: *he is about to be*: ozone. [1] 1. *Delusion* rubric: *strange*: *thing inside her*: ozone. [1] 1. *Delusion* rubric: *separated*: *body*: *mind are separated; body and*: ozone. *Delusion* rubric: *heart*: *absent; is*: ozone. [1] 1. *Delusion* rubric: *small*: *he is*: ozone.

Thuja: Mostly, I have successfully used the homoeopathic remedy *Thuja* to treat very simple cases of the wart virus in patients. *Thuja* have the *Mind* rubrics: *fear of others approaching them* and *insanity will not be touched*. Both of these are internal dialogues and responses one would expect from someone who has warts all over their hands or face. Warts on the face or hands can make people feel like they do not want to be touched or feel like they need to hide from society.

The underlying disturbance within the *Thuja* profile is fragility. *Thuja* have the *Delusion* rubrics: *the body is lighter than air, the body is delicate, body is brittle,* and *body is thin.* The *Delusion* rubrics: *their body will be dissolved* and *she can no longer exist* indicate a core disturbance underpinning *Thuja.*

Understanding the *Delusion* rubric: *body is dissolved* helped me understand the psychotherapeutic need in *Thuja* for the 'delusions of grandeur' which force them into believing they are *all powerful.* In a *Thuja* patient who consulted me, his fear of being eliminated was formed deep within his psyche when he was brutally attacked in his first sexual encounter. His first sexual encounter formed the primary 'never-well-since-event'. His crippling fear of being killed [*no longer exist*] every time he had sex in the future resulted in pre-emptive, self-protective erectile dysfunction. The self-deluding need to avoid his underlying fear of extinction created huge psychological 'delusions of grandeur'. He consulted me but left without taking a remedy because he believed that nothing was physically or mentally wrong with him. He also refused to take the homoeopathic remedy in case it changed him in some way.

Thuja fear attack. *Thuja* have the *Delusion* rubric: *body is in danger of coming in pieces.* [1] 1.

In the *Thuja* (case) written up in the *Case Companion* to *Homoeopathic Psychiatry*, the fear of no longer existing is the underlying psychological misrepresentation underpinning the development of the patient's Chronic Fatigue Syndrome and his mental and emotional breakdown later on in his life. His fear of being eliminated [*dissolved*] developed from the primary 'never-well-since-event' when he found out about nuclear extinction at a young age. His fear of nuclear extinction subsequently overwhelmed the patient with fear of his own extinction. A little while after finding out about nuclear extinction he was confronted with world poverty and starvation. He subsequently went on to develop food allergies as a child. The food allergies justified his reduced intake of food so he could become very *thin*. *Thuja* frequently develop psychosomatic empathic pathologies. *Thuja* have the *Delusion* rubric: *has lost the affection of a friend* – this rubric is reflective of a deep fear in *Thuja* of being *friendless* and isolated and *outcast*. As a result, *Thuja* often develop strong somatic empathic responses to others' suffering, especially animals. *Thuja* have the *Mind* rubric: *love for animals, and cats*. The development of the patient's Chronic Fatigue Syndrome developed from years of internal discord within himself.

Thuja have a profound contradiction between Stage one and Stage five. On the one hand *Thuja* manifest psychological 'delusions of grandeur' which allude to them being under God-like superhuman control, while on the other hand they have profoundly disabling psychological 'delusions of hypochondria' which cause them to feel that at any moment they will dissolve and die. The *Delusion* rubrics: *delicate*, *thin*, *about to die*, *diminished*, *disintegrating*, *emaciated*, are all examples of exaggerated predictions of physical decay.

The inconsistencies and contradictions between Stage one and Stage five in *Thuja* are evidence of self-deluding psychosis. Psychosis is a severe mental derangement involving the whole personality. Psychosis is the precursor to the destruction of 'ego' and involves a complete loss of contact with reality. *Thuja* need to believe they are all powerful to avoid their fears of extinction. Religious fanaticism is common in *Thuja*.

Thuja need a savior to save them from *diminishing*. *Thuja* have the *Mind* rubrics: *religious fanaticism, too occupied with religion, despair of religious salvation* and *reproaching oneself about one's own passion*. *Thuja* have the *Delusion* rubric: *is under superhuman control* and *she is all powerful*.

For the simillimum to be *Thuja* there has to evidence

that the patient is not aware of their own self-delusion. The psychological delusional stance of *Thuja* is locked in their unconscious mind. *Thuja* have the *Mind* rubric: *untruthful*. If *Thuja* are confronted in their conscious or sub-conscious mind with their underlying *disintegration* it will literally shatter a very *brittle* and fragile 'ego'. If *Thuja* are confronted by the homoeopath pointing out their denial, it will overwhelm them. I have experienced a few *Thuja* patients who have walked away from my consultations without taking the remedy because they did not think there was anything wrong with them. *Thuja* have the *Mind* rubric: *secretive*. [2].

In psychosis,[80] the mental derangement needs to remain hidden in the unconscious mind of the patient; to face the psychotic derangement would cause complete destruction. The simillimum will only be *Thuja* if the patient appears (to the homoeopath) mentally and emotionally fragile. *Thuja* will not believe *they* are fragile; they believe they are *powerful*. *Thuja* will acknowledge their physical fragility, but they will not acknowledge mental and emotional fragility.

1. Denial: *Delusion* rubric: *powerful: all powerful; she is*: thuj. *Delusion* rubric: *fancy, illusions of*: thuj. *Delusion* rubric: *superhuman; is: control; is under superhuman*: Thuj. [In relation to *Thuja* this rubric can be allocated to either God or the devil.]

2. Forsaken: *Delusion* rubric: *forsaken; is*: thuj. *Delusion* rubric: *appreciated, she is not*: Thuj. *Delusion* rubric: *friendless, he is*: Thuj. *Delusion* rubric: *outcast; she were an*: thuj.

3. Causation: *Delusion* rubric: *criminal; he is a*: thuj. *Delusion* rubric: *sinned; one has*: thuj.

4. Depression: *Delusion* rubric: *insane: he is insane*: Thuj. *Delusion* rubric: *worthless; he is*: thuj.

5. Resignation: *Delusion* rubric: *body: continuity of body would be dissolved*: thuj. [1] 1. *Delusion* rubric: *diminished: thin, he is too*: thuj. [1] 1. *Delusion* rubric: *body: pieces: coming in pieces; body is in danger of*: thuj. [1] 1. *Delusion*

rubric: *die: about to die; one was: Thuj. Delusion* rubric:
body: delicate, is: Thuj. [2] 1. *Delusion* rubric: *dirty, he is*:
thuj. *Delusion* rubric: *touched; he is: Thuj. Delusion* rubric:
flying: skin; out of his: thuj. [1] 1.

Inconsistencies:

1. Denial: *Delusion* rubric: *powerful: all powerful; she is*: thuj.

   Versus

5. Resignation: *Delusion* rubric: *body: delicate, is: Thuj.* [2] 1.

I have listed below an extensive list of rubrics which are
reflective of 'ego' disintegration. *Thuja* have numerous *Mind*
rubrics which reflect the same internal discord, for example:
disgust with his own body, aversion to be touched, and *always
washing her hands*. The psychotic patient can also develop
delusional disorders, disorganized thinking, hallucinations,
illusions, or paranoid delusional states.

- *Delusion* rubric: *bed: touch the bed when lying; as if she
  did not*: thuj.
- *Delusion* rubric: *body: brittle, is: Thuj.*
- *Delusion* rubric: *body: continuity of body would be dissolved*:
  thuj. [1] 1.
- *Delusion* rubric: *body: delicate, is: Thuj.* [2] 1.
- *Delusion* rubric: *body: immaterial, is*: thuj.
- *Delusion* rubric: *body: lighter than air; body is*: thuj.
- *Delusion* rubric: *body: pieces: coming in pieces; body is in
  danger of*: thuj.
- *Delusion* rubric: *body: ugly; body looks: Thuj.*
- *Delusion* rubric: *die: about to die; one was: Thuj.*
- *Delusion* rubric: *die: time has come to*: thuj.
- *Delusion* rubric: *diminished: thin, he is too*: thuj. [1] 1.
- *Delusion* rubric: *dirty: he is*: thuj.
- *Delusion* rubric: *divided: two parts; into*: thuj.
- *Delusion* rubric: *divided: two parts; into: which part he has*

possession on waking; and could not tell of: thuj. [1] 1.

- *Delusion* rubric: *double: being:* thuj.
- *Delusion* rubric: *emaciation; of:* thuj.
- *Delusion* rubric: *existence: longer; she cannot exist any:* thuj. [1] 1.
- *Delusion* rubric: *falling: height; from a: Thuj.*
- *Delusion* rubric: *feet: touch scarcely the ground: walking; when:* thuj.
- *Delusion* rubric: *floating: air, in:* thuj.
- *Delusion* rubric: *flying: skin; out of his:* thuj. [1] 1.
- *Delusion* rubric: *friendless, he is: Thuj.*
- *Delusion* rubric: *glass*[81]*: she is made of:* thuj.
- *Delusion* rubric: *glass: wood, glass, etc.; being made of: Thuj.*
- *Delusion* rubric: *ground: touch the ground; she would hardly:* thuj.
- *Delusion* rubric: *head: belongs to another:* thuj.
- *Delusion* rubric: *heavy; is:* thuj.
- *Delusion* rubric: *identity: errors of personal identity:* thuj.
- *Delusion* rubric: *influence; one is under a powerful:* thuj.
- *Delusion* rubric: *insane: he is insane: Thuj.*
- *Delusion* rubric: *intoxicated: is; he:* thuj.
- *Delusion* rubric: *legs: glass; were made of: Thuj.* [2] 1.
- *Delusion* rubric: *light: is light; he:* thuj.
- *Delusion* rubric: *move: he moves: to and fro; he moves: sitting and lying; when:* thuj. [1] 1.
- *Delusion* rubric: *outcast; she were an:* thuj.
- *Delusion* rubric: *people: beside him; people are:* thuj.
- *Delusion* rubric: *person: present; someone is:* thuj.
- *Delusion* rubric: *poisoned: he: has been:* thuj.
- *Delusion* rubric: *pursued; he was:* thuj.

- *Delusion* rubric: *seat: moving; seat is: to and fro*: thuj. [1] 1.
- *Delusion* rubric: *separated: body: mind are separated; body and*: thuj.
- *Delusion* rubric: *separated: body: soul; body is separated from*: thuj.
- *Delusion* rubric: *separated: world; from the: he is separated*: thuj.
- *Delusion* rubric: *strange: familiar things seem strange*: thuj.
- *Delusion* rubric: *strangers: seeing: Thuj.*
- *Delusion* rubric: *thin: body is*: thuj.
- *Delusion* rubric: *turn: she: had been turned: circle; in a*: thuj.
- *Delusion* rubric: *worthless; he is*: thuj.
- *Delusion* rubric: *wrong: something was wrong*: thuj.

- *Delusions: body: cut through: he is: Stram.* [2] 1.
- *Delusions: body: cut through: he is: two; in: Bell.* plat. stram.

Self-deluding: *Belladonna, Platina* and *Stramonium* all justify their need to resort to violence because they feel they will be attacked.

Belladonna have intense fear of the devil and intense fear that they are the devil. *Belladonna* are listed under the *Delusion* rubrics: *violent,* and *after vexation.* It is their violent, reactive rage which confirms their view that they *are* the devil. The *Delusion* rubric: *body cut in two* can be interpreted as an indicator of the underlying feelings of being destroyed by the devil from inside or from outside. It can equally be interpreted as a psychosomatic representation of the divide between the *great person* and the *devil* in the split personality of *Belladonna*. There is a stark split in the 'delusions of grandeur' and the 'delusions of hypochondria' in *Belladonna*. The *Delusion* rubrics: *body will putrefy*, *being sick*, *body cut through*, and *about to receive injury*, are all examples of *exaggerated* predictions of decay. *Belladonna* as a homoeopathic remedy is used for high fevers which are sudden and violent.

If there are stark inconsistencies between the obsessive psychological 'delusions of hypochondria' and the 'delusions of grandeur' then the constitutional remedy profile will be overwhelmed by anxiety and fear. This is why *Belladonna* on the one hand *see friends* and on the other hand suspiciously see *the devil taking them*. The simillimum will only be *Belladonna* if the patient is terrified of the illness destroying their body [*cutting them in two*]. *Belladonna* will only be the simillimum if the patient needs to delude themselves that they are well, when they are sick.

Belladonna believe they are *well* and *look beautiful*. The consequence of feeling terrified of sickness and unable to come to terms with the reality of *putrefying sickness* means that *Belladonna* become violent and delirious when they are sick. *Belladonna* become violent and delirious when they are sick because they are terrified that disease will destroy them.

Inconsistencies:

1. Denial: *Delusion* rubric: *things look beautiful*: bell. *Delusion* rubric: *well, he is*: bell.

   Versus

5. Resignation: *Delusion* rubric: *body*: *putrefy, will*: bell. *Delusion* rubric: *sick; being*: bell.

1. Denial: *Delusion* rubric: *great person, is a*: bell. *Delusion* rubric: *things look beautiful*: bell. *Delusion* rubric: *friend*: *surrounded by friends; being*: bell.

2. Forsaken: *Delusion* rubric: *home*: *away from home; he is*: bell.

3. Causation: *Delusion* rubric: *devil*: *Bell*.

4. Depression: *Delusion* rubric: *devil*: *taken by the devil; he will* be: bell.

5. Resignation: *Delusion* rubric: *body*: *cut through; he is*: *two; in*: stram. *Delusion* rubric: *body*: *putrefy, will*: bell. *Delusion* rubric: *injury*: *about to receive injury; is*: bell. *Delusion* rubric: *sick*; *being*: bell. *Delusion* rubric: *body*: *sink down between the thighs; body will*: bell. [1] 1.

Platina are listed in more of the *Delusion* rubrics pertaining to 'delusions of grandeur' than any other remedy profile. They obsessively need to maintain their narcissistic self-love when they are faced with illness. *Platina* are literally *cut through in two* between denial (delusions of cure) and hysteria (hypochondria). Underneath their 'delusions of grandeur' are several neuroses. Psychosis refers to loss of touch with reality. In neurosis the patient experiences anxiety. Neurotic tendencies may manifest as depression, acute or chronic anxiety, and/or obsessive-compulsive disorders. Emotional distress is often unconscious conflict and is expressed through various physiological, and/or mental and emotional disturbances (e.g., hysteria).

Platina are noted for several neurotic, psychosomatic, hysterical spasms and alternating states which come and go. *Platina* have the *General* rubrics: *alternating states, complaints accompanied by mental symptoms*, and *complaints gradually appearing and disappearing. Platina* experience extreme anxiety.

When *Platina* are faced with illness they turn to religious penance. I have found that several of my *Platina* patients, when they are sick or facing a life threatening disease, are drawn to the book, *Conversations with God*[82]. *Platina* have several undermining neurotic splits in which they appear divided and *cut in two*; on the one hand they believe that they are *strong* and *under superhuman control,* yet on the other hand everything appears to be *terrible* and under attack from *devils*. The *Delusion rubric*: *sees devils* and *all persons are devils* should not be interpreted literally. The definitive interpretation of these rubrics should be used as an indication of internal neuroses. *Platina* have several obsessive anxieties and hysterias. The 'devil' is generic for the 'evil persona' inside and outside. Alignment with God is extremely important to *Platina*. This is why they have so many *Delusion* rubrics of religiosity. *Platina* also have the *Mind* rubric: *religious affections, too occupied with religion, desires religious penance.* [2] 1. *Platina* call and *talk to spirits* (God) to save themselves from the devil inside and outside of themselves. *Platina* also have a self-punishing split inside of themselves in their obsession with, and repulsion of, their sexuality. *Platina* have a split between religiosity and their sexuality. *Platina* have the *Mind* rubrics: *religious affections, too occupied with religion, alternating with sexual desire, women become lascivious at every touch,* and *nymphomania.* [4]. The greater the need to align oneself with God, the greater the need to banish from yourself all signs of the devil inside. Self-punishment causes conflict, conflict in turn fuels anxiety. They maintain 'delusions of superiority' because they are undermined by a split between the delusional belief that they are *on a mission of greatness,* and fear of being *possessed by the devil.*

When they are sick *Platina* are extremely fearful of the illness inside themselves which they equate with the being *possessed by the devil.* Aside from the *Delusion* rubric: *possessed of a devil, Platina* have numerous *Delusion* rubrics which allude to their need to converse with God – *Delusion* rubrics: *talking with spirits, he is conversing with specters, ghosts, spirits,* and conversely, *sees devil,* and *devil is present.* It was not until I listed all the *Delusion* rubrics of grandeur for *Platina* that I understood the intensity of the need to preserve the psychological delusion that they are ultimately in control of the situation (life and death).

Conversely, fear of abandonment (for which they have numerous rubrics) is an undermining force which in turn fuels their need to maintain their numerous 'delusions of superiority'. *Platina* suffer from neurotic anxiety that they will be abandoned.

Platina fear *all persons are devils* and *that they will be choked in their bed at night* or *left alone in a strange land.*

The simillimum will not be *Platina* unless the patient is convinced that all illness will destroy them unless they are able to connect to 'their higher self' (God). The patient who is *Platina* needs to believe they are *strong* to avoid feeling anxious.

1. Denial: *Delusion* rubric: *superhuman; is; control; is under superhuman*: plat. *Delusion* rubric: *better than others; he is*: plat. *Delusion* rubric: *body: greatness of, as to*: Plat. *Delusion* rubric: *strong; he is*: plat.

2. Forsaken: *Delusion* rubric: *place: no place in the world; she has*: Plat. *Delusion* rubric: *strange: land; as if in a strange*: plat.

3. Causation: *Delusion* rubric: *devil: possessed of a devil: he is*: plat.

4. Depression: *Delusion* rubric: *terrible; everything seems*: plat.

5. Resignation: *Delusion* rubric: *body: cut through; he is: two; in*: plat. *Delusion* rubric: *dead: he himself was*: plat. *Delusion* rubric: *die: about to die; one was*: Plat.

Delusion rubrics of identification with God.

*   *Delusion* rubric: *help: calling for*: plat. [1] 1.
*   *Delusion* rubric: *talking: spirits, with*: Plat.
*   *Delusion* rubric: *superhuman; is; control; is under superhuman*: plat.
*   *Delusion* rubric: *better than others; he is*: plat.
*   *Delusion* rubric: *body: greatness of, as to*: Plat.
*   *Delusion* rubric: *exalted; as if*: plat.
*   *Delusion* rubric: *fancy, illusions of*: Plat.
*   *Delusion* rubric: *great person, is a*: Plat.
*   *Delusion* rubric: *humility and lowness of others; while he is great*: plat.

- *Delusion* rubric: *inferior; people seem mentally and physically*: entering the house after a walk; when: plat. [1] 1.
- *Delusion* rubric: *mission; one has a*: Plat.
- *Delusion* rubric: *noble; being*: plat.
- *Delusion* rubric: *proud*: plat.
- *Delusion* rubric: *religious*: plat.
- *Delusion* rubric: *superiority, of*: Plat.
- *Delusion* rubric: *wealth, of*: Plat.
- *Delusion* rubric: *looking: down; he was looking: high place; from a*: **PLAT**.
- *Delusion* rubric: *grow: larger and longer; he grew*: plat.
- *Delusion* rubric: *strong; he is*: plat.
- *Delusion* rubric: *tall: he or she is tall*: plat.
- *Delusion* rubric: *diminished: everything in room is diminished; while she is tall and elevated*: plat. [1] 1.

Delusion rubrics of being abandoned.

- *Delusion* rubric: *alone, being: world; alone in the*: Plat.
- *Delusion* rubric: *belong to her own family; she does not*: Plat.
- *Delusion* rubric: *appreciated, she is not*: plat.
- *Delusion* rubric: *disgraced: she is*: plat.
- *Delusion* rubric: *disgraced: family or friends; he has disgraced his*: plat.
- *Delusion* rubric: *enemy: everyone is an*: plat.
- *Delusion* rubric: *family, does not belong to her own*: plat. [1] 1.
- *Delusion* rubric: *forsaken; is*: Plat.
- *Delusion* rubric: *place: no place in the world; she has*: Plat.
- *Delusion* rubric: *strange: land; as if in strange*: plat.

- *Delusion* rubric: *neglected*: *he or she is neglected*: plat.
- *Delusion* rubric: *place*: *strange place; he was in a*: plat.
- *Delusion* rubric: *devil*: *all persons are devils*: **PLAT**.
- *Delusion* rubric: *choked*: *he is about to be*: *night*: *waking; on*: *Plat*.

Stramonium need to believe they are all powerful and under the influence of a powerful force because they have intense fear of the physical destruction of illness. *Stramonium* have numerous psychological 'delusions of abandonment', 'delusions of persecution', 'delusions of impending doom' and 'delusions of hypochondria'. Pre-empting their 'delusions of hypochondria' are 'delusions of persecution'. *Stramonium* believe they will be saved from their illness and death [*power of all diseases*] by the intervention of a higher power [*in communication with God*]. *Stramonium* need to align themselves with God to allay their overwhelming fears of being attacked.

When sick, *Stramonium* suffer from psychosomatic illusions and delusions that their body is dismembered. The 'never-well-since-event' or causation in any *Stramonium* case will have its root in victims of violence. Delusional paranoia arises from 'delusions of persecution' which results in a disproportionate or abnormal tendency to suspect others. Paranoia gives rise and justification to acts of retaliation and retribution.

Stramonium can be literally cut in two. On one hand their 'delusions of grandeur' can fuel and ignite their paranoid righteous retaliatory violence. And on the other hand their 'delusions of persecution' can fuel their paranoid 'persecution complexes' that they will be attacked, *cut in two* and *scattered* or *murdered and roasted and eaten*.

When *Stramonium* are sick or dying they can alternate between attacking their homoeopathic practitioner and fearing that their practitioner will attack them.

Ultimately, *Stramonium* will dismiss the services of the

homoeopathic practitioner because they have *power over all diseases* and do not need them. It is unusual to see *Stramonium* present in a consultation and not be arrogantly delusional. The simillimum will not be *Stramonium* unless the patient has a delusional split between needing the homoeopath, fearing the homoeopath, and dismissing the homoeopath. The somatic delusion that their *body is cut in two* is also symbolic of the spilt in their psyche between God and the devil. *Stramonium* have the *Delusion* rubric: *he is God, then he is the devil.* [3] 1. Often it is the case, that if 'God is on your side' in a battle, God can also punish and abandon you to the devil in the next battle. Consequently, *Stramonium* are never trusting of the homoeopath and the homoeopath in turn should expect from *Stramonium* suspicion and/or rejection.

1. Denial: *Delusion* rubric: *God: communication with God; he is in*: stram. *Delusion* rubric: *power. diseases; he had power over all*: *Stram.* [2] 1. *Delusion* rubric: *pure; she is*: stram. *Delusion* rubric: *influence; one is under a powerful*: *Stram.*

2. Forsaken: *Delusion* rubric: *alone, being: wilderness; alone in a*: stram. [1] 1. *Delusion* rubric: *dogs: attack him*: **STRAM**. [3] 1. *Delusion* rubric: *specters, ghosts, spirits: pursued by, is*: stram. *Delusion* rubric: *animals: devoured by: being*: *Stram.* *Delusion* rubric: *animals: persons are animals*: stram. *Delusion* rubric: *bitten, will be*: stram. *Delusion* rubric: *creeping things; full of*: stram. [1] 1. *Delusion* rubric: *cockroaches swarmed about the room*: stram. *Delusion* rubric: *cats: sees*: *Stram.* *Delusion* rubric: *devil: sees*: stram. *Delusion* rubric: *forsaken; is*: *Stram.* *Delusion* rubric: *suffocated; she will be*: *Stram.* *Delusion* rubric: *murdered: will be murdered; he*: *Stram.* *Delusion* rubric: *murdered: being murdered; he is: roasted and eaten; he was murdered*: stram. [1] 1. *Delusion* rubric: *persecuted: he is persecuted*: stram. *Delusion* rubric: *poisoned: he: has been*: stram. *Delusion* rubric: *wilderness; being in*: stram.

[1] 1. *Delusion* rubric: *injury: being injured; is*: **STRAM**. *Delusion* rubric: *snakes: in and around her.* stram.

3. Causation: *Delusion* rubric: *sinned; one has: day of grace; sinned away his*: stram.

4. Depression: *Delusion* rubric: *doomed, being*: stram. *Delusion* rubric: *joy: nothing could give her any joy*: stram. [1] 1.

5. Resignation: *Delusion* rubric: *body: cut through; he is*: Stram. [2] 1. *Delusion* rubric: *grave, he is in his*: stram. *Delusion* rubric: *die: about to die; one was*: stram. *Delusion* rubric: *Delusion* rubric: *body: scattered about; body was*: stram. *Delusion* rubric: *dead: he himself was*: stram. *Delusion* rubric: *disease: every disease; he has*: stram. *Delusion* rubric: *dying: he is*: stram. *Delusion* rubric: *sick: being*: stram. *Delusion* rubric: *head: disease will break out of head*: stram. [1] 1. *Delusion* rubric: *legs: cut off; legs are*: stram.

- *Delusions: hear, he cannot*: hyos. mosch. verat.
- *Delusions: blind; he is*: bell. hyos. mosch. stram. verat.

Self-deluding: These *Delusion* rubrics: *he cannot hear or see* (blind) reveal deep psychosis, self-denial and the refusal to face reality.

Moschus is a homoeopathic remedy derived from the perfume musk. Musk is a potent aphrodisiac. The purpose of an aphrodisiac perfume to the wearer and recipient is to erotically 'lift' or stimulate the senses, and then to overwhelm them and render them helpless to 'falling' for their own sexual desires and 'falling' for the sexual advances of others. The express purpose of a woman wearing a perfume, or a man wearing an aftershave is to fill the air with a waft of scent which they leave behind as they move through a room and past the man or woman of their desires. *Moschus* are the only remedy listed in the *Delusion* rubric which express this precise energy of seduction – *Delusion* rubric: *she was turning so rapidly that he perceived a current of air produced by the motion.* [1] 1. *Moschus* have the *Delusion* rubric: *elevated and he would fall.* [1] 1. The aim of an aphrodisiac is to render the wearer and recipient helpless to their desires.

My aim in *Homoeopathic Psychiatry* is to emphasize that *Delusion* rubrics always have a somatic and psychotherapeutic relevance to the remedy profile and to the substance from which the remedy is derived.

The psychodynamic, somatic application of a person without *fingers* is one who is helpless to resist advances, while the psychodynamic application of a person without *toes* is one who cannot escape sexual advances. The psychodynamic psyche of a person who is overwhelmed by the sexual advances of another is a person who has two minds [*heads*]. One head wants to stay and have sex and one head wants to leave.

Moschus as a homoeopathic remedy is used for fainting fits; especially applicable for the patient who feels like they are falling from a great height, or for the patient who is overwhelmed by hysteria. *Moschus* as a constitutional remedy profile carry this somatic fall within their psyche. *Moschus* are undermined in their pursuit of personal achievement by the lack of any *Delusion* rubrics of grandeur other than *floating in air*. The *Delusion* rubrics: *he cannot hear* and *he is blind* (see), and the *Delusion* rubric: *floating in air*, reveal a deep psychosis of self-denial and refusal to face the reality of failure (death).

Moschus fail to meet their own expectations and feel like they have fallen from elevated heights which they cannot achieve. *Moschus* exaggerate being *sick* and blame their lack of success on the opposition and *hindrance* of others. *Moschus* do not wish to acknowledge reality, that is why they have the *Delusion* rubrics pertaining to a refusal to *see and hear*.

What *Moschus* are refusing to acknowledge is within themselves; the *Delusion* rubrics: *two heads*, *being double*, *errors of identity,* and *she is some other person*, all allude to opposing forces. *Moschus* are hysterical. *Moschus* lack self-control. *Moschus* have the *Mind* rubric: *abusive and scolds until the lips are blue and eyes stare and she falls down fainting.* [2] 1. The underlying emotive fears behind hysteria can be varied, but the consistent theme in all patients with hysteria is that their symptoms will produce psychosomatic physical conditions. 'Somatization disorders' are imagined or 'medically unexplained' illnesses. Below I have listed the relevant *Mind* rubrics which add richness to the dilemma inside of *Moschus* to either surrender or flee. *Moschus* flee from and embrace sickness – *hypochondriacal anxiety – feigning to be sick. Moschus* flee from and embrace their sexuality – *sexual abstinence – hysterical lasciviousness. Moschus* flee from and embrace emotional control – *causeless anxiety – so angry he could have stabbed anyone.*

- *Mind* rubric: *anguish: causeless:* mosch. [1] 1.
- *Mind* rubric: *anxiety: hypochondriacal:* mosch.
- *Mind* rubric: *feigning: sick; to be:* mosch.
- *Mind* rubric: *hypochondriasis: sexual:* mosch. [1] 1.
- *Mind* rubric: *hypochondriasis: sexual: abstinence, from:* mosch.
- *Mind* rubric: *hysteria: fainting, hysterical: Mosch.*
- *Mind* rubric: *hysteria: lascivious:* mosch.
- *Mind* rubric: *perfume: loves to use perfume:* mosch.
- *Mind* rubric: *desire to play: buttons of his clothes, with the:* mosch. [1] 1. [The act of playing with the buttons on an article of clothing is a sexually provocative act of seduction.]
- *Mind* rubric: *gestures, makes: fighting with hands:* mosch. [1] 1. [The somatic act of fighting with one's hands is evocative of fighting to resist the desire to touch.]
- *Mind* rubric: *abusive: scolds until the lips are blue and eyes stare and she falls down fainting: Mosch.* [2] 1.

- *Mind* rubric: *anger. stabbed anyone; so angry that he could have*: mosch.

Moschus do not want to hear, or see, or face reality – they wish to *float in air*.

Moschus, when they are sick, will present with numerous feigned disorders which are imagined. Conversely, they will be also display hysterical neurosis and flee if you force them to face the fact or the *reality* that they are sick.

The simillimum will only be *Moschus* if the patient has a dissociative split [*being double*] in acknowledging reality. *Moschus* will only be the simillimum if the patient feels thwarted in life – *hindered by everyone else*. *Moschus* will only be the simillimum if the patient feels thwarted by their own lack of control over their anxiety, hypochondria and their anger – *Delusion* rubric: *she is some other person*. *Moschus* will only be the simillimum if the patient feels thwarted by their own lack of control over their body – *Delusion* rubric: *falling from a height* – *Delusion* rubric: *he cannot see or hear* – *Delusion* rubric: *his toes and fingers are cut*. A *Moschus* patient will not literally tell you that they have a psychological delusion that they will lose their fingers and toes, or they will become blind or deaf. A *Moschus* patient will say *I feel thwarted [hindered] at every turn in my life. Everyone and everything is standing in my way. I feel like I am free floating from a great height and that I am going to, all of a sudden, hit the ground with a big bang and then that will be the end of me. I can't seem to be able to grip on to reality. I can't seem to be able to make any move in one direction or another.*

1. Denial: *Delusion* rubric: *floating: air, in*: mosch. [This rubric can pertain to the need to dissociate from reality. Because *Moschus* have no other rubrics of grandeur which give them an inflated sense of power, this rubric pertains to avoidance and potential failure.]

2. Forsaken: *Delusion* rubric: *hindered: he is: everyone; by:* mosch.

3. Causation: *Delusion* rubric: *falling: height; from a:* mosch. *Delusion* rubric: *elevated: air, elevated in the: fall; and would:* mosch. [1] 1. *Delusion* rubric: *falling: elevated and would fall; he was:* mosch. [1] 1. [These rubrics can pertain to admittance of potential future failure or admittance of past failures (sins).]

4. Depression: *Delusion* rubric: *identity: errors of personal identity:* mosch. *Delusion* rubric: *double: being:* mosch. *Delusion* rubric: *person: other person; she is some:* mosch. *Delusion* rubric: *head: two heads, having:* mosch. [These rubrics all pertain to insecurity and anxiety about who one is in the world.] *Delusion* rubric: *falling: elevated and would fall; he was:* mosch. [1] 1. [This rubric can pertain to admission of guilt or predications of failure.]

5. Resignation: *Delusion* rubric: *hear, he cannot:* mosch. *Delusion* rubric: *blind; he is:* mosch. *Delusion* rubric: *sick: being:* mosch. *Delusion* rubric: *dead: he himself was:* mosch. *Delusion* rubric: *toes: cut off:* mosch. [1] 1. *Delusion* rubric: *injury: fingers and toes are being cut off; his:* mosch. [1] 1.

The Case Companion

In this section I present several cases[1] from my practice. In the case analyses I explain why each patient has set up the delusional state and why they need to maintain the misrepresentation of reality. I identify the *Delusion* rubrics used in the rubric-repertorisation and explain how the patient has used the psychological delusion to construct and to *maintain* their disease state. I unravel the significant 'never-well-since-events' in each patient's life and repertorise each poignant emotional event to give you an explanation of the causation within the case and an explanation of the rubric-repertorisation which justifies the use of the *Delusion* rubrics. These case analyses aim to give insight into the psychological modeling of why each patient has chosen to concoct a complicated system of excuses to justify their psychological delusions which help formulate their existing pathology.

Case Analysis: I use the following key points and headings in analyzing a case. Each individual case will dictate the particular order in which each point is discussed.

Rubric-repertorisation

Theme

Striking, or ***Peculiar* Signs and Symptoms; Organon 153**

---

1. To protect the patient's identity all names have been changed. I repeatedly use the names, Jane, Mary, Helen, John, David, Chris, and Peter. To protect the patient's identity the correct date of appointments have been changed. To protect the patient's identity locations have also been changed. To protect the patient's identity their date of birth has been changed.

Materia Medica

Follow-up Consultations

How, Why, and *When* **Causations – the 'Never-well-since-event'.**

Rubric-repertorisation – For example, if a patient says they are all alone in the world and they have no friends or family, it is either the *Mind* rubric: *forsaken,* or the *Delusion* rubric: *forsaken,* depending on the degree of delusional disturbance within the case.

It is good habit for homoeopaths to translate a patient's words into *Mind* or *Delusion* rubrics.

Theme – Every patient will have recurring patterns or themes in their lives. The theme inherent within the patient's story is an indication of whether the patient is predominantly preoccupied with disproportionate mental and emotional thoughts or feelings. The theme will resonate in one, several, or all of the five psychological stages. Each patient will have a tendency to be *predominantly* in denial, forsakenness and persecutory paranoia, guilt, depression, or hypochondria.

If you learn how to recognize these five psychological stages it will help you in the rubric-repertorisation and in finding the simillimum.

1. If the trauma inside your patient starts with martyrdom and/ or delusional belief in divine cure, then the simillimum is listed in Denial. If your patient unrealistically believes they are so *great* or *superior* that they will not die, then the simillimum is listed in all the *Delusion* rubrics: *immortality, in communication with God, under an all powerful influence,* or *being divine.*

2. If the trauma inside your patient starts with them feeling alone and abandoned, or singled out for punishment by their illness, then the simillimum is listed in all the *Delusion* rubrics: *forsaken* or *persecution.*

3. If the trauma inside your patient starts with them feeling

guilty and unrealistically responsible for their illness, then the simillimum is listed in the all the *Delusion* rubrics: *he is sinful, he has committed a crime* or *he has done wrong*, and is allocated to the section Causation.

4. If the trauma inside your patient starts with them feeling hopeless doom about being sick, or them feeling like they will never succeed in becoming well in life, then the simillimum is listed in the *Delusion* rubrics: *failure* and *he will not succeed,* and is allocated to the section Depression.

5. If the patient's trauma starts with hypochondria or delusional doom about being sick, or you feel that your patient is exaggerating their weakness or sickness then the simillimum is listed in the *Delusion* rubrics: *death*, and *disease* and is allocated to the section Resignation.

The advantage in identifying and understanding the psychological processing that your patient is moving through is that it allows you to narrow the remedies under consideration to the remedies listed in those particular rubric-categories.

Striking, or Peculiar Signs and Symptoms; Organon 153 – The inner disturbance is the core of our case-taking, and it is always reflective of what is unusual or disturbing to *your* (the homoeopath's) inner sensibilities. The homoeopath must identify what is disproportionate to reality in their patient's story. Hahnemann said in aphorism 153 of The Organon, that in the search for a specific homoeopathic remedy we should concentrate on "the *more striking, singular, uncommon and peculiar* signs and symptoms of the case".

The disturbance which reverberates with a *striking* symptom, will be when the patient reveals how they have constructed their mental and emotional outlook around the first *disproportionate* analysis of their lives.

In unraveling the significant events in the lives of your patients, and repertorising each poignant emotional event, the simillimum will be evident in every case once you identify the disproportionate interpretation of the patient's life. The key to unraveling your patient's story in case-taking is listening, asking the right questions, and finding the disproportionate disturbance or the *peculiar* interpretation each patient has developed around their trauma. I have been able to repertorise the *peculiar* signs and symptoms of the patient's case using the *Delusion* rubrics because these are the rubrics which resonate with disruption. I have found it invaluable in case-taking to be able to understand the significant psychological meaning and application of the *Delusion* rubrics.

Materia Medica – A prescription cannot be based solely on rubric-repertorisation.

The homoeopath must use Materia medica reference works to confirm their understanding of the simillimum.

Follow up Consultations – The follow-up consultation must confirm that the original prescription is correct.

If the remedy is the simillimum, the patient will often reveal the formation of their psychological delusions in the follow-up consultations. The patient must also indicate that they are free of previous pathology which has affected them on all levels – emotionally, mentally, and physically.

How, Why, and *When* **Causations** – The 'Never-well-since-event'. In these case-studies I emphasize repeatedly the need to understand the causation or the 'never-well-since-event'. Chronological events are crucial in case-development. They are important because they show us the cause and meaning of the '*how, why,* and *when,*' of the significant events in our patients' lives. The homoeopath needs to ask the patient "why do you think you are sick?" or "what event has happened in your life which you think has contributed to your illness?" or simply "tell me about your life and what has happened to you in your life". I prefer to ask the last question because then the patient will tell me about the events in their life which they think are crucial to their case. The first consultation is often on the conscious level. It is often not until patients have had several consultations that they are able to reveal deep traumatic events in their life which have formulated psychological delusions.

Until I discover the primary trauma in a patient's life, I am never totally sure of a simillimum prescription. **If the remedy is the simillimum,** the patient will often reveal in the consultation the formation of their psychological delusions in the follow-up consultations. The cure of, and from the simillimum will always elicit the 'never-well-since-event'.

It is what I refer to as the 'eye of the storm'. The 'eye of the storm' is when your patient reveals to you the primary traumatic event in their lives. The patient might not reveal the 'never-well-since-event' until the third or the fourth consultation. It occurs when everything stops in the case-taking, and you know you have arrived at the centre of your patient's internal storm.

Agaricus

Abstract:

This is a case of a woman who feels like she needs to be able to *exit* whatever world she creates. *Agaricus* have the *Mind* rubric: *making many bold plans* and the *Delusion* rubric: *enjoy to provoke out of body experiences.*

Keywords:

Incorrect judgement of size. *Alice's Adventures in Wonderland.* Parallel existence.

Case Notes:

First Consult: October 2001.

D.O.B. 1972.

Occupation: Events Manager.

Presenting Physical Complaints:

- Food bingeing and purging (Bulimia)
- Fluid retention and weight gain, especially problematic before her menses
- Fluid retention and weight gain, especially problematic proceeding emotional upsets, (especially with her mother)
- Sugar cravings

- Alternating diarrhoea and constipation

In the first consultation, the patient reports that she was concerned about her weight and fluid retention problems. When she is emotionally upset, she gains five to six kilos. She shows me a photo. The photo is a before and after shot from a visit by her mother. The difference is extreme. Preceding the visit she is clearly smaller in size. She assures me the difference on the scales was five kilos, from before to after the visit. She binges and purges on food, so her weight goes up and down after binges. She binges on sugar, ice-cream, cakes, and chocolate, usually after her mother's visits. She relays that her mother continually criticizes her, especially in relation to her size (she is not overweight).

She says she has a *yin/yang* concept of herself. *I become out of balance. I am too extreme with work.* She says, *I have no idea of 'how to do' an emotional life. I have a duality issue, always having two boyfriends and two jobs to choose from. I become overwhelmed and overwrought with hyperactivity. I become overwhelmed with speediness while working. I am continually overwrought about relationship choices. I don't know which man I should choose.* She does not tell her partners that she is seeing someone else. She often gets into relationships with men who are conservative, *boy next door types*, and at the same time she is in a relationship with a *bad boy type*.

She describes herself as a chameleon. She often feels like she has created *two parallel worlds*. She struggles with commitment. She always has two relationships going at the one time, so she does not have to make a choice. She becomes extremely bored being 'good'. Her parents are divorced. Her father left when she was three years old. She feels torn between them. She feels that her father has abandoned her, and that she is not able to have *control* over him. She fears she will end up repeating her mother's relationship patterning. Her mother is just about to leave her third husband. The patient is frightened about being alone like her mother.

She has a very good opinion of herself: *I have an almost magical or wondrous capacity to transform a company and make it great!* She describes herself as a *good leader, team organizer, and a good 'people person' at work.* She needs and likes to describe herself as financially successful in her own right.

Conversely, she is overwhelmed by a sense of helplessness. She is scared, and cautious about taking risks. She is scared of being alone. She is furious if she is contradicted by her partner. She describes herself as cautious and cowardly, but also boasts about how great she is, especially in business.

She is particularly averse to being contradicted by her mother, partner, or work colleagues.

Health History:

- She was born eight weeks premature
- Prolapsed bowel when toilet training at two to three years of age
- Nervous breakdown at twenty-one years old. At this time she experienced 'paralysis-like' symptoms similar to having a stroke on her right side. Her explanation of, or cause given for, her nervous breakdown is her mother's continual criticism of her weight gain
- At twenty-two years of age she developed hairs on her chest. The hairs upset her considerably
- Weight gain pre menses: six kilos

Rubrics Used: First remedy given: *Lycopodium* 200 C. 1 dose only.

- *Mind: adulterous: Lyc.*
- *Mind: ailments from contradiction:* **LYC**.
- *Mind: activity: desires activity: creative activity:* lyc.
- *Mind: ailments from neglected; being: father; by one's:* lyc.

- *Mind*: *ambition*: *increased; money; to make*: lyc.
- *Mind*: *boaster. rich, wishes to be considered as*: lyc.
- *Mind*: *bulimia nervosa*: lyc.
- *Mind*: *cautious*: *anxious*: **LYC**.
- *Mind*: *fear. alone, of being*: **LYC**.
- *Delusions*: *place*: *two places at the same time; of being in*: *Lyc*.

2nd Consult: November 2001

In the rubric-repertorisation, *Lycopodium* appeared to be the simillimum. However, *Lycopodium* made no difference to any of her symptoms. I gave her *Argentium nitricum* for her sugar cravings[2] and studied the case, again. I started at the beginning and analyzed all the original rubrics I had used. I studied notes from the first and second consultations, again.

Lycopodium has the delusion of needing to be in two places at the same time to increase their social importance. *Lycopodium* will also have two relationships going at the same time to alleviate their underlying insecurity. Their underlying insecurity is played out in the duality of their over-boasting performance, juxtaposed with their crippling inner doubt, lack of confidence, and fear of being alone. When *Lycopodium* has previously been the correct prescription, the patient's inner fear and doubt is profoundly eased. As a consequence, the 'in-your-face', over the top boasting normally associated with the *Lycopodium* persona also lifts. *Lycopodium* was not the correct prescription because nothing lifted or eased in this patient.

Lycopodium was an immediate surface prescription on my part. It clearly did not address the underlying conflict within this woman's psyche.

---

2 Second remedy given: *Argentium nitricum* 30 C. x 1 dose when needed for the sugar cravings. Rubrics used: Sweets, aggravation; Sweets, desire.

Notes from the 2nd Consult:

- Diet out of control; bingeing terrible
- Emotional distress and crying
- No confidence with work
- Sugar craving out of control
- Very bad Candida problems from the amount of sugar she has been having
- Rosacea around her nose and chin
- She reports she has been extremely up and down since the *Lycopodium*. (I suspect this existed before the *Lycopodium*. The prescription of *Lycopodium* has not addressed her need for polarity and change.)
- Very insecure over trust with her two boyfriends
- Huge confusion of the choice between her two current boyfriends
- She feels that she must *confess her duality in relationships*
- Huge confusion over two exciting and powerful job prospects
- She once again describes herself as *yin/yang*
- She says she is *totally disconnected to the world as if I am looking through a glass wall*
- *I am afraid everything will fall apart in my life*
- *I fear losing myself. I feel like I am creating an alternative world where I get to exist and have a fantasy world, and it exists parallel to my own. The parallel universe will have no cross over*
- *I have no exit valve*
- *I am afraid the choices I make will not be right*

My Observations:

- Duality

- Needs to be able to *exit* whatever world she creates
- Loquacious jumping from one subject to another
- Cheerfulness versus depression and lassitude
- A strong knowing that she is a *great person* versus paralytic ineffectiveness
- She displays determined purposefulness but clearly has a loss of control with food bingeing
- Dynamic business woman but conversely presenting as if on an emotional rollercoaster
- The need to create a parallel universe inside and outside is the key element which I have previously failed to address. This is the *peculiar* mental and emotional keynote
- *Lycopodium* has not addressed the conflicting self-destructiveness associated with her bulimia
- The correct prescription must address the frenzied need to binge and purge after any real or perceived criticism

New Physical Symptoms Given:
- Cold sweat on her legs. *They do not belong to me because they are so cold and have no feeling*
- Conversely, painful neuralgia of her feet
- Feeling of paralysis in her bowel; feels like when she was three years of age and unable to move her bowel. She previously had just mentioned diarrhoea and constipation
- The previous prescription had failed to address her history of paralysis. This is a *peculiar* physical keynote

3rd Consultation: December 2001

The *Lycopodium* has not made no difference to any of her symptoms; equally, the *Argentium nitricum* has not made any difference to the sugar cravings.

Remedy given at the third consultation: *Agaricus* 30 C., once a week for 4 weeks.

Case Analysis: I used the following key points and headings in analyzing this case, to arrive at the correct prescription of *Agaricus*.

1. **Rubric-repertorisation**
2. **Theme**
3. *Striking*, or *Peculiar* **Signs and Symptoms; Organon 153**
4. **Materia Medica**
5. **Follow-up Consultations**
6. *How*, *Why*, and *When* **Causations — the 'Never-well-since-event'.**

1. Rubric-repertorisation

- *Mind: ailments from: criticized; from being*: agar.
- *Mind: ailments from: reproaches*: agar.
- *Mind: anxiety: alternating with: cheerfulness*: agar.
- *Mind: bulimia*: agar.
- *Mind: chaotic*: agar.
- *Mind: cheerful: alternating with: sadness*: agar.
- *Mind: childish behavior[3]: Agar.*
- *Mind: company: desire for: alone agg.; when*: agar.
- *Mind: courageous*: agar.
- *Mind: cowardice*: agar.
- *Mind: delirium: gay, cheerful: alternating with: sadness*: agar.
- *Mind: egotism: reciting their exploits*: agar. [1] 1.
- *Mind: hatred: persons: offended him; hatred of persons who*: agar.

---

3 Vermeulen explains this dichotomy in *Synoptic Materia medica*. "Intoxication with fly-agaric is characterized by cheerfulness and loss of self-control, which is followed by lassitude and depression."

- *Mind: injuring himself: frenzy causing him to injure himself:* agar. (Re: bulimia.)
- *Mind: loquacity: changing quickly from one subject to another:* agar.
- *Mind: pities herself:* agar.
- *Mind: plans: making many plans: bold plans:* agar. [1] 1.
- *Mind: self-control: loss of self-control:* agar. (Re: bulimia.)
- *Mind: self-denial:* agar. (Re: bulimia.)
- *Mind: size: incorrect judgement of:* agar. (Re: correct assessment of her body size.)

- *Delusions: body: out of the body: enjoy to provoke out of body experiences:* agar. [1] 1.
- *Delusions: great person, is a: Agar.*
- *Delusions: hell: confess his sins at gate of; obliged to:* agar. [1] 1.
- *Delusions: legs: belong to her; her legs don't: Agar.*
- *Delusions: paralysed; he is:* agar.
- *Delusions: large: everything looks larger:* agar. (Re: body size.)

2. Theme

She describes herself as a chameleon. She needs to continually change worlds and environments accordingly. *Lycopodium* is also a plant remedy, however, *Lycopodium* did not address the underlying issue of paralysis. Nor did *Lycopodium* address the *peculiar* need to create an alternative parallel universe. *Lycopodium* have the *Delusion* rubric: *of being in two places at the one time.* This rubric pertains to 'delusions of grandeur' or self-importance.

Finding the simillimum is always about listening to the patient's words. In the first consultation she tells me she has *created two parallel worlds. Agaricus* have the *Delusion* rubric: *enjoy to provoke out of body experiences.* This rubric pertains to the need to create another experience. *Agaricus* have a psychological need to connect to a metaphysical experience outside themselves.

Themes of the Plant Remedies

- Sensitivity: plant remedies always have a strong need to find the right place to survive completely unaffected by others. Conversely, they also have the ability to change and adapt to new environments.

- Reactivity: plant remedies always have strong somatic pain sensations echoed in the emotional and played out in the physical and mental.

- Sensations: plant remedies always have strong sensations and opposite polarity in their lives.

A plant remedy will tell you that what others do to them always affects them. She had a nervous breakdown at twenty-one years of age, and at this time she experienced symptoms of paralysis similar to having a stroke on her right side. Her explanation of, or cause given for, her nervous breakdown was her mother's continual criticism of her weight gain. She is concerned about her weight and fluid retention problems. When she is upset emotionally, especially with her mother who criticizes her, she literally gains five kilos. She binges and purges on food; her weight goes up and down. She gets overwhelmed by, and overwrought with, hyperactivity in the work environment. She becomes overwrought about relationship choices. She has two men at the same time to match the two sides of her personality. The correct prescription must match the sensitivity to others' real or perceived criticism and abandonment. The correct prescription must match the frenzied need to change jobs, and boyfriends. The correct prescription must also match the frenzied bingeing.

Every patient will have recurring patterns or themes in their lives. The theme inherent within the patient's story is an indication of whether the patient is predominately preoccupied with disproportionate mental and emotional thoughts or feelings. The theme will resonate in one, several, or all of the five psychological stages. Each patient will have a tendency to be *predominately* in denial, forsakenness and persecutory paranoia, guilt, depression, or hypochondria. This patient alternates between psychological delusions that she is a great person, and persecutory sensitivity that she is being attacked. She has no control over her own body and her own bulimia.

The remedy must match the alternating psychological polarities of 'delusions of grandeur' and 'delusions of hypochondria'.

The *prominent* theme is her story of abandonment by her mother and father, and self-abandonment. This patient is self-destructive.

Agaricus have exalted hubristic delusions which cover up their fears of diminishing. *Agaricus* need to view themselves as great; this is reflected in the *Mind* rubric: *egotism, reciting their exploits*: agar. [1] 1., as well as in the *Delusion* rubric: *is a great person*. *Agaricus* have a strong need for materialistic proof of their grandeur and worldly success. This is not only reflected in the *Delusion* rubric: *is a great person*, but also in the *Mind* rubric: *incorrect judgement of size*. *Agaricus* feel threatened when they are sick, they feel like they will diminish in size, and lose their height and importance and that their own body will abandon them. If the homoeopath understands the rubrics associated with the remedies, and their importance, they will know that when *Agaricus* are sick they will present in the first consultation in a very depressed and *paralyzed* state. The grandness that is normally associated with the egotistical *Agaricus* is not what you will see. They will be in a very small and *diminished* state. If they feel threatened or shamed by failure they immediately feel as if they are diminishing and losing all power – *Mind* rubric: *looking down when looked at.* [1] 1. If challenged they feel as if they are losing their arms and legs in the world and they compensate for their feeling of vulnerability by being extremely nasty. *Agaricus* have the *Mind* rubric: *hatred of persons who have offended him*, and the *Delusion* rubric: *vindictive*. [1] 1. Their psychological need to connect to a metaphysical power outside themselves is paramount to finding their power in the world. *Agaricus* have the *Delusion* rubrics: *objects are enlarged, is under superhuman control*, and *enjoy provoking out of body experiences*. [1] 1. The psychodynamic polarity of expanding greatness and diminishing smallness is extreme in *Agaricus*. This *Agaricus* (case) solves the psychological dilemma of expanding and diminishing potency by creating two worlds. In each world she has a boyfriend. By having two partners and two worlds she is able to feel strong and *enlarged*, or 'larger than life'. Understanding the psychological processes that apply to illness, and understanding the rubric-analysis which I have outlined below, allows the homoeopathic practitioner to have a greater understanding of the remedies and the *Agaricus* patient.

1. Denial: *Delusion* rubric: *great person, is a*: *Agar.*
2. Forsaken: *Delusion* rubric: *legs: belong to her; her legs don't*: *Agar*. *Delusion* rubric: *arms: belong to her; arms do not*: agar. [These rubrics can reflect self-abandonment or they can be rubrics of hypochondria and be allocated to Resignation.]
3. Causation: *Delusion* rubric: *hell; confess his sins at gate of; obliged to*: agar [1] 1.
4. Depression: *Delusion* rubric: *paralyzed; he is*: agar.
5. Resignation: *Delusion* rubric: *body, diminished; is*: agar. *Delusion* rubric: *arms: belong to her; arms do not*: agar. *Delusion* rubric: *legs: belong to her; her legs don't*. *Agar.*

3. *Striking*, or *Peculiar* Signs and Symptoms; Organon 153

Agaricus can literally go from one extreme to another, and all their emotional feelings or experiences in life are very intense and very changeable. The homoeopathic remedy *Agaricus* is derived from a dilution of the *Fly Agaric* fungi, *Agaricaceae* family. *Agaricus* is a narcotic plant remedy which is intensely unstable. The *Agaricus* constitutions in my practice are highly strung about their health precisely because they suffer from extremely unexplainable or unusual physical pathology. This *Agaricus* (case) experiences changes in size which are truly profound. The *Delusion* rubric: *legs don't belong to her*, is indicative of self-abandonment and lack of self-control. Invariably, the sensations and disconnections to their feet or legs confirm the muscular, spasmodic nature of the physical effects of the narcotic, as well as the ludicrous mental intoxications of the narcotic. I am reminded of her prolapsed bowel when toilet training at three years of age. With her nervous breakdown at the age of twenty-one she experienced paralyzed symptoms similar to having a stroke on her right side, which mirror the narcotic nature of the remedy.

Alice's Adventures in Wonderland is a story of a rather curious dream had by Alice when she falls asleep one hot afternoon. *Alice's Adventures in Wonderland* is an extraordinary adventure. In her dream, Alice shrinks to ten inches tall, and then grows to more than nine feet high. She follows a white rabbit in a waistcoat down a rabbit-hole, nearly drowns in her own tears, seeks guidance from a caterpillar sitting on a mushroom, a cat assures her everyone is mad, the Queen and King from her pack of cards become real, and she nearly loses her head. We all have had a peculiar dream from time to time, that is after all the nature of dreaming, however, the uncanny resemblance of this dream to the effects of taking *Magic Mushrooms*[4], and the homoeopathic remedy *Agaricus* is startling in its accuracy. Homoeopaths have for years surmised the constitutional picture of Alice in the wonderful dream-tale of *Alice's Adventure in Wonderland* by Lewis Carroll. The fact that

---

4   *Magic Mushrooms* is the common name used to describe the psychedelic effects of consuming hallucinogenic mushrooms.

Alice repertorises so wonderfully as *Agaricus* is what continually stimulates the minds, and passions of all homoeopaths. Carroll writes, "Alice discovered that the Caterpillar was indeed right, one nibble from the right-hand side of the mushroom and she shrunk and one nibble from the left-hand side of the mushroom and she grew." Alice answers the Caterpillar, "I know who I *was* was when I got up this morning, but I think I must have been changed several times since then." "I can't[5] remember things as I used – and I don't keep the same size[6] for ten minutes together!"

- *Delusions*: *large*[7]: *everything looks larger.* agar.
- *Delusions*: *small*: *things*: *appear small; things*: agar.
- *Mind*: *mischievous*[8]: *Agar.*

---

5   Alice's speech indicates a continual hesitation or stammer. Alice frequently says "ca'n't" and 'sha'n't". *Agaricus* is noted as an excellent remedy for stammering. The author Lewis Carroll suffered with a stammer which was severe enough to prevent him from becoming a preacher in his younger years.

"*Agaricus* is mainly a neurological remedy with twitching, spasms, and even convulsions." "Grimacing of the mouth, especially on beginning to speak." [Morrison]

- *Mouth* rubric: *trembling of tongue.*
- *Mouth* rubric: *stammering.*
- *Mouth* rubric: *speech difficult.*

6   "One side will make you grow taller, and the other side will make you grow shorter."

7   After Alice eats the cake she grows into a rather large telescope like form. "'Now I'm opening out like the largest telescope that ever was! Good-bye, feet!' (for when she looked down at her feet, they seemed to be almost out of sight, they were getting so far off)."

8   Alice is unable to resist the temptation for adventure; she "was just going to leave the room, when her eyes fell upon a little bottle that stood near the looking glass. There was no label this time with the words "DRINK ME", but nevertheless she uncorked it and put it to her lips....before she had drunk half the bottle she found her head pressing against the ceiling, and had to stoop to save her neck from being broken. She hastily put down the bottle. saying to herself "That's quite enough – I hope I sha'n't grow any more – As it is, I ca'n't get out the door – I do wish I hadn't drunk quite so much!"

• *Mind: hysteria*[9]: *Agar.*

4. Materia Medica

Agaricus are extreme, and the highs and lows for *Agaricus* can be very confusing. They can literally be expanding and blowing up with "self-esteem, reciting his exploits; delusions of grandeur; exalted strength" [Vermeulen] and shrinking in size and bursting into tears with the next breath. The "excited and ecstatic states" [Morrison] of *Agaricus* also are able to fuel a personality picture that is brimming with "exalted strength" [Vermeulen] and "fearless"[10] passion for adventure. The effects of taking *Magic Mushrooms* as reported by Vermeulen: "rapturous visionary ecstasy", and "a feeling of well-being and enjoyment", are personality traits that I perceive in *Agaricus* patients which endowers them with an attractive "cheerfulness of spirit" [Vermeulen], and love of the extreme in life. Vermeulen, in *Prisma,* explains *Agaricus* as having a "disturbed sense of perspective". "Every little problem is exaggerated; small holes appear like frightful chasms; self-esteem, reciting his exploits; delusions of grandeur; exalted strength."

Agaricus can literally go from one polarity or perception of reality to another; all their emotional feelings or experiences in life are extreme lows or exalted highs.

---

9   *Delusion* rubric: *water: spoonful of water seems like a lake; a*: agar. [1] 1.

This *Delusion* rubric reflects the narcotic exaggerations of the remedy profile. *Agaricus* are also listed in the *Mind* rubric: *hydrophobia.* In the story, Alice finds herself in the extremely unusual predicament of nearly being drowned in the "gallons of tears" she shed when she grew as large as a telescope. She laments, "I wish I hadn't cried so much!.....I shall be punished for it now, I suppose, by being drowned in my own tears!"

10 Even allowing for the fact that Alice does check the bottle for the words "Poison"; her willingness to drink from the bottle that says "DRINK ME", and eat the cake that says "EAT ME", as well as her lack of hesitancy in following the Rabbit down the hole, certainly does markedly note an important rubric of *Agaricus,* which is the *Mind* rubric: heedless.

5. Follow-up Consultations

In the fourth consultation after the *Agaricus*, the distance between her and the world narrowed. In ascertaining the right prescription of *Agaricus*, I needed to see that the alternative states of being very large or very small had shifted.

I had given her *Agaricus* 30 C., 1 dose per week for 4 weeks.

Follow-up

Below is an abbreviated list of some of the wonderful feedback that I got from her consultations.

Fourth consultation

I am no longer having a conversation with myself about recognizing the world. I feel like I am not so foggy and I can see things. I don't feel as panicky with myself, and my own existence. I am not so hyped-up or as sad. I can feel more when I feel, if that makes sense. I feel like I can see myself more clearly in the mirror, and that maybe I can see how big I truly am. I have not been so needy of eating large amounts, and I haven't been purging even when I have eaten.

She reported:

- Diet not so out of control; bingeing less.
- Hardly any emotional distress and crying.
- Not so paranoid about her perceptions of herself.
- More confidence with work and belief in herself.
- More able to connect to the world.
- More able to concentrate.
- Doesn't feel so hopeless.
- Less anxious.
- Less hyperactive.
- Less cold and disconnected with her legs and feet.

- Less new hair growth on her chest.
- Less fluid retention.
- No change to the Rosacea and Candida infection.

Sixth Consultation

I have felt all my life that I am standing on the other side of a glass wall and I can't see to the other side. I can't get to my lovers or family or friends. There is no door, and I am very scared. I don't feel like there is the same distance between them and me anymore; I am not so lonely.

February 2005

All my life I have been paranoid over all my perceptions. I never believed I was right, nor did I think anyone else would believe me. I can now believe I was correct.

August 2005

She has started a relationship with *a man who is a 'stay-at-home, white-picket-fence man' who wants to marry 'the girl-next-door' and have children.*

I have got my diet together. I am not bloating any more. I do not binge, and I don't bloat up with fluid anymore. But at the same time I am realizing I can't do this relationship. I can't do this. I need to escape. I need excitement. I can see now what I do when I have felt trapped in the past. I have created a fantasy world in which to escape into. A world in which I can have adventures. I can't believe what you told me last time about what I have been taking because it is so true. I am Alice! (The last consultation I had showed her an article I was writing on *Agaricus*.)

February 2006

I have a New Year's resolution, how to have fun, and have balance as well.

When she arrived at this point, I knew that she was heading towards a healthy state of balance for *Agaricus*. It is important that we, as homeopaths, know that when healthy, an *Agaricus* (constitution) will still exist in two worlds.

I have worked with this woman from the first consult in October 2001, to April 2007. Although the doses of *Agaricus* have been repeated frequently, (listed below), I have not gone above the frequency of 1 M. I analyzed her emotional vulnerability, (in regard to her history of having a nervous breakdown), as being too precarious to deal with a much higher potency. Potency is, of course very much based on the individual homoeopath, but in my experience of *Agaricus* the very nature of the existence of two parallel worlds creates respect in me for the fragility of the underlying psyche of the patient.

- October 2001 *Lycopodium* 200 C. x 1 dose
- November 2001 *Argentium nitricum* 30 C. x 1 dose, as needed
- December 2001 *Agaricus* 30 C. x 1 week x 4weeks
- January to March 2002 consults monthly with *Agaricus* 200 C. each consult
- March 2002 Sulphur 30 C. 1 dose a day for 3 days [Candida; no difference.]
- 2 weeks later *Medorrhinum* 200 C. x 1dose
- 2 weeks later *Bacillinum* 200 C. x 1 dose
- April 2002 *Arsenicum album* 200 C. x 1 dose only. [Gastro virus; successful treatment.]
- May 2002 *Thuja* 200 C. 1 dose a week x 4 weeks. *Graphites* 30 C. 1/day x 3 days. [warts; successful treatment.]
- June 2002 *Agaricus* 1 M. x 1 dose only
- July 2002 *Kali bichromicum* 30 C. 3 doses a day for 3 days [Cold, chest infection; successful treatment.]
- 2 weeks later no remedy given
- October 2002 *Thuja* 200 C. x 1 dose

- November 2002 *Candida Nosode* 6 C. 1/day
- 2 weeks later *Carcinosin* 30 C. 1 dose a day for 3 days

  March 2003 to January 2004 there were 4 consultations in which I repeated *Agaricus* 30 C. 1 dose a day for 3 days.

The low dose prescription was aimed at treating the Candida and Rosacea infection; this was successful.

- March 2004 *Agaricus* 1 M. x 1 dose
- April 2004 Repeat *Agaricus* 1 M. x 1 dose
- May 2004 No remedy
- June 2004 No remedy
- September 2004 Candida infection returns. *Agaricus* 6 C. given continuously daily

  The low dose of *Agaricus* 6 C. daily has successfully rid the patient of her Candida and Rosacea infection; the above Miasmic and *Candida Nosode* treatments did absolutely nothing to the continual infection she was suffering with. I have listed the frequency of repetitions. The aim of listing the doses is to allow readers to see with this case in particular, that the one remedy only had to be used in various potencies to mirror the very nature of *Agaricus*.

  Agaricus has duality and continual movement between extremes, and between virtual worlds. It is only when I saw the somatic polarity of the true nature of *Agaricus* that I realized I had to match the potency of the remedy to the inner psyche of the *Agaricus* patient. *Agaricus* has extremes.

Dosing between a low potency and high potency matched and mirrored the nature of *Agaricus*.

The *Agaricus* constitutions in my practice suffer from extreme, inexplicable pathologies and polarities with all their physical complaints.

- October 2004 *Agaricus* 6 C. given continuously daily
- December 2004 *Arsenicum album* 200 C. x 1 dose [Gastro

virus: successful treatment.]

- Consults monthly from December 2004 to February 2006 with *Agaricus* 6 C. given continuously daily
- Next consult: August 2006 *Agaricus* 6 C. given continuously daily
- October 2006 *Agaricus* 1 M. x 1 dose. As well as *Agaricus* 6 C. given continuously daily
- November 2006 *Agaricus* 1 M. x 1 dose. As well as *Agaricus* 6 C. given continuously daily
- March 2007 *Agaricus* 6 C. given continuously daily
- April 2007 last appointment. *Agaricus* 6 C. given continuously daily

The following is a transcript from the video taken at the last consult in April 2007. Physically, she no longer suffers from any of the physical symptoms: chest hair, constipation, weight gain preceding her menses. She also has her bingeing and weight gain under control and has for the last few years not had to think about dieting or excessively exercising to lose weight. She no longer feels her legs are excessively cold and not attached to her body. Most significantly, she does not get emotionally upset when she is with her mother, and no longer increases in size when she is emotionally distraught. She has made a permanent commitment to one man, but has an affair when she is in London for business. The transcript below reveals how she has constructed her two worlds. When she has committed to one man in the past, she has immediately fallen in love with another man, whom she has used as an escape from the first man. She subsequently internalizes the struggle, which results in confusion, and self-punishing bingeing and purging.

Question: You have just said to me that you are afraid of not having an exit valve.

It is a suffocation feeling. There is not enough room for me to exist within the one linear life. There is not enough room, which is why I often set up that dual existence. (She is referring to the two relationships.)

So you feel like you have to expand?

Yes but I don't just do that in relationships. I do it in work and all facets of my life.

You have cried desperately before that you want to have a relationship in your life. We have arrived at this point many times before where you get the guy, he is going to live with you, and then you have to escape.

Well, I feel relieved. I know this is not rational thinking but I feel less concerned about it now, knowing he is coming to live with me. I am actually breathing again knowing I have the affair. It is like the affair and my boyfriend have compartmentalized into two separate things. So everything with my boyfriend is good in my mind, and that is separate to the fact that I have had an affair.

So, I think that for the first time you can see your parallel worlds?

Yes totally so clearly. I don't feel badly about it this time. I am not 'doing a judgment call' on myself. I don't feel bad about it.

Yes, that is called health.

Yes, but there has been so much moral judgment about it not being appropriate. I haven't been able to do it guilt-free before now.

Which I agree has caused you a lot of problems. Where do you express that degree of guilt?

I have turned it in on myself. The bingeing has completely destroyed myself. I am now binge-free, even in the most heightened situation that I am in at the moment. I have just come off a tour with the band, tired, on a bus with shitty food around and I feel great.

But is it not because you have had an affair? [She has had many affairs in the past.]

No.

Is it because you allowed yourself to exist in two parallel existences?

There is still a lot I have to work out. Is it okay if I have an affair if we live together? Is it okay if we have children together? I have to work out all those boundaries.

But what happens if you put a boundary on yourself?

Well I freak out. As soon as I let myself off the hook I feel better about my relationship with my boyfriend.

It is interesting that you have allowed yourself a parallel existence, and that you have stopped bingeing. You don't split off from yourself, you don't numb-out anymore, the bingeing is much less, and you are able to perceive the other universe. For the first time you are talking about the parallel world being outside of yourself, rather than all the splitting going inside of yourself where you would end up quite confused. You are not going up and down in weight six kilos, or puffing up and becoming emotionally traumatized.

Yes it is easier this time. I have been able to physically separate the worlds. My weight is consistent for the first time ever. The fact is, Liz, when I have that dual world operating, I can't stop it and I don't want to.

6. *How*, *Why*, and *When* Causations – the 'Never-well-since-event'

Agaricus exists in two worlds. It is important that homoeopaths know that even when healthy, *Agaricus* will still exist in two worlds. The difference is she can now calmly say *when I have that dual world operating I can't stop it and I don't want to*. This case is an important inner view of how *Agaricus* constructs parallel worlds.

They will continue to need two worlds regardless of whether they are a healthy, or an unhealthy, *Agaricus*.

This patient now sits in a healthy *Agaricus* state, which is one of knowing two worlds exist but she no longer feels she is losing herself by falling down a rabbit hole. The question remains as to why this woman created two parallel worlds. In homoeopathy, if we can delve into the original crisis or psychodynamic trauma in the patient's life that created the first delusional perception, we have the remedy profile, and we have the cure for the crisis in their existence and subsequent pathology.

She tells me in the very first consultation: *my parents are divorced. My father left when I was three years old. I am torn between them. I am fearful I will end up alone, like my mother who is now on to her third husband.* She says, *I feel like I am creating an alternative world where I get to exist and have a fantasy world and it exists parallel to my own. The parallel universe will have no cross over.* By choosing two worlds she is never forced to choose between parents, and by creating two partners she is also never forced to choose one or the other. All *Agaricus* have the resounding feature of having 'childish' behavior. In this case in particular, it is important to understand how 'childish' behavior manifests. As a child, she refused to allow her parents to separate. Instead, she separated herself so she could exist in two worlds. She has a nervous breakdown at twenty-one years of age and at this time she experienced symptoms of paralysis similar to having a stroke on her right side. She was literally shutting down one side. Her explanation of, or cause given for her nervous breakdown was her mother's continual criticism of her weight gain. Criticism will confront *Agaricus* with one reality or one world. With one reality she had no other world in which to run to, except for confusion and breakdown. If I was to apply somatic psychotherapy to this case, her right side which she shut down and paralyzed was her mother side. The 'never-well-since-event', which I did not listen to carefully enough in the first consultation was when she told me she was *torn between the two parents*. If a person is *torn* then this, by its very nature, has to become a precursor to internal conflict and future pathology.

Case Analysis

She told me in the first consultation, *I fear losing myself. I feel like I am creating an alternative world where I get to exist and have a fantasy world. I have no exit valve. I am afraid the choices that I make will not be right.* In the last consult she acknowledges her process when she says, *I have been able to physically separate the worlds. My weight is consistent for the first time ever. The fact is, Liz, when I have that dual world operating I can't stop it and I don't want*[11] *to. Agaricus* is much healthier and happier in two realities coexisting side by side. She is able to tell me, *I haven't been able to do it guilt-free before now.* Health is reflected in her cessation of self-punishing, purging, and bingeing.

In this *Agaricus* case, the woman presented herself in the case-taking as being invincible in business, which is the

---

11 The contrary and contradictory explanations and unrestrained outrageous protestations of Alice can easily be identified in the outrage this woman would have had over her mother's criticism of her weight. The Caterpillar calls out to Alice that he has something important to tell her. "Keep your temper", said the Caterpillar. 'Is that all?' said Alice, swallowing down her anger as well as she could." Alice does have a rather "thoughtless; reckless" [Vermeulen] side to her. *Agaricus* is highly spirited and easily "excited" [Morrison] and Alice is particularly adept at "putting her foot in her mouth", especially with the Queen who after this interchange threatens Alice with decapitation. "'Stuff and nonsense!' said Alice loudly. 'The idea of having the sentence first!' 'Hold your tongue!' said the Queen, turning purple. 'I won't!' said Alice." It also has to be noted that Alice's tendency "to put her foot in it", or her ability to "talk without listening", [Vermeulen] is a fine line between "unrestrained" [Vermeulen] and the rubric: *speech wandering*, and *mischievousness*, or *nervous anxiety*. Throughout the story, Alice has a tendency to mention to the poor mouse who saved her from drowning in her own tears, how wonderful her cat Dinah was because she caught a good many mice! At the Caucus-race she upsets all the birds with the same comments about her cat, and at the Mad-Hatter's tea party she offends the Dormouse and Hatter. Alice is too easily upset, and frequently comments, "I wish the creatures wouldn't be so easily offended!"

Delusion rubric: *she is a great person.* The reason this *Delusion* rubric is used in the rubric-repertorisation is that she presented with contradictory emotional fears around her stature, in the world. The *Delusion* rubric is also used because she presents a picture of her personality which is disproportionate to reality. The *Delusion* rubric underlying and undermining the case was loss of personal stature which are the *Delusion* rubrics: *everything looks larger,* and *legs don't belong to her.* The *Delusion* rubric: *everything looks larger,* mirrored her underlying inability to manage her size and control her food bingeing. The *Delusion* rubric: *legs don't belong to her* mirrored her continual fear of failure in relationships. Every time she failed in a relationship she felt she lost all grounding and believed she would never find her footing and validation in life until she found the right partner. This is the correct interpretation of the *Delusion* rubric: *her legs don't belong to her.* For a *Delusion* rubric to be correctly used, misrepresentations and misappropriate appraisals of reality have to be seen in the case analysis, otherwise the rubric used should be the *Mind* rubric: *fear of being alone, fear of business failure,* or *fear after eating.* In all of these *Mind* rubrics *Agaricus* is not listed. The patient says, *I fear losing myself. I feel like I am creating an alternative world where I get to exist and have a fantasy world and it exists parallel to my own. The parallel universe will have no cross over.* She uses her belief that she exists in a parallel universe as a delusion which allows her to have a relationship with a man in each universe. This is a psychological 'delusion of grandeur', or hubristic denial, which she has developed to support herself; it is an example of a psychological delusion being used advantageously to self-delude.

Agaricus have the *Delusion* rubric: *obliged to confess his sins at the gate of hell.* [1] 1. The psychological denial inherent within this *Delusion* rubric alludes to the fact that unless *Agaricus* are forced by someone else, they do not want to acknowledge their 'dark-side' [*sins*]. *Agaricus* have the *Delusion* rubric: *enjoy out of body experiences.* [1] 1. It is a mistake to assume that this *Delusion* rubric resonates with the energy of the hallucinogenic fungi. *Agaricus* have the *Mind* rubric: *self-denial.* [1] 2. [staph.] *Agaricus* have a strong psychotic split within their persona which allows them to dissociate from their body and indulge their personality in exalted hubristic visions. *Agaricus* have the *Delusion* rubric: *illusions of fancy*, and the *Mind* rubrics: *euphoria*, and *egotism, reciting their exploits.* [1] 1. Conversely, *Agaricus* have the *Delusion* rubric: *body is diminished*, and the *Mind* rubric: *biting himself.* The latter two rubrics reinforce the need within *Agaricus* to maintain hubristic visions of grandeur because they need to avoid their underlying fear that they will be diminished not only from outside themselves, but also from within. *Agaricus* have several *Mind* rubrics which collaborate: not only do they struggle to assert themselves, they are also involved in a self-punishing battle. Not only do *Agaricus* want to be out of their body [*Delusion* rubric: *out of body*], they want to self-destruct. The *Mind* rubric: *self-denial* will always indicate psychotic, self-destructive, addictive behavior. *Agaricus* have several *Mind* rubrics which corroborate this: *ailments from alcoholism – ailments from debauchery – ailments from punishment – ailments from sexual excesses – anger with himself – biting himself – bulimia – frenzy causing him to injure himself.* *Agaricus* have the *Delusion* rubrics: *he is intoxicated*, and *he is drunk.* Both of these *Delusion* rubrics indicate a strong psychodynamic need to split from their conscious mind. Not only do *Agaricus* transfer their metaphysical power outside of themselves, [*to a mushroom*], they also hand over control of their body. *Agaricus* have the *Delusion* rubric: *he is commanded by a mushroom to rip up his bowels.* [1] 1. *Agaricus* displays on the one hand, 'delusions of grandeur' – *is a great person* – and on the other hand, self-diminishing needs to dissociate themselves from their body – *legs don't belong to her.* This polarity indicates self-destructive tendencies. The purpose of identifying psychological behavioral patterning inherent within the remedy profile is it can then be applied to identifying the simillimum in case analysis.

Bibliography

Carroll, Lewis. *The Complete Illustrated Works of Lewis Carroll*. London, Chancellor Press, 1986. p. 24, 28, 39, 49, 53, 64, 112.

Morrison, Roger. M.D. *Desktop Guide*. Nevada City, CA, Hahnemann Clinic Publishing, 1993.

Schroyens, Frederik. M.D. *Synthesis*. London, Homeopathic Book Publishers, 1997.

Vermeulen, Frans. *Prisma*. Emryss Publishers, Haarlem, 2002.

Vermeulen, Frans. *Synoptic Materia Medica*. The Netherlands, Emryss Publishers, Haarlem, 1992.

Anacardium

Abstract:

This is a case of a woman who feels overwhelmed by her sins from past lives. She suffers from an internal struggle between her good and the bad self. *Anacardium* have the *Delusion* rubric: *the devil speaking in one ear, prompting to murder and an angel in the other ear, prompting to acts of benevolence.*

Keywords:

Clairaudience. Internal conflict. 'Spirit' opposing 'evil'. 'Delusions of grandeur'. 'Delusions of original sin'.

D.O.B. 1968.

First Consultation: November 2005.

Presenting Issue:

- She came needing control over her cravings for sugar
- Weight and diet issues
- Candida
- Food allergies
- A history of stomach bloating

Case Analysis: I used the following key points and headings in analyzing this case.

1. *How, Why,* and *When* Causations – the 'Never-well-since-event'
2. *Striking,* or *Peculiar* Signs and Symptoms; Organon 153
3. Rubric-repertorisation
4. Theme
5. Materia Medica
6. Follow-up Consultations.

1. *How, Why,* and *When* Causations – the 'Never-well-since-event'

First memory concerning her weight:

Her mother put her on a diet at three years of age. *She didn't want me.* She suffers with intense pain at being rejected, and feels continually criticized by her mother over being too fat. The messages she picked up about her diet from her mother and father were inconsistent. Her mother would restrict her food (even at the age of three) and her father would bring home hot chips for her to eat. She is now estranged from her father. Her father criticized her about her weight continually, and rejected her when she was a teenager because she *was too fat and shamed him.*

History: She has experienced a lot of pain around rejection because of her weight, and consequently her self image has suffered. She was not good at sport in school because of her weight. She felt abandoned by her mother at three years of age. She feels out of control with food, and like *I can never do anything right that will help me lose weight.*

Occupation: Administration job, but only works part time because her true calling is in her spiritual work.

Appearance and first impressions: Very sweet and nice. *My* *mum never let me be angry when I was little; she still won't let me be angry. I have never been allowed to have any feelings. I have not been allowed to feel.* She is dressed in sky blue with a matching blue bead necklace, and blue make-up. She is soft looking, long blond hair.

Her soft, sky blue appearance is in marked conflict with how she has described her evilness and feelings of self-hate and shame around her weight and body. *God is a c--t because I have this body.*

Hobby or passion: She is training with a spiritual guidance group. In the future she wants to work with *Spirit* (God.)

2. *Striking*, or *Peculiar* Signs and Symptoms; Organon 153

Presenting Trauma: Clairvoyant ability to see crimes that she has committed in her past lives. She feels overwhelmed by *how evil I am.* Feels *separate from other people in the world; they will never understand me. They will never understand me.* She trains with a spiritual teacher who helps her stay with 'Spirit' so she *can undo the karma in this life and know how to listen to Spirit. I hate my mother she was a bitch towards me but I love her.*

Case Analysis

As a practitioner, I avoid working with diet and weight issues. I tend to refer patients to a Naturopath, because when I concentrate on instructing patients on dieting practices I never succeed. I agreed to consult with this patient because she was sent to me by her spiritual advisor, who talked me into consulting with her. This case is a very good example of the simillimum addressing her feelings of hopelessness around her inability to succeed with dieting.

The simillimum in this case must cover abandonment issues, psychological perceptions of real and imagined persecution and, most importantly, delusions that she needs her communication with God because she has been evil.

Each patient will have a tendency to be *predominately* in denial, forsakenness, persecutory paranoia, guilt, depression, or hypochondria. The simillimum *must* have *Delusion* rubrics which match the delusional state of mind of the patient. The importance of understanding the five psychological stages within each constitutional remedy profile is that they provide psychological insight into how each constitutional remedy will behave when they are emotionally, mentally, or physically unwell. Each remedy profile will present in one, or all, of the psychological stages.

If the constitutional remedy that the homoeopath has chosen has *Delusion* rubrics allocated to Denial, the patient *must* display psychological 'delusions of grandeur'. The simillimum in this case must pertain to the delusion that she is able to hear 'Spirit' (God).

- *Delusions: voices: hearing: calling: his name:* anac. [1] 1.
- *Delusions: hearing: illusions of: Anac.*

If the constitutional remedy that the homoeopath has chosen has *Delusion* rubrics allocated to Forsaken, the patient *must* display psychological 'delusions of abandonment' or 'delusions of persecution'. The simillimum must cover her feeling that her mother did not want her. The simillimum must cover her feeling of being *separate from other people in the world.*

- *Delusions: outcast; she were an:* anac.
- *Delusions: separated: world; from the: he is separated: Anac.*

If the constitutional remedy that the homoeopath has chosen has *Delusion* rubrics allocated to Causation, the patient *must* display psychological 'delusions of original sin'. The simillimum must pertain to her belief that she is evil because she has committed crimes in her past life. The simillimum must cover her conflicting hate and love of her mother.

- *Delusions*: *devil*: *he is a devil*: **ANAC**.
- *Delusions*: *crime*: *committed a crime; he had*: anac.
- *Delusions*: *divided*: *two parts; into*: Anac.
- *Delusions*: *devil*: *speaking in one ear, prompting to murder. angel in the other ear, prompting to acts of benevolence; and an*: Anac. [2] 1.

If the constitutional remedy that the homoeopath has chosen has *Delusion* rubrics allocated to Depression, the patient *must* display psychological 'delusions of impending doom'. The simillimum must cover her feeling that she will never succeed in losing weight, and that she can never do anything right.

- *Delusions*: *succeed, he does everything wrong; he cannot*: Anac.
- *Delusions*: *worthless; he is*: anac.

If the constitutional remedy that the homoeopath has chosen has *Delusion* rubrics allocated to Resignation, the patient *must* display psychological 'delusions of hypochondria'. The simillimum in this case must address her feeling that she has been thwarted in her ability to be angry in life. The *Delusion* and *Mind* rubrics which pertain to not being *allowed to have any feelings,* must pertain to suppression.

- *Delusions*: *dead*: *he himself was*: anac.
- *Mind*: *destructiveness*: *emotions; destructiveness from suppressed*: anac.

The advantage in identifying and understanding the psychological processing that your patient is moving through, is that it allows you to narrow the remedies being considered to the remedies listed in those particular rubric-categories. I have no other information about this case other than what she has told above.

Just by following the psychological stages which I am proposing, I have easily found the simillimum and understood the disturbance in this case.

Her first memory concerning her weight was the grounding for the causation of *Anacardium.* Her mother put her on a diet at three years of age; this is a profoundly damaging age to restrict a child's food. She interpreted this as abandonment; *she didn't want me.* She suffered intense pain at being rejected, and she was continually criticized by her mother for being too fat. She was also rejected by her Father when she was a teenager because she *was too fat and shamed him.* This forms the grounding for her lack of confidence in relationships with men, as an adult woman. *Anacardium* finds God to communicate with because 'Spirit' will not reject her.

The only person who understands this patient is 'Spirit' (God). She has a delusion that she is aligned with God and not with any other mortal being on this planet, who she assumes will never understand her.

Whether her past lives are 'real' or not, the essence of the case is that she feels this trauma as a truth inside of her. She believes that she *committed those terrible crimes.* Whether I take this as reality now, or in a past life, or reflective of either a capacity or a desire to commit those crimes in this life is immaterial. The psychodynamic meaning of feeling guilty, and a *terrible person who has done evil things* has to be the basis of the repertorisation. It is also a strong possibility that she has processed her parents rejection of herself, and transferred this into past life crimes. It is possible that this woman is experiencing a type of psychosis.

More than likely she has voluntarily taken on this belief in the guise of a 'New-Age' philosophy so she can find an explanation for the cause of her current suffering. If the trauma inside your patient starts with them feeling guilty and unrealistically responsible for their illness, then the simillimum is listed in the *Delusion* rubrics: *he is sinful, he has committed a crime* or *he has done wrong.*

A *Delusion* rubric is used when there is an assumption or perception which is a misrepresentation of reality. It is important to allow the patient, to arrive at what they themselves believe to be the cause of their suffering. If the homoeopath interferes with this crucial process by debunking the concept of karma, then the homoeopath will not get to find out the information they need to be able to pick the *peculiarities specific* to that patient and not to the psychosis.

If you offer philosophy to the patient they will not offer you *their* explanation; *their* explanation is a gem which will indicate the simillimum.

If your patient says to you, with the intensity of the 'eye of the storm', that they know *why* they are ill, and they reveal their sins, and conclude that their illness is their *just desert*, then this is indicative of the psychological delusions of punishment. In psychiatry, self-inflicted exile or self-imposed punishment is a consequence or end result of a 'persecution complex'. In homoeopathy, 'delusions of self-persecution' are repertorised by using the *Delusion* rubrics pertaining to sins. If your patient believes that they truly *deserve* their illness and this is why they are sick, then this is representative of the *Delusion* rubrics of having *sinned* and *committed a crime*. If your patient believes in a system of just punishment for their sins, this is an indication of disproportionate retribution. If their reactions to their feelings of being bad are disproportionately an *over-reaction* and misrepresentation of reality, then it is important to consider the *Delusion* rubrics pertaining to *wrongs committed*. These rubrics are also important to consider for patients who believe that the reason they are sick is because they are essentially bad people [*evil*]. These are the *Delusion* rubrics of being *in communication with the devil* or *being the devil*, or *being evil*. This group of rubrics is crucial to case-taking for patients who believe that in some way *they* are the cause of their illness or misfortune. Self-persecution is commonly referred to as psychological 'delusions of original sin'.

Psychological delusions of guilt are fueled by a *disproportionate* reaction to crimes most commonly committed in childhood. This patient has transferred her crimes to a past life. The essence of avoidance and self-deluding is that it is a psychological technique which allows the patient to over-react to their sins. The disproportionate reaction is either used to their advantage, or used as self-destructive, self-punishing condemnation. Self-destructive depression and predictions of failure underpin and cover up the psychological delusions of self-blame and psychological 'delusions of original sin'. Self-destructive depression and predictions of failure advantageously protect the patient from having to acknowledge sins committed, or alliances made with the 'evil-side' of themselves.

Self-destructive behavior and self-blame will be maintained and nurtured because they help protect the patient from their innermost dark secrets about themselves. This patient needs to hold on to her beliefs because she is unable to face her fear that she is failing in this life to achieve her goal of losing weight. The role of the homoeopath is not to confront psychosis.

3. Rubric-repertorisation

1. Denial: *Delusion* rubric: *voices: hearing: follow, that he must*: anac. *Delusion* rubric: *voices: hearing: calling: his name*: anac. [1] 1. *Delusion* rubric: *hearing: illusions of*. Anac. *Delusion* rubric: *voices: hearing: distant*: anac. *Delusion* rubric: *sight and hearing, of*: anac. *Delusion* rubric: *superhuman; is: control; is under superhuman*: anac. [This rubric can pertain to God or the devil.]

2. Forsaken: *Delusion* rubric: *outcast; she were an*: anac. *Delusion* rubric: *enemy: surrounded by enemies*: Anac. *Delusion* rubric: *separated: world; from the: he is separated*: Anac. [This rubric in relation to *Anacardium* does not necessarily pertain to separation or abandonment – it can pertain to 'delusions of grandeur'. *Anacardium* have a

hubristic vision of persona: they believe themselves to be set apart from mere mortals who do not have clairaudience or clairvoyance.]

3. Causation: *Delusion* rubric: *devil: he is a devil*: **ANAC**. *Delusion* rubric: *devil: speaking in one ear, prompting to murder: angel in the other ear, prompting to acts of benevolence; and an: Anac.* [2] 1. *Delusion* rubric: *crime: committed a crime; he had*: anac.

4. Depression: *Delusion* rubric: *succeed, he does everything wrong; he cannot: Anac. Delusion* rubric: *worthless; he is*: anac.

5. Resignation: *Delusion* rubric: *dead: he himself was*: anac.

   • *Delusions: voices: hearing: calling: his name*: anac. [1] 1.

   • *Delusions: hearing: illusions of: Anac.*

   • *Delusions: outcast; she were an*: anac.

   • *Delusions: separated: world; from the: he is separated: Anac.*

   • *Delusions: devil: he is a devil*: **ANAC**.

   • *Delusions: crime: committed a crime; he had*: anac.

   • *Delusions: divided: two parts; into: Anac.*

   • *Delusions: devil: speaking in one ear, prompting to murder: angel in the other ear, prompting to acts of benevolence; and an: Anac.* [2] 1.

   • *Delusions: succeed, he does everything wrong; he cannot: Anac.*

   • *Delusions: worthless; he is*: anac.

   • *Delusions: dead: he himself was*: anac.

   • *Mind: destructiveness: emotions; destructiveness from suppressed*: anac.

4. Theme

Anacardium suffer loss of memory with any sort of performance anxiety. If their failure is observed they feel exposed to criticism and rejection. *Anacardium* avoid facing their fear of being criticized and avoid feeling vulnerable to their own lack of self-confidence by aligning themselves with, and relying on, their 'divine' (whether it be devil or angel) auditory intervention. This patient has not been able to come to terms with her inability to lose weight; she feels like a failure. She has transferred blame for this failure on to her sins from a past life. *Anacardium* are clairaudient and clairvoyant. *Anacardium* have the *Delusion* rubric: *of sight and hearing,* and the *Delusion* rubric: *hearing voices of dead people. Anacardium* also have the *Delusion* rubric: *someone is whispering to him.* [1] 1. It is extremely important to *Anacardium* that they do not show their weaknesses. Illness is viewed by *Anacardium* as proof of failure. *Anacardium* is a constitutional remedy profile which, historically, has not been associated with 'delusions of grandeur'. However, *Anacardium,* more than any other remedy, have profound 'hubristic denial' around illness. Illness threatens their perfectionist, hubristic vision of themselves as being 'one who is aligned with God'. (She refers to God as 'Spirit'.) If *Anacardium* fail by becoming sick, they believe this to be proof that they are aligned with the devil. In using the word devil, I am not assuming personage. The devil is used liberally and is a generic term for any belief in a supernatural power which is evil. Unless a patient is suffering from psychosis, they will not walk into your consulting room and declare they are the devil. *Anacardium* allude in the consultation to an internal struggle between the good part of themselves and the bad part of themselves. *Anacardium* rarely act on their 'evil' instincts. *Anacardium* are in conflict between the two sides of themselves, which is why they are always alluding to their guilt over feeling aligned with the 'devil' inside of themselves. *Anacardium* have the *Delusion* rubric: *divided into two parts.*

Hubris is an insolent pride, or alignment with the Gods, leading to nemesis. 'Hubristic denial' is the belief that God has bestowed upon one great powers of omnipotence. A patient suffering with 'hubristic denial' refuses to believe that they are sick or could die. In relation to disease, and impending death, a patient believes they will be cured by God. Often, they believe that they are so powerful they can cure themselves. 'Hubristic denial' is the denial of illness or impending death because one believes one *is* an omnipotent God. *Anacardium* believe that they are so powerful they can cure themselves. *Anacardium* also believe that God will cure them. If the patient does not continually allude to an urgent need to connect with a 'greater spiritual power' to overcome their shortfalls, then the simillimum is not *Anacardium*. The underlying dilemma which undermines *Anacardium* if they move out of denial, is having to face their psychological 'delusions of original sin'. *Anacardium* are divided into two contradictory sides. *Anacardium* believe that the devil within has caused their illness. *Anacardium* display an urgent need for a 'higher spiritual connection', but their ulterior motive to gain a 'free get-out-of-hell card'. Sankaran writes, in *The Soul of Remedies*, "Whereas Anacardium is known for its hard-heartedness, cruelty, want of moral feeling, a compensated Anacardium cannot be cruel even when the situation demands. He will, perhaps, be unable to kill even an irritating mosquito." The reason Sankaran refers to a "compensated *Anacardium*" is that *Anacardium* are motivated by a desire to be good in order to assure themselves of a passage into heaven. Sankaran also refers to the fact that *Anacardium* are not able to be confident of themselves. *Anacardium* fear that they cannot succeed without the power of either God or the devil (God or the devil is synonymous with any dominant power). *Anacardium* have the *Delusion* rubric: *he does everything wrong, he cannot succeed*. *Anacardium* self-sacrifice to others to deny their rage [*devil*]. Sacrificing your life to save others is akin to an assured passage into heaven. Self-sacrifice is the best way to wipe clean the slate of crimes or sins committed. Self-sacrifice contains an ulterior motive for *Anacardium*, it assures them they are not the devil. *Anacardium* wish to be seen in a good light.

Anacardium have 'hubristic visions' of persona. *Anacardium* have the *Delusion* rubric: *devil speaking in one ear, prompting to murder and an angel in the other ear prompting to do acts of benevolence*, [2] 1. *Anacardium* need to maintain their psychological delusions of 'hubristic denial' to feel assured that they *are* God and not the devil. The "compensated *Anacardium*" who allows themselves to be dominated by God-like acts of *benevolence* is compelled to martyr themselves to a greater cause because they are trying to avoid and deny their own devil-like rage. The "compensated *Anacardium*" trying to avoid their rage by sacrificing themselves can't help but fall victim to self-perpetuating rage. As *Anacardium* become more aware of the fact that they have allowed themselves to be tied to the *bier*, their vengeful, devil-like rage is overwhelmingly violent, and malicious. This is why *Anacardium* are trapped between two contradictory wills. *Anacardium* have the *Delusion* rubric: *body is separated from the mind*, and the *Delusion* rubric: *soul is separated from the body*. *Anacardium* alternate between 'hubristic denial' and devil-like rage which they feel victim to because they have fallen into a seductive trap: they have sold their soul to God and the devil for clairaudience and clairvoyance. Their 'hubristic denial' perpetuates self-sacrifice, and the self-sacrifice in turn perpetuates rage at allowing themselves to be self-sacrificed.

Anacardium have intense fear of their own hate and 'devil-like' rage which flares intensely if they are contradicted or criticized. *Anacardium* have the *Delusion* rubric: *surrounded by enemies*. This delusional paranoiac feeling of being surrounded by enemies leaves them open to being hypersensitive about all real, or perceived criticisms. *Anacardium* consequently over-react when they are criticized. This is why *Anacardium* are listed so prominently in the rubrics for the devil in one ear, and the angel in the other. *Anacardium* have the *Mind* rubric: *antagonism with self*. *Anacardium* avoid facing their fear of being criticized and avoid feeling vulnerable to their own lack of self-confidence by relying on their 'divine' (whether it be devil or angel) auditory intervention. *Anacardium* spend an enormous amount of time berating themselves for their 'devil-like' rage and hate, which they try to make up for by over-compensating with 'god-like' generosity. Guilt over their reactivity keeps them separate from the world – *Delusion* rubric: *separated from the world.* Separating themselves from the world allows them protection from being criticized and contradicted. As there is no peace from their internalized dilemma of the *devil speaking in one ear, prompting to murder; and angel in the other ear, prompting to acts of benevolence, Anacardium* solve the debate by avoiding the world. This avoidance then becomes a self-fulfilling prophecy for *Anacardium* as they then believe they have been abandoned (forsaken) because they are evil. The simillimum will only be *Anacardium* if the patient periodically needs to avoid people, especially proceeding any kind of dispute. If the simillimum is *Anacardium,* the homoeopath must perceive that the patient has approached their illness with the same internalized separation. The simillimum will not be *Anacardium* unless the patient indicates that they want to hide their illness. This patient has hidden her sins in her past lives.

Their self-destructive behavior is separating themselves from the world and remaining in self-inflicted exile. *Anacardium* are difficult to treat when they are sick because they do not want to talk about their illness, or acknowledge that they are sick. This is avoidance. Illness exposes them to criticism and illness is proof of their 'dark-side' [*devil*]. Disease and illness is also viewed by *Anacardium* as proof of their failure to succeed. Their dark secret or innermost fear is that they will not be recognized. *Anacardium* have the *Delusion* rubric: *seeing everybody's face in the mirror except his own.* [1] 1. *Anacardium* fear everyone else will be reflected in the mirror and not them. When they are sick *Anacardium* become *religious.* It is a mistake to assume the *Delusion* rubric: *religious* applies to institutionalized religious practices. *Anacardium* will align themselves to various 'New-Age' ideologies, firstly so they can assure themselves that they are 'seeking a cure', and secondly because they need to believe they are spiritual [*angel*]. *Anacardium* will not present as an evil person; they will see themselves as righteously 'good'. *Anacardium* prefer to hide (deny) their 'devil-side' from themselves and others; it is only if they are criticized that one sees the *devil* in *Anacardium*. The simillimum will only be *Anacardium* if the patient believes that they can cure themselves by being good. *Anacardium* have the *Delusion* rubric: *body is separated from soul*. The simillimum will only be *Anacardium* if the patient believes that it is their body which is sick not their 'true self' [*soul*].

The homoeopath must be able to detect that the patient is 'split' or in denial about the bad [*devil*] part of them which is sick. This patient aligns herself with 'Spirit'; this is how she has been able to transform herself into a 'good' person. The simillimum will not be *Anacardium* unless the patient shows signs of denial, as well as signs of exaggerated self-blame ('delusions of original sin').

The simillimum will only be *Anacardium* if the homoeopath can perceive that the patient believes that they and the homoeopath *will not succeed* in making them well. *Anacardium* have the *Delusion* rubrics: *he is worthless,* and *he does everything wrong, he cannot succeed.* On one hand, *Anacardium* are in denial about their illness, and on the other hand they are fatalistic, they believe they are already *in their grave*.

Materia Medica

Sankaran writes, in *The Soul of Remedies*, "The situation of *Anacardium* is that of a kind of child abuse. Over strict parents impose all their desires on the child and do not allow him to think or do anything on his own. He cannot take his own decisions, to the extent that he is not allowed even to decide what clothes he should wear. If he starts taking his own decisions or does not live up to the expectations placed upon him, he will be punished cruelly. So he tries to live up to these expectations by being obedient and angelic in his behavior, and by being excellent in his work. But he begins to develop a lack of self-confidence, and becomes nervous. He is irresolute, because the outcome of his decisiveness is usually a severe punishment. If the domination persists and he is compelled to put up with it, he starts reacting with cruelty, malice, want of moral feeling, and antisocial behavior. Here he may also develop a tremendous overconfidence with contempt for others. But *Anacardium* can be very hard and cruel, and at the same time have a lack of self-confidence. There are thus two sides to *Anacardium*. On the one hand he is good, angelic, obedient from fear of punishment. He is very orderly, fastidious, cannot rest till things are in their proper place. The other part of him is hard, malicious, violent, devilish, disgusted with himself. He becomes immoral, develops suicidal or homicidal tendencies, is abusive, stubborn and avoids the company of people. These two sides of *Anacardium* are constantly in opposition to each other: should he be an angel or a devil. *Anacardium* could be the wife of a selfish tyrant who rules with an iron fist, and does not allow her to take any decisions. She becomes irresolute, lacks in self-confidence, is confused – always has two wills. She becomes dull and very absent-minded (*Anacardium* have a marked absent-mindedness). She may be childish, idiotic and timid out of lack of self-confidence and fear. The fear can paralyze her thinking as can be seen when appearing for an examination."

"He is persuaded by his evil will to do acts of violence and injustice, but is withheld and restrained by a good will. His external voluntary is consciously excited by external influences, but his real will, in which is his conscience, restrains that and keeps him from carrying the impulses into effect. This can only be observed when its action is on a really good man. He has a controversy when his external will is aroused, but in an evil

man there is no restraint and he will not have this symptom."
[Kent]

"Anguish and apprehension as of imminent misfortune. He
is at odds with the world, and has little confidence in himself
being able to accomplish what is demanded of him. Internal
anguish, which did not allow him to rest, he troubled himself
about every trifle, as if it would cause great injury, with solicitude
about the future. He takes everything ill and becomes violent.
Timorous in all actions; he views everything more anxiously
and timidly, always thinks of being surrounded by enemies,
then he becomes hot, his blood seems to boil in his chest.
Passionate and contrary. Extremely passionate at a slight
offence, breaking out into violence." [Hahnemann]

Follow-up Consultations: January 2006, February 2006, April
2006, May 2006, and July 2006.

I had been treating her with an *Anacardium* 30 C., dry
pilule, 3 times a week. She had been doing extremely well with
her weight and sugar cravings on a this dose and frequency.
Her sense of rejection about her weight was greatly improved,
and she had started to lose weight and control her sugar
cravings. She had also employed the services of a personal
fitness trainer and had started, for the first time, to exercise.
The shame around her body was starting to lift. The shame
about her past life sins was easing; she had started to tell me a
bit more about some of the evil sins she had committed.

Follow up Consultation: July 2006

A catastrophe occurred for her, and I needed to increase
the dose. Her spiritual, clairvoyant teacher criticized her in
class *for being blocked to God's message*. After that class, I
needed to increase the remedy to *Anacardium* 1M. x 1 dose.
Anacardium suffer from extreme anger and rage if contradicted
or criticized. Her alignment with 'Spirit' [God] was the only thing
which validated her existence. *Anacardium* only know who they
are when they receive praise from the world for their actions.

Anacardium suffer from a fear that there is something wrong with them, and they continually need to strive to prove it is not correct.

• Tries to prove himself. [Vermeulen]

The need to align to the 'good' within *Anacardium* is what Sankaran refers to as "a compensated *Anacardium*".

Anacardium have the *Delusion* rubric: *sees everyone's face in mirror except his own.* [1] 1. This rubric reveals two aspects of *Anacardium*. On the one hand, their paranoia about not being recognized is so intense that they expect to see everyone's face but their own. On the other hand, *Anacardium* avoid seeing their own face because they want to avoid self-reflection and exposure. *Anacardium* suffer an intense fear of being found out to be evil. *Anacardium* believe they are outcasts and that no one will want them. The *Delusion* rubric: *sees everyone's face in mirror except his own* reflects internal, paranoid fears about rejection from the outer world, as well as self-rejection. Their paranoia about being rejected is so intense that they believe everyone will be noticed except them: *everyone's face in mirror except his own.* *Anacardium* also has the *Delusion* rubric, *he must go into the air and busy himself.* [1] 1. This rubric allows *Anacardium* to avoid inner reflection and self-confrontation. *Anacardium* have an intense fear of their own hate and devil-like rage which flares intensely if they are contradicted or criticized. *Anacardium* spend an enormous amount of time berating themselves for their devil-like rage and hate, which they try to make up for by overcompensating with God-like generosity. *Anacardium* have the *Delusion* rubric: *devil; speaking in one ear, prompting to murder and an angel in the other ear, prompting to acts of benevolence.* Guilt over their reactivity keeps them separate from the world – *Delusion* rubric: *separated from the world.* Separating themselves from the world allows them protection from being criticized and contradicted. *Anacardium* have the *Delusion* rubric: *his mother is dead. Anacardium* will in particular separate themselves from their mother. *Anacardium* have no peace because of their internalized dilemma of the *devil speaking in one ear, prompting to murder; and angel in the other ear, prompting to acts of benevolence.* They solve the debate by avoiding the world. This avoidance becomes a self-fulfilling prophecy for *Anacardium* as they then believe they have been forsaken because they are evil. Self-destructive behavior and self-blame will be maintained and nurtured because they help protect the *Anacardium* patient from their innermost dark secrets about themselves. Their dark secret is their innermost fear that they will not be recognized and that they are *worthless: seeing everybody's face in the mirror except his own.* Their self-destructive behavior is separating themselves from the world and remaining in self-inflicted exile – *she was an outcast.*

Homoeopaths look for the 'evil' *Anacardium,* but you will not see the 'evil' *Anacardium* until they have a crisis. A crisis for *Anacardium* will proceed criticism and exposure.

After that session with her spiritual teacher, she ceased all contact with her teacher. She sank into a severe depression, rolled up into a catatonic ball and was overcome with a desire to rage against her own faith in God. She sent me an email which said, *last night I felt like my solar plexus was hemorrhaging and I wonder if life will ever be any different for me.* Her rage towards, and venomous talk with, God was everything one would associate with *Anacardium. I feel like crawling under a rock and never coming out but I also feel like driving a car through God's front fence or smashing all the windows in God's house. The saddest part is that now it is fifteen years on and I am in exactly the same position I was fifteen years ago. I am curled up in the same room, wanting to die, and I am crying over the same things. I hate my jobs. I hate my car, and I hate where I live. I can't believe I have created a world of hate for myself, but there is no denying it now. No relationship. No one has ever chosen to love me. For fifteen years I have been caught up in this delusion, and even when I hated everything else in my life I still had Spirit.* (God). *It is the thing that has kept me going, but it is also the thing that has kept me trapped in this delusion. Maybe I am insane. It must take insanity to stick with a delusion for so long. That is it. I give up.*

Anacardium can present with contrasting personality reactions to criticism. On the one hand, they can be aggressive and arrogant over defending their rights, and then on the other hand they can fear any authority that questions their validity. If *Anacardium* are criticized *Anacardium* interpret this as God abandoning them. *Anacardium* suffer with intense fears of being 'left out in the cold', and shunned by the world. This aspect of *Anacardium* is often not understood; a compensated *Anacardium* will roll up in a catatonic ball and *give up*.

- Desire to rage against her own faith in God. *I feel like crawling under a rock and never coming out, but I also feel like driving a car through God's front fence or smashing all the windows in God's house.*

- *My mum never let me be angry when I was little; she still won't let me be angry.*

- Cannot succeed. *Last night I felt like my solar plexus was hemorrhaging, and I wonder if life will ever be any different for me.*

- Destructiveness and hate. *I hate my jobs. I hate my car, and I hate where I live. I can't believe I have created a world of hate for myself but there is no denying it now.*

- Separated. *No relationship. No one has ever chosen to love me. She didn't want me* (mother).

- With God: *I still had Spirit* (God).

- Rage and venomous talk with God, but under the powerful influence of God. *It is the thing* (God) *that has kept me going, but it is also the thing that has kept me trapped in this delusion.*

- Rage and venomous talk with God. *God is a c--t because I have this body.*
- Insanity: *Maybe I am insane. It must take insanity to stick with a delusion* (God) *for so long.*
- Cannot succeed: *That is it. I give up.*
- Devil: Overwhelmed by *how evil I am.*
- Devil: *committed those terrible crimes.*

I concentrate entirely on videotaping follow up consultations. I commence videos after the patient has taken the remedy for some time. In particular, I am always vigilant towards any new trauma which has sparked off their subconscious or unconscious memory because it is at that point I find the meaning and relevance of every *Delusion* rubric.

The following is a transcript from the videoed session after the one dose of *Anacardium* 1m.

Follow up on the August 2006

Question: How have you been?

Well, I have been sick for two weeks, which has been frustrating because I have been beating myself up about trying to figure out why I have been sick, because I think something must have been blocked. So after the first week of being sick and being angry about that, then I just sat still and then some past life came up and some karma. So it was releasing some stuff. Then at the end of last week, some other stuff came up that I have fear about now. I am always surprised when it comes up, but I know there is something. So fear came up, and I got to release that. I don't quite know where I am at because physically I am weak because I have been sick. I feel a bit stronger because there is always a relief when you let more of it out.

What was the fear in relation to?

I am organizing an event and it got rejected. The thought of putting it out there again to even more people and the fear of being rejected was even more fearful. But before it would have been too much to bear. But I felt it and cried and let it out, but I said okay I have to do it, [cries a little] *anyway it's that or nothing. So you see all the emotion is still there.*

So that is a big shift?

Yeh, I think it is too, because I felt before I couldn't even have considered it.

Question: Yes, before it was like I can't do this, I can't go back, I can't be that vulnerable, I can't be rejected again?

Yes and it is still there with Mary (her spiritual teacher). *There is still a bit of that there, but with this it is as if I felt that if it happens again I am not going to crumble to nothing this time.*

What have you done about Mary?

Well, I realized that the karma of that lesson is the same as from before. That I had sought to destroy in the same way before (past life) *and again someone that I loved, and so on an energy level I have spoken to her ethereally but I haven't done it; but I have apologized and....* (starts to cry)

So you see a part that wanted to destroy her?

Yes, and the repetition of the pattern. Yes. (Crying)

You could see that you had done that before?

Only last week. I could see the other life and this life, and yes the lesson is the same. The behavior is just repeating itself... (crying) *The hardest thing is it is not random. It might be easy if you can look back and say, I was a soldier in that life and I killed someone, and I know it is all karmic but the specific part that it is the people that I have loved the most* (crying, long pause) *it makes it hard....*(crying).

Last time we talked about the competition between you and Mary? So you can see the competition? At the same time as seeing your intense hurt at being criticized?

Yes.

When you first came to see me, we talked about how difficult it was to talk about what you had done, your collections of sins and evils. How do you feel about talking about the karmic play between Mary and you, now?

I don't have as much shame as I did. Even for me to be talking with the camera going is a huge thing, and to be able to even acknowledge that other people will see me for who I am, and not just in this life, and you know will make judgments around that. There is no way I could have done that before, and it is still terrifying but it's not as. Before, I was so ashamed that it would have been unbearable, and now I am forgiving of myself. (pause) I can see it from the higher. Don't know when you have got the lesson or can see it in the context of the bigger picture. For me I can accept it more, and I have more acceptance of myself, and the things that I have done, and I think because I understand more maybe it has made me who I am, and also what I have from this life. I am in a position of power to do something about all those things as well. Like maybe I have taken some power back, rather than just staying stuck in the shame. I think I will always be sad about those things that I've done, but hopefully as time goes on you, me, hopefully I will be able to reconcile them. I don't know whether that transforms you. I feel like the lessons of those things I can now use to make me a better person, more of the positive of who I am.

What are you going to do about this situation with Mary?

I haven't spoken to her yet as I am still scared of the rejection. She might say I don't want anything to do with you. But even that, just since last week, that could happen and I need to find the place where that will be okay if that happens.

When this happened, you totally dissolved and you were totally distraught. Where are you sitting with that, now?

I don't know how or why, but I am just in a different place, now, like I can do something, and even if I don't get the response from Mary that I would like, I have found something that I can do regardless, and so it won't be the end of me, and that is how it felt before. And it is different, it is not an ego thing where you are alright anyway, and that would have been the defense before. It is more of an internal knowing or sense that I am here, and that I do have the power to do something and I need to do it regardless, one way or the other.... (long pause and sigh). *Which is quite different.*

Where are you sitting with all the terrible things that you have done?

I think, it is like there is a part of you. Like, as if a child does something and you have this amazing forgiveness for whatever. But it is not the child in me that did them. So it is just acceptance that there are different aspects of me, and we all need to co-exist together. [Delusion rubric: *divided into two parts.*] *Hopefully, from this point forward I will have mastery over myself. Before I was so scared because I didn't have mastery, and I didn't understand that. That aspect of me would take control again, or be the overriding force.* [Delusion rubric: *devil speaking in one ear, prompting to murder, and an angel in the other ear, prompting to acts of benevolence.*] *And if you can't have influence over what you can't see or command? Now I have an intimacy with it now I have connected with it and know it and don't have that fear of it like I did.*

Where are you with your clairvoyance now, because you wanted to be finished with it?

Well, having dismissed and chucked it in the bucket, in the last few weeks I have had really clear pictures just without any effort; hilariously clear, it is pretty funny, and it's even that different, that it is more like that part of me. They all have equal importance, so the part of me which is that I have clairvoyance and clairaudience, and whatever, it seems right, and just as normal as any other aspect of me. And if I can accept the acceptance of what we call darkness, or the shadow, whatever the aspect is, the good and the evil part; in accepting that, I can accept the good as well, and the higher part of me... (she starts to cry with relief). *Because it wasn't getting a go either.*

Conclusion:

Anacardium has an angel, or God, or 'Spirit' on one side, and a devil on the other side and when they are in a healthy state they co-exist together in harmony, with neither having control over the other. As she says, *if I can accept the acceptance what we call darkness or the shadow, whatever the aspect is, the good and the evil part; in accepting that, I can accept the good as well and the higher part of me.* One month after this session she returned to her classes with her spiritual teacher, Mary.

The dose of 1 M. has only been repeated twice since then, September 2006, one month later, and again in November 2006. She continues to grow in emotional strength and forgiveness of her past life sins. She is now concentrating on *this* life. Most importantly for *Anacardium* is that she is not so intensely hypersensitive to being criticized. My experience of working with *Anacardium* when they are healthy is that they are comfortable with themselves; they do not continually strive to prove their worth. As she says, *I am in a position of power to do something about all those things as well, like maybe have taken some power back, rather than just staying stuck in the shame.* If they are criticized, *Anacardium* interpret this as God abandoning them. Healthy *Anacardium* know they can continue on from an internal recognition of self. They do not need recognition from the world, and they will not be plagued by shame or guilt, or delusions that they are evil, or from delusions that they have done something wrong. *And it is different, it is not an ego thing where you are alright anyway, and that would have been the defense before. It is more of an internal knowing or sense that*

I am here, and that I do have the power to do something, and I need to do it regardless, one way or the other.

Follow–up December 2006. I gave her one dose of *Anacardium* 200 C. in C4. potency.

This session was, and has been, the most significant session. She has been praying and hoping that her father would die. She believes that when he dies she will be released from the karmic power he has over her, and she will be able to find a man that will fall in love with her. Her father hurt her intensely when she was a teenager by telling her she was fat, and not attractive as a woman. The *Mind* rubrics: *hatred, hardhearted, malicious*, and *cruelty*, do not do justice to the rage and murderous coldness she has held for him. In this last session of 2006, she agreed to visit him on his death bed. She cried, because for the first time she acknowledged that he was also a good father who had loved her. She has not spoken to her father for five years. I am excited to see what the C4 potency of *Anacardium* moved inside of her. I had just learnt about the C4 potencies with Alize Timmerman, and this is the first time I have used them.

Follow–up, February 2007

• Return to the trauma and fighting with her spiritual teacher. *Anacardium* C 4 potency x 1 dose.

Follow–up March 2007

• Dreams of comforting her father

• Fear over starting a love relationship, attraction to a neighbor. The start of feeling it was possible to have someone attracted to her sexually. Wants to have a relationship

• Happier with herself, and her job, even though it is boring. (Her delusion of being aligned to God has continually created a conflict within herself as one worthy of being with *Spirit* ('delusion of grandeur'), and then the reality of being in a simple, lowly administrative job.)

Follow–up, May 2007

- Fear of potential financial loss over a promotional event she is responsible for. (She takes on a huge promotional event which will change the way people view the world. This is the *Delusion* rubric: *hearing voices that he must follow*.)
- Borrows money from her sports trainer

Follow–up July 2007

- She has collapsed over failure, the promotional event has failed. She was publicly humiliated

  Anacardium C 4 potency x 1 dose. Plus *Anacardium* 200 C. x 1 dose. Taken one week apart.

Follow–up, July 2007

Anacardium C 4 potency x 1 dose. Plus *Anacardium* 200 C. x 1 dose.

- She did not take this prescription.

She has suffered financial losses from the failed promotional venture. Consultations are stopped with me because of financial difficulties, and she has resigned from her job. She resigned from her job because her true path (she is told) is with 'Spirit'. (This is a 'delusion of grandeur'; she feels too special to work as an administrator. *Delusion* rubric: *hearing voices that he must follow*.) In this act she is attempting to transfer acknowledgment of personal failure. This is self-deluding. Psychological denial is adopted by the patient when they need to maintain their psychological delusion to avoid reality. *Anacardium* have the *Delusion* rubric: *he is separated from the world*. This rubric in relation to *Anacardium* does not necessarily pertain to separation or abandonment – it can pertain to 'delusions of grandeur'.

Anacardium have a hubristic vision of persona: they believe themselves to be set apart from mere mortals who do not have clairaudience or clairvoyance.

She has not been taking her remedy since July 2007. She stopped because 'Spirit' told her to. (This is a 'delusion of grandeur'. *Delusion* rubric: *hearing voices that he must follow*.)

Follow–up Last Contact: March 2008

The last contact was via email. Below is a copy of the email.

Ah, the time has come. I wondered when the karma would kick in and it just has. In another life you committed an act of betrayal that led to my downfall, and in this life we get to live it again in the hope that we will do it differently. I get the feeling you have a sense of this but I'll spell it out anyway. (*Anacardium* believe they possess auditory clairvoyance that allows them to see into future events.)

I assume you intend showing the video as part of your teaching while you are in the United Kingdom, which is why the karma has kicked in. I ask that you never show that video to anyone else for any purpose, that you hand the original tape to me and destroy any copies that have been made. Can you do that, Liz? In your head you will find a thousand reasons why it is an important part of your teaching and that it will serve a greater good. The reality is you will be in a battle between your conscience and your ego. It remains to be seen which will win. As you well know this is something I am very familiar with and I too am responsible for a significant act of betrayal in history so I know much of what I speak of. The dark forces work through man's ego and the more evolved you are the more subtle they get. The power is in your hands, Liz. You may want to ponder the following. Do fame and reputation always come at a cost and is this a price you are prepared to pay? Is the wounded child still trying to prove her worth? I judge you not, for where you now stand I have stood also. May the forces of light be with you.

The video tapes were of course destroyed. She sent a copy of the email (which she sent to me) to the personal trainer who was helping her with her fitness. He was the man who lent her money for her promotional event, which had lost money. She did not return the money. He was understandably confused by this email. I explained it as much as possible by informing him he would not be paid back the money because he had also been involved in karma with her in past lives. He said this was the first time he'd known someone to use this excuse for not repaying a debt!

To the Sports Trainer: *I have copied you in on this email as you are also part of this karma. When I asked the gods why I needed to include you, they said it is important that you know the truth of who we are. We are each imperfect humans trying to find our way in mastering the forces within. That is the process of life. No one is higher or lower. We each have talents and gifts as we each have challenges and struggles. In helping others we help ourselves. Our greatest teacher and our greatest healer is the one within.*

Anacardium suffer from anxiety about being judged or found out to be flawed. *Anacardium* are fastidious about every little detail in case they have failed to be perfect ('delusion of grandeur'). They are fearful of failure, of being exposed and the world finding out that they are flawed and evil ('delusions of original sin'). It is not until they are 'outed' in their failure that you see the rage and hatred that is associated with the constitution *Anacardium*. Until this email contact, I had considered this case a success. The fear of being 'outed' in this video became her subsequent focus because she had publicly failed in her previous venture. She needed to transfer the 'outing' on to me, and she needed to find a way out of having to pay back her financial debt to the personal trainer. The worst irony and sadness of this case is that I had no intention of showing her case, and if I did, I would have asked her a long time before my lecturing tour so she had time to think about how she felt about it being shown. I had always felt her tendency to go into psychoses made her too vulnerable. The transference of karmic blame on to me and the personal fitness trainer became a way out of having to acknowledge personal fault and failure.

This case highlighted for me the potential traps and damage we as homoeopaths can face in videoing our patients.

She requested that I must destroy the tapes by fire. I am reminded of all sinners being burned by the fires of hell. I had prescribed *Anacardium* because her relationship with *Spirit*, [God] and her mother were both filled with the polarity of the emotive words of love and hate, *God is a c--t because I have this body,* and *I hate my mother she was a bitch towards me but I love her.* It is this battle of *Anacardium* that is often not understood by homoeopaths. We look for the 'evil', but in fact we should be looking for the 'good' sweet *Anacardium* because it is the 'good', *Anacardium* that you will see in the first consultation, and in fact all consultations, until *Anacardium* have a crisis.

Follow–up, 2009.

I have heard through other patients that she is back with her spiritual advisor, and is continuing to do very well with her 'Spirit' and with her weight, so this encouraging.

Bibliography

Hahnemann, Dr. Samuel. *The Chronic Diseases.* New Delhi, B. Jain Publishers, 1995. pp. 277-281.

Kent, J. T. *Lectures on Materia Medica.* New Delhi, B. Jain Publishers, 1994. p. 103.

Sankaran, Rajan. *The Soul of Remedies.* Santa Cruz, Bombay, Homoeopathic Medical Publishers, 1997. p. 7.

Schroyens, Frederik. M.D. *Synthesis.* London, Homeopathic Book Publishers, 1997.

Vermeulen, Frans. *Synoptic Materia Medica.* The Netherlands, Merlijin Publishers, 1992.

Anhalonium

Abstract:

This is a case of a woman who knows she is the messenger of God. Her internal conflict is on the one hand fear of hubris, and on the other hand, fear that she will fail to be able to carry forth God's message. *Anhalonium* have the *Mind* rubric: *weakness of will* and the *Delusion* rubric: *of immortality.* *Anhalonium* is the link between the universal energy of God and the earthly plane.

Keywords:

Omnipotence and impotence. 'Delusions of grandeur'. 'Delusions of hypochondria'.

D.O.B. 1942.

Occupation: Practitioner of esoteric science.

First Consult: January 2007

Presenting Physical Symptoms and Illness:

- Positive Rheumatoid factor
- Hashimoto's
- Thyroglobulin (TG) antibodies
- Thyroid Peroxidase antibodies (TPO)
- Acne Rosacea

- Inability to manage weight, diet, exercise, food
- Inability to manage teaching timetables and work diary schedules
- Extreme heat and flushing
- Arthritis in hands and feet
- Unsteady on her feet
- Feels mentally vague and unable to regulate a food regime
- Hypoglycaemic
- Heat and skin rashes under her arms
- Complains of vague memory loss

Presenting Illness:

A prerequisite of an auto-immune disease such as Rheumatoid Arthritis, is that its pathology has to have its foundation in delusional disturbance. Auto-immune diseases produce anti-bodies which attack the body's own connective tissue and organs. The excess anti-nuclear anti-bodies subsequently become self-destructive. The rubrics that point to the correct remedy for the numerous auto-immune cases which I have treated in my practice are found within the *Delusion* rubrics because these are the rubrics which resonate with conflict, self-destruction and disorder; they match the very nature of the disease state. The primary trauma which caused the primary *Delusion* rubric is the causation in the case. Then *there must be evidence* in the case-taking of self-destruction and pathology which proves the need to use a *Delusion* rubric in the rubric-repertorisation. This is confirmed in the pending development of an auto-immune condition. You can only use a *Delusion* rubric in the case analysis if you can identify how the patient has used the psychological delusion as a revisionist misinterpretation of reality. You can only use a *Delusion* rubric in the case analysis if the four prerequisites have been noted in the patient's case-development.

My role in finding this patient's simillimum is to uncover the inner, self-destructive, 'never-well-since-event' which was the precursor to her auto-immune condition.

Case Analysis: I used the following key points and headings in analyzing this case.

1. *Striking*, or *Peculiar* **Signs and Symptoms; Organon 153**
2. **Rubric-repertorisation**
3. **Theme**
4. *How, Why,* and *When* **Causations – the 'Never-well-since-event'**
5. **Materia Medica**
6. **Follow-up Consultations**.

1. *Striking*, or *Peculiar* Signs and Symptoms; Organon 153

A prerequisite is to find the inner disturbance which is the core of our case-taking, and it is always reflective of what is unusual or disturbing to *your* (the homoeopath's) inner sensibilities. My aim in listing the rubrics used for each section is to construct a rubric repertory of the consultation which will enable you, the reader, to see one of the processes of case analysis which will be invaluable to your understanding of unusual cases.

This patient teaches a form of inner emotional work which enables her patients to be in touch with their own emotional consciousness and life purpose. Her work involves the mapping of several planes of consciousness to help her patients understand their own individual emotional mapping and behavior in the world. The 'sixth ray' she refers to is one of the categories of her levels of awareness or planes of consciousness.

Case Notes

Question: You were talking about your concept of the sixth ray can you tell me about that?

The sixth ray is about devotion and idealism. It is devotion to an ideal or personification of an ideal. It a can be devotion to a person, to a Guru or teacher. Joan of Arc would be an archetypical example, so there can be a martial element to the sixth ray, which would emphasize the idealistic nature, or there can be more of a personal devotional nature to it, like the student to the master. Having a strong counter dependence to the sixth ray, I realized my life's purpose is a sixth ray life purpose and that is not around devotion to a particular person but devotion to an ideal. A sense of what has to be done and an absolute commitment to making sure that it is done. And for a long time feeling somewhat embarrassed about that, wanting to deny that, but I think it is also about building the capability. The ideal is all very well and good, but if you don't have the strength of form to give it carriage in the world then it's just about smoke and mirrors. A lot of my life has been spent building the vehicle to enable the ideal to be in the world, to have expression in the world. The ideal that is at the seat of the sixth ray is about consciousness. It is about the unfoldment of human consciousness, towards a destiny of complete realization.

Striking, or *Peculiar* Signs

- Joan of Arc is her ideal, or the personification that she identifies with.
- This patient sees herself as having a similar life purpose to Joan of Arc.
- Joan of Arc is able to hear God talking to her. Joan of Arc has clairaudience.
- God tells her to go into battle to defeat the English. Joan of Arc resorts to military force to defeat the English i.e. *martial element.*

- She tells us: *my life's purpose is a sixth ray life purpose.*
- She tells us she has *devotion to an ideal.*
- *The ideal is all very well and good, but if you don't have the strength of form to give it carriage in the world then it's just about smoke and mirrors.* She is worried that her body will not be well enough to carry her on her journey.
- Her life purpose *is about the unfoldment of human consciousness towards a destiny of complete realization.* The patient is talking about how she is the messenger of a universal energy. She needs to be the link between the universal energy of God and the earthly plane.

It is important to note the rubrics for her alignment with Joan of Arc because this is an unusual personification to identify oneself with. In repertorising a case such as this it is important to listen to the patient's description of herself and repertorise on the basis of how she describes herself. She tells us her goal, like Joan of Arc's was towards *the unfoldment of human consciousness towards a destiny of complete realization.* What we know of Joan of Arc from history is that she had visions, and heard Gods message. When I ask this patient to describe herself she tells me that her life goal is aligned to Joan of Arc's. Then I should repertorise of what I know about Joan of Arc. The *Delusion* rubrics for the personification of Joan of Arc would be the following *Delusion* rubrics.

2. Rubric-repertorisation

- *Delusions*: *beautiful*: anh.
- *Delusions*: *fancy, illusions of*: anh.
- *Delusions*: *hearing: illusions of*: anh. [This rubric pertains to clairaudience.]
- *Delusions*: *visions; has*: [This rubric pertains to clairvoyance.]

- *Delusions*: *voices*: *hearing*: [This rubric pertains to clairaudience.]
- *Delusions*: *visions, has*: *wonderful*: [This rubric pertains to clairaudience.]
- *Delusions*: *immortality, of*: anh. [1] 1. (Her life purpose *is about the unfoldment of human consciousness towards a destiny of complete realization*. This is the *Delusion* rubric: *of immortality*. Hubris is an insolent pride or alignment with the Gods, leading to nemesis. 'Hubristic denial' is the belief that God has bestowed upon one great powers of omnipotence.)
- *Delusions*: *answers to any delusion*: anh. [1] 2. [aster.] [The meaning of this *Delusion* rubric is that *Anhalonium* are liable to be influenced or taken over by someone else, or desire another form. This rubric is about self imposed abandonment of the conscious self. *Anhalonium* desire decomposition of shape in the world. *Anhalonium* like the sensation that they are floating without form; transparent and able to be carried off into a non-material world. This *Delusion* rubric also means she can be easily swayed by any possible psychological delusion, or overwhelmed by mental and emotional instability. This confirms her doubt about *having the strength of form to give it carriage in the world*.]

The *Mind* rubrics to match her devotion to her ideal are:

- *Mind*: *euphoria*: anh.
- *Mind*: *fancies*: *exaltation of*: anh.

The following statement: *The ideal is all very well and good, but if you don't have the strength of form to give it carriage in the world then it's just about smoke and mirrors*, indicates a conflict over her ability (strength) to fulfill her quest.

The *Mind* rubrics that match her weakness of form are:

- *Mind*: *execution lost as the result of overpowering visual sensations*: anh. [1] 1.

- *Mind: will: weakness of: Anh.*
- *Mind: will: loss of will power: Anh.*

Immortality and omnipotence are the key words of an *Anhalonium* case. *Anhalonium* is the link between the universal energy of God and the earthly plane. Regardless of the nature of the trauma or disease, each individual *Anhalonium* patient will always be in a crisis which mirrors, or resonates with, the theme of immortality and omnipotence. In this *Anhalonium* case the woman is the messenger of God.

3. Theme

Anhalonium want to escape identifying with the external world by involving themselves in their inner spiritual clairvoyance and clairaudience. *Anhalonium* use divine auditory intervention to avoid emotional, mental, or physical interaction with the worldly plane. *Anhalonium* have the *Delusion* rubric: *merged with present eternity.* [1] 1. *Anhalonium* only experience conflict if they are *hindered*. *Anhalonium* experience all illness as a *hindrance* because they do not want to identify with their emotions, their mind, or their physical body. *Anhalonium* do not want to identify with their 'ego'. The 'ego' is the realistic rational part of the psyche. If a remedy profile has a weakened 'ego' then their psyche is under threat. *Anhalonium* choose to abandon their psyche, preferring *transparency* of the self. *Anhalonium* do not want to identify with their somatic 'id'. *Anhalonium* abandon their unconscious instinctual 'id', preferring an *out-of-body decomposition*. *Anhalonium* have the *Delusion* rubric: *body is immaterial*. *Anhalonium* do not want to be ruled by the conscience of the 'super-ego'. *Anhalonium* do not want to identify with the inspirational ideals and spiritual goals and conscience of the 'super-ego' which criticizes or prohibits any feelings or actions. *Anhalonium* identifies entirely with their *immortal* ethereal body. Their spiritual goal is to *merge in eternity* and not to strengthen their 'super-ego' on this earthly plane. *Anhalonium* have the *Delusion* rubric: *of immortality.* *Anhalonium* are in tune with the psychical energies of the soul. Because *Anhalonium* are in tune with the psychical energies of their soul they have no fear of death. *Anhalonium* know that their soul goes with them when they die. Disease is viewed as a *hindrance* because it forces them to become aware of their somatic body. *Anhalonium* will always be very agitated when they are sick because it forces them to re-enter their somatic consciousness. *Anhalonium* have the *Delusion* rubric: *parts of the body seem too large.* *Anhalonium* do not want to 'live in their body'. When they are sick they often complain that their body is cumbersome and irritating. If *Anhalonium* are forced by illness to 'live in their body' they often experience a *peculiar* 'persecution complex'. *Anhalonium* patients have often said to me: *I hate it when I am sick, it forces me to become aware of my body. People around me love it when I am sick because it makes them think I am just like them. I don't want to be like them. I think they all sit around looking at me, willing me to be sick so that I have to come back to this earthly plane. I feel surrounded and attacked.* This is the *Delusion* rubric: *sees faces scheming*, and the *Delusion* rubric: *snakes in and around her.* It is crucial that the *Delusion* rubrics are used in case analysis to psychosomatically mirror any emotive theme which is disproportionately paranoid. When *Anhalonium* are forced by illness to 'live in their body' they imagine that their body is forcing them to become aware of a somatic consciousness which they wish to discard. This is the psychodynamic meaning of the *Delusion* rubric: *parts of the body seem too large. Anhalonium* choose to connect to their *immortal* soul. *Anhalonium* have a psychic connection to a spiritual world, and actively disconnect themselves from an earthly, external world. Other *Delusion* rubrics to consider for *Anhalonium* would be, *out of the body, separated from the world*, and *decomposition of space and shape. Anhalonium* do not have any *Delusion* rubrics pertaining to self-blame or 'delusions of original sin'.

If your patient blames themselves for their illness, then the simillimum is not *Anhalonium*. *Anhalonium* does not necessarily blame anyone else, either.

1. Denial: *Delusion* rubric: *hearing: illusions of*: anh. *Delusion* rubric: *voices: hearing*: anh. *Delusion* rubric: *music: thinks he hears*: anh. *Delusion* rubric: *visions, has: wonderful*: anh. *Delusion* rubric: *visions, has: colorful*: anh. [1] 1. *Delusion* rubric: *sounds: color; are like*: anh. [1] 1. *Delusion* rubric: *transparent: everything is: Anh.* [2] 1. *Delusion* rubric: *seeing: herself*: anh. *Delusion* rubric: *space: decomposition of space and shape*: anh. *Delusion* rubric: *visions, has: beautiful: kaleidoscope changes; varied*: anh. *Delusion* rubric: *figures: seeing figures*: anh. *Delusion* rubric: *floating: air, in*: anh.

2. Forsaken: *Delusion* rubric: *faces, sees: scheming*: anh. *Delusion* rubric: *snakes: in and around her*: anh.

3. Causation: NONE.

4. Depression: *Delusion* rubric: *hindered; he is*: anh.

5. Resignation: *Delusion* rubric: *body: out of the body: Anh.* *Delusion* rubric: *transparent: he is*: anh. [These rubrics can pertain to hubristic visions of clairvoyance or to physical disassociation.] *Delusion* rubric: *large: parts of the body seem too large*: anh.

4. *How*, *Why*, and *When* Causations – the 'Never-well-since-event'

Question: Where do you think the blackness [shadow] comes from?

My earliest memory of my work in the world came in my adolescence, when I had a sort of a waking dream. I was on the hill where the Masonic temple stood and I was singing and they were listening and they (the Gods) were being moved. My singing had an extraordinary rightness and potency to it. There are numerous moments over my life of luminosity where the Gods came to dwell along side of my mere humanness. My difficulty was being able to embrace the grandeur as well as live with my human limitations and be who I am at the moment; which is certainly not God-like. So the bigness and the littleness and the gap in-between was a challenge to live with, and the sense of shame thinking it was something that I would ever do.

There is hubris in that. But secondly the shame that comes with the contrast with that vision and what I am actually capable of. It is not something that I am now living or grappling with, there is a depressive element in me. I am flawed.

Case Analysis

On the one hand she aligns herself to the potency of the luminosity of the Gods. *Anhalonium* is the only remedy listed under the *Delusion* rubric of *immortality*. *I was singing and they were listening and they were being moved my singing had an extraordinary rightness and potency to it. There are numerous moments over my life of luminosity where the Gods come to dwell along side of my mere humanness.* On the other hand, she identifies with her impotence: *my difficulty was being able to embrace the grandeur as well as live with my human limitations and be who I am at the moment; which is certainly not God-like.* There is a notable contradiction in what she has told us: *the shame that comes with the contrast with that vision and what I am actually capable of. It is not something that I am now living or grappling with, there is a depressive element in me. I am flawed.*

She aligns herself to God, but she is flawed and not able to live up to her ideal of being God. This is where her inner disturbance and inner conflict lies. In homoeopathy we do not prescribe on the basis of an event or particular disease; we prescribe on how the individual perceives and consequently internalizes that event, or how the patient experiences their particular disease. Each *Anhalonium* patient will conclude that they will survive any future potential assault if they were as one patient put it, *outside of my body, in tune with God and the universe.* A disturbance should be immediately noted by the homoeopath as unusual in the case if it is a *peculiar* and strange symptom of the case. The case notes transcribed below reflect how the patient has internalized trauma from her father's constriction and control in her childhood, and created the polar opposite of expanding her life purpose into the universal life purpose of attuning herself with the messenger of universal energy: God.

Question: What is the first conscious memory of being flawed?

It would have been maybe three or four years.

What was the event?

Dad was fixing up a house and there was a lot of tension in the house. Dad was a volatile individual, and there was a snake that came into the house and Dad's response to that. The fear that I went into. It wasn't so much the snake but Dad's response to that. It has either been inflated in my mind or it happened very closely to that event where we were jumping on one of the beds and my brother slipped between the bed and the wall and dislocated his shoulder or broke his arm. And once again Dad's response to that was once again the most terrifying thing. It was the omnipotence of the Gods to just sweep all, to lay waste to everything that had been built, and there is nothing you can do about it. Absolute helplessness in face of the annihilating storm; you cannot do anything about it.

But why were you flawed in that?

Well, it was my fault of course. [Laughs] *I suppose my impotence would have to travel with omnipotence. It's my omnipotence that says of course I am to blame if this is happening. I couldn't stop it, I couldn't make it okay.*

- *Delusions: immortality, of.* anh. [1] 1.
- *Delusions: separated: world, from the: he is separated: Anh.*
- *Mind: will: weakness of: Anh.*

She has no power or will power over the world: *it was the omnipotence of the Gods to just sweep all, to lay waste to everything that had been built, and there is nothing you can do about it.*

Anhalonium feel *separated from the world,* and believe they have been rejected by the world because they are so different. They also choose to *separate themselves from the world* to connect to the ethereal. *Anhalonium* have *wonderful visions* of the spirit world which are much more attractive to *Anhalonium* than this earthly world. *Anhalonium* will embrace death because they believe they are going to live forever in 'spirit'. If your patient is fearful about their fatal illness and death the simillimum is not *Anhalonium. Anhalonium* are not interested in, and do not cope with, the earthly plane of existence; they only feel depressed if they are *hindered* from leaving. *Anhalonium* feel like they are suffering by being forced to live on this earthly plane. They feel like they are waiting to die so they can be an *immortal* soul *merged in eternity. Anhalonium* have the *Delusion* rubric: *he had to wait.* [1] 1.

The *Mind* rubric, *loss of will power* indicates that within *Anhalonium* is an ability to have insight into their loss of will power, and insight into their desire for power when they align themselves to the immortality of God. Aligning themselves to God carries omnipotence and expansiveness. This reflects and explains the meaning of what is an unusual *Delusion* rubric: *answers to any delusion. Anhalonium* have the *Mind* rubric: *heightened awareness of body.* In *Anhalonium,* this awareness becomes intensely apparent when they have to face pain within a weak body that is on this world, not merged within the immortal, universal, omnipotent power of God. *Anhalonium* want to merge with the universal power of immortality.

5. Materia Medica

Anhalonium have to expand their reach and identity into the universe and into everything outside of their material world in order to have the sense that they will survive. *Anhalonium* is a drug remedy prepared from Peyotl, the cactus from which the phenethylamine mescaline is extracted. Sankaran, in *The Soul of Remedies,* writes, "The experience of mescaline is often one of merging with one's surroundings or the feeling of being one with the whole of existence, seeing oneself without boundaries. This experience implies immortality – what dies is the body; as the self is continuous with the whole of existence, it cannot be mortal." Immortality and omnipotence are the key theme words in an *Anhalonium* case. Sankaran says of this crisis within *Anhalonium,* "He starts living inside a bubble, isolated from the rest of the world but inside it, he creates his own universe." *Anhalonium* have the *Delusion* rubric: *he is separated from the world,* which reflects the struggle to stay on the earthly plane of consciousness.

When I studied homoeopathy, *Delusion* rubrics were interpreted as the flights of fancy of the unstable patient, or the presenting fantasies of the patient when they have a high fever. This astounding misunderstanding of the *Mind* section of the repertory is distressing to say the least. It is within our patient's disturbance that we find the *peculiar* symptoms that Hahnemann asked us to look for in aphorism 153 of The Organon. These disturbances are the *Delusion* rubrics.

The *Delusion* rubrics reflect our unconscious and subconscious; they are not relayed by our patients as part of their conscious, logical mind. The distinguishing characteristic of *Anhalonium* (which you will not see in any other constitution other than perhaps *Anacardium*) is that it is merged with the expansiveness of the subconscious and unconscious, as well as being acutely aware of struggling with the conscious world. This patient outlines the purpose and idealism of *Anhalonium*, and the struggle to be on the earthly plane, when she says, *a sense of what has to be done and an absolute commitment to making sure that it is done. The ideal that is at the seat of the sixth ray is about consciousness. It is about the unfoldment of human consciousness towards a destiny of complete realization.*

In *An Insight Into Plants*, Sankaran writes, "This is exactly the experience of *Anhalonium*. It has a lot to do with the mind expanding. There is talk of depersonalization and dissolving of the borders and yourself, expanding into the universe. The feeling is as if there is decomposition of shape. One's body is immaterial and enlarged and diminished. The merging of oneself with one's environment is basically a self-expansion. This is the main symptom of *Anhalonium*. In *Anhalonium* everything is getting narrow and shrinking and I have to expand or I will disappear." *Anhalonium* has a need to feel like they are expanding into the universe. Sankaran places *Anhalonium* in the Cancer Miasm and within the Cactaceae family. The sensation of Cactaceae is contraction, within the plant kingdom the theme is polarity and expansion. *Anhalonium* also has "confusion as to his identity, depersonalization, loss of self-knowledge and self-control, disassociation from or self-identification with environment." [Vermeulen].

6. Follow-up Consultations

Question: Do you think that since taking the homoeopathic remedy your grounding in dealing with the world is better?

Yes, I think so. What I would call the first ray element of will or power has found its right place in a way that it hasn't up till now. It is not nearly as shocking to a relatively sensitive personality vehicle as it used to be. So the personality vehicle has the strength to contain and hold that potency. The other thing that has happened since taking Anhalonium is that it is as though the masculine principle has taken its right place, which is absolutely standing in support of the feminine principle; absolutely making its commitment to serve the enduring values which are held, and ensuring that they get carried into the world. That is what Anhalonium has done. The impact on me is a much greater sense of capability and of authenticity, as there is a much greater representation in the outer world of what is being experienced in the inner world. As that more extroverted work goes forward I get feedback from the world that I would never get. It has opened parts of the world to me that I normally don't have access to. Left to myself I live a relatively introverted lifestyle, but that is not good enough for the work that I have to do and it's certainly not good enough for what Anhalonium is asking of me. So the fact that I have been able to adopt that stronger position is that I have met the world with a new face to different parts of life, with people whom I normally wouldn't speak to. Activities that I have had to engage in, that I am not used to, where I have had interesting and unusual responses from people that are very affirming. My instinct is not to speak about what I do for fear of thrusting it down people's throats, and that had to change and I think it is that masculine energy and the Anhalonium effect.

Is it fears of thrusting it down their throats or the fear of their rejection?

Well it's both, shame of the idea that I would attempt to persuade anyone of anything. That is a shameful thing to do. But also that would be times ten if I am rejected. Equally, if I am accepted, and if it is the result of convincing someone, either way I lose; the horror of it. So it has been a confronting thing to do the work that I do and bring it into the world and market it and confront it when it is too forceful.

Has the sense of shame and horror lifted inside of you?

Yes, it has in the sense that it hasn't stopped me, but the template is still there; the shadow is still there. That depressive element was as if somehow I could scuttle away and avoid my task, could say no and the cost was great, and it was only when I learnt how to say yes that the balance was achieved, of a particular sort. I am still in the process of achieving it.

So when you have students who are also in the Sixth Ray concept, how do you feel towards them?

I feel tender, deeply aware of its dangers, how you can put yourself into someone's clutches, and for it to be my clutches. So I feel protective of their right to choose of the absolute necessity of their separateness and time, conscious of the need to say yes to what they offer even though it's scary. It is scary to be offered devotion, not that it is done in an obvious fashion as it would be done in an old mystery school.

Do you think, since taking the remedy, there is less struggle over that degree of responsibility?

Yes, in that I don't think I would have created the opportunities in which they could offer in that way because I would not have wanted that responsibility. I am reserved in my acceptance of help, in part because I am needlessly independent but also because I don't want to enter into enslaving relationships with me as the slave, or me as the slave master. With the person offering help and so I am very alert to the quality that is in the individual because of that fact. All through my life, in one way or another, there have been several individuals drawn to me who want something of me, who want something of what I have to offer. There is a little straw that goes in and a suck, suck, suck, but nothing good that comes from that. From time to time, after running a weekend workshop or some other public piece of work, there would be people who would come up who would have that devotional element in them and want to be with me and offer themselves to that. That thing that happens after people have had an experience. I have found those experiences challenging. On the one hand there is a genuine experience there, but on the other hand there is a giant invitation to the pedestal, and I don't want followers; not interested it. It would prevent me from doing the work that I am to do, let alone all of the damage that can be created out of that. So it is how to say yes to the support in people, but no to that which would not serve life. That is the task.

So now you can see why I gave you the story of Galadriel and her struggle to not take the Ring? The temptation was so strong and yet she would not achieve what she had to achieve.

The funny thing is she knew! These are the sort of things I know because I reflect but in the doing of it, especially in years gone by, it was me finding my way through. Following my instinct, my intuition, saying no because I knew I had to say no without understanding why I had to say no. Also, whenever you have done a big piece of work, and have felt the expansion of the boundaries, [spreads her arms wide to express expanse] to that larger aspect of the self that comes into play, then there is the emptiness that has to be dealt with. Where there is emptiness and stillness required. Followers don't allow that. They want the archetype on tap, and they want to feed from that but the work is to access our tap to that, not to feed on others.

(*Anhalonium* have the two *Mind* rubrics: *forsaken feeling, isolation*, and *heightened awareness of body*. The constitution *Anhalonium* always resonates with the energy of what Sankaran identifies as "a total solitude and where they can identify themselves with not only a group or family but with the whole of existence.")

Do you think that since taking the remedy, the amount of time you have needed to rejuvenate yourself to go back out into the world is less?

Yes. I don't get much time these days, and yes I am still here. A few years ago I did what I call, fry my brains. I was doing an Easter Mediation and fried my brains in that I wasn't able to deal with the potencies of energies that I encountered. The result of that was I wasn't able to work in that way anymore. A lot more work had to be done, that sort of connection with that archetypal part of life had in the ordinary and the everyday, I think it has led to a safer progress, it has less bells and whistles but it has got those great moments of exaltation.

So, it would be interesting to see, in doing the workshops you are about to do, if you are able to hit that degree of exaltation and still be able to stay grounded and have some energy.

I would say that at the moment I am able to have quite a solid connection with the exalted in my work and to come back pretty quickly from it.

Has anything changed in relation to your business partner and how you have been able to work with her?

Yes. She has been coming into the world, more and more. She may well be an Anhalonium type. She is still grappling with not being able to stand with a clear form which can enable that.

(*Anhalonium* has the two *Delusion* rubrics: *separated from the world* and *he is transparent.*)

Sankaran states, in *The Soul of Remedies*, "Anhalonium comes from a situation where people experience a total solitude and feel they could lose their identity. In such a situation the only solution is being in the *Anhalonium* state, where they can identify themselves with not only a group or family but with the whole of existence. The experience of mescaline is often one of merging with one's surroundings or the feeling of being one with the whole of existence seeing oneself without any boundaries. This is the closest to the highest spiritual experience, as described in Hindu or Buddhist philosophy as oneness or non-duality of Spirit. This experience implies immortality – what dies is the body: as the Self is continuous with the whole of existence, it cannot be mortal."

Case Analysis

First Consult: January 2007 Remedy given dry pilule *Anhalonium* 200 C. 1/weekly continuous. The consultations are every six weeks.

Follow up: March 2007

- Rheumatoid factor now negative
- Hashimoto's. All Thyroid levels are now normal
- Thyroglobulin (TG) antibodies still high >500 normal range (<60) previously 25600.
- Thyroid Peroxidase antibodies (TPO) still high, indicative of idiopathic hypothyroidism
- Acne Rosacea is now less
- Inability to manage weight, diet, exercise, food. I needed to do a lot of counselling around food and exercise but she has started a food regime, weight management and exercise regime
- Extreme heat and flushing is now less
- Arthritis in hands and feet, greatly improved
- No longer unsteady on her feet
- Vague, unable to regulate a food regime (hypoglycaemic)
- Starting to regulate eating regimes
- Heat and skin rashes under her arms, improved
- Complaints of memory loss are not an issue now
- Complaints of vagueness no longer an issue

Follow up March 2008. Remedy has not changed. Dry Pilule *Anhalonium* 200 C. 1/week

- Rheumatoid factor still negative
- Hashimoto's. Thyroid Stimulating Hormone (TSH) increase

from 4.19 to 7.10 normal range (0.35-5.50). New Remedy given *Thyroidinum* 30 1/day.

- Thyroglobulin (TG) antibodies still high and increased to 2111 normal range (<60) previously 25600
- Thyroid Peroxidase antibodies (TPO) decreasing to 1119 they were 2282 still high indicative of idiopathic hypothyroidism. Normal Range (<60.)
- Acne Rosacea is much improved
- Now more able to regulate exercise and food management, and timetable management
- Extreme heat and flushing: still improving
- Arthritis in hands and feet: greatly improved, no pain

Follow-up Conclusion

The rubrics which point to the correct remedy for curing auto-immune cases are found within the *Delusion* rubrics because these are the rubrics which resonate with conflict. Disturbance and conflict in a patient will cause destructive pathology. Internal struggle is evident in chronic disease states. Physically, she has a thyroid auto-immune condition, Hasimoto's and Rheumatoid Arthritis. All auto-immune conditions are reflective of inner conflict. This conflict resonates across all levels of her life, not just on the physical. As *Anhalonium* she is enthralled with her life's work, and yet is struggling with managing its *carriage in the world. The ideal is all very well and good, but if you don't have the strength of form to give it carriage in the world then it's just about smoke and mirrors. A lot of my life has been spent building the vehicle to enable the ideal to be in the world to have expression in the world.* When she talks about her lack of form in the world, she is also talking about her physical struggle around practical matters of living and working. In this case, I have done a lot of counseling around how to eat, how to manage time, and the need for exercise. She has struggled to manage her time in her practice and in appointments with patients. She has now reduced appointments to a manageable and containable time slot of one hour, as opposed to two hour appointments. *Anhalonium* will lose themselves in their patients, and the fact that she can now put boundaries and time constraints around appointments for her patients is proof of her well being. She has also been vastly more productive in her writing, teaching, and commitment to completing her project around the levels of consciousness. She has been able, after one year of taking the remedy Anhalonium to work out a marketable method of teaching her life's work so that others can understand the complex nature of the levels of consciousness with which she identifies.

Follow up October 2009.

Remedy has not changed. Dry Pilule *Anhalonium* 200 C. 1/ week. *Thyroidinum* 30 C. 1/day.

- Rheumatoid factor still negative
- Hashimoto's. T4. TSH (Thyroid Stimulating Hormone) T3. Levels now all within normal ranges
- Thyroglobulin (TG) antibodies decreasing to 1608 normal range (<60) previously 25600.
- Thyroid Peroxidase antibodies (TPO) decreasing to 567, they were 2282, still high indicative of idiopathic hypothyroidism. normal range (<60.)
- Acne Rosacea is much improved
- Inability to manage weight, diet, exercise, food are still ongoing issues to address
- Extreme heat and flushing, still improving
- Arthritis in hands and feet, greatly improved, no pain

This case is ongoing. Her Thyroglobulin (TG) antibodies are still high, but they have decreased considerably (as above). Her Thyroid function tests (T4. TSH. and T4.) are now within normal range.

Bibliography

Sankaran, Rajan. *The Soul of Remedies*. Santa Cruz, Bombay, Homeopathic Medical Publishers, 1997. p.9.

Sankaran, Rajan. *An Insight Into Plants*. Santa Cruz, Bombay, Homeopathic Medical Publishers, 2002. p.143.

Schroyens, Frederik. M.D. *Synthesis*. London, Homeopathic Book Publishers, 1997.

Vermeulen, Frans. *Prisma*. The Netherlands, Emryss bv Publishers, 2002.

Arnica

Abstract:

This is a case of a man who feels like a severely traumatized child. He says: *I managed to stay off the ground and not have to go through any of the psychological and emotional difficulty that other people have gone through. I have remained Peter Pan. I am like a traumatized seven year old.* This patient is suffering from severe Catatonia as a result of Post-traumatic stress disorder. *Arnica* have the *Delusion* rubric: *floating in air* and the *Mind* rubric: *ailments from mental shock.*

Keywords:

Peter Pan Trauma.

Case Notes:

First Appointment 9/02/2009.

D.O.B. 1943.

Previous Occupation: Naturopath, Astrologer.

Presenting Symptom:

Medical diagnosis: Parkinson's Syndrome[12]. The patient

---

12 Parkinson's disease (PD) is characterized by muscle rigidity, tremor, a slowing of physical movement and, in extreme cases, a loss of physical movement. PD is the most common cause of chronic progressive parkinsonism, a term which refers to the syndrome of tremor, rigidity, bradykinesia and postural instability.

has a continual tremor in his arm and hand. He is slow to answer questions; physically it is hard for him to speak. He has lost the ability to hold a pen and write. His arm muscles are shortening. He is losing strength in his legs.

Counsellor's diagnosis: Post-Traumatic Stress Disorder. Catatonia[13].

Physical Rubric-repertorisation

- *Extremities: contraction of muscles and tendons: forearms: muscles: flexor muscles:* arn. [1] 1.
- *Extremities: cramps: wrists: writing agg.* arn.
- *Extremities: give way: lower limbs:* arn.
- *Extremities: trembling hands:* arn.
- *Mouth: speech: difficult: Arn.*

Case Analysis: I used the following key points and headings in analyzing this case to arrive at the correct prescription of *Arnica.*

1. **Rubric-repertorisation**
2. **Theme**
3. *Striking*, or *Peculiar* **Signs and Symptoms; Organon 153**
4. **Materia Medica**
5. **Follow-up Consultations**
6. *How, Why,* and *When* **Causations – the 'Never-well-since-event'.**

Below is a transcript from the first consultation in February 2009. In the text, I have highlighted recurring themes and

---

13 Catatonia is a syndrome of motor disturbances. This patient has an involuntary tremor of his right arm. Catatonia is associated with neurological conditions such as Parkinson's syndrome or stroke. Catatonia is also associated with psychiatric conditions such as bipolar disorder, schizophrenia, and post traumatic stress disorder. Catatonic patients will sometimes hold rigid 'frozen' poses for hours and will ignore external stimuli.

recurring words. In this case analysis I have added rubrics at the end of the relevant chapters.

Question: You have been diagnosed with the syndrome and not Parkinson's[14]? This is the syndrome and symptoms of Parkinson's without the diagnostic classification, from what I understand. What happened when you took the doctor's medication?

Absolutely nothing. It has been coming on slowly for about a year.

What are the symptoms you have other than the shaking?

I can't talk. The counsellor says I have complex Post Traumatic Stress Disorder. It is severe anxiety.

Did this come on with the breaking of the relationship?

Yes, it is quite substantially related to that. The breakdown of the relationship started about three years ago and it took about a year and a half to actually manifest. It has been eighteen months since we have gone our separate ways. Liz, I should have come earlier. I have been so ashamed of what is going on with me. I just want it to go away. I can't play guitar. I can't feel for anybody in any sort of meaningful way. To top it all off, about a year ago my daughter freaked out. She couldn't cope with me and abandoned our relationship again like she did when she was twelve. I felt so abandoned by the one person I needed support from the most. I just couldn't

---

14 I asked this question because the patient does not believe the medical diagnosis. He has taken the medication for PD and it has had no affect on his tremor, rigidity, bradykinesia and postural instability. It is common for patients when first diagnosed with a progressive disease to believe that the diagnosis is incorrect. It is important for the homoeopath to immediately note that the patient is in the first stage of psychological denial. The patient's answers indicate that he wishes to believe his counsellor's diagnosis, which is Post Traumatic Stress Disorder. If there is evidence of notable inner conflict, and evidence of self-destruction and pathology, this indicates that the rubric-repertorisation and case analysis must contain a *Delusion* rubric. A patient who is struggling to come out of denial or who refuses to believe they are sick is suffering psychological 'delusions of grandeur'.

believe it. Liz it was the combination of what my ex-partner did and what my daughter did. It was like punch, whack, and then sledge hammer. I can't take anymore. All I was asking from my daughter was understanding and tender loving care. In other words the roles got reversed and she couldn't cope with the roles getting reversed. I had always done that for her, too much in a way. Too much unconditional love, it doesn't help.

What did your partner do to you?

She started becoming abusive, firstly physically. When I put a stop to that she started being mentally and emotionally abusive. I didn't realize it was going on. I didn't realize the significance of it. I was just doing unconditional love as a way of coping in the relationship. It just went too far. The more I tried to love her through her difficulty the more abusive she got. She took advantage of my love and my kindness. It got worse and worse and worse, and she ended up projecting everything that was unsavory on to me. Convincing herself that was what I was doing. I just couldn't believe it. So ludicrous I laughed. She really used that. Then when I started standing up for myself she got really, really defensive. Liz, I don't know whether you know what a hate defensive mechanism is, but it's really destructive. I had no idea what hating was. She was harboring a hate mechanism from her childhood. She activated it to try to protect herself. She activated that hate mechanism against me. It tried to destroy me. She just took refuge in a hate mechanism. It was so undermining so cleverly subversive. She was able to turn me against myself. She made me doubt myself.

Rubric-repertorisation

- *Mind: ailments from; grief: Arn.*
- *Mind: ailments from: mental shock; from: Arn.*
- *Mind: ailments from: injuries, accidents; mental symptoms from: arn.*

- *Mind: answering: slowly*: arn.
- *Mind: anxiety: hypochondriacal: Arn.*
- *Mind: anxiety: health; about: own health; one's*: arn.
- *Mind: besides oneself; being: general; in*: arn.
- *Mind: delirium tremens: Arn.*

Question: In what way?

Blame myself just for things she was accusing me of. Making it sound so convincing. I just didn't have the psychological self-esteem or the emotional self-worth to cope with an onslaught like that. Then when I really started to stand up for myself and really question, really deeply, what she was doing, and the relationship, she just abandoned the relationship, ended the relationship. We were going okay for three of the six years we were together. Look, I thought we were going okay, but I have had so many realizations about my relationship with her. It is just appalling what I have come to understand. It's like I was in a three-way relationship, not just a two-way relationship. It was me and her and this other part of her. It was that she had a really abusive relationship within herself. She kept it so well hidden, I just couldn't see it. She kept it to herself, to her journal. She was journaling every day, sometimes three, four times day. She shared some of them with me. Before she got involved with me. About three years before she got involved with me, she got involved with a guy who, according to her was really, really, abusive. Really destructive. He nearly killed her, according to her. A couple of her family members tended to agree with that. This previous guy was so traumatic for her. Do you know what the Stockholm syndrome is? It is where you get so abused by someone that you go into an unnatural love and identification with them. That's what happened with her in relation to him. She got in touch with a part of herself that was unconditionally loving, and that she had never been in touch with before, so she didn't have a relationship with a part of herself. As distinct from myself. I have been in touch with that part of myself all my life. That was my survival, too much so. She only got in touch with it before I met her. It is a very powerful thing to have. She developed a weird relationship with that part of herself, the really abusive one, but I didn't understand that at the time. Neither did she, she knew it was weird. She described it to me sometimes. Liz, I believed it was impossible to have an abusive relationship with the higher self because I don't, and I didn't, have an abusive relationship with my higher self. So I just assumed that if someone was in touch with that it was a good relationship because that is how it was for me. I didn't know that people could have an abusive relationship with that part of themselves. I have come to understand that our higher self, spirit self, is actually our free will, our will. It's free for us to do what we want to do with it, we can vitiate our spirit. We can turn it into whatever we want to turn it into. We can have a really good, healthy, two-way relationship with it. I didn't know that then. So I assumed that the dialogue that she had with her spirit self was healthy, it was really unhealthy. It was like having a relationship with two people who were in a really unhealthy relationship with each other and I didn't realize that. She kept it really well hidden.

What has happened since the relationship? You have gone into a post-traumatic stress?

Yes, literally when she ended the relationship. We were living in the holiday house of her parents, but that is another story why we were down there. We should never have gone down there. I got asked to move out of there. I was looking for three months for a place to live and couldn't find one. I couldn't get even an approval on anything. Three solid months or longer. One day, when I was out looking for a place to live, I came back home and everything had been thrown out on the street. She got her brother and two other members of her family to pack up all of my stuff. I actually wasn't living in the house at that point. I was living in a self-contained flat at the end of the house, we had separated our living spaces so I wasn't bothering her. We were having nothing to do with each other, literally nothing to do with each other for three months. She threw me out on the street and made me homeless. That is what f***d me up. She didn't care whether I lived or died. Her hate just took over. I couldn't believe that someone who loved me could do that. I don't know whether this is a weird perspective, Liz I have come to understand that I hate defensive mechanisms. Defensive mechanisms only exist because of the vulnerability and the pain and the fear that someone has experienced around love. Love makes people feel so vulnerable. Some people just can't cope with that because of the way their childhood is or was, and they develop a complex mental hate mechanism to protect themselves from the vulnerability and fragility of love. But you already know that. I was completely oblivious to this. I didn't know what hate was. People would use the word hate, and would talk about an emotion. It is a really complex, mental defensive mechanism and it takes all the fear and all the negativity, all the pain that the person has, and links it all together as one single power base, as a weapon. It is the Darth Vader of the mind. It is truly fucking scary. She turned hers on me. I didn't even know what was going on. It is the Darth Vader of the mind. It is very f***ing destructive and can destroy people. I didn't know that. My ex-wife wasn't like that, she was just neurotic. I don't think I ever had come upon anyone like that before. I really should have trusted my first instinct. I met her at a permaculture course I was doing at Healsville. My first impression in the class room was that she is a weird ex-Christian. I didn't even know who she was. It turns out she was an ex-Christian. I worked it out before I even spoke to her, my first impression were right. I didn't know she was a f***ed up ex-Christian who was still caught in the cult. She was part of a really destructive Christian cult called the Dutch Reform Church of Australia. It has a real fundamentalist part (to them) that does love and hate together; it doesn't do love by itself; love and hate.

When did the shaking happen?

Exactly after I became homeless. I got put out on the street for about six months. I got so distressed I went and hammered on the Housing Commission door until they gave me a unit. One of the things that is coming to a head for me at the moment is because of where I live. There are only two good things about where I live, and there are a dozen things that are not good about it. The only two good things about it are that it is peaceful and quiet. They put me in a old people's housing commission because I was over fifty-five years of age. I just asked for a peaceful and quiet location. I didn't ask for that. I just asked for peaceful and quiet. Two have died already. I have a little garden out the back, a private garden. It is really private. They have just thrown a hand grenade in the middle of it three weeks ago. They have decided to totally redevelop and renovate all the units and the grounds for the next three weeks. They started by cutting down four really big trees, paint all the units, put in night lighting and footpaths. They didn't ask anyone if they wanted this. Just forcing this on people. So it has become a construction site.

So are you going to lose your backyard?

No, I am not going to lose it. It is very interesting that they are going to put a high fence around it. I was screaming at them, no you don't. I don't want it. But Liz for the last three weeks there have been chain saws and bulldozers. It is just going on every day. This is going to go on for the next two and half months. It is really doing my head in. I have been to the housing commission and I have said, heh! you can't do this to me I am not well. I got my therapist to write me a letter. They have to do something about this. Relocate me for the duration. I put that application in last week. I don't know whether they can do that. The woman at the Housing Commission said that they don't even have a policy to cover this, if they start working and it is adversely affecting someone's health. That is how insensitive they are. Really, the one thing that has been working for me there is that in the morning I just do yoga and chanting, quietly working in the garden. Slowly trying to get my head together to recover from this trauma and two and a half years of abuse before that. I can't do that anymore because these people start work. That really quiet time between eight and ten o'clock is all gone now. There have been times when I have been out, and I start packing, and I have to come back home because that is the only safe place I know. I can't do that at the moment. Noises and people hammering is just terrible, just terrible. I feel like I am homeless again. They have taken my home away. It took me six months to feel like I had a home when I first moved. It is a dog box of a place. It is really very disgusting, really. Hardly any natural light. At least I had a roof over my head. I felt like I was getting better, really. Getting down to the bottom of things.

What are the other symptoms other than your tremor and voice?

A loss of emotional feeling. I have got massive anxiety, my anxiety is just way, way, over the top. I am pretty sure I am depressed. I can't feel anything for any music that I know and love. I have just lost myself, Liz. My ability to just appreciate anything. I didn't think anything could ever do that to me. What is going on inside of me is that I need to deeply grieve. It is so deep, so horrible, I can't go there. I started to go there when I first moved down here. When I first got a roof over my head, my own place, but it is just so excruciating. Just the grief. What she did to me, it is not just about that. It has really, really shocked me. I didn't realize I was doing this but I had a lot of blinkers on, and a certain amount of rose colored glasses on. I know everyone does that to cope. To understand what Mary had done, to not blame myself for it, I had to take all my blinkers off and all my glasses off. I got the answers that I needed from my own wisdom about what she had done how she had blamed me for the whole thing, scapegoated me. Literally crucified me. Physically, emotionally and mentally. Literally, those three things. That is why there are three crosses on Calvary. Cardinal, fixed and mutable, astrologically. Physical, emotional and mental. She literally crucified me on all those three levels. I just didn't know. I have had to wake up to what has happened. It has woken me up to the way the world works, the way it operates, the way people are. The way the system is out there. I have been, as a Sagittarian, in a helicopter twenty-five meters above the ground, that is the way I coped. Connecting, but sort of above it all, like a lotus, but not in it. Not really getting affected by it. Therefore, not psychologically and emotionally learning, because I wasn't out on the street. That is the only way I could cope, and to be unconditionally loving, which kept me up there. But that is all over. I can't do that anymore. She brought me down so badly. I just crashed, crash landing, just smashed.

And the shame that you talked about when you first came in?

I just have so much shame about the condition I am in.

Do you think you are sick, or do you think this is Post-Traumatic Stress Disorder?

That is an illness.

Yes, I know, but do you think you have the start of Parkinson's or do you think this is trauma?

I think it is trauma. I really do, because when I am in a safe place and I start feeling that everything is okay, this calms down. [Referring to tremor.] It is not Parkinson's. When I have a Reiki, it stops completely, especially when she uses Reiki on my head. When I get excited about anything in a positive way, or negative way, it just gets worse. It is like, I saw a child once, it was a long time ago, it might have been a child at the student clinic, maybe one of the festivals I working at when I was a naturopath. This woman was talking about her child with her naturopath, who I was sitting next to. She said that her child couldn't cope with any excitement at all, he would go haywire when overexcited. In fact, he couldn't get overexcited. He would go haywire and just start shaking. It is what I am doing. A traumatized child, not a traumatized adult. My counsellor said it has taken me a while to understand this, but you have a regressive pool going on. I said to her, I don't think I am an adult who is traumatized, because psychologically and emotionally I never became an adult. I never went through adolescence. Literally, Liz. I never went through adolescence. Staying above it all by using love and big heart to do so. I managed to stay off the ground and not have to go through any of the psychological and emotional difficulty that other people have gone through. I know it sounds weird. So, I have remained Peter Pan. Really immature in a child-like and innocent way. Not a horrible or weird way, just in a really child-like and innocent way. My ex-partner just stomped all over me. It turns out she actually admitted this one day, that she was really abusive to her children. She had to go and get help to stop herself from doing it. I think she just did the same thing to me because she could get away with it, and get away from all the abuse and self-deception she was doing, dumping everything on me. I was just too naive, too innocent to even know what was going on. I am like a traumatized seven year old.

1. Rubric-repertorisation

- *Delusions: floating: air, in: arn.*

Question: Why seven?

I don't know. I have said that a few times even to my counsellor. Not sure I just put an age to it.

What happened when you were seven?

I got dragged over here to Australia. I got dragged away from my home and my country. Away from people who really love me, who were my grandparents, my cousin Mary, which I remember. I came to this country, and the only way I could do it was to do unconditional love. I couldn't cope with the stress, psychologically and emotionally, I didn't even try. My motus operandi was survival. Be as open and loving and kind to everyone as possible, including all the people who were bastards.

Rubric-repertorisation

- *Mind: estranged: family; from his:* arn.

Question: Did you also feel the shame with your daughter when she said she didn't want to have anything more to do with you?

Yes, I felt like I was being treated like I was an abuser, like there was something disgustingly wrong with me. She sent me an email that was judgmental, critical, shaming, and blaming, because I told her off about something one day. She lost it so badly. She sent me an email that was vitriolic. I was so shocked I was unable to write back to her. I replied to her email by voice mail. I spoke my truth that way and she got worse, she disowned me basically. She sent me one letter that I started to read. I was so shocked by how horrible it was, I had to stop reading it. I had to get the counsellor to read it. She read the rest of it and I asked her to tell me whether there were any redeeming features in it at all, and she said you don't need to read this, she has just wiped her hands of you. I just don't know how I can live with that. It is really doing me in, more so that Mary because I actually understand how her head took over. I actually understand what is going on with my daughter, but there is nothing I can do about it.

What did you say to her?

I told her off and asked her to please ring me up. I asked her to get back to me in person, don't just text me. Because it was crucial. I told her off about texting me and not being personal, and she just lost it. There was obviously stuff going on for months before that. The condition I have been in was asking of her unconditional love and she couldn't do it. It triggered *off too much stuff about the way she had been abused by her mother. I didn't say anything about that to her, but just the condition I was in and the role reversal just confronted her. She just didn't want to be honest about it and she just dumped it on me. She started accusing me of manipulating her and controlling her, blaming her. I just can't believe it. It is so mind f***ing, Liz. She is shaming and blaming me, and in her letter she is saying I am blaming her. How do people do that when they are blatantly doing the very thing they are accusing the other person of doing? What I needed in my recovery was unconditional love, to know I was loved unconditionally. I wasn't expecting her to be there every weekend. Just to have her tender loving care and support. She managed it for about two months and then she couldn't cope with it anymore. She withdrew, became critical, starting making excuses. Liz, I was sixty-seven last year and she didn't even contact me for my birthday. Ring up or do anything. It was really hurtful. It was the most hurtful thing I have had anyone do to me. It was treating me like I was a child abuser and she had just woken up to it. She is not even accusing me of that. But what I am and what I am going through is a huge threat to her life to the way she does her life with her partner and her brother, who is still in her life. I represent the truth of how she was forced by her mother to eliminate her father from her life. She was so emotionally abused, she had to get me out of her life when she was eleven and twelve. Her mother couldn't cope with shared parenting. The only way Helen was going to have a happy parent during her teenage years was to have her mother and no-one else. She didn't understand that. She actually blamed me for not wanting to have me in her life. She couldn't blame her mother. She has done it again because she doesn't want to face what she did to herself when she was twelve. I wasn't confronting her with anything. I was just traumatized. What she is demanding of me at the end of the email she sent me was, she said, all I want from you dad is your unconditional love, nothing else.*

She didn't even say 'your love' she said your 'unconditional love'. Love is unconditional. She wants my love but she doesn't want me. She wants me to be like a spirit, like a saint without any personality, no humanness. She just wants my love, she doesn't want me, she said that in her email. When I answered her email, I told her that is not on. I can't do that, it is unhealthy. It is taking my love. It is misusing my love, which is what abuse is. She hated that truth. That is why she wrote that other letter disowning me. If I was strong enough, Liz, I would just forget about her. Start developing a new life for myself. But I am not. I am like a severely traumatized child. I can hardly look after myself. I have obsessive compulsive thinking going on and am compulsively in the garden all the time. I can't leave it alone. If I am at home, I am out in the garden all the time, but not in a healthy way. I had an episode of that when I was a child, about ten or eleven. I just remembered. I had a terrible, terrible nightmare about being on a ship in a battle. I woke up traumatized by it. My parents had to take me to the doctor I was so traumatized by it. I was about ten or eleven years old and I became compulsive about my clothing. For weeks and weeks afterwards, my clothing had to be perfectly folded at the end of my bed. If I thought it wasn't, I had to get up and check that it was. It could go on for hours. I think I got given some medication. I am obsessively obsessing in my mind about Helen and sometimes about Mary. I worked my way through a lot of that by journaling, when I could write. I think I did too much journaling. I put too much energy into what happened with Mary and what she actually did. It is literally a book, hundreds of pages, called a 'letter to Mary'. I started to letter and got to 110 pages, and started again, and got to 120 pages, and started again with a whole new perspective on things. Eventually, I couldn't hold a pen still, particularly after Helen and what she did. I know it might not have been a completely healthy relationship between me and my daughter. I think she represented too much of the feminine, too much of my mother for it to be healthy. It was really different when Mary came along. I transferred all my love of the feminine to her, away from my daughter. As a consequence of that, I was able to reconnect with my daughter, and start getting a relationship going. That suited her, then. She could have a relationship at a distance without having to resolve anything, and just be social and loving to some extent. When I got really traumatized and needed a lot of support, it held a mirror up to her. Our spirit is like a mirror to ourselves psychologically and emotionally. Mary accused her spirit self, who she got a lot of guidance from, a number of times, of being abusive to herself. I was too naive to know what was going on. It was actually her being abusive to it, not the other way around.

Rubric-repertorisation

- *Mind: dictatorial: talking with air of command*: arn.
- *Dreams: death: dying: he has to die*: arn. [1] 4. (lach. nit-ac. sil.)
- *Mind: sensitive: noise, to: Arn.*

Question: Other than the garden, what other obsessive things have you got going on?

Obsessive or compulsive?

Both

I just have to escape from where I live. I feel claustrophobic and trapped there. It is pretty isolating. It is a long way from Melbourne. Doing the garden is good for me but it is over the top. I don't know when to stop. I have a couple of friends who I am compulsive about wanting to connect with, but that is natural. I don't want to be alone, but at the same time I am ashamed of being with people. I was compulsively masturbating for a while but I stopped doing that about six months ago. I lost all feeling for it, which is really disturbing.

(Off-camera, he tells me that he has been obsessing about the noise the pigeons make in the mornings. He can't stand it to the point that he goes out in the mornings and throws stones at them.)

2. Theme

Every patient will have recurring patterns or themes in their lives. The theme will resonate in one, several, or all of the five psychological stages. If the trauma inside your patient starts with them feeling alone and abandoned, or singled out for punishment by their illness, then the simillimum is listed in the *Delusion* rubrics: *forsaken* or *persecution*. The advantage in identifying and understanding the psychological processing that your patient is moving through is that it allows you to narrow the remedies being considered to the remedies listed in those particular rubric categories.

- *Ashamed.*
- *I can't feel for anybody in any sort of meaningful way.*
- *I felt so abandoned by the one person I needed support from the most.*
- *It was like punch, whack, and then sledge hammer.*
- *It tried to destroy me.*
- *She started becoming abusive.*
- *I just didn't have the psychological self-esteem or the emotional self-worth to cope with an onslaught like that.*
- *A loss of emotional feeling.*
- *I have got massive anxiety, my anxiety is just way, way, over the top.*
- *I am pretty sure I am depressed.*
- *I can't feel anything for any music that I know and love.*
- *She literally crucified me on all those three levels.*
- *I managed to stay off the ground and not have to go through any of the psychological and emotional difficulty that other people have gone through.*

- *Really immature in a child-like and innocent way.*
- *I had a terrible, terrible nightmare about being on a ship in a battle. I woke up traumatized by it.*
- *I am like a traumatized seven year old.*

Arnica suffer from persecutory illusions as well as fanciful illusions. The *Delusion* rubric: *illusions of fancy* alludes to the need to create in one's fantasy a grander vision of the world which one aspires to, i.e. one's ideal world. In the Introduction, I outlined a simple rubric-repertorisation of the character of Lars, from the film *Lars and the Real Girl*. The character of Lars is a good example of psychological modeling being adopted because it is advantageous. Lars sets up a delusional relationship with a life-like plastic doll, which he names Bianca. His underlying need for the delusion is based on his fears of the future loss of a real girlfriend because his own mother died giving birth to him. To avoid the loss of a real wife, he has a relationship with a life-like plastic doll. With the help of a psychologist, he is able to slowly unravel his need for the psychological delusion. He then allows the plastic doll to die so he can be released from the relationship and fall in love with a real girl. In the analysis of a *Delusion* rubric (in case-taking) you have to see and understand, within the case and within the nature of the constitutional remedy profile, why the patient needs the delusional state. Lars's psychological delusion is needed to avoid grief. The rubrics for Lars would be the following, to confirm the remedy *Arnica*.

- *Delusion* rubric: *fancy, illusions of.*
- *Delusion* rubric: *visions, has; fantastic.*
- *Mind* rubric: *fear: touched; of being.*
- *Skin* rubric: *coldness.*
- *Skin* rubric: *coldness; sensation, of.*
- *Delusion* rubric: *dead: persons, sees.*
- *Delusion* rubric: *die: about to die; one was.*

In taking Lars's case, the above list of rubrics appear in the order in which they are revealed in the film. The first rubric, the *Delusion* rubric: *illusions of fancy*, is a psychological 'delusion of grandeur' which allows the patient who is suffering with grand visions of persona to create a vision of their expectation of the world. Lars's fanciful illusions allow him to imagine that the life-like plastic doll called Bianca is a real girlfriend. The next piece of information we find out about him is his fear of being touched. The patient needing *Arnica* is fearful of being approached, fearful of being touched, and their whole body is over-sensitive. Lars wears several layers of clothing to protect him from being touched. Lars experiences being touched as cold and physically painful, as well as being emotionally painful. *Arnica* have the *Mind* rubric: *fear of being touched* and the *Skin* rubric: *coldness on skin*. *Arnica* is a homoeopathic remedy commonly used to treat shock. The Lars character is a beautiful portrayal of the remedy *Arnica,* and if Lars was my patient in a homoeopathic consultation I could surmise that he has been in emotional shock since his mother died giving birth to him. Although I would prescribe *Arnica* for shock, I would only prescribe it on the basis of the above five rubrics in the rubric-repertorisation. I would not assume anything about Lars being in shock about his mother's death until Lars tapped into his unconscious in the follow-up consultations and revealed that element in the case analysis. I would also repertorise the case systematically, chronologically compiling the above rubrics in the precise order in which they were revealed in the case-taking. This is case-development. The psychologist in the film did not uncover his unresolved grief about his mother's death, or his overwhelming fear that a future real wife could die in childbirth until several consultations had occurred. *Arnica* also have the *Delusion* rubric: *one was about to die*, and *sees dead persons*. Both of these rubrics reinforce his fear of having a real relationship with a real girl. If Lars gets close to someone, the psychological delusion is that they could die; this is the meaning of the *Delusion* rubric: *he sees dead persons.* In a homoeopathic consultation, the same process unfolds. It is not until the follow-up consultations that I compile all the rubrics, or understand all of the patient's delusional needs for the *Delusion* rubrics attached to a particular remedy profile. Although I might surmise that Lars could have been in shock since his birth, I would not use the *Delusion* rubrics: *one was about to die,* and *sees dead persons,* in the rubric-repertorisation until Lars revealed his fear of a real future wife dying.

Lars's *illusions of fancy* enabled him to believe that the lifelike plastic doll, Bianca, was a real girlfriend, and although this was obviously a self-delusion, it was advantageous to him to be able to imagine that Bianca was real. The profoundly touching aspect of the film is that everyone in his small town goes along with his psychological delusion and does not confront or try to dispel his illusions. Psychological denial is adopted by the patient when they need to maintain their psychological delusion and illusion to avoid reality. The simillimum will only be *Arnica* if the patient needs to create an illusory fantasy to help them escape reality. *Arnica* need to rely upon their fanciful illusions because they are undermined by persecutory illusions of ill health and death. If there are contradictions and inconsistencies between Stage one ('delusions of grandeur') and Stage five ('delusions of hypochondria') then the remedy profile will contain undermining illusory and delusionary psychoses and neuroses. The simillimum will only be *Arnica* if the patient is undermined by their own persecutory illusions and delusions. *Arnica* suffer exaggerated persecutory fears and delusional beliefs that others are pursuing them in order to harm. *Arnica* also suffer exaggerated fear about diseases, and obsessive fear that they are going to die. A psychosis is a severe mental derangement. The *Delusion* rubrics which cover psychoses are the *Delusion* rubrics: forsaken, depression and resignation. All these *Delusion* rubrics emphasize the threat that the world poses to the 'ego'. All these *Delusion* rubrics contain the 'delusions of abandonment', 'delusions of persecution', 'delusions of impending doom', and the 'delusions of hypochondria', in that order. *Arnica* is a homoeopathic remedy which is commonly used for shock because inherent within the psychological profile is the need to dissociate from reality. *Arnica* have the *Delusion* rubric: *floating in air*. The *Delusion* rubric: *lumps in bed* confirm the depth of their sensitivity. *Arnica* is a remedy which should be used for the patient who is suffering from dissociative trauma as a result of having experienced Post-Traumatic Stress Disorder. The simillimum will only be *Arnica* if the patient presents with dissociative psychoses. The simillimum will only be *Arnica* if the patient presents with physical neuroses. Lars was terrified of being touched. This particular presentation will not be the specific for every *Arnica* case, but the patient must show evidence of psychosomatic physical trauma. Freud analyzed a neurosis as a conflict between the 'ego' and the 'id'. Neuroses relate to psychosomatic conditions, and psychoses relate to mental conflict between the 'ego' and the external world. The simillimum will only be *Arnica* if the patient presents with psychosomatic trauma. *Arnica* shroud themselves in psychosomatic neuroses as a way of protecting their psyche from coming in touch with the shock and trauma that they have experienced in the past. *Arnica* also envelop themselves in psychoses to protect themselves from the shock and trauma that they expect to experience in the future. The patient needing *Arnica* is fearful of being approached, fearful of being touched, and their whole body is over-sensitive, and over-reactive to all outside influences. The 'never-well-since-event' in an *Arnica* case must contain evidence of emotional, mental, or physical, abuse or trauma. *Arnica* enshroud themselves in fanciful illusions in order to create a fantasy of a grander [*fantastic*] vision of an ideal world. The homoeopath working with *Arnica* must be patient because the trauma is enshrouded in their unconscious, traumatized past, and is not accessible to their subconscious or conscious mind. The action of the simillimum will slowly unravel the psychodynamic need to create and maintain their illusions and delusions. The action of the simillimum will slowly heal their traumatized psyche. The action of the simillimum will also slowly unravel their need to create and maintain their numerous psychosomatic neuroses.

As a consequence of having no 'delusions of original sin', or no concept of personal guilt or self-blame, *Arnica* experience trauma more intensely than a lot of other remedy profiles. *Arnica* are often left feeling confused as to why they have been singled out for persecution. This patient is a bewildered, traumatized child.

1. Denial: *Delusion* rubric: *floating*: *air, in*: arn. *Delusion* rubric: *visions, has*: arn. *Delusion* rubric: *visions, has: fantastic*: arn. *Delusion* rubric: *fancy, illusions of*: arn. *Delusion* rubric: *well, he is*: **ARN**.

2. Forsaken: *Delusion* rubric: *dead: persons, sees*: arn. *Delusion* rubric: *dead: corpse: mutilated corpse*: arn. *Delusion* rubric: *arrested, is about to be*: arn. *Delusion* rubric: *bed: lumps in bed*: arn. *Delusion* rubric: *images, phantoms; sees: frightful*: arn. *Delusion* rubric: *mutilated bodies; sees*: arn. *Delusion* rubric: *thieves: seeing*: arn. *Delusion* rubric: *churchyard: visits a*: arn. *Delusion* rubric: *objects; about: lean forward and about to fall; high places*: arn. [1] 1.

3. Causation: NONE.

4. Depression: *Delusion* rubric: *council; holding a*: arn. [1] 2. *Delusion* rubric: *succeed, he does everything wrong; he cannot*: arn. *Delusion* rubric: *objects; about: lean forward and about to fall; high places*: arn. [1] 1. [This rubric can pertain to predictions of failure or persecutory paranoia.]

5. Resignation: *Delusion* rubric: *disease: incurable disease; he has an*: arn. *Delusion* rubric: *die: about to die; one was*: arn. *Delusion* rubric: *heart: disease: going to have a heart disease and die; is*: arn.

3. *Striking*, or *Peculiar* Signs and Symptoms; Organon 153

I said to her, I don't think I am an adult who is traumatized because psychologically and emotionally I never became an adult. I never went through adolescence. Literally, Liz. I never went through adolescence. Staying above it all by using love and big heart to do so. I managed to stay off the ground and not have to go through any of the psychological and emotional difficulty that other people have gone through. I know it sounds weird.

So I have remained Peter Pan. Really immature in a child-like and innocent way. Not a horrible or weird way, just in really child-like and innocent way. My ex-partner just stomped all over me.

Arnica is a homoeopathic remedy which is commonly used for shock because inherent within the psychological profile is the need to dissociate from reality. *Arnica* have the *Delusion* rubric: *floating in air*. When a patient says that they managed to *stay off the ground,* this should be repertorised as the *Delusion* rubric: *floating in air*. *Arnica* dissociate to protect themselves from further shock, hurt, and pain. The most unusual statement this patient has made is that he had arrested his development into adulthood to avoid experiencing further trauma. *Arnica* do not want to grow up. Inconsistencies between *Delusion* rubrics pertaining to grandeur, and *Delusion* rubrics pertaining to destruction in the rubric-repertorisation indicate that the constitutional remedy has a vested psychological, delusional interest in suppression and denial. If the patient displays evidence of disproportionate disturbance and contradictions, this will often be an indication of future pathologies which the homoeopath must be able to identify and predict in the treatment. The constitutional remedy profiles which contain inconsistencies indicate that the patient will have a vested interest in maintaining their illness. Pathology has its foundation in delusional disturbance. This is acknowledged in the modalities of psychiatry and homoeopathy. The homoeopath must be aware of the patient's destructive need to maintain their illness. Under every self-delusion is a specific need to maintain the denial. Homoeopaths need psychological foresight to unravel the various processes of psychological denial. If we develop this foresight, it not only helps us to understand the development or causation within the constitutional remedy, it also helps in the management of the patient. Psychological insight comes from understanding the *Delusion* rubrics which are *peculiar* to a remedy profile. The *Delusion* rubric: *lumps in bed* confirms the depth of their sensitivity; they do not want to feel. When a *Delusion* rubric has only one or two remedies,[15] it should be weighted heavily in the rubric-repertorisation.

Arnica is a remedy which should be used for the patient who is suffering from dissociative trauma as a result of having experienced Post-Traumatic Stress Disorder. *Arnica* presents with dissociative psychoses and with physical neuroses because they do not want to grow up into an adult world which involves adult feelings.

Arnica are often confused about the adult[16] world.

---

15 The *Delusion* rubric: *lumps in bed,* lists only two remedies: *Magnesium carbonicum* and *Arnica.* Within the remedy profile of *Arnica,* this rubric pertains to disproportionate sensitivity: emotionally, mentally, and physically. Within the remedy profile of *Magnesium carbonicum,* this rubric pertains to the need for security in their home, and specifically in their bed. *Magnesium carbonicum* have the *Mind* rubric: *fear something will happen, the warmth of the bed ameliorates.*

16 Volker Schlöndorff's film, *The Tin Drum* tells the story of a Oskar Matzerath, who is born with a discriminating intellect beyond his years. As he witnesses, and is overwhelmed by, the hypocrisy of his mother's affair with her cousin Jan, he rejects both parents, and on his third birthday decides to stop growing. Oskar says in the film, "that day, thinking about the grown-up world and my own future, I decided to call a halt. To stop growing then and there and remain a three-year-old, a gnome, once and for all". On his third birthday, Oskar deliberately falls down the stairs and never grows again. Whenever the world around him becomes too overwhelming, Oskar lashes out with piercing screams that shatter glass and tyrannically pounds on his tin drum. Oskar is not an innocent or cute updated version of Peter Pan. Oskar is angry. As Oskar witnesses the hypocrisy of his mother's affair with her cousin Jan, he decides to stop growing. Vermeulen writes that *Arnica,* "wants to know better than everybody; no one can take him up. Disdainful and imperious. Opinionated". Oskar is the wide-eyed, discriminating bystander who judges and condemns all for their hypocrisies. Phatak writes that *Arnica* sheds tears after rage. Oskar is the

This patient holds on to a concept of child-like, innocent, unconditional love.

4. Materia Medica

Phatak writes that *Arnica* experience "fear; of being struck or touched; or approached; of space; on awakening; of crowds, public spaces. When spoken to, answers slowly with effort. Mentally prostrate and apathetic, but physically restless; says nothing ails him. Hopeless: indifferent. After rage sheds tears and makes exclamations. Sensation of being good for nothing". Vermeulen writes in *Prisma*, "starting from sleep, caused by frightful dreams, after an accident or injury; awakes in terror; horror of instant death. ..Obstinate and headstrong resistance to other people's opinions. Would like to quarrel with everybody. Up against the whole world. Wants to know better than everybody; no one can take him up. Disdainful and imperious. Opinionated." This patient is incensed and reacts to his daughter's texting. *Arnica* have been traumatized by the world. For the simillimum to be *Arnica,* the patient must display continual, disproportionate reactions to all trauma. An *Arnica* patient is incensed by injustice and hypocrisy.

I told her off and asked her to please ring me up. I asked her to get back to me in person, don't just text me. Because

traumatized bystander who is witness to all the hypocrisies and atrocities of the Second World War, the Holocaust, several love affairs, the Russian invasion, and the world of postwar Europe. It is to Oskar's advantage to maintain the stature of a child. Oskar needed to remain a child to punish his mother. Oskar instigates the death of his Uncle Jan (his mother's lover, and his biological father) and his father. At the age of twenty, when he was finally orphaned and free of all his parents, he decided to grow again. He was hit on the head with a rock, fell down into the grave of his father and started to grow again. Oskar is an *Arnica* constitutional profile. *Arnica* is often traumatized as a child, they do not want to grow up into an adult world which involves adult feelings.

Arnica have the *Mind* rubrics: *ailments from anger, ailments from mental shock, refusing to answer, audacity in children, howling with anger, violent,* and *weeping, whimpering.* *Arnica* have the *Mind* rubric: *desire to be carried.* Oskar needed to remain a child to entrap his mother.

it was crucial. I told her off about texting me and not being personal, and she just lost it.

5. Follow-up Consultations

March 2009.

There have been several short, follow-up phone consultations. These are the notes from the March follow-up:

Due to the patient's health, he has not been able to drive to Melbourne to have a face-to-face consultation. The patient has been taking *Arnica* 30 C. daily continuously.

He reports he is now aware of the trauma to his psyche. *I feel like I am in chronic stage fright. I have been shot out of the sky. I am now coming face to face with evil, the person who loved me was evil. I have a desire to kill anyone who would hurt me. I have been undermined by her.*

All my life, I have not been nurtured. I now realize what a profound effect leaving my home was, when I was seven. I now know why you have given me Arnica. I have been in an expected state of shock ever since then. I have attracted abusers to me because that is what I felt. I was used to being traumatized. I now can identify inside of myself how threatened I feel. I have been fighting off demons all my life.

Follow-up Consultations

The first face-to-face follow-up consultation was the 9th February 2010. The patient's first appointment was on the same date one year earlier. *Arnica* pertains to trauma. Patients who have experienced trauma often live their life unconsciously attuned to superstitious synchronicity. The patient needs obsessive compulsive behavior or superstitious rituals as forms of protection.

The patient is now able to talk in a clear voice. He still has the tremor. The catatonia is significantly less.

Patient: *Someone said to me, you're very mentally or psychologically fragile aren't you? I thought about it for a moment and I said, no I am not psychologically fragile, I am physically fragile, to the point where it is terrifying for me to be relating to the physical world in the harsh way that it works. I am okay in the bush, but anything to do with the physical society is terrifying. It is dangerous for me because I am so fragile at a physical level. I said to someone, I think I said it to you that last time I saw you, I am so fragile that if I had a car accident and I got knocked* (bangs his hands together) *it would knock me out of my body, and I would be gone. I feel like I have this very tenuous hold on my physicality. I am the complete opposite of robust, and I don't even know what the word for it is. I have been looking for a word for it. Fragile comes close to it. Do you know?*

Vulnerable?

No it's not vulnerable. Vulnerable means the ability to be open. It is like a translucent skin. I have translucent skin, physically. I have never been able to cope with the harshness of the physical world of sport. When it got competitive I couldn't compete with it. I am not robust. On the basketball field when I crashed into someone I would be on the ground knocked out and they would be standing there wondering 'Gee I wonder what happened to him?' The shock of it was too much. I can be very easily physically traumatized. Psychologically traumatized as well, but that is from lack of experience and naivety. That is because I live in the helicopter and not down on the street, where you learn psychological lessons, and develop ego. I presume that psychological is very connected to the physical, but I am learning psychological stuff. I hate the psychological jungle out there. There is more lethal jungle than used to exist.

Are you dealing with the psychological better?

I don't know because it is foreign territory. To develop ego in the world. I lived completely without it. I was talking to a friend on the weekend at the Black Saturday commemorations, and listening to her story about what she had been through in her life, aside from the Black Saturday bush fires. I don't understand how she survived. She has a psychological toughness. I don't understand how someone can develop that. Some of it is good for her, and some of it cuts her off from people; 'I am an island unto myself'.

It protects her and you don't have that?

No. What I am doing is a really reactive rather than responsive thing. 'Stay right way from me. Don't come near me. Don't talk to me.' I am totally intolerant of anyone I don't know coming anywhere near me. I am wary of even people I know. It is not just about my physical fragility. Although it is the physical fragility which is making me terrified and that fright, I car.'t fight against, compete or fight against the brutality of the way people are. At the moment I can't fight, so that is why I am doing freeze, which is catatonia. It is happening because of the physical fragility of being affected by physical realities around me. There is also another thing.

My reactiveness or defensiveness, instead of protectiveness which I don't have, means my mind is coming up with reactivness which is ridiculously over the top. That frightens me just as much as the physical fragility.

Can you give me an example?

I went to the chemist a few days ago. They had given me the wrong brand of medicine and I didn't want this substitute brand and they didn't ask me whether I wanted this brand. They made every excuse in the book to give the real one. I was getting more and more angry. I started swearing. I knew they could replace it. I was throwing a f***ing tantrum. I am really scared I am going to get physically violent because of it and then I am really in trouble aren't I, Liz? I won't survive the consequences of court cases and cops. I don't have the natural protectiveness which isn't reactive to protect me. I tend to not stand up for myself because I don't know how to protect *myself in a natural way. I have no self-confidence. The user term in Australia which is derogatory, is spineless. I have got no spine to stand up to the ugly people and the competitive people and the aggressive people. I don't have an eighth of the strength they are using to lord it over me. So I get really defensively reactive. It is really negative. It has the potential to cause me problems. I have to keep it under control when I am out there dealing with society. Consequently, I stay right away from society as much as possible. My fridge is often empty because I don't want to go shopping. The whole energy is harsh, the way it is set up is harsh. I don't want to have to deal with people in the world. Then I go to St Andrews market and then there are a different breed of people there and after a while I start breathing again. I don't think I can develop the robustness, the self-confidence and ego to not get affected. Because three years ago I got forced to the bottom of the heap because of the circumstances that I am in. It is starting to affect my health. I feel like my life is threatened. I don't have enough life support. I am going into freeze mode. I feel like I am in so much danger because I am not able to take care of myself the way that I need to. I am going into catatonia.*

How are you going with the tremor? I think your voice is much better.

The tremor is worse with the catatonia. The voice is hard. On the weekend I had to force myself to speak. I was mute, but I must admit it was a group of people who I didn't like. When they asked me what I did, and I said I teach astrology, they ridiculed astrology for twenty minutes. It would have taken too much energy, which I didn't have to stand up for myself. I just went mute. They would have stomped all over me if I would have spoken out. The shaking is happening all the time. It is a reaction to the catatonia going on inside. The more frozen I am, the more muted I am, and the more unable I am to speak, the more the shaky I am. Interestingly, the more negative I am to suggestions from people, even stuff I know that is good for me. I can't even motivate myself. So when the catatonia is severe, the frozen feeling is severe. I can't make a meal for myself. I know I need to eat. I can't do yoga. I can't run because I am uncoordinated. It has been really good to come to an understanding about what is going on for me. That it is catatonia. The more I find out that catatonia is an extreme end result of pretty severe trauma, and stress. A feeling that you are completely disempowered and trapped. That your life is threatened by the situation. That is the only reason why the non-organic related catatonia, the trauma related catatonia, happens in people.

I don't know if I told you this on the phone, but the only thing I can find on the internet in the medical is Atavan, which I already take. It is a band-aid. Catatonia is not a psychotic response, and it is not a psychotic reaction either. It is a somatic response. The anti-psychotics that they give people are to prevent psychotic reactions from happening; just in case. Because they are terrified that someone who is catatonic will get out of control.

But you can see, that is also what you are worried about. When you start to feel really threatened, like what happened in the chemist. Because the more you are becoming aware of the degree of trauma that is there, then the more you are aware of new presenting traumas. Whereas when I first saw you, you were not aware of the affect of the trauma.

No.

Now you are much more aware of the trauma. It is hard because now you are aware of the threat of all new situations. The fear is *as* intense in that moment so therefore you are really scared. But when you first saw me you were actually more terrified and more fearful. You were not aware of it, and also I don't think you had any way of coming out of it. I think you come out of it now, but when you go back into a situation which is really scary, it gets more scary. Does that make sense?

Yes. It gets scary for two reasons. One, my physical fragility is so acute and my psychological fragility is so acute, that people can just do someone thing which is really harmful to me. On Christmas day I sat down at the piano at my friend's place and I just played around with a little bit of stuff, but I am so uncoordinated I couldn't play anything. After a while I gave up because it was too hard, and I stopped. The next day my friend said to me, 'I heard you on the piano yesterday. You were sounding good but then you stopped. Did you stop because you were really self-conscious of everyone in the lounge room in the next room? I said, 'Not at all. I stopped because I suffer from really severe existential stage fright. Whenever I do anything in the world that brings any attention to me I get terrified.' When I told him that he instantly, without deliberately meaning to do it, I know he didn't deliberately mean to do this, he started laughing uncontrollably, really hysterically. God it really hurt. Then he realized what he was doing he stopped and said, 'I am sorry I didn't really mean to do that.' Then he asked me more about the existential stage fright. Then when I explained it more, he started laughing again. It was really hurtful, but he didn't mean to do it. I just had to up and leave and said, 'I can't cope with this, I will see you tomorrow or the next day.' It took me three days to get back to him. Our friendship was on the line. I asked him to really think about why he did this. He said, 'I have already thought about it mate. It disturbed me.' He said, 'I had never experienced anyone who could be terrified about just existence itself. It was such a shock the only way I could deal with it was to laugh.'

I have always had life threatening trauma.

Is that from the trauma of being taken out of your home?

No. That was being taken away from my tribe.

Do you remember the dream that you had when you were a little kid, when you were going to die? You woke up and became obsessive after that. Is that the first time you experienced that existential trauma?

That was the first time. So do I think that had to do with being taken away from my home. Yes I do, because Australia is an alien landscape for me. I am constantly in this landscape. I was down at the port where we came to Australia. There was an English frigate in the harbor but we got there at four o'clock when it was closing. I was walking away and the mid-shipman called out and said would you like a tour of the ship. He gave me a personal tour of the boat after normal tourist hours. They were doing normal things like getting dinner ready and stuff. In the space of an hour I heard every single accent from the British Isles. So comforting. I cannot tell you. I felt so wonderful just being there. I was just crying after awhile. I said this ship feels like back home. It feels like England. I felt this incredible longing and sadness, and loss, and connection again to where I come from. I walked back out into Australia which I can't relate to; the thinking, the people, the society, the culture. The only place I felt safe here was at Confest. (Back-to-earth festival.)

There are two things about the catatonia which are contributing to it: the existential stage fright, the terror about being in the physical world, and my fear about how I deal with it, because it is getting worse. The reaction is getting worse. I have to deal with people who I don't know and people who are nasty and horrible.

And you are more aware of how that makes you feel?

Absolutely.

You know that innocence that you have talked about with Mary? That innocence is not there anymore.

No it is not. She stomped all over it. It is really sad. I am deeply sad about the loss of that. I don't mind losing my naivety, but I do mind losing my innocence. It was an important part of myself. I need ego. Really I just don't want to develop ego in the world. Most ego that people have is corrupt. They have corrupted their energies. Most ego is defensive rather than naturally protective. If there was some way I could learn how to naturally protect myself. But that needs self-confidence, and self-esteem, psychologically, and self-worth, which I hardly have any of at the moment. I used to have a lot of it. Mary abused it and stomped all over it, and then my daughter did it. They were all the good parts of me.

Hence the tremor. Mary and Helen.

Yes, I think it contributes to it. I think Helen more than Mary because I am completely powerless to do anything about how she treats me. Helen has an agenda going on about me. I have been used as the scape-goat, and discarded. There is nothing I can do about that. I think this personal disempowerment began with the situation to do with Helen. When I got into the relationship with Mary I was weakened, and Mary's defensive mechanism totally overwhelmed me. Helen said she wanted my love, but she didn't want me. That is so abusive.

Are you still grieving as deeply?

Yes, I think I am. Well, when she was born I dedicated my life to her and her protection. That is the sort of person I am. I made a vow that I would do everything to protect her. Almost to the point I would give my own life for her. She took me up on it. Not consciously, unconsciously. You asked, 'Am I as deeply grieving about her?' No.

The answer is no?

No. I don't think I am. I have gone deeper into the struggle for survival, and the existential issue that was there before Helen came along.

Case Analysis

This case will be ongoing for many years. His Parkinson's Syndrome has not progressed in the one year period of treatment. I have included this case in the Case Companion because it is important to see the progression of the simillimum. The simillimum will always unpeel trauma layer by layer. In the first session he was suffering Post-Traumatic Stress Disorder as a result of his abusive relationship with his partner. He was also suffering from grief about his daughter's rejection of him. In the first consultation he was stuck in a deep, catatonic, traumatized state. He found it hard to speak and would remain frozen for prolonged periods of time. Now the catatonia is not present all of the time. He is now able to say, *I said no I am not psychologically fragile, I am physically fragile, to the point where it is terrifying for me to be relating to the physical world in the harsh way that it works. I am okay in the bush but anything to do with the physical society is terrifying. It is dangerous for me because I am so fragile at a physical level. I said to someone, I think I said it to you that last time I saw you. I am so fragile that if I had a car accident and I got knocked* (bangs his hands together) *it would knock me out of my body and I would be gone.* Arnica has the remedy profile of the psychological and physical state associated with catatonia. He is now aware of his physical and psychological fragility.

This patient has been extremely traumatized in his life. Now he is able to unravel his history of abuse, and has gone back to the origins of his catatonia: his childhood. When he is feeling safe, he is able to stop the tremor in his right arm. He is now more aware of the existential shock and trauma that he has experienced all of his life. Similarly to the character Lars, he was not aware of the catatonic state he was in. Now it feels and appears harder for him because he is aware of the threat from all new situations. It is important to know and understand the unpeeling of the trauma and shock which is inherent in an *Arnica* constitution. If I panicked and thought that he was now more traumatized, I might have been tempted to change the remedy. He is now able to say, *I have always had life threatening trauma.*

In this last session, I increased the *Arnica* to a 200 C. potency daily.

6. *How*, *Why*, and *When* Causations – the 'Never-well-since-event'

The 'never-well-since-event' in *Arnica* has to involve childhood trauma. *Arnica* have the *Delusion* rubric: *sees frightful images, phantoms.* Until I discover the primary trauma in a patient's life, I am never totally sure of a simillimum prescription. It occurs during a consultation when everything stops in the case-taking and you know you have arrived at the centre of your patient's internal storm.

I had an episode of that when I was a child, about ten or eleven. I just remembered. I had a terrible, terrible nightmare about being on a ship in a battle. I woke up traumatized by it. My parents had to take me to the doctor I was so traumatized by it. I was about ten or eleven years old and I became compulsive about my clothing. For weeks and weeks afterwards, my clothing had to be perfectly folded at the end of my bed. If I thought it wasn't I had to get up and check that it was. It could go on for hours.

Arnica is a constitutional remedy which has its origins in trauma. It is extremely important when listening to a patient that you listen to the *cause and effect* of the trauma, and not to the presentation of the after-effect of the trauma. The rubric-repertorisation has to be formulated upon the *event*.

The homoeopath should not build the case analysis around the obsessive compulsive after-effects of the nightmare. The keynote effect of the trauma is shock. Obsessive compulsiveness over his clothes is how this patient tried to reconstruct his life in an attempt to regain control and order. The rubric-repertorisation should include only these rubrics.

- *Mind*: *ailments from*: *mental shock; from*: Arn.
- *Mind*: *ailments from*: *fright*: arn.
- *Mind*: *besides oneself; being*: *general; in*: arn.
- *Delusion* rubric: *images, phantoms; sees*: *frightful*: arn.

- *Delusion* rubric: *images, phantoms; sees*: *night*: arn.
- *Delusion* rubric: *die*: *about to die; one was*: arn.

Conclusion

Arnica is a remedy for shock. He says, *It is like a translucent skin. I have translucent skin, physically. Arnica* have no protection in the world. This patient has just started to emerge from his catatonia; he is now starting to feel.

Bibliography

Phatak, Dr. S. R. *Materia Medica of Homeopathic Medicines.* New Delhi, Indian Books & Periodicals Publishers, p. 66.

Schroyens, Frederik. M.D. *Synthesis.* London, Homeopathic Book Publishers, 1997.

Vermeulen, Frans. *Prisma.* Emryss Publishers, Haarlem 2002. p. 167.

Baryta carbonica

Abstract:

This is the case of a woman who did not speak until she was ten years of age. She made a decision very early on in her life that there was no success in speaking up. The *Delusion* rubric: *he does everything wrong, he cannot succeed*, is meant to be taken literally in this *Baryta carbonica* case. This woman needs to be overweight to get people to abandon her. This is the *Delusion* rubric: *forsaken*.

Keywords:

'Shaken Baby Syndrome'. Slow to develop. Self-fulfilling prophesies. 'Delusions of abandonment'.

Case Notes:

D.O.B. 1958.

Occupation: Special Aid Teacher

Presenting Physical Complaints:

- Repeated colds
- Low energy from the repeated colds
- Suffers with the cold and gets chills easily
- Overweight

- Binges and overeats. (I know, from members of her family who consult me, that she hoards and hides food, even though she lives alone)
- Kidney-function problems: diagnosed from Kidney Function Blood Test.
- Diabetes Type 2, developed in her early 30s. No medications. Her doctor wants her to lose weight. Blood-sugar reading of 7.4
- Polycystic Ovarian Disorder (P.C.O.D.) diagnosed at 25 years of age. (Weight problems can also be caused by P.C.O.D.)
- History of respiratory immune diseases, bronchitis, and asthma. She now lives in the country to avoid city smog
- High Blood Pressure: 150/100

First Consultation: April 2006

First memory of Trauma: She had Meningitis when she was seven years old. Her mother has reported that she was *never the same after this*. This event was significant, as her father was away and her mother was sick, so no one visited her in the hospital. This is her first conscious feeling of abandonment. After she was released from hospital, she had to catch the tram home. She says, *this was actually good as it gave me time to think before I got home about the fact that no one visited me*. At seven years of age, when this event happened, she had still not learnt how to speak, and although speech classes commenced at five years of age, she could not talk until she was ten years of age. She would have been unable to explain how she felt, or to communicate to the nurses and doctors in the hospital. Until she reached the age of ten, her older brother was the only person in the family who knew what she wanted, he was her voice and *he would translate my every need*.

Details of the Case: She has considerable trouble reading for longer than thirty minutes, and this is an issue in her work. She suffers low energy. Speaking is very slow, and she is slow to respond to questions. There was a history of violence toward her mother by her father, in her childhood. Her parents separated when she was ten years old, and divorced when she was thirteen years old. She was sent to boarding school at fifteen years of age. Boarding school was something she wanted as it allowed her to get away from home and *find security within the school community*. She tells me that her mother said she was extremely frustrating as she *was stubborn and difficult, as a child, and slow to learn scholastically.* Although speech and reading were delayed, she was always very good at mathematics. In her private life, outside of work, she is involved in pastoral care within the church; *the church provides a worthwhile way of contributing to a community.* She is currently studying theology so she can eventually work in pastoral care. (This study is practical study, not academic study.) She tells me that her services to the church are so highly valued that it would not be possible for the bishop to cope without her helping him. She says, *I am the only person who understands and gets on with the bishop.* She describes herself as the one who is *able to approve of people who come to the church.* She says that her boss at work says that she is such a special person, that she is *way too special and sensitive and gifted to be working in the public service,* and that she should work in the church helping older people. She is more socially confident visiting older parishioners.

> The most important aspect of taking a patient's case is not the *actual* truth of the situation, rather how the patient has relayed or embellished their story. I often consult with several members of a family. I never concern myself with whether a particular story is 'correct'. I never believe one version of the story over another. I am only interested how and why the patient has embellished their story. How a patient describes their childhood trauma will be told through the eyes of a child.

She is extremely shy. She says she suffers from 'social embarrassment' and lacks confidence in all social and work situations. She feels that she is continually criticized and laughed at because of her size. She does admit to hoarding food and hiding food in her cupboards, *just in case my blood sugar falls and I need to eat straight away.* (I have heard from her family members that this is a habit which she has had since childhood.) She does not believe that it is possible for her to lose weight because the type of weight she has *is flabby and not possible to change.* She believes that she will always be rejected and *picked on* because of her weight. She says, *my mother and father and other brother have rejected me because of my weight, they find me an embarrassment to be with.* (I have also been told that she was particularly sensitive as a baby, and would scream uncontrollably at any noise. She was so sensitive to noise that her mother found it difficult to use saucepans in the kitchen because the process of taking them out of the cupboard would cause considerable distress.)

Case Analysis: I used the following key points and headings in analyzing this case.

1. **Rubric-repertorisation**
2. **Theme**
3. *Striking*, or *Peculiar* **Signs and Symptoms; Organon 153**
4. **Materia Medica**
5. **Follow-up Consultations**
6. *How, Why,* and *When* **Causations – the 'Never-well-since-event'**

1. Rubric-repertorisation

- *Mind: answering: reflecting long: Bar-c.*
- *Mind: concentration: difficult:* **BAR-C**.
- *Mind: confidence: want of self-confidence:* <u>**BAR-C**.</u>
- *Mind: cautious: anxious:* bar-c.
- *Mind: development of children: arrested: Bar-c.*

- *Mind: fancies: exaltation of:* bar-c.
- *Mind: reading: unable to read: children, in:* bar-c.
- *Mind: secretive: Bar-c.*
- *Mind: slowness:* **BAR-C**.
- *Mind: sensitive: noise, to: slightest; to the:* bar-c.
- *Mind: speech: inarticulate:* bar-c.
- *Mind: speech: childish:* bar-c.
- *Mind: studying: difficult: Bar-c.*
- *Mind: timidity: bashful: Bar-c.*
- *Mind: forsaken feeling:* bar-c.

- *Delusions: criticized, she is: Bar-c.*
- *Delusions: forsaken; is:* bar-c.
- *Delusions: robbed, is going to be:* bar-c.
- *Delusions: succeed, he does everything wrong; he cannot: Bar-c.*
- *Delusions: wrong: suffered wrong; he has: children; in:* bar-c.
- *Delusions: fancy, illusions of:* bar-c.

- *Generals: cold; taking a: tendency:* <u>**BAR-C**</u>.
- *Generals: cold; becoming: after: agg.:* **BAR-C**.
- *Generals: cold: air: agg.:* **BAR-C**.
- *Generals: history; personal: pharynx; inflammation of: Bar-c.*
- *Generals: flabby feeling: Bar-c.*

2. Theme

Minerals
- need structure
- need security

- need stability and suffer from the feeling they lack stability
- need position
- lack confidence
- worry if they lose security
- feel alone if they do not belong to a group or organization

Her need to create stability, structure, and family support through the church and school community are the themes of a mineral remedy. Her need to hoard and hide food indicates underlying insecurity. Her vulnerability to cold is a mineral theme.

Key Themes

- *no one visited me*
- *find security within the school community*
- *contributing to a community*
- *slow to learn scholastically*
- *he would translate my every need*

The following transcript echoes the themes of overprotection, and the need for protection. These are the early developmental themes of a mineral remedy.

Question: What do you think were the things that stopped you developing as a child?

My older brother, who took such good care of me. He's a born leader, so it was because he could do all these things better than me. So he did it. But that is only a tiny aspect of it. The other aspect of it was almost like he was the leader, he was the boss. He didn't do it in a nasty way, actually, a very affectionate way, but it didn't allow me to develop. He talked for me, he was my voice, but like he is one of the most intelligent and capable people you could ever meet, but because of this I was smothered. Allowing something to happen is one thing, smothering is another.

Baryta carbonica are weighted heavily in all the rubrics of being forsaken. I have listed ten of them below, in Forsaken.

This *Baryta carbonica* (case) was abandoned in hospital as a child but it was not until very recently, after a long time of taking her constitutional remedy, that she realized her obesity was the tool she used to reinforce societal rejection of her as an 'obese person'. *Baryta carbonica* blame themselves and hate themselves because they believe their *body looks ugly*. All the psychological delusions of being forsaken and neglected in *Baryta carbonica* are complicated, enmeshed psychological avoidance techniques which become self-fulfilling prophecies of self-inflicted abandonment.

Baryta carbonica are the only remedy listed in the *Delusion* rubric: *beloved friend is dying*. *Baryta carbonica* fear that everyone they become close to will abandon them. The world is a particularly unsafe place for *Baryta carbonica*; they have the *Delusion* rubric: *every noise is a cry of fire and she trembles*. [1] 1.

1. Denial: *Delusion* rubric: *fancy, illusions of*: bar-c. [This rubric pertains to idealism. In relation to *Baryta carbonica* it reinforces what they have *not* achieved as distinct from what they *have* achieved.]

2. Forsaken*: Delusion* rubric: *abused, being*: Bar-c. *Delusion* rubric: *laughed at and mocked at*; *being*:** BAR-C**. *Delusion* rubric: *forsaken; is*: bar-c. *Delusion* rubric: *criticized, she is*: Bar-c. *Delusion* rubric: *dying: friend is*; *beloved*: bar-c. [1] 1. *Delusion* rubric: *robbed, is going to be*: bar-c. *Delusion* rubric: *laughed at and mocked at*; *being: street*; *whenever she goes into the*: bar-c. [1] 1. *Delusion* rubric: *people*: *seeing people*: *looking at him*: bar-c. *Delusion* rubric: *wrong*: *suffered wrong; he has*: bar-c. *Delusion* rubric: *watched, she is being*: Bar-c.

3. Causation: NONE. [*Delusion* rubric: *body*: *ugly*; *body looks*: bar-c. This rubric is allocated into 'delusions of original sin' because *Baryta carbonica* blame themselves over their looks.]

4. Depression: *Delusion* rubric: *succeed, he does everything wrong; he cannot*: *Bar-c*. *Delusion* rubric: *walking*: *knees, he walks on his*: *Bar-c*. *Delusion* rubric: *small*: *body is smaller*. *Bar-c*. [The last two rubrics can be allocated to depression and failure, or resignation to illness and death. They indicate feelings of helplessness or inability to do anything about one's situation.]

5. Resignation: *Delusion* rubric: *die*: *about to die; one was*: bar-c. *Delusion* rubric: *legs*: *cut off; legs are*: bar-c. *Delusion* rubric: *sick*: *being*: bar-c. *Delusion* rubric: *walking*: *knees, he walks on his*: *Bar-c*. *Delusion* rubric: *body*: *ugly; body looks*: bar-c. *Delusion* rubric: *small*: *body is smaller*. *Bar-c*.

3. *Striking*, or *Peculiar* Signs and Symptoms; Organon 153

In deciding if the remedy was *Baryta carbonica*, the *Mind* rubrics which I chose in the first consultation confirm the correct prescription. The following transcript outlines the striking *Delusion* rubrics of the case which come to light in the follow-up consultation, which further confirm *Baryta carbonica* as the remedy.

In this consultation she cries a lot and tells me a lot about the history of her inability to speak until she was ten years of age, and how her brother was her voice. She tells me about her father, and how violent he was to her mother.

Question: What do you think the fact that your parents were in conflict had to do with the way you perceived the world?

The thing that comes instantly to mind was that I wasn't allowed to speak out.

If you were allowed to speak out what would have happened?

Probably violence.

Do you have a memory of consciously thinking that?

When I was about seven. But intuitively when I was two; but I can't tell you anything about that. My father was bashing my mother a fair bit, and I can remember my father putting some hooks up on the kitchen sliding door, and anyway I indicated to my father about the hooks (she would point; she could still not talk) *and he said "You don't have to worry about that". They were so high none of us kids could actually reach it. Anyway very shortly after that my father went in, put the hooks on so we couldn't access the kitchen, and starting laying into my mother.*

So what decision do you think you made about yourself, or your mother or your father at that particular time?

I felt that I couldn't help my mother.

What did you feel about that?

Very helpless, I was just too little, I just can't do anything. But one of the things that came out of it was I made up my mind on that particular day that I would always go into bat for the little people.

The *Delusion* rubric: *he does everything wrong, he cannot succeed*, is meant to be taken literally in this *Baryta carbonica* case. This rubric is reflective of a patient's inner psychological delusional belief that they cannot succeed. This is the case of a child who did not speak until she was ten years of age. The decision she made very early on was that there was no success in speaking up. *Baryta carbonica* feel unable to enact change of any kind. *Baryta carbonica* have the *Delusion* rubric: *walking on his knees*. All three remedies listed in this rubric [*Bar-c*. bar-m. med.] lack the ability to self-actualize.

The *Delusion* rubrics which match her overwhelming feeling of being too little to speak are:

- *Delusions: forsaken; is*: bar-c.
- *Delusions: succeed, he does everything wrong; he cannot*: *Bar-c.*

- *Delusions*: *wrong*: *suffered wrong; he has*: *children; in*: bar-c.
- *Delusions*: *walking*: *knees, he walks on his*: *Bar-c.* [2] 3. [bar-m. med.]

The inner disturbance is the core of our case taking, and it is always reflective of *what is unusual or disturbing to the homoeopath*. *Baryta carbonica* have the *Delusion* rubric: *illusions of fancy*. The *Delusion* rubric: *illusions of fancy*, alludes to a psychological 'delusion of grandeur'. A patient who is suffering *illusions of fancy* has grand visions of persona: their expectations of what they can achieve, or what they *have* achieved, or who they are in the world, are exaggerated. This *Baryta carbonica* patient has a strong need to embellish her role within the church. If a patient has a strong need to exaggerate, then the homoeopath has to be alerted to an underlying psychological delusion.

With this *Baryta carbonica* (case), what I am particularly interested in is the patient's delusional stance and how she sets herself up to be repeatedly abandoned because of her obesity. She stays obese so that people will abandon her, as her mother and father did when she was young. In the consultation, she tells me: *I need to be overweight to get people to abandon me*; *it is also proof they will abandon me*. This is the *Delusion* rubric: *forsaken*; in particular, the *Delusion* rubric: *being laughed at and mocked*. Although it is true that society rejects obese people, she has used her body as self-fulfilling proof of future abandonment. The psychological delusions of being *forsaken* are always maintained to help the constitutional remedy profile avoid exaggerated self-blame or 'delusions of original sin'. It is always easier to blame others. Exaggerated delusions of self-blame are psychological delusions which each patient wants to avoid. The best way to avoid self-blame is to redirect blame on to the world, your bodies health, or God for abandoning you. This is why a particular remedy profile will need to maintain their 'delusions of persecution' or their 'delusions of abandonment'; they wish to avoid personal involvement. *Baryta carbonica* have no personal 'delusions of original sin'. They do have the *Delusion* rubric: *body looks ugly*. This rubric is allocated into 'delusions of original sin' because *Baryta carbonica* blame themselves over their looks. *Baryta carbonica* use their looks to test someone's love. *Baryta carbonica* lack self-confidence to the extent that if they are sick, it adds to their fear of being looked at; therefore they view illness as a threat. Rejection based on how they look reinforces their 'delusions of persecution'. *Baryta carbonica* are not listed in any significant 'delusions of grandeur', or 'hubristic denial' rubrics. If you have a patient who presents with psychological delusions of denial about their illness, the constitutional remedy cannot be *Baryta carbonica*. When sick, *Baryta carbonica* do not fall into psychological denial; instead they collapse into the stages of projected abandonment and self-abandoning predictions of failure and decline. This patient felt unable to protect her mother, and she feels unable to change her weight problem. *Baryta carbonica* feel mocked and hopelessly wronged, and unable to enact change of any kind – *Delusion* rubric: *walking on his knees*. Their only psychological delusion and perceived sin is that their body looks ugly; hence their fear of ridicule. The *Delusion* rubric: *being laughed and mocked at,* is a self-fulfilling prophecy of self-condemnation and expected abandonment. *Baryta carbonica* feel self-defeated because they feel guilty for their *body looking ugly*. Over-reacting is self-deprecating and self-deluding. The *Delusion* rubric: *forsaken* will be used by each constitutional remedy profile as an emotional avoidance or self-deluding denial, which will be adopted and destructively nurtured by the patient to justify *continually* feeling hurt and abandoned by friends or family. In the case-taking it is important to understand, firstly, how the patient has used the psychological delusion in a disproportionate way to misinterpret reality. Secondly, it is crucial to understand why the delusional stance is maintained by the patient and why and how it is advantageous to the patient to delude themselves that they are alone. Thirdly, it is essential to understand the conflict *specific* to the constitutional remedy profile which explains the disproportionate need to maintain a misinterpretation of reality. Lastly, it is important to understand why the remedy profile needs to maintain the psychological delusion of being abandoned.

If a patient has a conflicting interpretation of reality, it is important to understand the nature of what they need to avoid.

Identifying delusional inconsistencies is synonymous with identifying the simillimum in the case. This woman needs to hoard and hide food even though she lives alone. *Baryta carbonica* have the *Delusion* rubric: *is going to be robbed.* *Baryta carbonica* in particular hoard food because they are fearful it will be taken away from them. *Baryta carbonica* have the *Delusion* rubric: *is forsaken,* and the *Mind* rubrics: *borrowing from everyone, desire to nibble,* and *impelled to touch everything.* I have heard from her family members that her hoarding and hiding of food preceded boarding school. The cure of chronic disease is the cure of the delusional state. With every remedy we choose for our patients, we must see the level of the *Delusion* rubrics and we must understand how they come into our patients' lives. The transcript above captures that moment of reflection and inner change and knowing in the follow-up consultation, which is reflective of the homoeopathic cure of a trauma state. The simillimum brings to the surface the psychodynamic process of the original trauma. Cure in the treatment of chronic disease is reflected in the change to the psychodynamic crisis, which was reflected in the psychological delusional state. I always like to see this development of the *Delusion* rubrics in the follow-up consultation.

4. Materia medica

Rajan Sankaran, in *The Soul of Remedies,* writes, "*Baryta carbonica* is totally dependent on others, almost like a cripple or an imbecile. 'Delusion that he walks on his knees' and 'Delusion that a beloved friend is sick and dying' show the crippled, dependent feeling of *Baryta carbonica* and his fear of losing this support. There is a feeling of total incapacity to take on responsibilities or do one's own work. *Baryta carbonica* has anticipatory anxiety because of this feeling of incapacity. The patients are totally irresolute and depend completely on someone else to take decisions for them."

5. Follow-up Consultations

Treatment:

Diet advice re: avoiding carbohydrates and sugars. I advised a high protein, low glycaemic diet, and exercise.

Remedy: *Baryta carbonica* 30 C., one pilule dry by mouth, daily, and continuous.

Second Consultation: June 2006.

- Blood pressure is now 130/75
- Normal kidney function test recorded
- No change to blood-sugar readings; still 7·4
- Noticeable weight loss. (I do not have the scale reading from before treatment, but I am estimating by size that she has lost five kilos)
- Has now enough energy to walk thirty minutes at a brisk pace, *most days*
- Now not needing to sleep so long: eight hours; before, ten to twelve hours
- Less cold physically
- Had a cold, recently

Her energy is considerable stronger, and her kidney function and blood pressure are now normal. She has a cold, but it has not gone to her chest like it would normally. All of the above changes can be attributed to diet and exercise changes. The change to her personality is profound. She has reported that she is now able to read for up to two hours at a time. She is noticeably quicker to answer questions. She also reports that she is far less shy at work, and is now able to talk to people. Her colleagues at work have noticed a big difference in that she is able to converse about what she feels and thinks about things. In this consultation, she is very touched by the profound difference in her ability to read, and her newly found ability to talk. Interestingly, she reports that her intuition is far less.

Question: What do you mean by "my intuition"?

I used to get by with my intuition. Now I find that I have a lot more of the logical part of my brain. I still have my intuition, but I also have a part of me which is able to think.

Below is a transcript from a videotaped session with the patient. The fact that she agreed to being filmed shows an incredible difference in her degree of social confidence. The interesting aspect is that the patient is learning how to operate in the world from an analytical framework, and not from her intuition. Initially I was worried about this, but the patient is in fact now developing an intellectual capacity to assess situations, as well as being able to fall back on her intuition.

Question: What are the sorts of things that have been going on?

I have bought an investment unit. So I have had a lot going on. [sighs]

Did that bring up some anxiety?

Absolutely. I have had some of my work colleagues saying settle down, you are doing the right thing. Even my solicitor has been saying I am doing the right thing. Perhaps some of it is because of the treatment my intuition has gone down, and I am faced with making a big decision without relying on what I used to rely on, my intuition. Now I think that more logical analysis has come into things, that I am not quite trusting that yet. So I am a little bit nervous. But I am in some ways taking far more things in my stride. Yes, a tad anxious. Secondly, my normal security people were away [bank manager, solicitor], *so I had to do a fair bit by myself. So yes, very anxious.*

So what are the differences people have noticed about you?

What I was I really noticing is that I could sit down and read. Before, I could kind of sit down and read but it was always a bit of a struggle, but now I can sit down and read, and wow! Is this like everyone else just reads! This is amazing. Before, if I had to really concentrate, I could read for about half an hour, then I had to have a sleep. Now I can read for a couple of hours, and it doesn't affect me at all, which is amazing. Absolutely phenomenal. So my library has increased.

My doctor (she visited her doctor in the previous week, who now works as a spiritual healer) *has noticed my immune system is far better. I don't struggle between visits* [three months between visits]. *I have far more energy. Another thing I am noticing is, that while everyone is wearing jumpers, I am not! I used to always rug up. I am not anymore, which is amazing. What my friends are saying is that I tend to be able to focus on what they are saying a lot more, not that I didn't focus before, but they just feel like I am listening a lot better to what they are saying.*

Do you think you are more outgoing?

I think I am a bit more assertive.

In what ways?

For instance, if I am not happy with the situation, I will say so, not in a nasty way. I am saying what I think far more. One of the things that I have noticed is that within my role within the parish, I am visiting and talking to people much more, things like that. So I suppose I am stepping out of my security zone a bit more. I don't know if shy is the right word. I don't think I am as self-conscious. Not that I went out to hide things, it's just that I didn't have the confidence to just do it.

Fourth consultation: November 2006

Feels like she is getting a cold. This did not develop. [*Baryta carbonica* have a tendency to catch colds frequently.]

When I left last time, I was thinking I was too harsh about my brother, but now I think, no, I wasn't. We had a family meeting, and I realized that he wouldn't listen to what I thought were good and valid questions and points that I made, and he wouldn't let me speak. I feel like saying to him, you know I can speak too. I have subsequently realized I don't need a protector as much as I did. I also asked mother about when I was a baby, as you can't remember that time can you? She said I used to cry a lot, apparently I was very bad with loud noises, and that father used to shake me very badly. After she said that she became very quiet and wouldn't talk any more about it. (Please note that even if the mother had realized this was a problem, she herself was a bashed wife.) But I have worked out the reason I wouldn't have spoken was to avoid being shaken. This last year has had a lot going on for me, emotionally. There have been a lot of changes. I now know I need to consolidate next year, and lose the weight. (Currently 103 kilos.)

6. *How*, *Why*, and *When* Causations – the 'Never-well-since-event'

In the fourth consultation, I am shocked into realizing that the patient's delayed speech and learning difficulties were more than likely the result of Shaken Baby Syndrome. Shaking a baby can produce speech disabilities and learning difficulties.

Her father had been extremely violent towards her mother. According to her mother, her father had shaken her violently as a baby to stop her from crying. The *Materia medica* on *Baryta carbonica* is relatively well known, so I have chosen only to concentrate on the relevant and insightful *Materia medica* to help explain this case. Philip Bailey in *Homeopathic Psychology* notes, "In some cases there was physical trauma to the head during birth (or subsequently)." Bailey also notes that it's "remarkable that individuals with longstanding brain damage can recover a great deal of function after the remedy is taken." This has been proven correct in this case.

Case Analysis

This woman is going forward in her life in leaps and bounds. The intensity of what she would like to say to her bother — *you know I can speak too* — is reflective of the essence of the case; she can now literally speak for herself. This has been a beautiful healing of *Baryta carbonica*. She is attending exercise classes three days a week, and I know that her newly found mental and emotional strength will strengthen her resolve to get the weight off, and get her blood-sugar levels back to normal. Bailey notes: "*Baryta* has a tendency to dig in his heels and say no when asked to do something. This is partly due to insecurity. *Baryta* feels instinctively that he is not properly 'equipped' to deal with the complexities of the world, and one of his strategies is to resist change of any kind." The *Baryta carbonica* in this case is now considering a possible job or career change. She has bought an investment property by herself, and is studying homoeopathy! The insecurity Bailey acknowledges within *Baryta carbonica* is no longer undermining her confidence. She is no longer *too little*.

Follow-up Consultation: November 2007.

I have now increased the remedy to a 200 C. potency given monthly. Consults are approximately three monthly.

The patient now has enough confidence to branch out and look for other work. She has started full-time study in homoeopathy.

Follow-up Consultation: September 2008.

I increase the potency to a single dose of 1 M. dry pilule.

Her confidence continues to grow, and she is coping with study quite well. Her struggle with her weight waxes and wanes, but in this area she has made a big breakthrough as she has come to terms with why she feels she needs the weight.

Baryta carbonica is a slow-to-progress remedy profile. Her weight has increased, and her blood sugar levels have now increased to eight. This is a process consistent with the energy of *Baryta carbonica*; slow and steady and in her own time. Every profoundly overweight person will have a different interplay with themselves and overeating. If the patient realizes the exact mental and emotional triggers around food bingeing, it is an important breakthrough which, in my experience, always leads to change.

This patient's breakthrough takes us back to the start of the case, to the first *Delusion* rubric: *forsaken*. This is the law of cure and it will happen in all cases if the simillimum is correct. Proof of cure is cure of the psychological delusion layers within the case. She tells me in the last consult that her obesity is needed so people will abandon her, as her mother and father did when she was young. She tells me *I need to be overweight to get people to abandon me*; *it is also proof they will abandon me*. This is the *Delusion* rubric: *forsaken*. The reason why it is important to know the disturbance in a case is because any severe disease state is always a reflection of our inner angst. With this case, what I am particularly interested in is the development of the stance she takes as a child which formulates this disturbance. The destruction is the delusional stance, and how she sets herself up is to repeat abandonment through her obesity. We, as a society, reject obese people. Destruction to her own health though obesity, and the subsequent disease of diabetes, is self-destructive and self-abandoning. This is what we can now see coming to the surface; this is cure of the psychological delusional state because the deeper layers of *Delusion* rubrics are now surfacing.

- *Delusions: forsaken*: bar-c.
- *Delusions: criticized; that; she is*: Bar-c.
- *Delusions: imagines; laughed at; she is*: **BAR-C**.
- *Delusions*: *watched; she is*. Bar-c.

In case analysis, and understanding cure, we must know what we want to change and what we expect to change inside of our patients. The above *Delusion* rubrics reflect what she has realized about her weight. She eats obsessively to be watched, so she can be *forsaken* or abandoned and rejected or *laughed at*. If the patient uses abandonment as a psychological delusion, and perverts it into an often complicated system of psychological avoidances or self-delusions, then the person has a *Delusion* rubric in their case. The simillimum will always bring evidence of the psychological delusions to the surface in the follow-up consultations, and this is cure of the delusional state. Cure and change of the psychodynamic crisis, as reflected in the *Delusion* rubric is what this patient is now seeing reflected back to herself in the mirror of her own life. She is now starting to understand the excuses and self-deluding avoidances she has created around her weight issues.

Follow-up Through her homoeopathic studies she has decided that she is not constitutionally *Baryta carbonica*. This is not an unusual occurrence. Homoeopathic students will periodically switch from remedy to remedy in their exploration of homoeopathy. The *Baryta carbonica* prescription could also have been reflective of a 'layer' which needed lifting in her case-history. This case is still ongoing.

Bibliography

Bailey, Philip, M. M.D. *Homeopathic Psychology*. Berkeley, California, North Atlantic Books, 1995, pp.35-36.

Sankaran, Rajan. *The Soul of Remedies*. Santa Cruz, Bombay, Homoeopathic Medical Publishers, 1997. p. 25.

Schroyens, Frederik. M.D. *Synthesis*. London, Homeopathic Book Publishers, 1997.

Lac humanum

Abstract:

This is the case of a woman who believed her 'karmic journey' in life was to save her sister's life. She sacrificed herself to her sister, her mother, her baby, and husband. This is a case of *Lac humanum* finding independence.

Keywords:

Oedipus complex. Self-sacrifice. Fibromyalgia. Empathic over-identification.

D.O.B. 1963.

Details of the Case:

The first consultation occurs directly after I consult with her older sister. The sisters present with the *exact* same health history.

When I compare this woman's health history with her sister's health history, I notice that this patient has been diagnosed with *every* single health complaint six to twelve months after the older sister has been diagnosed.

Furthermore, they are on the exact same prescription medications; even down to the dose. I gave her older sister *Carcinosin*. Other than this patient being extremely thin and having a history of eating disorders, everything else in their medical history is the same.

First consult: June 2006

Reason for consult:

- Fibromyalgia
- Post-natal Depression
- Disorder of Initiating and Maintaining Sleep (DIMS) after the birth of her child

Medical History:

- Immunizations: Not Chicken Pox. Rubella, Measles, TB, Whooping Cough, Diphtheria, Polio
- Allergies: Sulphur-based drug, Pethidine. Opiates, Medical Tape, Cat-gut stitches
- Anorexia nervosa and Bulimia, 1987-91
- Basal Cell Carcinoma, 1988, left leg
- Keloid skin
- Cystitis and Kidney infection, 1994
- Menses ceased June-November, 1998, and February-November 1999
- Glandular Fever. Diagnosed 1991 and 2004
- Severe Sinusitis – surgery Septoplasty June, 1999. Surgery repeated November 1999
- Pregnancy Termination 1993
- Polycystic Ovarian Disorder (PCOD) diagnosed 1994
- Hypoglycemic
- Chronic Fatigue Syndrome (CFS)
- Smoker 5.5 yrs; ceased 1995
- Fibromyalgia, 2002
- Neural Mediated Hypotension, 2002
- DIMS. The first episode in 2002
- Anaemia, 2002
- Cystitis May 2005

- Continual bronchitis and sinus infections. She is on a weekly dose of antibiotics
- DIMS after the birth of her child
- Breast Feeding. Baby is 9 months old
- Post-Natal Depression

Current Medications:

- Endep 10mg
- EES Erythromycin 400mg 3 times a week
- Panamax Paracetamol 500mg 2/day as needed
- Nilstat 500,000 IU 3 times a week
- Zoloft 100mg 1/day
- Dalacin C. 150mg. 3 times a week, for Chronic infections

She is *notably* thin. I start my rubric-repertorisation from the *only* distinguishing and individualistic pathology that she has, which her sister does not have. In homoeopathy, the psychological delusion is viewed as an exaggeration of personality status which indicates an abnormality or an illness. This patient is suffering from an exaggerated perception of herself as being fat. A *Delusion* rubric applies to the case analysis when a patient misrepresents and misinterprets reality in a disproportionate way, consistent with the psychiatric definition of a psychological delusion.

- *Delusion* rubric: *body: ugly; body looks: fat; too:* Acer-cic. lac-h.

This case, however, is extremely fascinating, as the patient has an amazingly strong empathic sharing of her older sister's emotional, mental, and physical health. I remark on the phenomena to the patient. As a student of homoeopathy I was taught not to ask leading or inquiring questions which would cross the boundaries of psychotherapy. If you don't ask leading questions you will struggle in the rubric-repertorisation. In the Cases, I emphasize repeatedly the need to understand the causation or the 'never-well-since-event'. I asked her, "What is going on between you and your sister? I am asking because I am confused. You have the same health history?"

The patient relays a past life story told to her by her clairvoyant guide and teacher. She and her sister were also sisters in the second World War; their parents were arrested by the Nazis and they were left to fend for themselves. Her older sister died in her arms, and she died next. *I was not able to save her* (sister) *and take away her death. In this life, my journey is to share in her* (sister's) *pain and help save her life.*

Presenting Issue:

She describes herself: *I am currently exhausted. My baby is sucking my life from me, and I cannot relate to him* (baby) *anymore. I feel nothing. I have no love to share with him* (baby) *or my husband; I feel nothing.*

She finds her husband irritating because he does not understand the support she needs with the baby.

He has no idea how it is for me; (cries) *I am alone with my baby.*

Family Background:

Her father was diagnosed with Bi-Polar depressive disorder.

I remember making a conscious decision to become my mother's friend and counselor. I sacrificed myself to help her. She needed me. She would talk to me for hours, and unburden her heart to me. I now do that for my baby, and he (baby) *is sucking the life out of me. I am here and my journey in this life is to save my sister's life, and to save my mother's life; to complete the Karmic lesson from the last life; to give myself. I am still there for my mother – now she shares all her burdens with me. I have nothing but hate for my father, and his lack of love and support for us.*

This patient alternates between martyring herself to save her mother and sister, and feelings of bewilderment as to why she has been abandoned and left alone with her baby. She is trying to resolve her guilt by continuing to martyr herself.

Her course of action is a self-fulfilling prophecy. The more she martyrs herself by looking after her mother, her sister, her husband and her baby, the less likely it is that she will receive the attention and care she needs as a new mother. It is her 'duty' and 'fate' in this life to look after them and save them because she failed in her last life; this is the 'original sin'.

Case Analysis: I used the following key points and headings in analyzing this case.

1. *Striking*, or *Peculiar* **Signs and Symptoms; Organon 153**
2. **Rubric-repertorisation**
3. **Theme**
4. **Follow-up Consultations**
5. *How*, *Why*, and *When* **Causations – the 'Never-well-since-event'.**

1. *Striking*, or *Peculiar* Signs and Symptoms; Organon 153

She describes herself as skinless, with no identity of her own. I ask myself, what is the *Delusion* rubric for this? Someone who has not yet developed an identity or persona is a baby.

- *Delusion* rubric: *born into the world*; *he was newly*: cori-r. lac-h. olib-sac. plut-n. symph.

In the first consultation, I noticed that she wore lots of different crystals on her wrists. I asked her in the first consultation why she liked them. She replied, *they are my friends* and that she *eventually wanted to work with her friends*. It was not until the follow-up consultation that I understood that the crystals were a replacement for not having a mother to mother her. Initially, in the first consultation, I looked up the *Delusion* rubrics: *unwanted by friends,* and the *Mind* rubric: *forsaken feeling, sensation of isolation.*

- *Delusion* rubric: *friend: unwanted by friends: Lac-h.* [2] 1.
- *Mind* rubric: *forsaken feeling: isolation; sensation of:* abies-c. aids. allox. *Anac. Androc. Anh. Arg-n.* arist-cl. *Bit-ar.* camph. cann-i. cann-s. carb-an. carc. choc. coca coli. cortico. crot-c. cygn-be. cypra-eg. cystein-l. dendr-pol. des-ac. dioxi. falco-pe. fl-ac. galla-q-r. *Germ-met. Ham.* hippoc-k. hura. *Hydrog.* irid-met. *Kola.* lac-ac. lac-del. lac-h. lac-lup. lap-la. loxo-recl. lyss. mang-p. marb-w. merc. musca-d. **NAT-SIL.** *Oncor-t.* op. ozone phasco-ci. pip-m. plac. plat. *Plut-n.* polys. *Positr.* psil. psor. puls. pycnop-sa. rad-br. **RUTA.** sal-al. sal-fr. stram. *Symph.* tab. taosc. thuj. *Vanil.* vip.

  Prescription: *Lac humanum* 30 C. 1/day, dry pilule, continuous. *Lac humanum* 200 C. 1/week, continuous.

2. Rubric-repertorisation

- *Delusions: alone, being: always alone; she is:* Lac-h.
- *Delusions: body: ugly; body looks: fat; too:* lac-h.
- *Delusions: born into the world; he was newly:* lac-h.
- *Delusions: crime: committed a crime; he had:* lac-h.
- *Delusions: wrong: done wrong; he has:* lac-h.

- *Mind: ailments from: neglected; being: mother; by one's:* lac-h.
- *Mind: anger: alternating with: repentance; quick:* lac-h.
- *Mind: despair: life, of:* lac-h.
- *Mind: despair: pains, with the:* lac-h.
- *Mind: forsaken feeling: isolation; sensation of:* lac-h.
- *Mind: orphans:* lac-h.

3. Theme

In this *Lac humanum* (case) the patient needs to maintain her feelings of aloneness and being abandonment because they protect her from her overwhelmingly disproportionate feelings of guilt for not being able to save her sister in their last life together. Her abandonment is reminiscent of Jesus declaring on the cross, *Father my God why have you abandoned me?* *Lac humanum* has an inner conflict between living as a self-determined individual in a group and feeling beholden to the group.

The theme in the remedy profile of *Lac humanum* is the group versus self. When she explains that she decided to abandon herself to looking after her mother because it was an act of love, she says: *I sacrificed myself to help her; she needed me. She would talk to me for hours, and unburden her heart to me. I love her dearly and I did it with love, but it was at a cost; I know that now.* This reflects the importance of the group versus her self-importance. It also explains another crucial aspect of *Lac humanum*. *Lac humanum* have one rubric of grandeur, the *Delusion* rubric: *he was newly born into the world.* *Lac humanum* are the 'milk of human kindness'. They have sacrificed themselves so that life will continue. *Lac humanum* are the only remedy listed in the *Delusion* rubric: *as if she is nesting.* *Lac humanum* are the savior and the mother and nurturer of the human race.

Lac humanum have the *Mind* rubric: *Oedipus complex*[17]. *Lac humanum* will always develop an overprotective, symbiotic relationship with one parent, and a hate relationship with the other. *Lac humanum* project on to the parent whom they hate,

---

17 Oedipus Complex is a son's largely unconscious sexual attraction toward his mother accompanied by jealousy toward his father. Austrian psychiatrist Sigmund Freud first used the term. Oedipus is the hero of the ancient Greek play *Oedipus Tyrannus,* by Sophocles, which tells the story of how Oedipus was abandoned at birth by his parents and returned as an adult to kill his father and marry his mother. Freud suggested that if this complex is not resolved in the young child, it contributes to neurosis in later life. Swiss psychologist Carl Jung suggested that such feelings were not restricted to boys but that girls could also experience a similar complex.

all their psychological 'delusions of persecution'. *Lac humanum* will be convinced that the parent whom they hate is injurious to them and to the rest of the family. She says: *I have nothing but hate for my father, and his lack of love and support for us. Lac humanum* always equate abandonment with *injury*, this is why the list of abandonment rubrics below are a mixture of being *alone, friendless* and *neglected,* as well as being *poisoned* and about to receive *injury*. This association relates to the fact that they are *newly born into the world*; a baby themselves who needs to be protected. They will always hate the parent who has abandoned them, and they will always encourage a symbiotic love/mothering/Oedipal relationship with the other parent. It is possible to see the co-dependent symbiosis of an 'Oedipus complex' when this *Lac humanum* patient says of her relationship with her mother: *I sacrificed myself to help her; she needed me. She would talk to me for hours, and unburden her heart to me.*

Lac humanum continue to stay alone and maintain the situation of being alone, because they have exaggerated and disproportionate feelings of having committed 'wrongs'. Once *Lac humanum* acknowledge all 'wrongs', they sink into disproportionate depressive reactions to their 'crimes'. *Lac humanum* have disproportionate feelings of being *worthless*. Saving humanity is more important to them than saving themselves. *Lac humanum* have the *Mind* rubric: *detached from ego.* [1] 1. *Lac humanum* justify their predetermined martyrdom and self-actualized abandonment because they are *too ugly and fat* to be worthy of individualization. When *Lac humanum* are sick they question whether they are worthy enough to save. A *Lac humanum* patient will more than likely quibble over the cost of the consultation because they feel unworthy of spending the money on themselves rather than on their family. *Lac humanum* have the *Delusion* rubric: *face distorted*, as well as the *Delusion* rubric: *body looks fat and ugly. Lac humanum* have the *Mind* rubric: *anxiety about food.*

[1] 1. *Lac humanum* believe that when they are sick they are too *ugly, fat* and *distorted* to be included in the human family. *Lac humanum* also have the *Mind* rubric: *aversion to being watched.* [1] 1. They will feel *unwanted by friends, alone,* and *friendless.* *Lac humanum* deals with the separation by over-mothering humanity. If your patient feels alone and separated from others and yet continues to care for others, then the simillimum could well be *Lac humanum. Lac humanum* perpetuate being alone and abandoned because they struggle to ask for help in their lives.

1. Denial: *Delusion* rubric: *born into the world; he was newly*: lac-h.

2. Forsaken: *Delusion* rubric: *alone: being: always alone; she is*: Lac-h. *Delusion* rubric: *body: ugly; body looks: fat; too*: lac-h. *Delusion* rubric: *betrayed; that she is*: lac-h. *Delusion* rubric: *friend: unwanted by friends*: Lac-h. [2] 1. *Delusion* rubric: *friendless, he is*: lac-h. *Delusion* rubric: *neglected: he or she is neglected*: Lac-h. *Delusion* rubric: *poisoned: he has been*: lac-h. *Delusion* rubric: *violence, about*: lac-h. *Delusion* rubric: *injury: about to receive injury; is*: lac-h.

3. Causation: *Delusion* rubric: *crime: committed a crime; he had*: lac-h. *Delusion* rubric: *wrong: done wrong; he has*: lac-h.

4. Depression: *Delusion* rubric: *worthless; he is*: lac-h. *Delusion* rubric: *unreal: everything seems unreal*: lac-h. *Delusion* rubric: *body: ugly; body looks: fat; too*: lac-h. [This rubric pertains to being depressed with oneself or self-rejection.]

5. Resignation: *Delusion* rubric: *face: distorted*: lac-h. [1] 1.

Themes of *Lac humanum*

*   Sense of isolation
*   Responsibility and a strong sense of duty
*   Am I the baby or the mother?

- Forsaken
- Loss of self confidence
- Difficulties in childhood – unable to separate from the mother. *I am still there for my mother, now she shares all her burdens with me.*
- Dependence on the group versus independence
- "A need to put the world close to home in order." [Vermeulen] *I am here and my journey in this life is to save my sisters life and to save my Mother's life; to complete the Karmic lesson from the last life; to give myself.*
- Lack of self confidence; she describes herself as, *skinless with no identity of her own.*
- "They have a sense of isolation with the world. They become detached, and have a sort of numbness to life." [Vermeulen]
- "My survival depends on my ability to get approval. A struggle to live up to expectations. Survival depends on choices made by someone else." [Notes from a Shah case 2004 that I attended in India.]
- Conflict of the right to exist
- Selfless
- Having a conscience
- Conflict of the right to exist – her empathic somatic sharing of her sister's illness confirms this conflict
- Irritable cursing anger at not being nurtured
- No ego / self / identity.

Clinical Themes of *Lac humanum*

- Hormonal imbalance
- Breast disorders, low milk supply
- Post-Natal Depression

- Mood swings: indifference, detachment. The patient describes this detachment when she says, *I am currently exhausted. My baby is sucking my life from me and I cannot relate to him anymore. I feel nothing. I have no love to share with him or my husband; I feel nothing.*
- "Indifference to everything." [Vermeulen]
- Eating disorders

4. Follow-up Consultations, one month later, July 2006.

Question: You said you have had some dreams?

Very vivid, very animated, quite a lot of details, lots of action. The main gist of the dreams was: I was being accused of something that I hadn't really done, or pleaded my case, or convinced people that I didn't do that. And in a more recent dream I was concerned for others welfare. And they were judging me.

What were they judging you for?

Quite a weird scenario; someone rang the door bell and asked if this was where the sausage sizzle was. I said no, and then they wanted to come in and use the phone. I knew this was not right, and he was trying to force his way in, and then the next scene was the whole street standing there and saying he wasn't wrong, he wasn't bad, and you should not have treated him that way. And then my husband came in my left side and I said, look can't you convince them? And he said of course she was right. The other dream was my baby and us on the beach, and the water was coming in and I said we have to go back, and my husband said, no it is alright. Then the water came up to my baby's neck, and it was like, well you haven't heard me, you didn't listen to me, you didn't hear my truth.

Dream Themes

First Dream:

- Accused
- Concerned for her welfare
- Misjudging me
- The man in the dream wants to force his way in

Second Dream:

- Protect her child
- *You didn't hear my truth*

Rubric-repertorisation

- *Mind*: *anger*. *contradiction; from*: lac-h.
- *Mind*: *fear*. *attacked; fear of being*: lac-h.
- *Delusions*: *betrayed; that she is*: lac-h.
- *Delusions*: *neglected*: *he or she is neglected*: *Lac-h*.

When the patient is retelling dreams which resonate on the same level as the simillimum, I know that I will always discover the 'never-well-since-event'.

The following transcript is from a videoed session. I asked to video the session because in her initial relaying of the dreams in the first few minutes of the consultation, she had told me that in the dreams she was starting to find her ability to stand her own ground when she reprimand her husband for not hearing her truth. In the following transcript, she uses those exact words when she says that she can now stand in her own power.

Question: How does that relate to the difference in how you have been feeling since you last saw me?

I noticed more a standing in my own shoes, a standing in my own power. Able to access and verbalize what is right for me, or what I need to say no to, or finding that I do have the energy to challenge the conversation or fight the argument.

Before, it was too exhausting to do so. It has come without thinking. It has bypassed the conscious thinking processes. I would think: I should do this, or why am I allowing myself to do this – perhaps manipulated? Now I think: no I am not doing this, and it is without any guilt, it is just this is the way it is. It's so nice. It's great. I have to say it's like some wonderful cocktail when you have taken a few sips.

So there has been a little more emotional strength, and has that correlated to having more physical strength?

Before, I found that the Fibromyalgia and the muscles are more noticeable, but I have realized just recently that I have been able to physically do more. I can pack more into the day. I am very rarely still, now. I have been able to do loads of washing. There are so many things that I want to do that I haven't been able to do before.

Has anything changed in the way you are relating to people?

There is a change with my husband. In standing in my own power. He would be on the couch and I am in the kitchen, and he would say, do you have to do that now? And I say, yes I do because otherwise I have to get up tomorrow and do it, so deal with it! Before, I would have done it more quietly so as not to disturb him. With the Fibromyalgia I would drop things and bang, and now I have more control over things, and I am telling him it's not happening, get over it. Now I have the energy to confront things; whereas I didn't have the energy to do that. I have fully held my space. It is sitting more in my centre; that's very new.

Do you think you are feeling as depressed?

No. [Laughs a lot.]

What does it feel like to not have to be so sensitive to other people?

Good. Very good. Overdue. Like a breath of fresh air. It is still too new to say that, but that is how it feels. That's not to say I don't care, or that I am not sensitive to others, but it's a process of claiming back me first, and caring and thinking about me, then look at the rest of the world. Scary because it's new and different. I don't think I have ever felt that. And I get excited when I say, No deal with it, and I think wow! That just came from nowhere – wow! Like I stand taller.

To go back to your dream what do you think was playing out in the dream?

Feeling unworthy, and it is something I have had since I was a child.

Can you remember when it was played out?

I can't remember, but my feeling is it was as a wee small person. My father said up until a certain age you were like the sunshine; you light up and you light everyone else up, and then one day the clouds came over and you disappeared. I think it was realizing my external environment. Realizing my parents were not happy in their marriage. And there was an element of fear there, so I started to feel their relationship and feel responsible for taking away their pain or woes, and how that affected my sister. So I felt that I must have in some way done something, so I should try to do something to make them all happy. Responsibility for other people's pain and woes, because I remember thinking I will be everyone's sunshine. I spent a lot of time with mum, sharing a lot of stuff that was inappropriate for a child, because she was unhappy. I was mature enough to say yes you can share that with me, and I did too much of that and not being a child. There was a sense of achievement to compensate for the home environment, a need to prove yourself because something is shaky. My real desire is now to have worth for me and not to be preoccupied with them.

This is very different from when you first came to me, because you said the reason you wanted to be well was so you could be a wife and a mother.

I remember. It is amazing. It's amazing.

The reason you told me you took the anti-depressants is that you didn't want to be miserable for your husband or baby.

Yes, but I wasn't able to say then that I wanted to feel stronger for me first and foremost which is what I would say now. Huge shift, Liz.

How many cold and sinus infections since you have seen me?

Probably two. But I have not had to go near any antibiotics, which is why I do this to you [she bows] to those amazing tablets, as I didn't really ever think I would get off those antibiotics. Because I also needed such a strong antibiotic as well, and this has been such a persistent upper respiratory weak area that I have had for years. That is why I love them. I love those two bottles. The light looks different. Standing forward again.

What do you think you lost when you became your mother's counselor?

I think I lost my identity. My precious time to discover the individual without stress; those child years. I had to become responsible. I didn't have time to allow myself to feel things. I love her dearly, and I did it with love, but it was a cost. I know that now.

5. *How, Why,* and *When* Causations – the 'Never-well-since-event'

- *I didn't feel good enough – I, me alone, was not enough – not worthy*
- My parents were not happy in their relationship – *I am responsible for their pain*
- *I must in some way have done something, so I must do something to make them all happy*
- Loss of her childhood years – had to grow up

- *I didn't have time to allow myself to feel things*
- *I think I lost my identity*

Case Analysis:

Causation: Lack of nurturing by the mother.

- *Mind*: *ailments from*: *neglected; being*: *mother; by one's*: lac-h.

Lac humanum have an inner conflict between living as a self-determined individual in a group, and feeling beholden to the group. She says, *I think I lost my identity. My precious time to discover the individual without stress; those child years I had to become responsible.*

Lac humanum are the savior, mother, and nurturer of the human race.

In the first consultation, I noticed that she wore lots of different crystals on her wrists. I asked her in the first consultation why she liked them. She had replied *they are my friends* and that she *eventually wanted to work with her friends*. In this follow-up consultation I asked her to explain further.

Question: Last time, I asked a bit about what you now want to do?

I was talking to an acupuncturist, who was talking about patients who come in and leech her room. I asked, do you have crystals to help with that? She said, tell me more! So I was off. It is a nightmare with set-up money.

What sort of work do you do?

It would probably be a bit of an amalgamation of crystals and energies, and initially finding out where they are at, spiritually. How crystals would help with that.

Tell me again what you were telling me last time – why you like crystals?

Vibrational energy.

But what do they do for you?

They talk to me and awaken my energy. They take you different places, as well. They can be programmed to be sources of energy to be pulled in, to take out, to heal. They are like my friends. I feel an instant harmony and happiness.

How do they protect you?

Because in essence they are pure. Unconditional love quality. They are not negative in source and in origin. They are my friends, they are familiar to me. They make me feel like I have met lost friends, like home. Where we come from, from a spiritual place, and where we go to after this life. They talk to me.

This is a repeat of the energy of the case. She had no mothering. This is the *disturbance* in the case. The crystals give her unconditional love: they are her origins, they are her mother, they talk to her, they are her home.

Conclusion

She consulted with me for two years, every eight to twelve weeks, depending on financial considerations. The prescription was *Lac humanum* 30 C. 1/day, dry pilule, continuous. The *Lac humanum* 200 C. 1/weekly was also continuous[18]. Her mental and emotional health is now excellent. Physically, the fibromyalgia is no longer an issue. Physically, she is left with continual sinus infections only if she gets a cold or flu, which are now infrequent. She has blocked sinus passages from

---

18 The *Lac humanum* 30 c. daily prescription is working in this case as a 'Drainage remedy'. In 1950 Dr Leon Vannier, a French homoeopath, wrote *La Pratique de L'Homoeopathie.* If a Constitutional remedy is given in high-potency to a patient who has not been given preparatory homoeopathic treatment, a sudden aggravation of his or her condition may occur. Vannier regards this as an 'eliminatory crisis': a sudden elimination of toxic substances which overwhelm the organism. According to Dr Vannier an acute aggravation can always be prevented by using what he calls *Drainage treatment.* In this case I have had the patient on a Drainage potency of the simillimum as well as a *Delusion* potency of the simillimum. De Ruyter, E.A.A.A.D. *Computer Homoeopathy and a Summary of Dr. Leon Vannier's Theories on the Paratuberculous and Paracancerous States.* self-published, Australia, 1994, pp.46-48.

a history of repeated sinus infections and past surgery. She is currently waiting to have surgery on her sinus passages. She has also been advised that if she could move away from Melbourne (which has a high pollen count) that her sinus infections would lessen considerably. She and her husband are looking to relocate to Queensland, which is much warmer. She is no longer her mother's counsellor. She has broken all ties with her sister, much to her mother's distress. Her mother is also a patient. Her mother comes to have consultations with me regularly, every six weeks, since 2005. I would like her to return so that I could try to unblock her sinuses. However, the surgeon says that they need to be scraped out because they are completely blocked. Money is also a consideration. She is much happier *not having anything to do with her sister. She continually drained me. I was never going to be happy or well as long as she held me back. She is a constant drain on my health. We are, as our wee family, much happier not having her destroying our marriage. I decided I have helped her all that I can.* Her sister continues to have consultations, but her life circumstances has been exhausting for the whole family. I cannot expand further of those circumstances, as I do not have permission to do so. However, it is important to note that the fact that this woman separated from her family of origin, in order to flourish in her own immediate *wee family,* is an indication of *Lac humanum* health. She also decided that she only wants to have one child.

She wants to concentrate not only on loving her family, but on finding out who she is as an individual.

Bibliography

Vermeulen, Frans. *Synoptic Materia Medica 2.* The Netherlands, Merlijin Publishers, 1992. pp. 538-540.

Medorrhinum

Abstract:

This is a case of a woman who feels like she wants to flee from her own life. *Medorrhinum* abandon themselves and avoid all responsibility even for living and preserving their life.

Keywords:

Suicide. Implosion and explosion. Depression. Mood swings. Passive-aggressive ineffectualness. 'Night Owl'. 'Delusions of impending doom'.

Case Notes:

First Consult: April 2004

D.O.B. 1961.

Occupation: Conceptual sculpture artist and musician. Conceptual around the themes of space, form, objects within space, and existence. Her work focuses on *the themes of body as reflection of identity, as a woman bleeding and in tune with the functions of birth and procreation. For example: I collect old, used tampons and use these in my sculptures. I construct work around the theme of the moon and the emotional and physical phases of energy. The theme of my body, being a black woman as reflection of identity is also a resoundingly emotional and political statement in my work.* She describes herself as a *struggling artist with no money. I struggle with conventionality and routine.*

- **Job**: Artist's model
- **Hobby**: Yoga
- **Single mother**: She has one son. She struggles with responsibility and would often like to run away. *I have a desire to flee.* She has very little support from the father
- **Mother**: African
- **Father**: 'White' Australian
- **Migrated to Australia**: She was eight years of age when she came to Australia. She was brought up in an 'all white' suburban area of an Australian capital city. Her mother denied her African heritage and her father denied her blackness
- **Brother**: Famous television personality (She emphasizes both her brother's successes to highlight her families perception of *her* failure to achieve economic status.)
- **Brother**: Public servant, also financially successful.

First Impression: She has very *passionate* alternating feelings; *from black depression about her existence to elation about life.* She has *passionate anger* and very strong political ideas. She describes herself as a *radical feminist.* She has been treated by another homoeopath with *Anacardium* for suicidal depression. Although I am able to perceive duality, the simillimum is not *Anacardium. Anacardium* are able to self-actualize, and this woman is struggling with existence.

Presenting Physical Complaints:

- Hormonal extremes, premenstrual tension
- Struggles with her smoking habit
- Struggles with eating too much sugar
- Candida

- Mood swings
- Depression
- Strong suicidal feelings
- 'Night Owl': struggles with inability to sleep at night before 3 am
- Finds it hard to get her son to school each day
- Skin acne: < premenstrual

I write letters that will hurt and then I burn them. My dad wrote such letters and sent them. I have learnt not to send such things. Here I feel I have a sense of boundary. I have terrible reactions when on the few occasions I have hit my son. I live in fear of repeating the trauma I experienced as a child and as a young adult. I experienced physical violence from my dad. I experienced desperate sarcasm as a child and physical violence from my mother as a young adult.

There is great anxiety about not being able to sustain the façade of functioning and coping. Albeit only just most of the time and sometimes not at all, great anxiety about collapsing. Overwhelming sense of loneliness because I am so extreme this alienates me from many, though I don't feel that extreme. I alternate between trying to be a good girl so as to be accepted as a normal citizen and then I get really angry, deeply resentful about towing the line, conventions etc. Mostly this anger is ultimately towards myself for allowing myself to be manipulated. I want to be braver, to have more courage to accept myself to be myself in all her complexity. Anger about doubting my intuition, being called upon to justify my intuition, to explain it. I do not shy away from my inner self. I fantasize about life as a hermit. I enjoy solitude. I suffer if I don't get enough time alone. I really want to reach a place where I can accept my complexities. Perhaps I will accept that I am not who I wish to be; a calm, contented, trusting person.

Definitely attacking, critical when overwhelmed or pressured, then when the pressure is sustained over time I implode; loss of meaning, suicidal. I have a profound sense of being broken, of having been so for such a long, long time. My grief and rage express a loss of a self I remember somehow, somewhere. She says of her inability to cope: *I doubt my inability to accept and to function in society's construct of reality and my inability to conform to this construct is what disturbs me. Control, convention, escape.* She says of her concern around the issue of suicide: *How do I reconcile meaningless, purposelessness, so as to avoid suicide?* This woman is struggling with abandonment from society, her family, and from herself.

She struggles with her *right* to continue to exist. This patient is imploding and exploding with a crisis of self-examination.

Case Analysis: I used the following key points and headings in analyzing this case.

1. **Rubric-repertorisation**
2. **Theme**
3. *Striking*, or *Peculiar* **Signs and Symptoms; Organon 153**
4. **Materia Medica**
5. **Follow-up Consultations**
6. *How, Why*, and *When* **Causations – the 'Never-well-since-event'**.

1. Rubric-repertorisation:

- *Mind: ideas: abundant: uncertain in execution; but*: med. [1] 1.
- *Mind: cursing: restrain himself in order not to curse; has to*: med.
- *Mind: expressing oneself: desire to express oneself: Med.*
- *Mind: activity: desires activity: creative activity: Med.*

- *Mind: ailments from: discords; parents; between one's:* med.
- *Mind: despair: criticism; from the smallest: Med.*
- *Mind: fear: insanity:* med.
- *Mind: postponing everything to next day: Med.*
- *Mind: responsibility: aversion to: Med.*
- *Mind: suicidal disposition: sadness, from:* med.
- *Mind: temper tantrums:* med.
- *Mind: weak character:* med.
- *Mind: wild feeling in head: Med.*
- *Delusion* rubric: *crime: committed a crime; he had:* med.
- *Delusion* rubric: *torture: rid her mind of the torture; she must do something to:* med. [1] 1.
- *Delusion* rubric: *insane: become insane; one will:* med.
- *Delusion* rubric: *business: accomplished; business could never be:* med. [1] 1.
- *Delusion* rubric: *die: time has come to:* med.

2. Theme

When consulting I make a list of themes to help me find the essence of the conflict and inner disturbance in the case.

- *I write letters that will hurt and then I burn them.*
- *I enjoy solitude.*
- *I suffer if I don't get enough time alone.*
- *Definitely attacking, critical when overwhelmed or pressured.*
- *Overwhelming sense of loneliness because I am so extreme this alienates me.*
- *I implode; loss of meaning, suicidal.*
- *I alternate between trying to be a good girl, and then I get really angry and resentful about towing the line.*

- *Mostly, this anger is ultimately towards myself.*
- *I want to be braver, to have more courage to accept myself.*
- *Anger about doubting my intuition. I am being called upon to justify my intuition.*
- *I have great anxiety about collapsing.*
- *How do I reconcile meaningless, purposelessness, so as to avoid suicide?*

For the majority of the cases, the relevance of each of the *Delusion* rubrics will throw light on the underlying guilt and the overwhelming effect that the concept of original sin and the expulsion of Adam and Eve has had in our psyche. Every patient who has issues around abandonment will always present with the assumption of original sin. This case is based on the concept of the 'delusions of original sin'.

This suicidal case reverberates with a crisis of self-examination which reflects the *Delusion* rubric: *he has committed the unpardonable sin*. Guilt about the right to exist is a core underlying theme within *Medorrhinum*.

Medorrhinum struggle intensely with inner questioning and doubt about their motives because they appear, even to themselves, to be extremely unstable. The contrasting themes within their nature mean that they are extremely reactive and go into flight from themselves, as well as over-react and go into flight from all other constraints or social expectations. *Medorrhinum* have the *Mind* rubric: *aversion to responsibility,* and the *Mind* rubric: *restlessness, must constantly move, goes from one room to the next*. Their reactivity is evident in the *Mind* rubric: *has to restrain himself in order not to curse*. *Medorrhinum* condemn themselves and throw themselves into the fires of hell, especially with *despair from the smallest criticism*. *Medorrhinum* have numerous *Delusion* rubrics pertaining to paranoia: *hearing voices behind him, someone whispering behind him,* and *sees faces looking from behind bed and furniture*. This *Medorrhinum* (case) highlights the seriousness with which they take their *unpardonable crimes.* *Medorrhinum* will be tormented by their sins, which is why *Medorrhinum* are the only remedy listed in the *Delusion* rubric: *she must do something to rid her mind of the torture.* When sick, *Medorrhinum* are totally sure that they deserve to die. *Medorrhinum* have the *Delusion* rubric: *time has come to die.* When *Medorrhinum* have even the smallest of health problems, like acne or a boil, they will seriously evaluate whether they should continue to live and whether they are worthy of your attention and care. Self-deluding is evident in the way *Medorrhinum* abandon themselves and avoid all responsibility even for living and preserving their life – *Delusion* rubric: *life was unreal. Medorrhinum* will choose to condemn themselves to die rather than take responsibility for getting themselves out of the hell and torment they are in. Their passive-aggressive ineffectualness becomes a procrastination and crippling undermining of their own self-confidence. This is self-deluding behavior which they continue because it helps them avoid responsibility. It is important to identify the psychological steps a patient will move through as they struggle to acknowledge, or resign themselves to their illness. *Medorrhinum* religiously and righteously condemn themselves for their perceived sins; this is why they have the *Delusion* rubric: *going to hell because he had committed an unpardonable crime. Medorrhinum* have strong, self-defeating, psychological 'delusions of persecution' which need to be acknowledged when you are treating them, as they desire death so they can avoid the responsibilities involved in living. A neurosis indicates an inability to have a rational or realistic objective view of one's life. *Medorrhinum* have no personal 'delusions of grandeur'; all their power is transferred outwards on to their 'spiritual guides' who stand beside them *caressing their head. Medorrhinum* struggle to separate their psyche from the influences of others. This instability perpetuates their numerous 'persecution complexes'. 'Transference neuroses' are a conflict between the 'ego' and the 'id'. The realistic 'ego' in *Medorrhinum* is undermined. The unconscious and unfettered 'id' in *Medorrhinum* is suppressed by their disproportionate 'delusions of impending doom'. *Medorrhinum* have the *Delusion* rubrics: *being doomed*, and *something dreadful has happened.* [1] 1. The 'id' is unconscious and is not restricted by social conventionality. The 'id' is unrestrained, selfish self-gratification. *Medorrhinum,* for all their supposed social unconventionality, restrain their own 'id', *cut their own legs off,* and surrender personal power into persecutory paranoia because of their exaggerated 'delusions of original sin'. The 'never-well-since-event' or causation in a *Medorrhinum* case will always come from an over-exaggerated reaction to an *unpardonable crime.*

1. Denial: *Delusion* rubric: *religious*: med. *Delusion* rubric: *caressed on head by someone*: *Med.* [2] 1. *Delusion* rubric: *hand*: *smoothing her; felt a hand*: med. [1] 1. *Delusion* rubric: *women*: *bedside; by*: med. [1] 1. *Delusion* rubric: *hearing: illusions, of*: med. *Delusion* rubric: *people*: *seeing people*: med. [These last few rubrics can allude to hubristic illusions or to paranoid 'delusions of persecution'.]

2. Forsaken: *Delusion* rubric: *persecuted*: *he is persecuted*: med. *Delusion* rubric: *people*: *beside him; people are*: *Med. Delusion* rubric: *people; behind him; someone is*: *Med. Delusion* rubric: *faces, sees*: *looking from behind bed and furniture*: med. [1] 1. *Delusion* rubric: *faces, sees*: *wherever he turns his eyes, or looking out from corners*: med. *Delusion* rubric: *people*: *behind him; someone is*: *whispering*: med. [1] 1.

3. Causation: *Delusion* rubric: *hell*: *going to hell because he had committed a unpardonable crime*: med.[1] 1. *Delusion* rubric: *crime*: *committed a crime; he had*: med.

4. Depression: *Delusion* rubric: *doomed, being*: med. *Delusion* rubric: *anxious*: med. *Delusion* rubric: *insane*: *become insane; one will*: med. *Delusion* rubric: *trembling*:

he was trembling: *without trembling; but*: med. *Delusion* rubric: *torture*: *rid her mind of the torture; she must do something to*: med. [1] 1. *Delusion* rubric: *intoxicated: is; he*: med. [This rubric pertains to unconsciousness.] *Delusion* rubric: *happened; something has*: *dreadful has happened; something*: med. [1] 1. *Delusion* rubric: *unreal*: *life was unreal*: med. *Delusion* rubric: *business*: *accomplished; business could never be*: med. [1] 1.

5. Resignation: *Delusion* rubric: *die*: *time has come to*: med. *Delusion* rubric: *legs*: *cut off; legs are*: med.

Medorrhinum have the *Delusion* rubric: *seeing persons*. On the one hand, *Medorrhinum* fear they are *seeing people* who are judging them, and on the other hand they believe the people they see are proof that they are connected to a greater mystical force that is protecting them. *Medorrhinum* are so intent on avoiding societal expectations that they are always paranoid about someone judging them. *Medorrhinum* have numerous *Delusion* rubrics which highlight their inner instability over real or perceived rejection. *Medorrhinum* have the *Delusion* rubrics: *persecuted, watched, spied on, poisoned,* and *pursued*. *Medorrhinum* withdraw into an inner world in which they are able to align themselves with a mystical inner conviction that God is *a delicate hand that has smoothed* their psyche. *Medorrhinum* have the *Delusion* rubric: *she was smoothed by a delicate hand*. *Medorrhinum* do not have any hubristic delusions of personal grandeur. God, for *Medorrhinum,* is a mystical *woman standing beside their bed whispering guidance*. *Medorrhinum* have the *Delusion* rubric: *talking with dead persons*, and the *Delusion* rubric: *caressed on head by someone*. [2] 1. *Medorrhinum* have the *Delusion* rubric: *women by the bedside*. Transference is characterized by unconscious redirection of feelings on to another person. All the *Delusion* rubrics for *Medorrhinum* which pertain to communication with God transfer hubristic power on to spirits. *Medorrhinum* quite often create sculptural representations of their 'spirit guides'. *Medorrhinum* have the *Delusion* rubric: *delusions about imaginary objects*. This *Medorrhinum* (case) is a sculptor who concentrates her work around the imagery of women. *Medorrhinum* have the *Delusion* rubric: *women by the bedside*. The dead women who are *talking* and *whispering* and *smoothing the head* of *Medorrhinum* are their ancestral guides. With no hubristic 'delusions of grandeur' allocated to their own persona, *Medorrhinum* struggle with self-actualization. *Medorrhinum* transfer inner knowledge and personal power to the dead.

3. *Striking*, or *Peculiar* Signs and Symptoms; Organon 153

She says of her inability to cope: *I doubt my inability to accept and to function in society's construct of reality, and my inability to conform to this construct is what disturbs me. Control, convention, escape. Medorrhinum* are the only remedy listed in the *Mind* rubric: *abundant ideas but uncertain in execution.* [1] 1. *Peculiar* to *Medorrhinum* is their inner knowing that they cannot construct their psyche around societal conventionality[19]. This

19 "An overwhelming sense of inner emptiness often disturbs *Medorrhinum*, so much so that they think they are going insane. *Medorrhinum* are driven by a need to experience intensity. The drive to cover up inner weakness and conflict brings about anxiety that is unique to *Medorrhinum*. If you do not have a point of reference, there are always unlimited horizons you can travel to. *Medorrhinum* can appear to others to lack self-control. If someone else tries to enforce controls or their concepts of conventions in the form of taking responsibility, *Medorrhinum* are likely to want to escape. If, inside of themselves, *Medorrhinum* know they do not have a solid grip on reality, they will push in the opposite direction to make sure all possible weaknesses are covered up. At the time *Medorrhinum* are feeling most unsure and vulnerable, they will often act as if nothing scares or affects them. *Medorrhinum* are extreme in everything. It is possible to either catch them on the flight out of themselves when they present as the extrovert, or on the flight into themselves when they present as the introvert. The essence is the same; they have to always be exceeding all limits. If you do not have an orientation point or boundary that contains you, then you will always alternate between extremes. The character Smilla in the novel *Miss Smilla's Feeling for Snow*, by Peter Høeg, is a *Medorrhinum*. At one point in the book she is faced with the possibility of imprisonment. *Medorrhinum*

woman is a sculptor of destruction. She creates sculptures of discarded menstrual tampons and old bones. She dismembers her bodily functions, and societal functionality.

4. Materia Medica

Sankaran, in *The Soul of Remedies,* writes, "The feeling of incapacity in *Medorrhinum* is represented by anxiety of conscience as if he were guilty of a crime, by fear as if someone was behind him, and a constant inner anxiety and restlessness."

She describes herself as *definitely attacking, critical when overwhelmed or pressured, then when the pressure is sustained over time I implode; loss of meaning, suicidal. I have a profound sense of being broken, of having been so for such a long, long time. My grief and rage express a loss of a self I remember somehow, somewhere.*

The psychological process of bargaining, or of trying to be good is masking the underlying delusional belief in punishment for being bad. She outlines this dilemma when she says, *I alternate between trying to be a good girl so as to be accepted as a normal citizen and then I get really angry, deeply resentful about towing the line, conventions etc. Mostly this anger is ultimately towards myself for allowing myself to be manipulated. I want to be braver, to have more courage to accept myself, to be myself in all her complexity.* A *Delusion* rubric can only be used in the case if you can see a conflicting struggle which is *self-punishing* in your patient's psyche. If your patient believes in a system of just punishment for their sins, this is an indication of disproportionate retribution. If their reactions to their feelings of being bad are disproportionately an *over-reaction* and misrepresentation of reality, then it

cannot deal with being restrained or imprisoned, and her inner knowledge that this would send her over the precipice of sanity into insanity is the core of *Medorrhinum* struggle with their grip on sanity. Lalor, Liz. *A Homeopathic Guide to Partnership and Compatibility.* Berkeley, California, North Atlantic Books, 2004. p.p.193-195.

is important to consider the *Delusion* rubrics pertaining to *wrongs committed.* Self-persecution is commonly referred to as psychological 'delusions of original sin'. Self-destructive depression and predictions of failure underpin and also cover up the psychological delusions of self-blame and psychological 'delusions of original sin'. Self-destructive depression and predictions of failure advantageously protect the patient from having to acknowledge sins committed, or alliances made with the 'evil-side' of themselves. Self-destructive behavior and self-blame will be maintained and nurtured because they help protect the patient from their innermost dark secrets about themselves. The simillimum in a suicide case has to resonate on the level of the patient's internal psychodynamic crisis. *Medorrhinum* have abandoned themselves. She describes this loss when she says, *over time I implode; loss of meaning, suicidal. My grief and rage express a loss of a self, I remember somehow, somewhere.* The anxiety of conscience that Sankaran notes within *Medorrhinum* is the precursor of their internal restlessness. *Medorrhinum* choose to abandon themselves rather than face their internal demons.

5. Follow-up Consultations

The following is a transcript from a videoed session, 18/9/06. This session was recorded after the patient being on *Medorrhinum* 200 C. 1 dose a week for four months. The last four months had been particularly traumatic because of a relationship breakup with a boyfriend who she described as her *soul partner in life.* I had been treating her for two years, so it has been a long case. Up until the recent trauma, the dose started at 6 C. then 30 C. potency. It had been low to deal with the physical symptoms of premenstrual hormonal swings and the instability of her depression. Up until recently, I have given six doses of 200 C. over the three years of treatment to deal with particular suicidal setbacks. The significance of this session is that for the first time she has been able to know and acknowledge her shame and fear about existence. I contribute this breakthrough to the consistent high dose of the remedy, but also to a visit from her father where for the first time he acknowledged she was telling the truth. The effect of this will absolve a *Medorrhinum* (case) of original sin.

Patient: (She starts the conversation after explaining that she had started to cry when her father was visiting.)

There was my dad and there was this thing that once again I am too emotional for this family. I am really obviously f***ed up here as nobody wants to know or it's that thing of we know something is wrong but we are not going to go there. I guess there was a little girl in me that wanted my mummy and daddy to say: is everything okay? So my dad is explaining all these things and I just have these huge tears coming down my face and he just ignores it for quite a while. (Laughs.) *Hilarious. This is how he deals with it. And then he said do you want to talk about it?*

I said there is not much to talk about. I am in really deep grief. David, my beloved, and I have split up and I am completely devastated. It is because he has an addiction. (Heroin.) *And then he started talking about my mum. He and mum are waiting for me to kind of understand that I need goals. He asked me about work like to you ever have any goals, do you ever think you should get some material things. I walked into the kitchen and yelled back how dare you ask me whether I ever think about getting anything. Of course I do, I've just finished this degree.* (Fine Arts, Sculpture) *And then we went on. He talked about how he has all these successful children except me. You know you just have to accept. But I have been affected, my confidence has been affected, and I am definitely working on it and getting a whole lot better. But you need to understand that when I was very young, about sixteen and about to leave school, about to go into the world with this passion and joy after everyone has been saying you can do whatever you want; well what I wanted to be was something you couldn't handle. Your own fears and stuff. So I finally said about the dumb nigger thing right;* (her father had said all she was going to be good for was playing the dumb nigger) *and he was totally shocked and said I would never have said anything like that. I said you f***ing did say that and I said to him, here it was this time of the day, and we were here, this street. I saw all this truth flash across his face. And all power to my father, as he has got older and mellowed and acknowledged things, he sort of did this internal stuff and acknowledged well I have done some really crazy things. Written crazy letters to people and said some incredible things so there is all likelihood I have said this to my daughter.*

What effect do you think it has had to tell him?

It's eroded it; it's held it back. I feel like that is what this new feeling is like you know what I don't give a f**k about what other people think, what their problems are. This is what my passion is, this is what one of my gifts is. You know when I hear music and feel passion I am able to dance and feel alive so this is a gift to me. He wrote an email basically apologizing for having said that all those years ago and that he and mum were waiting for me to come down from the mountain (laughs). *He talked about how proud he is of his children. This is all very new for my father, to express his emotions like that. You can't stay frightened of being here.*

So the fear of being here comes from where?

I think that it is a response, a learnt thing I have acknowledged as a sensitive child, as most children are sensitive to the energetic world coming from people, so I think from a very early age there was this thing about being a show off, about being told not to be in terms of being an expressive person. Learning about being frightened of being. My experience of coming here as a child was being teased and isolated because of my color, which of course had never happened in Africa. So you have a choice to totally disappear, to not drawing attention to that, or go into denial, so of course that is what I did. So I remember going back to Africa and my mother's family and realizing that was what I had done. So it was this terrible grief and this terrible shame, and like a counter shame and denial that came from shame. So I go from this memory of this sixteen year old girl who is going like this, (expands her arms) *and then her family, my father's fear, taking that in.*

What do you think shame can make someone feel?

Shame can make people want to die. It can make you not want to be alive, you're not worthy of being here. So there is something intrinsically wrong.

You are talking about your actual appearance?

Yes there is anger around that realization, grief around that realization. Also recently there has been a joy because of letting it go, and an understanding that it's not me. (Laughs.) *And that is also sad, and that also brought up a lot of compassion, and I am glad my dad has cried about this because he has been carrying this even if he hasn't been consciously aware that he has.*

So your dad coming was quite powerful in this conflict between white and black, and the fact that he acknowledged it because he hasn't acknowledged it before?

Yes that is the whole story.

Do you remember the poem you gave to me a long time ago? The first three lines *She doesn't belong anywhere... but everywhere ...and nowhere* expresses the integral dilemma of existential alienation within *Medorrhinum.*

Yes this is me. I can still recognize this. [Cries] *The murderous rage I have spoken to you about this before, all of those things they are still in me. She is hate, she is fear*

And the basis of those feelings is the issue of shame?

Yes. For me shame is where the fear about being has come from. It's so fearful and shame is fear and I am fearful of it; it's so nebulous. It's boundless, like a big cloak it is hard to find the beginning and the end of where it is sourced. You know that feeling of late, of having that feeling come over me, of allowing myself to be here.

6. *How*, *Why*, and *When* Causations – the 'Never-well-since-event'

In the transcript the patient refers to a conscious thought and inner psychodynamic crisis.

The 'never-well-since' crisis of conflict about the right to exist is the precursor of *Medorrhinum*.

Learning about being frightened of being. My experience of coming here as a child was being teased and isolated because of my color, which of course had never happened in Africa. So you have a choice to totally disappear, to not drawing attention to that, or go into denial, so of course that is what I did. So I remember going back to Africa and my mother's family and realizing that was what I had done. So it was this terrible grief and this terrible shame, and like a counter shame and denial that came from shame. So I go from this memory of this sixteen year old girl who is going like this (expands her arms), *and then my father's fear, taking that in.*

This is a *Medorrhinum* (case) in conflict with her right to exist as a result of absorbing her parents' conflicts about race and color. She is, in her mother's eyes a 'half-caste', and in her father's eyes, 'a black nigger'. She has absorbed shame from her mother's denial of her own black African heritage. She has absorbed her father's desire for her to hide her blackness in 'white Australia'. The result is *Medorrhinum*. She says of herself: *definitely attacking, critical when overwhelmed or pressured. Then when the pressure is sustained over time I implode; loss of meaning, suicidal. I have a profound sense of being broken, of having been so for such a long, long time, my grief and rage express a loss of a self.*

Case Analysis

In the first consult the patient said: *How do I reconcile meaningless, purposelessness, so as to avoid suicide?* The disturbance that is peculiar to *Medorrhinum* is the delusion that *someone is behind him.* This means that not only is the concept of original sin tormenting *Medorrhinum;* they also think they should be questioning their own right to exist. Someone looking over their shoulder will point out the dichotomy of their existence. Cure for *Medorrhinum* is when they know and feel inside of themselves that they have the right to exist. This patient now knows this when she is able to say: *you know that feeling of late, of having that feeling come over me of allowing myself to be here.*

Bibliography

Sankaran, Rajan. *The Soul of Remedies.* Santa Cruz, Bombay, Homoeopathic Medical Publishers, 1997. p. 133.

Schroyens, Frederik. M.D. *Synthesis.* London, Homeopathic Book Publishers, 1997.

Muriaticum acidum

Abstract:

This is a case of a woman who feels like she is unable to make the decision to live or die.

Keywords:

Eczema. Destruction. Dissociation. Suicide. 'Frozen Inertia'.

D.O.B. 1957.

First Consultation: 2003.

Occupation: Psychotherapist.

Presenting Issue:

- Eczema (dermatitis) covering her entire body
- < back and torso++
- < legs +++
- Covering her arms, face and hands
- Cracked and dry, as well as wet and weeping skin
- Weeping, clear fluid and yellowish sticky fluid
- Itching, day and night
- Thick hardened patches of skin on her torso
- Dry patches as well as blisters on her back and stomach
- Small patches of raised red rash-like bumps

- Considerable loss of skin and scaly. When she took her clothes off to show me her skin, large pieces of skin fell on to the floor
- Strong moldy smell
- Dry and greasy patches
- Hot parts of skin and cold parts of skin
- < Hot and cold water, and weather
- Red and inflamed skin, plus pale areas
- Her legs were swollen with the start of cellulitis
- Fluid filled blisters on her legs
- Inflamed sections of skin on her legs which looked like they were starting to become infected

Every homoeopath reading the above list of symptoms will immediately realize that this patient had every possible symptom of eczema. There was not one single individual characteristic of her skin presentation on which I could repertorise. She had dry and wet, weepy and cracked, with aggravations from hot and cold, and raised, fluid filled blisters as well as small raised rashes. This case filled me with terror. All homoeopaths will privately admit to fearing treating eczema cases because they are so hard to treat; not only is it difficult to find the right remedy, it is very hard to stop aggravations. Her skin was already so angry and worrisome that I was very scared of aggravation, especially considering her legs already looked like they were starting to develop cellulitis. This case is a very good example of cure from the constitutional simillimum. My prescription was based entirely on her inner disturbance. In these cases I emphasize repeatedly the need to understand the causation or the 'never-well-since-event'. In homoeopathy we do not prescribe on a disease state or the miasmic presentation of the disease state, we prescribe on how the patient has interpreted those events or that disease state in a *peculiar* and individualistic way. This eczema case reconfirmed for me how unique homoeopathy is in this approach. Disturbance within a patient can cause conflict and pain which can eventuate in a physical illness or mental and emotional illness which is reflective of the intensity of the conflict. The reason it is important to know the disturbance in a case is because a severe disease state can often be a reflection of our deep subconscious struggles. This disturbance can form the foundation of our inner angst and the basis of future pathology.

I asked her, what event had happened in her life which contributed to her skin?

- *I have been depressed all of my life but I think that what has caused me the most amount of grief is that my sister committed suicide. At the time when it happened I didn't feel or think anything about it. I was at work when I found out. Everyone else around me was upset and I just sort of thought oh well, and then I went into a meeting. I sort of have been like that ever since. I am not really here. There is a part of me that gets things done but it is quite separate from me.*

- She goes on to say there is a spiritual side that knows and then a *fearful aspect of me is the one that feels stuck, immobilized and doesn't know how to, it goes into freezing, and inertia. I disappear.*

- *I suppose I have always called it disassociating.*

- *It is not me that is making the decision to do with anything in my life.*

- *I get really depressed when I get a cold.*

- *I still struggle with feeling scared. Fear of survival, how am I going to survive. I go into the fear then I just want to disappear. There is an underlying, deep, ancient feeling that I can't look after myself; that I can't survive.*

- *I feel like a failure that is what it feels like.*

- *I struggle with life.*

- *I don't want to be here.*

- *Even if you are right take the blame.*
- *I give myself a hard time.*
- *I still feel I am in pain and suffering a lot.*
- *There is a sadness I carry around with me all the time. It is not mine. It doesn't belong to me. It is my mother's, I know it. I really got in touch with my mother and my sister; you know the one who died. I carry their spirit with me. We all do the same thing – we push people away – and my sister who committed suicide, I mean that is the ultimate, pushing away or pulling back. We don't push people away, we disappear, it has the same effect.*
- *I still feel like I am in pain and suffering a lot. I can feel it a bit that I am not in as much pain as I was but I would have thought by now I wouldn't be in so much pain.*

Case Analysis: I used the following key points and headings in analyzing this case.

1. *Striking*, or *Peculiar* **Signs and Symptoms; Organon 153**
2. **Rubric-repertorisation**
3. **Theme**
4. **Materia Medica**
5. *How*, *Why*, **and** *When* **Causations – the 'Never-well-since-event'**
6. **Follow-up Consultations**.

1. *Striking*, or *Peculiar* Signs and Symptoms; Organon 153

First Impressions: This woman is not here. She is empty, there is not a person in her psyche. She has dissociated. She is fearful of existing and feels inadequate in being able to make decisions for herself. Most importantly, she is struggling to make the decision to live or to die.

She is stuck in a *frozen inertia;* she has *disappeared.* The simillimum has to cover the following *striking and peculiar* statement.

- *It is not me that is making the decision to do with anything in my life.*

My first impression was that the remedy had to be a Universal Kingdom[20] remedy because those remedies have

---

20 Themes of Universal Kingdom Remedies: Jenni Tree © 2006. Notes from her Melbourne conference.

- Magnesium
- Sol Luna
- Polaris Venus
- Fire
- Hydrogen
- Ozone
- Mobile Phone
- Wind – South west wind
- DNA
- Polystyrene
- Vacuum
- Positronium
- Time
- Connection and disconnection from self, concerned only with the outer appearance.
- Separation from self through hereditary – Miasm, allopathic drugs.
- No Integration with self or humanity – unable to connect with the outer world.
- Deep depressions.
- Connection to their journey / process / purpose.
- Drifting without purpose.
- Survival need to move, grow, continue and surge with life.
- Being in control of their direction in life.
- Dissolution.
- Darkness.
- Death of soul and self.
- Timelessness.

the same themes of disconnection and disassociation. The
first *Delusion* rubric which I looked at was the *Delusion* rubric:
emptiness.

Delusions: *emptiness; of*: am-c. *Calad.* cann-i. **COCC**.
Gels. germ-met. *Ign.* irid-met. *Kali-c. Kola.* lac-loxod-a. *Mur-
ac.* oena. ol-eur. *Olnd.* ozone. petr-ra. *Plat.* plut-n. **PULS**. sars.
SEP. stann. stry. *Sulph.* tritic-vg. *Vanil. Zing.*

The Universal Kingdom remedy listed in the above
rubric is *Ozonum*. However, *Ozonum* fluctuate between the
contradictory states of powerful grandeur[21] and failure. This
patient has no 'delusions of grandeur'. Equally, it is not a drug
remedy like *Cannabis indica. Cannabis indica* delight in their
belief in their omnipotence[22]. She is severely depressed and
unexpressive of all emotions. But her skin is angry. There is
clearly an underlying destructive pathology which is literally

---

- Infinity.
- Perfection.
- Tranquility.
- Effortless / calm / centered / integrated.
- Impersonal.
- Objective about life.
- Power and influence on consciousness.

21 *Ozonum* refuse to take responsibility for their internal abandonment [*emptiness*].
Ozonum can't afford to acknowledge their vulnerability because it would
require them to give up their 'delusions of grandeur' that they are *powerful*.
Generally speaking, the human race cannot acknowledge that we need to give
up our excesses of living to protect our vulnerable ozone layer. The simillimum
will only be *Ozonum* if the patient shows signs of psychotic behavior [*heart is
absent*]. *Ozonum* are indifferent to their own *abyss* and indifferent to others.
Ozonum are *connected to the devil and are arrogant towards those who strive
for purity, light and love.* [1] 1.

22 *Cannabis indica* delight in their belief in their omnipotence. They believe they
are a heavenly queen in a beautiful cathedral listening to choirs of angels.
Cannabis indica will have contradictory responses if they have to face illness.
On the one hand they can believe they are so great that they cannot possibly
die – *Delusion* rubric: *body covers the whole earth.* On the other hand they can
sink into over-exaggerated fears of being *annihilated* and *diminished* by their
disease.

breaking and tearing her skin to express itself. However, she is so dissociated from herself that she does not feel as if she is even in control of her own thoughts or decisions. The only part of her which is expressive is her skin. 'Dissociation'[23] is a normal response to trauma. If the patient dissociates, they can distance themselves from the feelings which are overwhelming them.

This patient has no relationship between herself and the world. She says that she has a *fear of survival.*

I go into the fear then I just want to disappear. There is an underlying, deep, ancient feeling that I can't look after myself; that I can't survive. I feel like a failure, that is what it feels like. I struggle with life. I don't want to be here.

2. Rubric-repertorisation

- *Delusions*: emptiness; of: am-c. *Calad.* cann-i. **COCC.** *Gels.* germ-met. *Ign.* irid-met. *Kali-c. Kola.* lac-loxod-a. *Mur-ac.* oena. ol-eur. *Olnd.* ozone. petr-ra. *Plat.* plut-n. **PULS.** sars. **SEP.** stann. stry. *Sulph.* tritic-vg. *Vanil. Zing.*

- *Delusions*: die: about to die; one was: **ACON.** agn. alum. am-c. ant-t. *Arg-n.* arn. ars. asaf. asar. bar-c. bar-m. bell. cact. calc. cann-i. caps. caust. cench. *Chel. Croc.* cupr. gels. glon. graph. hell. iris-t. kali-c. lac-d. *Lach.* lil-t. lyc. lyss. mag-p. magn-gr. med. meli. merc. mur-ac. *Nit-ac.* nux-v. petr. phos. *Plat. Podo.* positr. psor. puls. pyrus raph. rhus-t. ruta sil. stram. sulph. tab. thea *Thuj.* v-a-b. verat. *Xan.* zinc.

- *Delusions*: sleep: going to sleep; he were: asar. lappa merc-act. mur-ac. plat.

I used the above three *Delusion* rubrics for the rubric-

---

23 'Dissociative disorder' on the other hand is a far more complex disorder in which the patient creates multiple personalities which allow their psyche protection from what they perceive to be potentially traumatic situations, within and outside of themselves. This patient has no indicators of 'dissociative disorder'.

reportorisation. *Platina* repertorised the highest. Once again this patient is not *Platina*[24] because she has no 'delusions of grandeur'. *Muriaticum acidum* is a homoeopathic remedy derived from hydrochloric acid. It is highly corrosive. This woman is struggling on all levels, emotionally, mentally, and physically to be able to hold her psyche intact. Her spirit is corroded.

3. Theme

All the acids have themes of loss of money, or family; loss of pleasure in life; humiliation and shameful feelings of being a failure; dissociation and trying to forget. Acid remedies are cut off from themselves and the world; they struggle to be able to relate. Dr. Massimo Mangialavori notes that, "Muriaticums have a terrible problem of relating. In Muriaticums you will see a severe depressive attitude along with a strong sense of rage that can't come out. Their anger is silent, dwelling and constantly digging into their soul and can't be solved. Muriaticum + acid makes it worse. *Muriaticum acidum* do their best to *not* come out of this situation." Mangialavori lists loss, trying to forget, and significantly needing their *disease as a structure* as some of the main features of the acids.

Learning how to recognize these five psychological stages it will help you in the rubric-repertorisation and in finding the simillimum.

I did not write up *Muriaticum acidum* in the *Rubric-categories* of *Homoeopathic Psychiatry*. This case has far more relevance because it highlights the need to match the simillimum to the psychological stages that your patient is displaying. *Muriaticum acidum* have no psychological 'delusions of grandeur'; nor does this patient. *Muriaticum acidum* have no psychological 'delusions of original sin'; nor does this patient.

1.   Denial: NONE.

---

24 *Platina* are listed in more of the *Delusion* rubrics pertaining to 'delusions of grandeur' than any other remedy profile.

2. Forsaken: *Delusion* rubric: *images, phantoms; sees: ever changing: past to present:* mur-ac. [1] 1. *Delusion* rubric: *images, phantoms; sees: frightful:* mur-ac.

3. Causation: NONE.

4. Depression: *Delusion* rubric: *sleep: going to sleep; he was:* mur-ac. *Delusion* rubric: *emptiness; of: Mur-ac.*

5. Resignation: *Delusion* rubric: *die: about to die; one was:* mur-ac.

The patient says in the first consultation, *there is a sadness I carry around with me all the time. It is not mine. It doesn't belong to me. It is my mother's, I know it. I really got in touch with my mother and my sister; you know the one who died. I carry their spirit with me. Muriaticum acidum* have the following *Delusion* rubrics. *Muriaticum acidum* have 'delusions of persecution' that they carry with them the spiritual energy of their past and present relatives.

- *Delusion* rubric: *images, phantoms; sees: ever changing: past to present:* mur-ac. [1] 1.

- *Delusion* rubric: *images, phantoms; sees: frightful:* mur-ac.

Mangialavori writes that the "acids are an extremely fragile or weak structure, which recognizes they have a huge inability to do anything in life, and that they have really poor tools to go through life with." *Muriaticum acidum* go through life disconnected *as if asleep.* The patient describes this state of inertia as *one that feels stuck, immobilized and doesn't know how to, it goes into freezing, and inertia. I disappear. Muriaticum acidum* have the *Delusion* rubrics: *of emptiness,* and *he was going to sleep.* When I asked this patient what was the cause of her eczema, she related the present pathology to the trauma of her sister's suicide and to her inability to live her life. She herself is stuck in a *frozen inertia;* a kind of living suicide of her own. She says, *I disappear.*

Mind Rubrics of *Muriaticum acidum*

- *Mind*: *ailments from death of loved ones*: *parents or friends*; *of*: mur-ac.
- *Mind*: *business*: *incapacity for*: mur-ac.
- *Mind*: *confidence*: *want of self-confidence*: *self-depreciation*: mur-ac.
- *Mind*: *sadness*: *gloomy*: mur-ac.
- *Mind*: *morose*: mur-ac.
- *Mind*: *weary of life*: mur-ac.
- *Mind*: *absorbed*: mur-ac.
- *Mind*: *brooding*: mur-ac.
- *Mind*: *delirium*: *muttering*: *Mur-ac.*
- *Mind*: *discontented*: *himself, with*: mur-ac.
- *Mind*: *discouraged*: mur-ac.
- *Mind*: *fear*: *misfortune, of*: mur-ac.
- *Mind*: *grief*: *silent*: *Mur-ac.*
- *Mind*: *irresolution*: mur-ac.
- *Mind*: *prostration of mind*: *Mur-ac.*
- *Mind*: *succeeds, never*: mur-ac.
- *Mind*: *stupefaction*: mur-ac.
- *Mind*: *stupor*: *Mur-ac.*
- *Mind*: *talking*: *himself, to*: mur-ac.

4. Materia Medica

Sankaran states, "The main theme of an acid is struggle followed by collapse: exertion and exhaustion. The theme of struggle and collapse is clearly expressed in certain symptoms common to all the acids: hurry, industry, the feeling that their efforts are unsuccessful, fear of failure, and also fatigue, indolence and indifference."

Clarke describes the corrosive nature of *Hydrochloric acid*. Clarke writes, "The distinctive features of *Mur.ac* are: Muscular prostration from blood-poisoning going on to paralysis, finally of brain or heart. Burning is a great feature in its symptomatology, as its escharotic powers might suggest – ulcers (especially their margins), eruptions, piles, varices, stomach, and abdomen. It sours the excretions and makes them acrid. Offensive secretions, offensive breath and body-smell; and it is indicated in fevers of all kinds, exanthematous, typhoid, puerperal as well diphtheria, when these symptoms with the mental and paretic state are present. The mucous membranes are dry, bleeding, cracked, and ulcerated."

Mangialavori lists the themes of *Muriaticum acidum* as, "a strong sense of impotence. You will see a severe depression and anger along side of impotence."

5. *How*, *Why*, and *When* Causations – the 'Never-well-since-event'

This *Muriaticum acidum* patient was born into an established, wealthy family. She was brought up with the expectation that her father would provide for her, and that her husband would become her provider after she had married. There was never the expectation that she would ever have to work or know how to provide for herself. When she was in her early twenties, her father made numerous financial blunders and lost the family fortune. She has been angry with him ever since but because he died a broken man, her grief has remained silent and the anger over the loss of the family wealth has remained unexpressed. She was brought up with the expectation that she would always be able to move in the wealthy circles. She was married to wealthy men, but both marriages failed. She has not known how to financially manage her marriage settlements. Her relationship with her mother is *toxic*. *She put herself into a nursing home at the age of eighty and decided she didn't want to look after herself anymore. To me she still had a few years in which she could have looked after herself.* She describes her mother as a *narcissist who is only interested in herself.*

In all my patients with the element of *Muriaticum,* the theme of the mother will be transferred to the symbolic provider in their life. The *Mind* rubric: *silent grief* and the premonition of the death of the mother, or provider, in their lives are the 'never-well-since-event' which can immobilize *Muriaticum.* As homeopaths we are similar to psychotherapists in the sense that we are concerned with identifying the psychodynamic trauma or the 'never-well-since-event'.

It is not until *Muriaticum acidum* confront the theme of betrayal of trust and faith to do with the mother or provider in their lives that they then act to overcome the *acid* theme of struggle and collapse, and the feeling that their efforts are unsuccessful. The simillimum resonated with the destructive and corrosive internal rage which manifested in her skin.

Dose: *Muriaticum acidum* 30 C., one dose a day, dry pilule and continuous.

6. Follow-up Consultations

I treated this patient from 2003 until 2009. Her first consult was on the 2/12/2003. By the 1/7/2004, her skin was perfect. I have continued with this patient in a counselling role, which has focused entirely on educating her in self-assertion and self-actualization. She has monthly consultations. Over the years her skin has flared periodically, but it has always responded to *Muriaticum acidum* 30 C., three doses a day as needed. I have then returned to *Muriaticum acidum* 30 C., one dose a day, continuously for six years. Her skin breaks out in patches of eczema whenever she has to take antibiotics. There have been three occasions: after an abscess on her tooth, after an unexpected cellulitis infection on her leg, and after she had a kidney infection. All illnesses have proceeded failed relationships. Her skin also threatens to break out in response to traumas in her life. She has never had any severe outbreaks of eczema since her first consultation. With each illness (mentioned above) I have increased the dose to *Muriaticum acidum* 200 C. x 1 dose, and have kept her on the daily dose of 30 C. The following is a transcript of one of those traumas. The man she has been in a relationship has just told her he will not live with her and he will not support her financially.

This session was in August 2007.

Question: Would you please tell me again what you were saying about your process?

It feels as though, – I might have said this to you ages ago, I am sort of aware that I have said this to others – it is not me that is making the decision. There is a part of me that just gets things done. There is a part of me that knows how to do things but it seems to be quite separate from me at times. In terms of giving that part of me a name, I suppose in the later years I come to terms with the fact that there is that spiritual self, the one that knows how to do things. But there is that other aspect of me, the one that sort of gets stuck, that doesn't know how to make decisions. It is not that it doesn't know how to, it goes into this freezing, inertia, and disappear. I call it disassociating.

(This is nearly word for word what she said in her first consultation with me in 2003.)

How is it with Peter and the decisions you are making with that, where are you up to with that? (I ask her about her relationship because I know that this has to be the cause of her present setback.)

We have, (she corrects herself to *I have,* I suspect the decision has been his) *I have come to a place where I have to accept his process. It takes two people to have a relationship, so if I am in a relationship with Peter I am very aware of his process. To honor his process I have to relinquish the higher dream of my relationship with him which is to live together.*

I thought initially that I didn't think that I could do that, be in a relationship with him and not live with him, because it is in every aspect of me. It is in my dream, it is a paradigm, it is culturally. Everything I have ever dreamed of is that the way to be in a relationship for me is to be living together. So I have had to accept his process and really see for myself whether he was leading me down the garden path or – whether? I have really thought about my issues with co-dependency, or what part of me is hanging on to this relationship with him, and there is an aspect of that. However, what I really see is that the qualities that I was attracted to in him in the first place are still there, they are still in place, they are still there. It is a good relationship if you take away my need. Actually my desire, belief, my want of living with him. Put that aside, we actually have a good relationship. We share spiritual beliefs, art and culture together, they are two big issues for me. So rather than feeling deprived or feeling angry by what I can't have, which is wanting to live with him, I am turning it around in terms of being grateful about what I actually do have. Which is pretty healthy functioning; I am aware of that. But to then see how much of that is kidding myself. Like giving myself, oh well! There is so much good in this relationship. I think the hardest thing is giving up the dream. But that is my process. But I have been really honest with him, and that in itself has been an amazing process. I have really cried, especially with the worst of this cold, because I get very depressed when I get a cold.

(It is true that she now knows what she feels and is able to express that, but her ability to support her own needs is still vulnerable to disintegration and destruction. She has allowed his need to corrode her own dreams and cultural (Italian background) aspirations of living with someone. When she talks about feeling *deprived and angry*, that is what she feels. She is a psychotherapist who has a strong identification with 'New-Age' processes. Consequently, she sees that *she has turned it around* so that she can have *healthy functioning*. I perceive that she has suppressed her own needs and desires. Suppression is the core cause of all skin complaints.)

How it is with your work?

Good I have about fifteen clients now a week. My goal is to have twenty. I still struggle with feeling not confident, with feeling scared. That is something that is so old with me, my fear of survival. The thought of living on my own just brings it all back up again. Because, now I have to move out. Can I manage? Just the thought of it! I can feel that fear. So that is what happens. I just go into the fear and I just want to disappear.

So Peter definitely wants to be by himself?

Yes, for now. That is what I was talking about, me honoring his process and his need to be by himself after a thirty year marriage. And maybe it is about me learning to be by myself.

How do you feel about surviving and about being by yourself?

Well that is the thing that holds me back. There is an underlying, deep, ancient feeling that I can't look after myself. That I can't survive. I don't survive. I don't want to.

Last Saturday I had a day like I hadn't had for years. It is coming to terms with the fact that I have to move on and that I have to live on my own. I just withdrew. I had been to the art fair and I had dipped into a former world. I found it hard to come back. It is not so much regret as I feel like a failure. That I have got to this age and stage of my life and I don't feel like I can look after myself. [Mind rubric: succeeds, never.]

Feels very young. I can't survive. And every single person says, well you are earning money aren't you? And I go, yes. But I don't think I am making enough. There is absolutely no security in it all. (She is referring to her job as a psychotherapist). Mind you I have lived so long without any security anyway. (Laughs).

The whole thing about living with the man is that feeling of living with security. It just feels easier for me I don't want to have to live my life so hard. The tears are really close. It just feels like my life is so f**king hard. Hard work being me. I am exhausted by it well you know my immune system is exhausted. I struggle with life. I am still struggling. Now when I am in that state it is interesting because I can now compare me being in that state from before.

(This is an important process because here she can now allow herself to stay present enough to feel. She is no longer disappearing.)

So I was in it with the understanding, and that in some ways is even more bloody painful. I was aware of being in this state and thinking it is not fair to the others and then I thought bugger it. That is when I disappear and push everyone away from me. And nobody is my friend and I don't relate to anybody and I just isolate. Total victim position. It is a bit of a game but I still can't come back from it.

So, in that victim state do you want to live?

No! That is what I am saying to you. I have not experienced that for a while. I did when Peter and I broke up. No, I was like that in December.

How much has your skin been flaring up?

A lot. It flares up. There is that underlying feeling which just doesn't go away, so it is deeply connected to that fear. It comes back with cold. My system can't fight it off, my system can't fight it off and it comes back on my lips and on my hands. It isn't on the rest of me and it isn't on my legs.

Follow-up Consultations

The session transcribed below was in October 2007. This was a difficult session in which her anger surfaced. She was very angry towards me because she felt I couldn't possibly understand how hard it is for her not to be able to find somewhere to live. Her relationship had broken up, she needed to rent a flat, and she found herself in the situation of not having enough money to rent a flat which would match the image of who she was. She was extremely angry about it being so hard for her to know how to live independently. Every time she got close to becoming aware of how she felt the *pain of feeling* overwhelmed her. She would continually say, *the pain of feeling is disintegrating me, it is destroying me.* There were several times during the period of her treatment when she became overwhelmed at how hard it was for her to not dissociate from herself. At those times I increased the frequency of the *Muriaticum acidum* 30 C. to three doses a day. I have learnt from experience that high frequency, low potency has been the best way to effectively manage severe skin conditions which are associated with mental and emotional psychological dissociation.

This case emphasizes that with acid remedies the healing process can be *very* long. As a student of homoeopathy, I was taught that you give the right remedy and three months later the patient is cured. This case has been ongoing for six years.

Question: So what is happening?

Well I feel like I am caught between a rock and a hard place. It feels like stasis. It feels really stuck. I am still looking for somewhere to live. I had no idea it was going to be this difficult. Apart from the fact that it is not a process I enjoy, I have managed to overcome that by talking to myself and say, well other people feel the same, but it brings up a lot of stuff around why am I doing this again in my life? How I don't have a base. I am ungrounded. I don't feel secure in anything in my life and that is a really painful place to be. It is very competitive, and you have a whole lot of people going for the same property and I have never been good at competition. I expect things to be easy. I don't expect to fight. It is mustering up that sort competitive nature. I don't want to fight. (Cries.) There is so much in my criteria about needing so much to be able to feel safe. The decision is so painful. I feel like disappearing. That is my fallback position. That is where I go. Now I know I can't do that, so the struggle is constant, it is 24/7. I feel trapped. I feel stuck, same thing. I can't make it happen. This is not about my decision making process. I have no choice. I am forced to make a decision based on my earning capacity. So now when I talk about it, I realize it is not about me not being able to make a decision. I can't afford to get a two bedroom flat. I feel like I want to move forward energetically, but because of the financial restrictions I can't. Then I pull back and disappear. Then I can't stay there because that feels so painful. It feels like a tortoise. It is like sticking my head out and not being able to do anything and then feeling this horrible pain of being stuck. And then disappearing again into the shell into the depths of something to protect myself. But that is no longer a good place to be, but because I am so much more aware that that is not a good place to be, that is where the real pain is now. I can't feel good here and I can't feel good out there. Then of course, the old thoughts of really not being here start to surface again. (Suicide.) Then when I start thinking of that as a way out, that is no longer a way out either. Then I start to think I am depressed. There is no respite. When I wake up and when I go to sleep it is with me. The only time it is not is when I am with clients. Which is a miracle. Which makes me think I am not totally depressed. I do get out of bed. I do get ready. But it is a struggle. Then I try to reframe this and think, well I just need to enjoy this process. Then it overwhelms me, and then I am aware of how hard it is, and it is a struggle.

How does it feel to not have someone to take care of you?

I don't know how to answer that. I can answer from the young part of me. It feels lonely. But I don't need someone to take care of me. I can look after myself. But then I do. I oscillate. I am such a paradox in that way. Will I be a victim or won't I be a victim? Am I a victim or am I not a victim? I have told you before people see me as being very competent, which I am.

But I am not very competent at certain things, like money. That is why I haven't got any. That is not the reason why I haven't got money. See I can sit here and have this duel. I have not wanted to have money because I haven't wanted to take care of myself. When I had the opportunity to have money, I either lost it or gave it away, refused in some way to take ownership.

What is money symbolic of?

Dad – love. I worked that one out ages ago. That was the only way he showed us he loved us. He was so remote in his love. He controlled us all through money and provided for us. He was a good father because he looked after us, and we got the very strong message that you can't do it yourself, we needed him for that. We didn't get to learn anything about it because that was his domain. Well, some children rebel against that and they do brilliantly. My father didn't understand about money, that is how come he lost it. Which was a joke because we had it. He wouldn't listen to anyone's advice. That aspect of my father must be in me too because he must have had a fear of some sort. He has been dead for ten years. There was something he couldn't hear. He had friends telling him what to do with his money and the opportunities for my father to invest were amazing. I don't know if I need to let go of that.

Case Analysis

In this session above she is clearly distressed and crying, but she is present in her feelings. She has not disappeared.

It is important to know and understand a patients psychodynamic patterning so that you can know when to respond homoeopathically. It is a mistake to assume that if a patient confronts their own avoidance or self-deluding that this will not be a painful process.

Her old suppressive technique of 'New-Age' reframing is no longer working. She is no longer able to suppress her own feelings. This is the start of health. Skin problems have their origins in suppression. Suppression is avoidance.

In case-taking, the homoeopath needs to understand the excuses and avoidances which maintain the patient's psychological avoidance of reality. Psychological denial is adopted by the patient when they need to maintain their psychological delusion to avoid reality. *Muriaticum acidum* have the *Delusion* rubrics: *of emptiness,* and *he was going to sleep.* She has needed to go into freezing inertia, and disappears to avoid her feelings. The deceptive motivations which form the basis of this mental and emotional need will fall into two categories; avoidance or self-deluding denial. If the patient has a psychological delusion, then the patient also has a *need* for the delusional stance.

Muriaticum acidum is a remedy picture trapped between the corrosiveness and destructiveness, of an *acid,* and the moral self-examination of the *muriaticum* mind. Sankaran states that the theme of *acid* is a "constant struggle, the patient is so exhausted that a small setback like the proverbial straw that broke the camel's back, leads to a state of collapse."

Follow-up Consultations – from the same session on October 2007.

Question: Why is it so hard to stay disappeared?

I am more aware that I have disappeared. So in actual fact I have not disappeared. (Laughs.) *So that is good.*

So you are aware of the struggle now?

I have always been aware of the struggle but now I am feeling it. I wouldn't be me for quits. There is just this long suffering. I really identify with my sister. No wonder I was the only one who was understanding of her suicide. Her note said that she couldn't bear the pain any longer. I don't disappear so much anymore even when I am depressed. I have greater awareness. It is so weird because when I really think about it I don't find enjoyment. It is like the other is much bigger and it overrides. But what is different is that I don't stay there. Many years ago I would have been in what is called a sulk or a mood and not been able to get out of it. I haven't given up. [Mind rubrics: morose, brooding.]I want to give up but I haven't.

Again that is Muriaticum acidum. That is the struggle, to die or not to die. Which is the same as to be or not to be, to be all of me which is to be present. This process of looking for a place to live is really scary because being means being, then I be, and then I don't get what I want. In the past that classic of no effort put in, means that nothing happened. It is a safer place because you justify to yourself, well I didn't try anyway. I am not like that anymore.

So it is much more painful?

Yes it is much more painful. [Laughs.] *Can I please go back to the other?* [Laughs.]

Case Analysis

At this point, the patient has let go of her need for psychological avoidance. She was able to find accommodation which is affordable and suitable for her psychotherapy practice.

Last Consultation Notes: Case Analysis

She reports she feels *better about herself. I like myself much better. I have a feeling of being okay. I am now responsible for my own aloneness. I feel lonely but I don't go into depression and give up on life. I am able to feel loneliness and have hope as well. I can now speak up for myself and ask for myself in my relationship now. I now realize I have two things going in relationships; passiveness versus expansiveness. The way I used to assert myself was to explode into lots of disintegrating pieces and float around in emptiness. I can now fit myself into containment. I am now good enough to be able to do things for myself. I never realized how angry and hurt I was. Now I can be alone and know I will be okay. The irony is that now I have a relationship which I think will work but it is up to me continuing to express my needs to get it to work. I now know that I never used to express myself. I used to just disappear, disassociate from myself. There were advantages in the dissociative state. I could avoid the pain of not being loved. Because I never knew how to live with that much pain. I didn't know how to live with the anxiety and insecurity about money and with no support. I can now feel here and supported inside of myself. I am now no longer self-destructing myself to enable myself to disassociate. 'To be or not to be' – hopelessness versus acceptance and etermination. I now know why you gave me Hamlet[25] to read.*

---

25 *Muriaticum acidum* is personified in the character of Hamlet in the play, *The Tragedy of Hamlet, Prince of Denmark*, written by William Shakespeare. The profile that identifies Hamlet as *Muriaticum acidum* is his inability to act. Hamlet is perceived as a man tormented by his own indecisive inertia, which eventually drives him into insanity and depression. I repertorised Hamlet as mirroring the psychological inertia of the destructive elements of *acidum* and *muriaticum* within the remedy picture of *Muriaticum acidum*. Hamlet pontificates, "To be or not to be"; this is the remedy profile of *Muriaticum acidum*.

The play opens with the ghost of Hamlet's father telling Hamlet he was poisoned by Hamlet's Uncle, Claudius, who has since married Hamlet's mother, and entrenched himself on the throne of Denmark. Hamlet is confronted by the ghost of his father. The ghost commands Hamlet to avenge his murder, but to not blame or hurt his mother, Gertrude who has subsequently married Claudius. Instead of instinctually reacting, Hamlet is overwrought by the responsibility of his father's request for revenge. Previous to hearing the news of his father's murder, Hamlet had returned home distraught over his mother's hasty and seemingly adulterous marriage to his uncle, Claudius. If Hamlet had been a constitutional remedy picture motivated by revenge, he would have acted immediately and instinctively to avenge the crime committed against him and his family. Instead, Hamlet procrastinates. He is torn between doubting his sanity, and the vision of his father's ghost. He procrastinates over his rage towards his mother's disloyalty. Hamlet displays a depressive inability to act and avenge his father's murder. Hamlet is clearly not a play about proactive decision-making. It is instead a long drawn out dialogue that concentrates on the psychological debate within the tortured mind of a person under extreme emotional stress, who is forced by his inertia to consider his own madness. As homoeopaths, we are always looking for the 'never-well-since-event' that distinguishes the case as a particular constitutional remedy. As homoeopaths, we need to know why the person reacted to a particular stress in their life in the way they did. It is the answer to this question which will always indicate the simillimum. The question I am asking is: what is it within Hamlet that forces him into inertia and insanity that also distinguishes and mirrors the remedy profile of *Muriaticum acidum*? And, why is it that Hamlet is rendered inactive by what would have to be considered an instinctual human emotion of revenge.

The *acids* have an affinity for weakness, collapse [*Mind* rubric: *never succeeds*] and prostration [*Mind* rubric: *discontented with himself*]. Hamlet is consumed with anger and internal grief but he is unable to act. Hamlet pontificates on [*Mind* rubric: *brooding*] his fate for five acts until he is able to find the courage to act. Ironically, even then it is not until he accidentally slays Polonius that he is forced to flee to England to seek help for the kingdom of Denmark. In the meantime, he is 'afflicted' with internal debate [*Mind* rubrics: *muttering, talking to himself*] to the point where he doubts his own madness and the vision of his father's ghost [*Delusion* rubric: *sees images, phantoms, past to present*].

Muriaticum has an affinity for the psychodynamic preoccupation with the incestuous love of the mother. Hamlet is in a morose stupor, unable to even respond vengefully to the ghost of his father. He is beside himself with suicidal grief, which focuses more on the adulterous loss of his mother to Claudius, than the murder of his father. It is not until Hamlet confronts his mother with her adultery that Hamlet is able to act. Hamlet, up until this point, is frozen [*Mind* rubric: *stupefaction*] in his own procrastination [*Mind* rubric: *prostration of mind*] and inertia. Consumed with grief and rage over the loss of his mother to Claudius, he accidentally stabs Polonius, mistaking him for Claudius. Even though in Act I, Scene II, Hamlet declares, "Frailty, thy name is woman!" he still debates the ethical nature of the vendetta for several more acts of the play. Before Hamlet is confronted with the ghost of his father at the start of the play, he curses his mother: "She married. O, most wicked speed, to post with such dexterity to incestuous sheets!" Sankaran defines the theme of *muriaticum* as the "theme of betrayal of trust and faith". The *Muriaticum* element has an affinity for the psychodynamic premonition of the loss of the mother. Within *Muriaticum* the obsessive psychodynamic [*Mind* rubric: *silent grief*] of the loss of the mother is so all consuming, the person is thrown into a *morose stupor*.

Hamlet is so overwrought (at the end of Act I Scene V) with the prospect of action, he curses, "O cursed spite, that ever I was born to set it right!" (*Muriaticum acidum* as a constitutional profile would contemplate a situation so thoroughly that any course of action would be conceived to be beyond their capacity. Subsequently, he would not be able to instinctively react with rage and murderous revenge for such a heinous crime committed against his own father. Hamlet, rather than trust his vision of his father's ghost, sinks into *moroseness*. Motivated by his own doubt and "madness", Hamlet uses a group of visiting actors to re-enact his father's murder.

Hamlet, discontented with himself, [*Mind* rubric: *discontented with himself*] and corrosive in his own indecision, sinks into a depressive neurosis that doubts his own sanity. Hamlet doubts his own sanity and declares "the spirit that I have seen may be the devil". By Act III Scene I he laments, "To be, or not to be: that is the question: whether 'tis nobler in the mind to suffer the slings and arrows of outrageous fortune, or to take arms against a sea of troubles, and by opposing end them. To die: to sleep." Hamlet eventually does kill the King, but only by default. The Queen accidentally drinks from the poisoned cup meant for Hamlet; and it is only as the Queen is dying and only when he himself has been fatally stabbed by the poisoned arrow in his duel with Laertes, the son of Polonius, who he had previously accidentally killed, that Hamlet stabs the King. Hamlet, in the final duel with Laertes, who is seeking redemption for

I used to go into an inactive state of inertia. My life is about a lesson in survival. At the age of fifty plus now and to have no house and maybe no partner who can look after me and to still feel able to be here and not dissociate is incredible. I used to think about not being here. If I made myself small and avoided responsibility no one would notice me and I would not notice me.

The 'never-well-since-event' in her life had been the loss of financial support when her father had lost the family fortune. Her sister's suicide had exacerbated and helped to confirm that she could not survive. She is now doing much more than surviving; she continues to grow and develop within relationships and within her role as a successful psychotherapist.

Bibliography

Clarke, John Henry. M.D. *A Dictionary of Practical Materia Medica.* New Delhi, B. Jain Publishers, 1994. p. 508.

Mangialavori, Massimo. Dr. Notes from the first Koiné degree seminar in Bologna, 3-9 October 2005. Complied by

Polonius's death, admits his "madness" in his plea for pardon; "his madness is poor Hamlet's enemy". Hamlet in comparison to Laertes comes across as a dithering coward. Laertes acts instinctually and impulsively.

It is firstly the collapse and indolence of the *acid* and secondly the *muriaticum* theme of betrayal within Hamlet's emotional make-up of *Muriaticum acidum* that forces him to spend five acts of a play debating with himself over the correct moral and ethical considerations of one course of action over another, to the detriment of his own sanity and survival. Had Hamlet not been so focused on, and consumed with his *muriaticum* perceived theme of betrayal of trust and faith directed at his adulterous mother, he would have been able to act upon the call for vengeance by the ghost of his father. But *Muriaticum acidum* have no 'delusions of original sin', therefore they have no evidence that they are capable of committing an act of revenge. *Muriaticum acidum* have the *Mind* rubrics: *silent grief, want of self-confidence, self-depreciation, prostration of mind, never succeeds,* and *talking to himself.*

In Act III Scene IV, when Hamlet confronts his mother, he is once again visited by the ghost of his father who pleads with Hamlet to "speak to her". It is not until Hamlet has to plead with his mother to repent and "confess yourself to heaven", we see him prepared to act and come out of his inertia.

Deborah Vidal, *Self Destructiveness*. Matrix, 2006. pp. 74-77.

Sankaran, Rajan. *The Soul of Remedies*. Santa Cruz, Bombay, Homoeopathic Medical Publishers, 1997. p.127, p.159, p.164.

Schroyens, Frederik. M.D. *Synthesis*. London, Homeopathic Book Publishers, 1997.

Shakespeare, William. *Shakespeare: The Complete Works. Volume III*. England, Heron Books, 1995. pp.482-574.

Natrum sulphuricum

Foreword

For the summer edition of *Homeopathy in Practice* 2008, I published an article on *Natrum sulphuricum* entitled: *Oedipal Conflict and Self Destruction*. In that article I wrote the following: "Vermeulen makes a note in *Synoptic Materia Medica* that *Natrum sulphuricum* is in 'NONE' of the *Delusion* rubrics. *Natrum sulphuricum* is listed under the *Mind* rubrics for remorse and anguish, and under the *Mind* rubrics for suicide even though *Natrum sulphuricum* has no delusional crisis of self. The *Delusion* rubrics pertain to a crisis of self examination; with *Natrum sulphuricum* their fate is sealed; there is no debate or crisis of self examination. *Natrum sulphuricum* anguish is a "realistic" and "objective" [Vermeulen *Prisma*] foregone conclusion and proof of remorseful guilt; consequently the anguish and anxiety about their right to existence is overwhelming. *Natrum sulphuricum* knows with "realistic" knowing they are guilty; it is this assumption of guilt that fills them with mania, alternating with depression, and anxiety. With *Natrum sulphuricum* the *Mind* rubric: *fear of misfortune*, and the *Mind* rubric: *never succeeds*, is the foregone conclusion and proof of their powerless in relationship to life."

I was wrong in this article. *Natrum sulphuricum* does have a *Delusion* rubric. I have come to the conclusion that if there is anguish, there is inner conflict and there *has* to be an underlying *Delusion* rubric. I have finally found the *Delusion* rubric for *Natrum sulphuricum*; it is the *Delusion* rubric: *one will become insane.*

In the process of writing *Homoeopathic Psychiatry*, I have gone through every *Delusion* rubric. Although *Natrum sulphuricum* are not listed under the main *Delusion* rubric heading (Vermeulen is correct in this) *Natrum sulphuricum* is listed under the *Delusion* rubric: *one will become insane* and the *Delusion* rubric: *she is disgraced.* This *Delusion* rubric explains so clearly why *Natrum sulphuricum* are *so* worried about not succeeding, and why *Natrum sulphuricum* alternate between depression and mania about their state of mind. The *Delusion* rubrics reflect and mirror the psychodynamic trauma inside the patient and have always been an invaluable explanation of the underlying crisis in my patients' lives.

I am very happy to have finally found the *Delusion* rubrics for *Natrum sulphuricum.* Finding their *Delusion* rubrics is crucial because they indicate and explain any future stance, which is a disproportionate disturbance in any *Natrum sulphuricum* case. This disproportionate disturbance will often be the primary source of future pathologies.

Natrum sulphuricum struggle with their validity. The first case describes the inability of a business man to cut a deal for himself which favors his business without being overcome by anxiety and remorse about his staff's needs, as opposed to his own. In the second case, the man struggles to enjoy his wealth and musical career. He is overcome by guilt because his fellow musicians are not as fortunate, and he is overcome by guilt because his mother had to give up *her* musical career.

All my *Natrum sulphuricum* cases, whether they are men or women, are crippled by internal self-doubt and remorse, and question their actions. The underlying fuel for that anxiety is the *Natrum sulphuricum Delusion* rubric: *she is disgraced.* In the first case, the man says: *There was another level of pressure that I shouldn't feel unhappy because I am so fortunate. Most people in my situation should feel happy, and that was excruciating for me to try and reconcile.* In the second case, the man says: *But even there, with the person I am playing with there, is guilt over the situation I am in.*

When the remedy is taken, the *Sulphuricum* part of the remedy profile strengthens, and the man or woman becomes empowered with a *Sulphuricum* need to succeed creatively *for themselves*. *Sulphur* does not suffer with internal conflict over success. In fact, *Sulphur* are well known for their wonderful 'delusions of grandeur'.

The *Natrum* part of the remedy is the dominant player in an unhealthy *Natrum sulphuricum*. The *Natrum* part of the remedy martyrs, holding them with guilt and inner insecurity and fear of not succeeding. The *Natrum* part of the remedy is the precursor to their feeling sensitive about being reprimanded as children.

In the two *Natrum sulphuricum* cases, both men remained loyal to not succeeding because that was the psychological programming from the mother. In the first case, the sense of failure is expressed in his conflict over learning: *I hid under the toilet, and that's the moment that sticks in my mind where there was conflict between my parents and how they should raise me, and how that made me feel. I was why they were unhappy. I was not achieving what I should. I was terrified to learn from then on, whether it was spelling or reading.* The second case, after taking the remedy, also identifies this conflict when he tells his mother: *I have the right to love someone other than my mother, and that is what hurts her. When I say my partner is number one in my life, and you and my relationship have changed. I am making that choice now and I am telling you that you and my relationship have changed.*

The *Natrum* salt is aligned to the mother; the *Sulphuricum* has been abandoned or disowned by the father. The first person that dominated or suppressed was the mother, and the first person who they felt unworthy towards was the mother. The first person *Natrum sulphuricum* have responsibility to is their mother. The first person for whom *Natrum sulphuricum* experiences remorse, is their mother. The first relationship in which *Natrum sulphuricum* feel they have failed is with their mother.

If we can delve into the original crisis that created the first conscious sense of self, we have the remedy profile, and we have the cure for the psychodynamic crisis, and subsequent pathology. The *Sulphuricum* alignment in both cases has either been abandoned by an absent father, or the mother[26] has

26 This *Natrum Sulphuricum* oedipal theme is explored by the writer D. H. Lawrence in what is supposedly the most autobiographical of his works, *Sons and Lovers*. *Sons and Lovers* is the story of a young man, Paul Morel, struggling to fall in love with a woman other than his mother, Mrs. Morel. Paul Morel is tied to his mother by his "strong feelings of responsibility and guilt" [Sankaran]. Guilt is the psychodynamic crisis of emotional remorse in *Natrum Sulphuricum* which ties them to the mother. Sankaran says of *Natrum Sulphuricum*, "Since they make a lot of effort to maintain the relationship, they can be dominated or suppressed, taken advantage of, or scorned. Though they resent this internally, they are so dependent on the relationship that they allow themselves to be made use of and treated badly, all the while feeling not too good about themselves, unworthy." The domination and suppression Sankaran refers to is evident in both my *Natrum Sulphuricum* cases. Mrs. Morel in is a woman who turns her hope and love towards her sons to help heal her broken heart when her husband fails to meet her expectations. When "her own bitterness of disillusion was hardest to bear; when her faith in life was shaken, and her soul felt dreary and lonely. She made much of the child, and the father was jealous. At last Mrs. Morel despised her husband. She turned to the child; she turned from the father."

"Paul was dissatisfied with himself and with everything. The deepest of his love belonged to his mother. When he felt he had hurt her, or wounded his love for her he could not bear it."

"'And I've never – you know, Paul – I've never had a husband - not really.'

He stroked his mother's hair, and his mouth was on her throat.

'And she [Miriam] exults so in taking you from me – she's not like ordinary girls.'

'Well, I don't love, mother,' he murmured, bowing his head and hiding his eyes on her shoulder in misery. His mother kissed him a long, fervent kiss.

'My boy!' she said, in a voice trembling with passionate love.

Without knowing, he gently stroked her face."

Lawrence writes of Paul Morel: "He had that poignant carelessness about himself, his own suffering, his own life, which is a form of slow suicide." The essence of feeling hopeless is the *Mind* rubric: *never succeeds*. Paul Morel subjugates his love and becomes powerless to the mother. My first *Natrum sulphuricum* case was not able to negotiate with his staff or a business partner because, he says, *I have not wanted to disappoint. When I talk about these flashes of me being a child, feeling like I don't want to disappoint, but there is more than that; it is about how that made me feel. It would make me feel hopeless.* In the second case the patient can see how he subjugates himself proved the stronger force. *Natrum sulphuricum* subjugate their own power within any relationship; whether it be with business partners or with a lover. Sankaran says the sensation of *Natrum sulphuricum* is one of feeling "scorned, disgraced, insulted or not appreciated" by the person they love. Sankaran makes the observation that "when the relationship is not successful, they go into a stage of deep sadness and become melancholic, which is usually unexpressed and internal." The source of the internal anguish and guilt inside of *Natrum sulphuricum* which causes them to feel so crippled is their feeling that they will never succeed. *Natrum sulphuricum* have the *Mind* rubric: *never succeeds*. The first case describes the source of his feelings of failure: *My mum, who was a special education teacher, told me I had a learning disability but I think it was more based in*

---

with his music partner when he says: *How it plays out for me is that she will flippantly say, 'Don't leave me,' so don't book your own work and be more successful than me. So again, I restrict myself. Not anymore.* In both cases the *Natrum* relationship with the mother his the causation.

"'You know, mother, I think there must be something the matter with me, that I *can't* love.'

'I even love Clara, and I did Miriam; but to *give* myself to them in marriage I couldn't. I couldn't belong to them. They seem to want *me*, and I can't ever give it them.'

'You haven't met the right woman.'

'And I never shall meet the right woman while you live,' he said."

Paul is torn and locked in his feelings of love and loyalty to his mother to such an extent that he can't love another woman as long as his mother is still alive. Paul is unable to love another woman other than his mother, and in knowing the helpless bind he is in, sinks into "poignant carelessness about himself." [D. H. Lawrence]

"When the relationship is not successful, they go into a stage of deep sadness and become melancholic, which is usually unexpressed and internal." [Sankaran] "*Natrum Sulphuricum* patients feel that nothing ever works: 'Succeeds never.'" [Sankaran]

Bibliography

D. H. Lawrence. *Sons and Lovers*. Hertfordshire, Wordsworth Editions Limited, 1993. p. 14. p. 186. p. 188. p. 224. p. 305.

Sankaran, Rajan. *The Soul of Remedies*. Santa Cruz, Bombay, Homoeopathic Medical Publishers, 1997. pp.147-148.

fear of failing my parents' expectations which has led to my own expectations of how I live my life, and there has been that conflict. In the second case, the patient describes the history of the development of remorse and guilt when he says: *Doing the wrong thing, yes I just heard my mother saying you have to be a good boy. 'I betrayed her', was a word she used to use. And still she would say that, and it still operates for her.*

Natrum sulphuricum Case One:

Presenting Issue: Anxiety in running his business. He is unable to assert himself as the boss. Mood swings. He feels tired and exhausted with the responsibility of his staff. He is unable to create strong boundaries between himself and his staff. He keeps wanting to get his staff to have consultations with me, and *I will pay for them* (which is not appropriate) because he is so concerned about their health. He is an obsessive compulsive cleaner.

D.O.B. 1964.

This patient has been consulting me for counselling since he was sixteen years old. His first consultation for homoeopathic treatment was in July 2002. I had previously given him *Natrum muriaticum* which had helped his tendency to martyr himself and put his staff's needs above his own. His underlying anxiety and obsessive compulsive disorder had not changed on the prescription of *Natrum muriaticum.* Because he had consulted me for counselling I dealt only with those issues in the psychotherapy sessions. This was clearly not satisfactory. I now call myself a homoeopath, not a counsellor. If I have two roles with a patient it does not work because the counselling role can mask the simillimum.

Increasingly, I become aware that although the *Natrum* was clearly working in his case I did not feel that the *muriaticum* was the correct prescription.

In August 2006, I changed the remedy to *Natrum sulphuricum* on the basis of his consultation with me. In that consultation he admitted that he had never wanted to run the business he had. After so many years of consulting with him this was a revelation not only to he himself, but to me as well. He felt pressured by his father and mother. He was torn between guilt over his family and what *he* wanted to do. He told me, *the only time I have been truly happy was when I was designing and building my first shop. It is not the business or the shops that I am interested in. I never wanted to run retail outlets. I have only ever been happy when I was creating the design of the shop. I am not academic. I don't want to do business. I have an enormous amount of guilt over my family and the Italian expectation to run businesses. I am not achieving in business. I am a failure and I am always crippled by the feeling that I will never succeed. I want to express myself manually. I loved building my first shop. I want to do garden design or design interiors. I want to be creative. I have never told you this Liz because Italians are not meant to be creative manual laborers.* This is a typical *Natrum sulphuricum* passive-aggressive internal battle. *Every day I absolutely loathe how my life is. I am extremely sad and depressed and I can't see the point anymore. But if I give up business I will disgrace myself in my eyes and in my family's eyes.*

Case Analysis

Natrum sulphuricum is a homoeopathic remedy which is commonly used for mental confusion arising from physical injuries to the head. *Natrum sulphuricum* have the *Mind* rubrics: *confusion of mind after injury to the head* [3], and *mental symptoms from injuries to the head.* [2] 1. Within the profile of *Natrum sulphuricum* is evidence of a desire to remain unconscious. *Natrum sulphuricum* wish to obliterate their psyche. *Natrum sulphuricum* as a constitutional remedy profile is traditionally thought of as a strong suicide remedy. *Natrum sulphuricum* are the only remedy in the two *Mind* rubrics:

loathing life, must restrain herself to prevent doing injury, and *suicidal thoughts, must restrain himself because of his duties to his family*. [3]. 1. *Natrum sulphuricum* feel overwhelmed by the seriousness of responsibility. *Natrum sulphuricum* have the *Mind* rubrics: *too much sense of duty, never succeeds*, and *taking responsibility too seriously*. *Natrum sulphuricum* choose to maintain the belief that they cannot cope [*insane*] to avoid the fact that too much responsibility can make them feel like they will not *succeed* [*disgraced*]. The *Mind* profile of *Natrum sulphuricum* is abandonment of life [*suicide*] and abandonment of all belief in the self. The psychodynamic theme in the *Delusion* rubrics attached to *Natrum sulphuricum* is unconscious self-effacement. *Natrum sulphuricum* have a delusional need to deface [*disgrace*] themselves – they unconsciously sabotage everything they attempt. *Natrum sulphuricum* is a remedy profile for a patient who displays passive-aggressive behavior. *Natrum sulphuricum* have the *Mind* rubric: *strongly attached to others,* and conversely they have the *Mind* rubrics: *aversion to his wife*. *Natrum sulphuricum* will sabotage their relationships (including their relationship with the homoeopath) because they are frightened of becoming dependent. Passive-aggressive behavior is passive, sometimes obstructionist resistance to following through with expectations in interpersonal relationships. It can manifest itself as learned helplessness, or deliberate failure to accomplish requested tasks for which one is responsible. The passive-aggressive person 'defends himself' from others by retaliating with passivity and unconscious sabotage. Passive-aggressive behavior can manifest as a destructive need to deliberately sabotage relationships by withholding intimacy. What underpins passive-aggressive behavior is a deep feeling of rage (in the unconscious mind) which is transferred on to anyone upon whom one becomes dependent. The 'never-well-since-event' in all *Natrum sulphuricum* cases arises from abandonment in childhood. For many constitutional remedy profiles, abandonment is part of their 'never-well-since-event'. The *specific* and *peculiar* interpretation (aphorism 153) of a particular trauma by an individual patient is the inner disturbance which is the core of our case-taking. This disturbance is always reflective of what is *unusual* or disturbing to the homoeopath's inner sensibilities. *Natrum sulphuricum peculiarly* interpret abandonment shamefully. *Natrum sulphuricum* have delusional feelings of shame [*disgraced*] over being abandoned. Understanding this helps explain why *Natrum sulphuricum* need to withhold intimacy. Intimacy is disproportionately associated with feeling abandoned; acknowledgment of abandonment is associated with acknowledgment of shame. In turn, feeling disgraced is proof of never succeeding in life. Never succeeding is continually reinforced because whenever they take on responsibility they are overcome with the pressure of the responsibility and subsequently collapse.

A *Delusion* rubric is used only when there is an assumption or perception which is disproportionate to reality. If the trauma inside your patient starts with them feeling *intense* hopeless doom about being sick, and/or always being sick, or feeling that they *will never succeed* in becoming well, then the simillimum is listed in the *Delusion* rubrics of Depression. These are the *Delusion* rubrics: *he cannot succeed, everything will fail, he does everything wrong, he is trapped, he is ruined, he will become insane,* and *being doomed,* to list just a few. Psychological 'delusions of impending doom' are disproportionate assumptions about future failure.

The need to believe that one is unfortunate in life is usually based on exaggerated psychological delusions of being evil, wrong, or bad. This is the reason that Causation, or 'delusions of original sin', precedes Depression in the five stage psychological model. If a patient needs to hang on to the belief that they are unfortunate, then they need to deflect responsibility for their situation from themselves. Commonly, patients will blame their unfortunate circumstances on past life laws of karma, fate, or God who is testing their faith, or God who is punishing them for past sins. These varying ideologies are covered in the *Delusion* rubrics of Depression because underpinning their assumption that they deserve punishment is the need to believe that they are *doomed* and are *unfortunate*. (Aside from believing that one is ill-fated, the other reason why a person may not be able to achieve 'self-actualization' is that realistically they do not have the capacity to solve their problems. This is not necessarily delusional and is covered in all the *Mind* rubrics of Depression).

In the case studies of *Natrum sulphuricum*, I specifically concentrate on the delusional belief in failure. The need to believe one will always fail is an all consuming problem which causes future pathology. The *Delusion* rubrics of Depression resonate with disturbance because *Natrum sulphuricum* wish to maintain their depression and their belief that they will *always* fail and they will *never* succeed. The delusional belief in failure is self-destructive. To an outsider, or to the homoeopath observing the patient suffering 'delusions of impending doom', it is not always reflective of reality. A patient can maintain a perception of themselves as a failure whereas in reality they are very successful. The *peculiar* reason why a patient continues to need to believe they will not succeed will always indicate the simillimum.

The purpose in understanding the five stage psychological analysis of the *Delusion* rubrics is to highlight the specific *peculiarities* of a remedy profile. The constitutional remedy profiles which are profoundly consumed by 'delusions of impending doom' have no 'delusions of grandeur' or denial processes which are able to create a 'hubristic illusion' of success. The *Natrum sulphuricum* patient who has no delusional belief in cure or no hubristic denial process in place within their psyche will be more likely to sabotage their success and their medical or homoeopathic treatment.

1. Denial: NONE.
2. Forsaken: *Delusion* rubric: *disgraced*: *she is*: nat-s. [This

rubric can pertain to abandonment or admission of guilt.]

3. Causation: *Delusion* rubric: *disgraced: she is*: nat-s.
4. Depression: *Delusion* rubric: *insane: become insane; one will*: nat-s.
5. Resignation: NONE.

Mind rubrics for *Natrum sulphuricum*

- *Mind: ailments from: honor; wounded*: nat-s.
- *Mind: ailments from: injuries, accidents; mental symptoms from*: **NAT-S**.
- *Mind: aversion: wife, to his*: nat-s.
- *Mind: doubtful: recovery, of*: nat-s.
- *Mind: estranged: family; from his*: nat-s.
- *Mind: estranged: wife, from his*: nat-s.
- *Mind: fear: suicide; of: Nat-s*.
- *Mind: injuring himself: fear to be left alone, lest he should injure himself: Nat-s*.
- *Mind: insanity: periodical*: nat-s.
- *Mind: kill; desire to: herself; sudden impulse to: Nat-s*.
- *Mind: loathing: life: injury, must restrain herself to prevent doing herself*: **NAT-S**. [3] 1.
- *Mind: love: family; for*: nat-s.
- *Mind: responsibility: taking responsibility too seriously: Nat-s*.
- *Mind: sadness: suicidal disposition, with: Nat-s*.
- *Mind: sensitive: reprimands, to: children; in*: nat-s. [1] 5. [carc. med. sacch. staph.]
- *Mind: succeeds, never*: nat-s.
- *Mind: suicidal disposition: grief; from: Nat-s*. [2] 1.
- *Mind: weary of life: unworthy of the gift of life: Nat-s*. [2] 4. [carc. naja plat.]

Case Analysis

Natrum sulphuricum are a remedy profile which suffer from fear of abandonment [*estranged from family*.] Both *Natrum sulphuricum* cases were crippled with anguish as a child when they were rejected by their mother. Insight into any issues around abandonment always present with the *Delusion* rubrics of having being cast out of paradise. *Natrum sulphuricum* have the *Delusion* rubric: *she is disgraced*. The two cases, previous to taking the remedy, struggled to assert their right to be assertive; they were crippled by fear of rejection. *Natrum sulphuricum* have the *Mind* rubric: *sensitive to reprimands in children*.

The 'never-well-since-event' for *Natrum sulphuricum* will always have its origins in feelings of being reprimanded.

Follow-up Consultation: August 2006.

The following is a transcript from the videoed session one month after taking one dose of *Natrum sulphuricum* 200 C. x 1/week x 3 weeks.

Question: Can you talk to me about the feelings that you came to me with last visit?

I was feeling torn and locked up. I couldn't feel happy, I was stuck with something I couldn't control, which was a business outcome, to the point that it was crippling. The relationship was the expectation of what I should have achieved and not being able to feel satisfied with what I had achieved. I was feeling anxious, not happy. What I was confronted with was feeling torn with a feeling I should be happy with the privileged life that I feel that I have and the feeling which was not those things. That was another level of pressure that I shouldn't feel unhappy because I am so fortunate. Most people in my situation should feel happy and that was excruciating for me to try and reconcile. Four weeks since I have seen you and I feel vastly different. I feel happier and I don't feel as hard on myself.

I have a lot more perspective about the conflict I found myself in. I feel lighter.

Has it had a cross-over effect into your relationship?

Nothing is as black.

I meant in terms of the degree to which you need to have things controlled?

With myself I don't feel as neurotic so I definitely feel I am not trying to control the house as much. Things that would normally drive me crazy aren't driving me up the wall as much. Not so obsessive. (He is an obsessive compulsive cleaner in his house which puts a lot of emotional strain on his wife; especially because she is a *Medorrhinum* who reacts to control.) *Normally I would have to go to yoga three times a week and I haven't been in three weeks.* [Laughs.] *I am just not as hard on myself. I am not working so hard and not exercising, which are normally the things I would have to do to try and hold on to myself. I am feeling like if I sleep in, it's okay. I am working because I want to, not because I feel guilty because I should. These are huge for me. Of all the homoeopathic remedies that I have had* (previously *Natrum muriaticum*) *this is the one that is working the best.*

Yes, that is what I was looking for. So the question of over-responsibility and guilt is still an issue of carrying the whole thing.

So, that is a good thing. Yes, I don't. A staff member would call me and I would go into a tail spin; obsessively there and then. I am able to keep my perspective on my own terms, and that is a very empowering thing, it takes far less energy. I feel lighter about my staff. One of the things I do is obsess on issues. It comes from Dad, it's a trust thing. I am not needing to control that so much, the roof is not going to fall in, and it allows me to do what I want to do. I don't have to shift my focus. I feel protected. I feel stronger to be able to say no. Almost like it is okay to defend yourself.

What is the fear that comes up if you say no?

Consequences; the fear, anxiety. Disappointing the person who I am saying no to. Extreme anxiety. Loyalty. I am definitely able to stand my ground more if I think about the negotiations in my life lately.

But what is the anxiety?

This is why I feel so happy. I am not actually feeling anxious, and I am getting a buzz out of the negotiation. It is about what I want. I have not wanted to disappoint. When I talk about these flashes of me being a child and feeling like I did not want to disappoint, but there is more than that. It is about how that made me feel. It would make me feel hopeless.

Where did the disappointment come from?

Disappointment came from disappointing my parents. Not doing what they thought I should be able to do. Now in my own business I disappoint myself by not doing what I thought I should be able to do. I want to understand the anxiety and where it came from. The feeling of disappointment because you are getting what you want.

Is it guilt?

Yes, of course it is. See, I always pride myself on cutting the deal they can be happy with, and I can be happy with. Sometimes, I had an overwhelming feeling in the last three weeks. I was feeling like people were shafting me. It is almost like I want to seize examples so I can get what I want.

Tell me about the first time you felt you were going to disappoint your parents.

I remember clearly. I was chased into a bathroom and my dad and my mum arguing over whether I should or shouldn't be able to spell something, and I hid under the toilet. That is the moment that sticks in my mind where there was conflict between my parents and how they should raise me, and how that made me feel was that they were unhappy, and I was not achieving what I should. I was terrified to learn from then on, whether it was spelling or reading. To this day, I don't know how to spell. I sit in my office and scream out how do you spell the most basic words. My mum, who was a special education teacher, told me I had a learning disability. But I think it was more based in fear of failing my parents expectations, which has led to my own expectations of how I live my life, and there has been that conflict. I have been aware of those things all my life, but at the moment I feel less conflict and more peace.

Case Outcome: Case-Development

Presenting Illness: He was diagnosed with Crohn's disease in April 2007.

- Crohn's Disease
- diarrhoea
- pain, cramping
- bleeding

I recommended that he immediately start my Irritable Bowel diet, which is low fibre, and carbohydrate foods separated from fruits and sugars. His bowel needed a chance to recover from being irritated by high fibre foods. I took him off all wheat and cow's milk products.

I have been treating this man since he was sixteen years old, so I was extremely upset at his diagnosis. On the one hand I was distraught for him, and on the other hand, I felt confronted that after many years of successful treatment on *Natrum sulphuricum* for his obsessive compulsive behavior, I had obviously *not* been able to find the simillimum which would have prevented this disease. Whether he would have got this disease when he was sixteen, which is common, and I had been able to delay the onset, is unknown. My self-doubt proved incorrect.

This case has showed me that *potency* of the simillimum must *also* resonate with the patient. I dropped the *Natrum sulphuricum* to a 30 C. potency 1/day.

He has been in remission with his Crohn's ever since. I have experienced personally in my life with my own health and in many patients' lives, that the simillimum will cure auto-immune conditions. The primary trauma which caused the primary *Delusion* rubric is the causation in the case; this is why in this case I continuously emphasize the need to understand the causation or the 'never-well-since-event'.

Prescription: *Natrum sulphuricum* 30 C. daily, dry pilule continuously, and *Natrum sulphuricum* 200 C. weekly.

This patient's Crohn's disease is in remission. I have been treating him continuously for four years. I have him on *Natrum sulphuricum* 30 C. daily, and *Natrum sulphuricum* 200 C. weekly, continuously, since April 2007. He has sold his business, is now working for himself in interior design, and is much happier. His relationship is much happier because he is less obsessive about housework. His relationship with his partner is much improved because he finds he is able *to be more open and loving*. They now have a four year old child. He was always terrified that he would damage his child because of his obsessive compulsiveness around the house; that has not eventuated. His relationship with his mother has changed considerably. He feels less indebted to her, and panders less to her fears about his potential failure in business. He still has consultations with me, but only when he notices that his anxiety has resurfaced. At those times I give him *Natrum sulphuricum* 1m. x 1 dose. In 2009 I had only one face-to-face consultation with him.

Follow-up: November 2009.

In November 2009 his gut started to become inflamed. His diarrhoea had not started again, but he had small, and thinner than normal stools. He had no bleeding but his stomach area was extremely sore to touch, and hard. He was experiencing urinary frequency at night. I was worried, as he was, that the Crohn's had returned, or that his bowel had a blockage from scar tissue. I had not noticed, because he had not been having face-to-face consultations with me, that he had failed to renew his prescription of the *Natrum sulphuricum* 30 C. daily remedy. He had not taken this prescription for ten months. He had remained on the *Natrum sulphuricum* 200 C. weekly. One week after recommencing the *Natrum sulphuricum* 30 C. daily remedy his gut pain ceased, and his stools have returned to normal size and frequency. The frequent urination at night ceased after one week.

Case Analysis

The *Natrum sulphuricum* 30 C. daily prescription is working in this case as a 'Drainage remedy'. In 1950 Dr Leon Vannier, a French homoeopath, wrote *La Pratique de L'Homoeopathie*. This work has been translated into English by E.A.A.A.D. de Ruyter. If a Constitutional remedy is given in high-potency to a patient who has not been given preparatory homoeopathic treatment, a sudden aggravation of his or her condition may occur. Vannier regards this as an 'eliminatory crisis': a sudden elimination of toxic substances which overwhelm the organism. According to Dr Vannier an acute aggravation can always be prevented by using what he calls *Drainage treatment*. In this case I have had the patient on a Drainage potency of the simillimum as well as a *Delusion* potency of the simillimum.

Natrum sulphuricum Case Two:

Presenting Issue: Anguished guilt about his right to be a musician.

D.O.B. 1952.

Presenting Illness:

- Eczema on his face
- Eczema on his eye lids
- Eczema on the back of his neck
- < heat at night in bed
- < dry
- Itching, hot+++, dry, scaly eczema.
- First Consultation: March 2005. Prescription Given: *Sulphur* 6 C. 1/day
- Second Consultation: April 2005. Slight improvement in his skin. No change mentally and emotionally. Prescription Given: *Sulphur* 30 C. 1/day
- Third Consultation: May 2005. Slight improvement in his skin. No change mentally and emotionally. Prescription Given: *Sulphur* 30 C. 1/day. *Bacillinum* 200 C. 1/week x 4 weeks
- Fourth Consultation: June 2005. Slight improvement in his skin. No change mentally and emotionally. Prescription Given: *Sulphur* 200 C. 1/week. *Thuja* 200 C. 1/week x 4 weeks
- Fifth Consultation Phone Consultation: Late June 2005. Marked improvement in his skin. No change mentally and emotionally. Prescription Given: *Sulphur* 200 C. 1 x 3 doses in a 24 hour period
- Sixth Consultation Phone Consultation: Late July 2005. Marked improvement in his skin. No change mentally and emotionally. Prescription Given: *Sulphur* 200 C. 1/day. 3 days on the remedy. 3 days off x 3 cycles
- Seventh Consultation: August 2005. Marked improvement in his skin. No change mentally and emotionally. Prescription Given: *Sulphur* 200 C. 1/day. x 3 doses. Then *Sulphur* 200 C. x 1 dose, *Calcarea carbonica* 200 C. x 1 dose, then *Lycopodium* 200 C. x 1 dose

- Eighth Consultation: August 2005. Re-examination of the case

Once again there has been a marked improvement in his skin, but as soon as he becomes anxious, his skin goes back to what it was like originally. The *Sulphur* has improved his skin but the prescription has changed nothing mentally or emotionally. *Sulphur* is *not* the simillimum.

Prescription Given: *Natrum sulphuricum* 200 C. x 1/week.

I reconsidered his *Natrum* hurt from his mother, and his *Sulphur* abandonment from his father. The predominant mental and emotional aggravation in his case is his crippling anxiety and depression, and strong belief that he will not succeed as a musician. I give *Natrum sulphuricum* not yet truly knowing or understanding his psychodynamic trauma or 'never-well-since-event'.

If this prescription is correct, I know the action of the simillimum will reveal that trauma in a subsequent consultation.

Mind rubrics for *Natrum sulphuricum*

- *Mind*: *doubtful*: *recovery, of*: nat-s.
- *Mind*: *responsibility*: *taking responsibility too seriously*: Nat-s.
- *Mind*: *sadness*: *suicidal disposition, with*: Nat-s.
- *Mind*: *succeeds, never*: nat-s.
- *Mind*: *weary of life*: *unworthy of the gift of life*: Nat-s. [2] 4. [carc. naja plat.]

Ninth Consultation: March 2006.

It has been a long time between follow-up consultations because he has been overseas. Thankfully, this has not been a problem. He is markedly much happier. He reports that he has less grief around his mother. He also reports that he is *hanging on to rage and anger less*. This is the first time that he has named his feeling towards his mother as *grief*. He believes that he has been in *deep despairing grief ever since my father left*. It is not until this consultation that I discover that he views the difficulties that he has in his marriage as stemming from his inability to love. He perceives that his mother has 'demasculinised' him. He believes that he was not allowed to love anyone other than his mother; but because he refused to love her, he has been unable to love anyone else. His loyalty to another woman means that he is no longer loyal to his mother. His loyalty to his father meant that he was no longer loyal to his mother.

- *Mind*: *suicidal disposition*: *grief*; *from*: *Nat-s.* [2] 1.

Consultation: August 2006.

Between March and this consultation in August, I have been slowly increasing the dose. The following is the transcript from a videoed session one month after taking three doses of *Natrum sulphuricum* 10 M. (The patient was meant to take one dose only. But he took one dose a day for 3 days. On the third day I had a premonition to ring him. I then explained it was one dose only and not to take anymore!)

In the cases I emphasize repeatedly the need to understand the causation or the 'never-well-since-event'. The first consultation is often on the conscious level. It is often not until patients have had several consultations that they are able to reveal deep traumatic events in their life which have formulated psychological delusions. Until I discover the primary trauma in a patient's life I am never totally sure of a simillimum prescription.

The simillimum will undo the layers of psychological delusions.

Question: What is the difference with how you feel?

I feel a lot calmer, less agitated. Less stress on my system.

There was an inner agitation that would fuel my inner response to whatever I was doing.

Any difference to how agitated your skin feels?

No.

It looks less irritated.

Yes. (He has eczema on his neck and face which flares up when he fears whether he will succeed as a musician.)

Any difference to how agitated it is with your sleep at night, itching with getting hot?

Yes, it is not as hot.

What have you noticed you are less agitated about?

Last time we met, we talked about the situation I am in. I have just sat with that. I have been observing that I am less agitated with that. I can just relax into where I am without feeling guilty about where I am.

Can you give me an example?

Yes. I met with my younger brother whose girlfriend has just left him. He lives in a remote town in Western Australia. He has confessed that he had a drug and alcohol problem and he was in really bad shape, and normally that would make me feel guilty. I would pay his bills, fines, do you need some money, that sort of thing, because I can. Then I came home and spoke to my partner, and she said, well isn't it interesting the choices that he has made and the choices that you have made. Same situation of when your father left, and how your mother was, but you have made different choices.

Just being around the house, and I really love it and just feeling blessed. (He is in a very good situation financially, and has not, up until now, been able to allow himself to enjoy it or feel worthy of having so much wealth.) *So mainly around my family that the guilt has been there, and my mother of course.*

So you have been able to enjoy your house more?

Yes, the whole life style, it has been good. The guilt fuels most things that I do.

Have you seen your mother?

Yes. I rocked up with my suitcases and she was feeling anxious. She doesn't know how to behave around me, and we talked about the letter I wrote her. It was quite good I stood my ground with her, and called her on a number of things in the past that I had had to deal with silently on my own. When she said your father this, and your father that, and she would follow up with you are just like your father. I said just hang on a minute you said this, and this, you can't say that. This is what I am talking about and this is the effect it has on me. And I called her on it about four or five times. It was good to say those things to her. It got to the point where we were talking about the music. We were talking about choices, and I said that these are some of the choices that I make. I said to her the most tragic thing is that you gave up your music, and she said well your father made me give up the music. And then I said, one of the reasons I haven't been doing things with the music is that I feel guilty. I broke down and said I can't do this because you were not able to do it. She was hugging me and she said, stop this don't be stupid I want you to do well, I want you to succeed. It was good for me to be able to say that because I got to that really sobbing state, and it really surprised me. I felt good because I was able to stand my ground around her, and call her on a few things.

Is it because I am filming? It seems to me that you are able to answer the questions a lot quicker?

It is not the filming. It is that I am able to know what I feel. I am a lot clearer. I can be more responsive to my partner, and I can hear her without getting agitated. It is easier and more joyful. She would say something, and then the voice in my head would get agitated. Now I can say, you are not in competition with her, you don't have to do the opposite[27]. That was operating quite fiercely.

Is there a difference with your music?

But even there, with the person I am playing with, there is guilt over the situation I am in. How I could use the money, I am not using it, but I could use that. Guilt over my talent. I pull it back a bit when I play with her. I noticed I would do that.

So guilt means you have done something wrong; do you think that is right? What does guilt mean?

I find that really hard to answer. It is more like a judgment like they are in a worse situation, and I am in a better situation. I can't answer that for some reason.

So when you think of your mother, can you think back into your childhood? It is hard because you have just started to identify the layers of guilt, but can you think back into your childhood, and can you remember when you became aware of feeling guilty?

I would associate that with when I was fifteen or sixteen, when I would have contact with my father, when letters would come from him, and she would get the mail, and she would throw it at me, and she would die to want to know what was in it[28]. And she would say, you having contact with your father is like sticking in the knife, and then withdrawing it. And that is when I started to feel guilty about whether I should I have communication with him after he has just left us. I took on the guilt because I was one of the only members of the family who was having contact with him. The years leading up to him

---

27 *Natrum sulphuricum* is a remedy profile for a patient who displays passive-aggressive behavior. *Natrum sulphuricum* will sabotage their relationships because they are frightened of becoming dependent. The passive-aggressive person 'defends himself' from others by retaliating with passivity and unconscious sabotage.

28 Passive-aggressive behavior is passive, sometimes obstructionist resistance. Passive-aggressive behavior can manifest as a destructive need to deliberately sabotage relationships by withholding intimacy.

leaving were filled with turmoil, and I always blamed my mother for driving him away. When he left I felt the rug was pulled out from under me. I lost the stabilizing force in my life. Then I started to feel angry with her, as I felt she made me feel guilty for still corresponding with him.

So if you start to feel guilty you feel agitated and angry?

Uncomfortable, I wouldn't say angry.

So what do you think guilt is?

I don't know. My mind goes blank. I can't answer that.

So, what are other words you would associate guilt with?

I blank.

There seems to be a strong relationship between what you want and guilt. You feel guilt over wanting to pursue your music, over not looking after your family; you feel guilt over enjoying your house and wealth.

Yes, but less and less.

You look less agitated about it as well.

Yes, and that is what friends have said. I look less agitated, softer, and more open.

What has guilt got to do with enjoyment?

For me it stops me from enjoyment, it is disabling.

So in society, when you hear the word guilt, what is it associated with?

The legal system. With people doing the wrong thing. Argh! Nice work Liz. Doing the wrong thing. Yes, I just heard my mother saying, you have to be a good boy. I 'betrayed' her. That was a word she used to use. And still she would say that, and it still operates for her. When I had my father stay recently for a family thing, she said I betrayed her by putting my father up, and putting her up in a pub. I said mum, it wasn't a pub, it was a very flash hotel. 'Oh well,' she said 'he was in your house'. I have the right to love someone other than my mother, and that is what hurts her. When I say my partner is number one in my life, and you and my relationship has changed, I am making that choice now and I am telling you that you and my relationship have changed.

So, what you were saying with your music partner is that if you become first fiddle over her then you are betraying her?

How it plays out for me is that she will flippantly say, 'Don't leave me', so don't book your own work and be more successful than me. So again, I restrict myself.

Not anymore.

Case Outcome:

This patient has given up trying to succeed at becoming a *famous* musician; he plays and records albums now for pleasure. Before, he was so driven to become 'famous' that he was not able to enjoy his success. He consulted me for three years, every six weeks. He still gets herbs and Omega oils from me for his skin, when required. The last dose of *Natrum sulphuricum* was in December 2008 and I gave him a 10 MM x 1 dose. He says he has not needed another dose from me since. He has been studying psychotherapy and wants to become a therapist. He is still struggling in his relationship with passive-aggressive patterning, *but he is able to see* (consciously know) *what he is doing, and work on his issues in therapy.* In 2009 he asked me a few times how I think he is going. At the end of each discussion, he has decided that he has *a good handle on the situation.*

It is very important to allow *Natrum sulphuricum* time to find their own footing in life. Their passive-aggressive behavior has its origins in over-control, specifically from their mother. As a female homoeopath and therapist working with *Natrum sulphuricum,* I am always hyper-vigilant to the need to avoid counter-transference.

Natrum sulphuricum choose to maintain the belief that they cannot cope [*insane*] to avoid the fact that too much responsibility can make them feel like they will not *succeed* [*disgraced*].

When healthy, *Natrum sulphuricum* are able to support themselves.

Bibliography

De Ruyter, E.A.A.A.D. *Computer Homoeopathy and a Summary of Dr. Leon Vannier's Theories on the Paratuberculous and Paracancerous States*. Self-Published, Australia, 1994, pp.46-48.

Sankaran, Rajan. *The Soul of Remedies*. Santa Cruz, Bombay, Homoeopathic Medical Publishers, 1997. p. p.147-148.

Schroyens, Frederik. M.D. *Synthesis*. London, Homeopathic Book Publishers, 1997.

Vermeulen, Frans. *Synoptic Materia Medica*. The Netherlands, Merlijin Publishers, 1992. pp. 281-282.

Vermeulen, Frans. *Prisma*. The Netherlands, Emryss bv Publishers, 2002. p.937.

Sepia

Abstract:

This is a case of a woman who fears exposure. *I am always looking, watching anticipating things that were going to expose me. Maybe that is like the squid going into the shark's mouth?*

Keywords:

Depression. Smoke and mirrors. Hiding. *Sepia* subterfuge and escape. 'Delusions of persecution'. 'Delusions of abandonment'. Neglect. Independence and dependence.

D.O.B. 1955. Single mother.

First Consult: October 2006.

Presenting Issue:

- Fibroid (no physical symptoms of excessive bleeding)
- Premenstrual tension for ten days preceding her menses
- Feels wired and manic
- Wretched
- Angry
- Tired
- Unable to sleep
- Unable to go out of the house and face people

- Crippling depression
- Overwhelmed with managing the house and her child
- Only starts to feel better once the menses have stopped

Her biggest concern is her inability to leave the house in the ten days preceding her menses. She is terrified of seeing people.

My life is a masked life. If I have a facade I can do this. I am hiding. I am always behind a smoke and mirrors facade of being socially perfect. I am socially conventional but inside I am a fragmented person. She is overwhelmed and crippled by an inability to cope emotionally, mentally, or physically with her duties as a single mother. This is only crippling in the premenstrual period. She feels *so sick that it is not possible to function.* She feels confused to the point of feeling like she *can't understand even the most basic things. I have a lot of fears that I can't do this. I can't live up to the challenge of being a single parent. I need to hide so that others and myself can't see myself. If I go out when I am like this then it is obvious to everyone around me that I am not coping. Every time my period finishes I then feel like I have to start again and rebuild who I am as a person.*

Prescription: *Sepia* 30 C. 1/dose a week. I initially gave her *Sepia* daily but she rang me three days after the consultation complaining that she was worse. I dropped the remedy back to a weekly dose and I have kept her on this dose for eighteen months. She is extremely sensitive and her premenstrual depression has been so crippling that any higher dose, or higher frequency, has resulted in aggravations.

Case Analysis: I used the following key points and headings in analyzing this case.

Rubric-repertorisation

1. **Theme**
2. **Follow-up Consultations**

3. **Materia Medica**
4. *Striking*, or *Peculiar* **Signs and Symptoms; Organon 153**
5. *How, Why,* and *When* **Causations – the 'Never-well-since-event'.**

1. Rubric-repertorisation

- *Delusions: people: seeing people*: sep.
- *Delusions: sick: being: work; and for this reason will not*: sep.
- *Delusions: emptiness; of:* **SEP**.
- *Delusions: understand: not understand anything; she could*: sep.[1] 1.
- *Delusions: air: suspended in the air*: sep. [1] 1. [This *Delusion* rubric pertains to feeling ungrounded or not able to deal with realistic practical matters in life.]
- *Delusions: anxious*: sep.
- *Delusions: learn: anew everything she wished to do; she would have to learn*: sep.[1] 1.
- *Delusions: laughed at and mocked at; being*: sep.
- *Mind: abstraction of mind*: **SEP**.
- *Mind: company: aversion to: sight of people; avoids the*: Sep.
- *Mind: confusion of mind: menses: before*: Sep.
- *Mind: duty: aversion to: domestic duty*: SEP.
- *Mind: duty: too much sense of duty*: Sep.
- *Mind: fear: approaching; of: others; of*: sep.
- *Mind: mania: menses: before*: sep. [1] 2. [cimic.]
- *Mind: mania: menses: during*: Sep.
- *Mind: secretive*: Sep.

- *Mind*: *suicidal disposition*: *despair, from*: *miserable existence; about his*: *Sep.* [2] 2. [ruta].
- *Sleep*: *disturbed*: *menses*: *before*: agg.: sep.
- *Sleep*: *dreaming*: *menses*: *during*: agg.: sep.

2. Theme

Sepia is a homoeopathic remedy derived from a sea creature. *Sepia* is derived from the ink that cuttlefish squirt out when they sense that danger is present. If cuttlefish feel hemmed in or threatened, they need to quickly create a subterfuge so they can escape. The theme of escape and subterfuge runs through the presentation of the emotional, mental, and physical complaints. The *Delusion* rubric: *seeing people*, can be interpreted as one's feelings of persecution and potential threat, or it can be interpreted as a sign that one will be saved. *Sepia* fear being exposed. They feel they need to protect themselves from potential threat. *Sepia* fear being looked at and mocked. *Sepia* alternate between illusions or idealized perceptions of hope that they will be saved, and psychological 'delusions of persecution' that they will be attacked or persecuted. The duel interpretation of the *Delusion* rubric: *seeing people* highlights an inherent polarity within their psyche. The theme is dependence versus independence. When *Sepia* are sick, it is easy for them to feel anxious and ungrounded and unable *to understand anything*. *Sepia* appear extremely foggy and confused when they are sick (especially with all hormonal changes). This is indicative of their psyche somatically mirroring the murky ink of the cuttlefish. The *Delusion* rubric: *seeing people* highlights an inherent polarity within their psyche. *Sepia* see people who are their saviors and they see people who are potential attackers. Often the distinction will be determined by hormonal changes and periodicity.

1. Denial: *Delusion* rubric: *people*: *seeing people*: sep. *Delusion* rubric: *doctors come; three*: sep. [1] 1. *Delusion*

rubric: *witches; believes in*: sep. [1] 1. *Delusion* rubric: *calls: someone calls: sleep; someone calls him during*: **SEP**. [3] 1. [These rubrics can pertain to *doctors* or *witches* or *specters and ghosts* coming to save them, or illusions of people coming to *mock* them.] *Delusion* rubric: *fancy, illusions of*: sep. *Delusion* rubric: *visions, has*: sep.

2. Forsaken: *Delusion* rubric: *people: seeing people*: sep. [This rubric can pertain to perceptions of saviors or attackers.] *Delusion* rubric: *laughed at and mocked at; being*: sep. *Delusion* rubric: *poor; he is*: Sep. *Delusion* rubric: *robbed, is going to be*: sep. *Delusion* rubric: *starve: family will*: Sep. *Delusion* rubric: *unfortunate, he is*: sep. [This rubric can pertain to feeling abandoned, or feelings of depression and failure.] *Delusion* rubric: *air: suspended in the air*: sep. [1] 1. *Delusion* rubric: *alone, being: graveyard; alone in a*: sep. *Delusion* rubric: *neglected: he or she is neglected*: sep. *Delusion* rubric: *poisoned: he: has been*: sep.

3. Causation: NONE.

4. Depression: *Delusion* rubric: *anxious*: sep. *Delusion* rubric: *understand: not understand anything; she could*: sep. [1] 1. *Delusion* rubric: *unfortunate, he is*: sep. *Delusion* rubric: *emptiness; of*: **SEP**. *Delusion* rubric: *learn: anew everything she wished to do; she would have to learn*: sep. [1] 1. *Delusion* rubric: *run: backward; he was chased and had to run*: sep. [1] 1. [This rubric pertains to ineffectual actions.]

5. Resignation: *Delusion* rubric: *sick: being*: sep. *Delusion* rubric: *strain herself; she could easily*: sep. [1] 1. *Delusion* rubric: *faint; he would*: sep. *Delusion* rubric: *sick: being: work; and for this reason will not*: sep.

3. Follow-up Consultations

First Follow-up Consultation:

- Feels less cloudy
- More open to others and the world. Not feeling so threatened but feels more aware of how exhausted she actually is
- She also feels like she is aware of her depression more

My Conclusion: The fog of the *Sepia* confusion is lifting and she is aware of how she feels emotionally, mentally and physically.

Second Follow-up Consultation:

- Her depression is considerably better
- Feels more aware of herself
- More aware of how she needs space and freedom

This consultation is a good counselling session focusing on her constitutional profile. I give her a copy of my book *A Homeopathic Guide to Partnership and Compatibility* so she can read the profile of *Sepia* as the threatened cuttlefish swimming in an ocean.

Third Follow-up Consultation:

- Less depression and her premenstrual tension is manageable
- She has started to realize she needs to get back out into her garden
- She has started to develop her creative side and has got back into her craft work
- She reports she feels very relieved to understand that if she creates space and creative freedoms and independence in her life, they will contribute to her feeling less threatened about society and potential new partners

My book has explained her whole relationship history; from the profile of the *Sepia* harridan, to the *Sepia* woman alive in her garden, to the *Sepia* single mother trapped and depressed at home, feeling alone and isolated. She now understands her dilemma in relationships; her need for space, and her need for support. She also understands the reasons behind her crippling, overwhelming depression which has trapped her when the support in the relationship becomes over-controlling.

She has managed to change the constraints of her life so she is able to have more creative freedom and space for herself as a healthy *Sepia* woman.

This case is a good example of how understanding the nature of a constitutional remedy picture has helped a patient decide to take a new direction in their life which is more harmonious with their constitutional remedy profile.

When she read my book, *A Homeopathic Guide to Partnership and Compatibility,* and the profile picture of *Sepia* which I have used as the Materia medica, below, it greatly eased her internal distress. I have found that if I give *Sepia* patients understanding of themselves as a threatened sea creature, the understanding of the fear which they struggle with all of her life then becomes the first step towards compassion for themselves. Self-acceptance and understanding then allows a patient to construct their life so they can avoid internal and external conflict.

4. Materia Medica

I have used my own book for the Materia medica. The simillimum will only be *Sepia* if the patient has a need to create dependency and a need to create independence. My portrayal of *Sepia* in *A Homeopathic Guide to Partnership and Compatibility* is the only Materia medica which emphasizes this dilemma.

Sepia present with converse polarities. The healthy *Sepia* is self-actualized, and the unhealthy, ungrounded *Sepia* struggles to realize independence: the theme is dependence versus independence.

• Healthy *Sepia* are nonconformist

- Need to find meaning and purpose in life – through career, occupation, or creative outlet
- Freedom is crucial to feeling happy and secure
- The *Sepia* love of space and freedom is often expressed in a love of dance, movement, or exercise
- Often feel better if they are busy and active; even feel better if they rush around and clean the house
- Healthy *Sepia* are creative and passionate
- Need physical and emotional space to feel alive
- All gender role expectations of wife and mother will threaten *Sepia* women
- Unhealthy *Sepia* are irritable and defeated
- When they feel distraught, can often present as typical nagging harridans
- Unhealthy *Sepia* look and feel overburdened and exhausted
- React to restrictions with anger
- Feel emotionally disconnected if they feel overburdened
- The cuttlefish need to create subterfuge has parallels in *Sepia* feeling cut off and detached
- Premenstrual tension, anger, and weepy depression are all worse if *Sepia* feel overburdened
- Indifferent to everything when depressed and passionately creative when healthy
- A *Sepia* woman who is able to walk away from family is healthy. *Sepia* often stay feeling overburdened out of a strong sense of duty; this is the type of self-suppression that will eventually lead the *Sepia* woman into crippling depression. It is, of course, far healthier for *Sepia* to know that some independence will prevent the need to walk away in the first place. [Lalor]

The Emotional Need for Freedom within *Sepia*

Sepia is the only constitution that I discuss exclusively from a female bias. *Sepia* women need independence and freedom in relationships if they are to remain healthy. The difference between the healthy and unhealthy *Sepia* women is so marked it is crucial for *Sepia* women to understand their emotional need for freedom. In my clinical practice I see far more unhealthy *Sepia* women than unhealthy *Sepia* men simply because it is far easier for a man in this society to walk away from family commitment than it is for a woman. *Sepia* needs to be unhindered physically and emotionally to be able to be healthy. Successful relationships for *Sepia* have to be with a partner who can allow them independence; otherwise, they sink into depression. If they are controlled or dominated they become ungrounded and out of touch with themselves. The homeopathic remedy *Sepia* is derived from the ink cuttlefish squirt out when they sense that danger is present. If cuttlefish feel hemmed in or threatened they need to quickly create a subterfuge so they can escape. Cuttlefish like to swim alone; they do not collect in groups. *Sepia* also need to be able to go off and swim alone. Their need for independence and space is essential.

The Emotional Legacy of the *Sepia* Woman

Sepia women feel they do not have many successful relationships. In relationships they struggle to try to balance their need for a career with their husband's and children's needs. Even if *Sepia* is not married the expectations and demands of a partner are seen as a struggle. *Sepia* will feel they are trying to be all things to all people. This, of course, means they will feel absolutely exhausted and worn down. *Sepia* is striving for her own self-realization and, in her mind, children and a partner can be seen as a hindrance in that process. It is not that she does not love; it is she does not love with the same dependency so many women project on to their children and husband. *Sepia* do not identify themselves first and foremost as mother and wife, and feeling forced to love and give makes

Sepia women feel the need to escape. The *Sepia* woman is grounded in herself, but only if she is emancipated from the passive role of wife and mother.

Sepia become distraught in relationships when they feel controlled or trapped. An unhealthy *Sepia* woman will turn into a complaining, nagging harridan. *Sepia* suffer from terrible fatigue and exhaustion when they feel threatened. The *Sepia* depression is particularly visible before their menses, and this is when *Sepia* are most likely to express feelings of being threatened or hemmed in. Their restlessness is so extreme they can become completely disconnected from themselves and their family. There is such confusion in their depression it gets translated as complete apathy, and they cannot find their grounding. Premenstrual *Sepia* have such strong emotional extremes they can literally be laughing one moment, crying the next, or imploding or exploding with rage the next. [Lalor]

5. *Striking*, or *Peculiar* Signs and Symptoms; Organon 153

Eighth Follow-up Consultation:

I concentrate entirely on videotaping follow-up consultations. I commence videos after the patient has taken the remedy for some time. In particular, I am always vigilant of any new trauma because it is at that point I find the meaning and relevance of every *Delusion* rubric. The prescription has been *Sepia* 30 C. 1/dose a week. After this consultation, I increased the dose to *Sepia* 30 C. 1/dose a day. The weekly dose has held her premenstrual tension in check and she has continued to improve for the last eighteen months. Trauma will bring to the surface the psychodynamic conflicts which match the *Delusion* rubrics. The following transcript is taken from a video of the eighth consultation. I only ever increase dose or frequency when a new traumatic event in a patient's life sparks off old underlying trauma. I chose this transcript because it explains the *Delusion* layer of *Sepia*. *Sepia* feel constantly like they are being *chased and had to run backwards*. This rubric indicates how *Sepia* feel exposed and threatened, always in dread of a perceived attack. If attacked or threatened, they are forced to run backwards. This *Delusion* rubric gives us great insight into the crippling depression and hopelessness *Sepia* suffers. She says, *I avoid seeing people. Even with you now I feel like you should be able to feel it. If I go out and try and fake it I feel so out of touch with who I am. I'd rather just sit with who I am than fake it. Even with my son I think there has to be some way for me to be who I am. This week I stayed in bed for three days. I felt exhausted, flat, unable to move.*

What I am particularly interested in teaching is the moment in each case in which the *Delusion* rubrics come into play. The first consult is often on the conscious level. In the first consult I like to be able to see the development of the *Delusion* rubrics even though at the time of the initial prescription I might not know fully *'how, why, or where'* they developed. In the subsequent consults I get to see through the homoeopathic effects of the simillimum into the subconscious and unconscious of how patients have constructed their life. When the patient takes their simillimum, i.e. the remedy which matches their disturbance, I have to see proof, in the subsequent consultations, of the layers of how they have constructed their story, or patterning which governs their actions and perceptions of the world.

She says in this consult, *now I feel like I have stepped out from that illusion. I feel stripped bare. I feel really exposed. Everything is very plain, like taking off rose-colored glasses.* This is the unveiling of the delusion layer of *Sepia*. The theme of escape and subterfuge runs through the presentation of *Sepia*. The presenting trauma in her life, which she talks about in the transcript below, is how to resolve her romantic involvement with an old lover. The effect of taking the remedy has meant she no longer hides herself in the smoke of her own life. Depression is a state in which the patient shuts down and hides from their feelings. Depression is a suppression of feelings. In case management, it is important to know how the delusion layer will be stripped away. We have to know the process and meaning of the delusion layers in homoeopathic case management. If she describes the process as, *like taking off rose-colored glasses*, then I need to be there to help her feel protected. Because they are a sea creature, *Sepia* will feel very vulnerable and exposed when they emerge out of their fog and depression. She expresses this fear of exposure when she tells us: *I say I have been in a sort of a fantasy land, out of touch with reality, but one of things that I have struggled with all my life is that I am hyper-vigilant that I am always looking, watching anticipating things that were going to expose me but not hyper-vigilant to the things that were actually going to harm me. Maybe that is like the squid going into the shark's mouth.*

Question: Do you remember a while ago that we were talking about the dreams you were having where you would wake up covered by a dolphin? The feeling that you're talking about now is that similar?

Ahh, yes. Like this is just reality. Cold, wet, boring. [Makes a gester of being squashed under a dolphin.] *Heavy, flat reality.*

The dreams that you are having now, are they like that?

No. The David dreams [ex-partner] *are shuffling though real life events that actually happened, that I didn't see realistically at the time, or that I did but I let my anxieties and panic distract me from them and kept going anyway, and now it's like I am reliving them. I am shuffling through the memory bank, seeing him realistically for what he is doing, who he really is. It's like reality shuffling by me in my subconscious, then I wake up from them and I am relieved that it is not reality. But I have this really flat feeling, like this is what he was really doing, what was actually happening. It is like once I had one insight into who he was I had to go – back though the years when I had hoped it was otherwise, or even blamed myself maybe it was me? I am not even attributing blame now I can just see it happening in a realistic way.*

It is flat and boring and it is not romantic or idealized. I am having other dreams as well really confronting dreams in which I am walking down the street and an ordinary guy in a blue shorts and tee shirt walks up to me and fumbles with a knife and stabs me and I see it all happening in the second. It is just about to happen and there is nothing I can do about it. I am waking up every night having some really confronting dream of harm or violence.

That is always done to you?

Also to my son. It is almost like in the dream I am floating along la la la and then right there, bang, something really horrible happens, bang, and I can feel the knife go into my solar plexus. It is just like I am going along, and then someone can have mean intent to me but I see it just as it is too late. I do wonder if I haven't been in some sort of fantasy land, and I haven't been realistic about real harm that has been in close proximity to me and maybe to my son. I think a lot of what I have gone through it quite negative and destructive. I was in close range to someone who really was heartless.

And taking away the house, students and sitting there with Peter, [her son] just the two of you, how does that feel?

I feel stripped bare. It's just me now. The dreams I have been having of going along and then something really violent and shocking happening, I wake up from them stripped bare, just me. I don't have anything to buffer me from reality. It is just me. Even when I walk down the street now, I am looking out for danger. I feel like I am much more realistic now as to what people can be like in real life, the harm that can be there. Sitting alone in the house with myself and Peter at school, it feels very flat, very ordinary. I question my motivation about everything. Why do I care if I clean it or not, all the memorabilia I am going through; I ask why do I keep moving it around, why do I care? I even question the value of keeping photos. Some photos, why would we keep all of those photos. I have things from my school days, and they almost make me feel sick to look at them. Why not get rid of anything? Nothing I have got is worth anything, nothing could I sell. I have nothing to insure, and when you don't have a home and possessions around you, all I have is me and my child and some furniture and books. I have found this more confronting because in the other house where I had all those students that I had to churn out a meal for I was living way beyond my socio-economic means. Like what we talked about, the smoke and mirrors. I think that since Peter was born, I just kept trying to think of ways to create the illusion that we were a family living in middle class Australia. And that is not what is happening for me. It is not who I am. Now I feel like I have stepped out from that illusion. I feel stripped bare. I feel really exposed.

Is that what you meant when you said before that the depression is palpable, that people can feel it?

I avoid seeing people. Even with you now, I feel like you should be able to feel it. If I go out and try and fake it, I feel so out of touch with who I am. I'd rather just sit with who I am than fake it, even with my son. I think there has to be some way for me to be who I am. This week I stayed in bed for three days. I felt exhausted, flat, unable to move. It is a worry for me to feel like this because nothing much gives me pleasure. It feels like for me that is the definition of depression. When I am stripped bare of everything, I am not sure of what I want to do. I knew I wanted to come here today and see you, but any other day of the week I feel quite lost. I am surprised that this is what was on the other side because when I last cancelled the appointment with you I was exhilarated. I am getting out of here, I am simplifying everything, I was lightening my load. There is no escape anymore. One superhuman effort after another, after another, that is the story of my life. Even the circumstances of Peter's conception up, until very recently I had a very romantic version of who his father was, that it was love child.

When you first came to see me you said your whole life was about this smoke and mirrors and about escape?

Avoiding being exposed. It is all gone now.

And now you are sitting in exposure.

The stage lights are off. The smoke machines are turned off. The mirrors are laid flat. There is not one prop around me, it is just me alone. I use the analogy of addiction like I am going cold turkey because part of me believed the illusion as well. I thought I was happy. I thought I liked being that busy and exhausted.

Feeling so exposed, do you feel safe?

I don't feel safe with people. I feel safe with you. I feel safe with my son. But no, I woke up this morning thinking, no I don't actually feel safe. In the dreams they are saying to me, you don't feel safe on the street. Just walking along the street in your favorite red dress. I say I have been in a sort of a fantasy land, out of touch with reality but one of things that I have struggled with all my life is that I am hyper-vigilant, that I am always looking. Always watching and anticipating things that were going to expose me, but not hyper-vigilant to the things that were actually going to harm me. Maybe that is like the squid going into the shark's mouth? Now all I see is the sharks. Now what I realize is that I was sleeping with the shark for four years. He didn't have my best interest at heart. It is interesting when I think back about that dolphin dream. The dolphin landed on me like that, but the dream I was having when the dolphin landed on me was I was in the Garden of Eden. It was all happy, beautiful fruit trees all covered in fruit, and then bang – there it was. The dolphin was jumping from one level to another, then it landed on me.

Everything is very plain, like taking off rose-colored glasses.

Are you still seeing your therapist?

I couldn't sit there any longer. I started to tell her the things that I am telling you today. Finally, I started to tell her about taking off the rose-colored glasses and she said, I don't think things are that dire, and I couldn't sit there anymore. I felt betrayed. I had used the smoke and mirrors analogy with her, and when I finally told her how confronting I was finding sole parenting, and in fact being a mother, in the last fifteen minutes of the session with her she didn't want it to be true. I feel relieved I don't have to keep going into that room. I thought if I went there long enough I could crank up the mirrors, and if I worked long enough at that sort of therapy, even for two years after the separation, I could have some great insight that would shed light on the problem with David. Two different sorts of therapy: I have done one for ten years before Peter was born, and then six years, and part of me thinks it only took me so far. I mean, when I first came to see you I was ill, I could barely function.

After I had videotaped her, she reacted intensely to the exposure and asked me to destroy the tapes. This is not an unusual response from a remedy which is a sea creature. Exposure and being seen is very difficult, which I should have realized.

In the following consultations, the patient is extremely well. She is feeling no longer overwhelmed or shut down. When she says: *I mean when I first came to see you I was ill, I could barely function,* it was not an exaggeration. Now her premenstrual tension is barely noticeable. In this case in particular, I have been able to develop a lot of understanding about how the fish feel when I have frightened them snorkeling in the ocean. I have also understood how exposed *Sepia* feel by being videotaped.

Key Words Used in the Consult:

- Hiding
- Illusion smoke and mirrors
- Stripped bare, exposed
- Lost
- No escape
- Superhuman effort
- The mirrors are laid flat
- Alone
- Isolated
- No one bears witness
- I don't feel safe on the street, not safe with people

Themes of the Sea Creatures[29]

- Feeling alone and isolation: *There is no escape anymore. One superhuman effort after another, after another. That is the story of my life.*

- A need for solitude versus feeling exposed when they are alone: *There is not one prop around me, it is just me alone. I use the analogy of addiction like I am going cold turkey because part of me believed the illusion as well. I thought I was happy. I thought I liked being that busy and exhausted.*

- Feeling detached, lost in the fog [ink] of their own creation: *When I am stripped bare of everything I am not sure of what I want to do.*

- Feeling spied on and observed or watched: *What I have struggled with all my life is that I am hyper-vigilant, that I was always looking, watching anticipating things that were going to expose me.*

- Feeling unprotected: *Maybe that is like the squid going into the shark's mouth. Now all I see is the sharks. Even when I*

---

29 *Corallium, Sepia, Ambra grisea, Murex, Spongia, Elaterium, Homarus.*

walk down the street now I am looking out for danger.

- Need to hide at home, or in gardens, or in creative work: *I think that since Peter was born, I just kept trying to think of ways to create the illusion that we were a family living in middle class Australia. And that is not what is happening for me. It is not who I am.*

- Feeling vulnerable to attack: *It is almost like in the dream I am floating along la la la and then right there, bang, something really horrible happens.*

- Dependency versus their need for independence and freedom to swim alone: *It is interesting when I think back about that dolphin dream. The dolphin landed on me like that, but the dream I was having when the dolphin landed on me was I was in the Garden of Eden. It was all happy, beautiful fruit trees all covered in fruit and then bang there it was. The dolphin was jumping from one level to another, then it landed on me.*

Sepia have the *Delusion* rubric: *something else comes from above which is pressing the chest.* [1] 1. Her dolphin dream is a recurring dream. Sometimes the dolphin is smothering her, while in other dreams the dolphin is making love to her and she is in the Garden of Eden. *Sepia* have recurring themes in their dreams of being raped and attacked, or amorously aroused. If a patient refers to their dreams, then it is important to include those dreams in the rubric-repertorisation. The problem with using the *Dream* rubrics in the repertory is that it is often impossible to find the specific dream rubric which matches a patient's *peculiar* dream. Dreams mirror the subconscious and unconscious mind. A patient's memory will reside in their conscious mind, and it is more than likely that the patient is aware and able to verbalize their trauma. If the patient is not aware of the memory they are trying to avoid, the memory will often reside in their subconscious or unconscious mind. Their memory block is often a complicated system of psychological avoidances to cover up their mental and emotional trauma.

If I can't find a particular *Dream* rubric, I use the *Delusion* rubrics. If the patient has a psychological delusion, then the patient also has a subconscious or unconscious memory of the delusional stance, and this memory will often manifest in recurring dreams.

- *Dreams: ghosts: fighting with ghosts:* sep.
- *Dreams: rape: threats of rape:* sep.
- *Dreams: rousing the patient:* Sep.
- *Dreams: pursued, being: run backwards, must:* sep. [1] 1.
- *Dreams: amorous: erections: with:* sep.

Her dream highlights the conflict between the need to be dependent versus the need for independence: *It is interesting when I think back about that dolphin dream. The dolphin landed on me like that, but the dream I was having when the dolphin landed on me was I was in the Garden of Eden. It was all happy, beautiful fruit trees all covered in fruit and then bang, there it was. The dolphin was jumping from one level to another, then it landed on me.*

This dream is a good example of the *Striking*, or *Peculiar* paradox of *Sepia* relationships and of their life in general. Dependency in relationship is associated with being smothered, like when the dolphin landed on her. Dependency on the homoeopathic practitioner brings to the surface the same dilemma; this is why *Sepia* have the conflicting *Mind* rubrics: *fear doctors,* and *aversion to homoeopathy,* versus the *Delusion* rubrics: *three doctors come,* and *believes in witches.*

Dependency on the homoeopathic practitioner brings to the surface their 'delusions of hypochondria'. The underlying, psychodynamic, somatic feedback loop that *Sepia* are embroiled in is a negative reinforcement and it is self-deprecating. *Sepia* undermine their power to support themselves financially in this world. *Sepia* were undermined as infants; they in turn, then undermine themselves by not taking their own energy seriously. *Sepia* have been unsupported and they, in turn, struggle to believe their own body will support them. This is why *Sepia* have numerous hypochondriac *Delusion* rubrics alluding to not being strong enough to work. *Sepia* have the *Delusion* rubric: *he would faint*, and the *Delusion* rubric: *she could easily strain herself*, and the *Delusion* rubric: *being sick and for this reason will not work*.

6. *How*, *Why*, and *When* Causations – the 'Never-well-since-event'

The homoeopathic practitioner will be viewed as their 'God' who is able to save them. This is the psychodynamic application and relevance of the *Delusion* rubric: *three doctors come*. *Sepia* disproportionately over-react to their illness; this is why they need not one, but *three doctors* to attend to them. *Sepia* are also listed in the *Mind* rubrics: *fear doctors,* and *aversion to homoeopathy*. It is normal to struggle with the acceptance of disease and death, but *Sepia* struggle with their *dependence* on their health practitioner. *Sepia* disproportionately depend on their health practitioner and conversely react negatively to becoming dependant on their practitioner. The essence is the internal struggle for independence. *Sepia* are listed in the *Mind* rubric: *antagonism with self*. *Sepia* struggle to survive unsupported in their life in general. Conversely, they struggle to *allow* themselves to be supported. A *Delusion* rubric is only used if you can see a misinterpretation of reality which prevents the person from making a correct assessment of reality. The *Delusion* rubrics of the psychological 'delusions of grandeur' become relevant in case-taking when the patient presents with an unrealistic belief that they can depend on someone else to save them. The psychodynamic relevance of the *Delusion* rubric: *three doctors come*, and the *Delusion* rubric: *illusions of fancy*, is that it indicates an exaggerated belief in cure, as well as an exaggerated assessment of the gravity of their illness. If there is an exaggerated belief in cure or need, then underneath it are numerous *Delusion* rubrics of being forsaken. If there is an exaggerated assessment of the gravity of their illness, then the fear of losing support will also be exaggerated. This is why *Sepia* have numerous rubrics pertaining to persecution and abandonment. The most potent is the *Delusion* rubric: *he or she is neglected.* *Sepia* feel ungrounded and unsupported in life, particularly around their inability to survive financially in the world. *Sepia* have the *Delusion* rubrics: *he is poor,* and *family will starve.* The *Delusion* rubrics: *family will starve, going to be robbed,* and *he or she is neglected,* are *Delusion* rubrics which indicate psychological 'delusions of deprivation'. In *Sepia,* the psychodynamic struggle to survive in the world and become a self-actualized person, has its causation in neglect and starvation as a baby. *Sepia* struggle their whole life to have their needs met. The psychodynamic trauma inside *Sepia* which undermines them, or leaves them floundering in *starving emptiness,* is that they do not believe they can have their needs met in a relationship, or in life, because they literally do not know how to verbalize or understand those needs. *Sepia* have the *Delusion* rubrics: *she would have to learn anew everything she wished to do,* and *she could not understand anything.* Both of these *Delusion* rubrics indicate that the 'never-well-since-event' in a *Sepia* case has its foundation in the early, pre-verbal years of their life. If the first needs of the infant are not met, then the infant presumes that their needs will remain unmet for the rest of their lives. It was not until the last consultation with this woman that she told me that her mother had suffered from terribly crippling post-natal depression. Her mother was often not able to feed her, and would leave her in the backyard for long periods of time unattended. She said, *now I understand why when it comes to asking for what I need in life that I feel completely speechless. I am unable to ever voice how I feel or what I want in any relationship or in any work situation. I always feel like I am going to be smothered, and that I will never have my most basic needs met. I have always felt like I didn't even*

*know how to ask. I must have spent long periods of time crying
and alone. I must have given up in the end and stopped crying.
Now I understand why I let everyone control me like they are
better than me, and why I always think I can never do what
they have been able to do. Even in my relationship, I never
felt I deserved or could even ask for the financial support that
most single women receive. I have not got a single penny from
his dad* (her son's) *at all. I was never fed or looked after as a
baby.*

Case Analysis

Sepia are confused and unrealized in their emotional
independence, and in particular in their financial independence.
The *Mind* rubric: *antagonism with self*, indicates the degree
to which *Sepia* feel unsupported, even within themselves and
towards themselves. Interestingly, *Sepia* do not have any
psychological 'delusions of original sin'. Their internal battle
is about whether to accept and trust the support offered from
the world, not about whether *they* have personally caused the
unsupported dilemma they find themselves in. *Sepia* struggle
to acknowledge any wrong doing. The biggest undermining
fear which causes *Sepia* pain is the fear that others will laugh at
them, particularly when they don't know how to do something.
Sepia have the *Delusion* rubric: *being laughed and mocked at,*
and *she could not understand anything.* [1] 1. *Sepia* have the
Delusion rubric: *suspended in the air.* This rubric should not
be taken literally; rather it is indicative of the psychodynamic
trauma within *Sepia* which is caused by lack of support. *Sepia*
often appear unable to enact effective change. *Sepia* have the
Delusion rubric: *he was chased and had to run backwards.*
[1] 1. The psychodynamic interpretation of this rubric indicates
that *Sepia* feel as if they can always be potentially defeated.
Furthermore, all effort to enact change [*escape*] is self-
defeating because it is ineffective [*backwards*]. *Sepia* are often
noted for their confusion and inactivity if they are depressed.

Their depression is not the cause of their confusion. Their depression arises as a result of feeling defeated in their attempts to enact change. *Sepia* have the *Delusion* rubric: *delusions of emptiness*. *Sepia,* aside from feeling empty and unsupported, literally feel crushed if they are over-controlled. *Sepia* have the *Delusion* rubric: *something else from above which is pressing the chest.* [1] 1.

This woman is now employed. She now works outside in a kitchen garden which she has creative control over. She is financially independent. She no longer suffers from premenstrual tension. I have consulted with her once, in 2009, when she was feeling overwhelmed by her father's illness (lung cancer). I did not prescribe any homoeopathics because she only felt like she needed to take some B vitamins to help her with energy. I agreed because her tiredness and sadness was in proportion to the dynamic that was happening and was an expected response to his illness. When she was consulting me, her consultations were paid for by a benefactor. The owner of the kitchen garden is the benefactor who paid for her consultations with me. This arrangement constitutes a 'supported independence' which is harmonious and sympathetic to *Sepia* and with their struggle between dependence and independence. Her benefactors, after having read my book, *A Homeopathic Guide to Partnership and Compatibility,* understand *Sepia.*

She said in her last consultation with me, *it is funny Liz, but now I am financially independent and I can now pay for my own sessions with you. But now I feel like I am well, and don't need you anymore. I can now work and have control over my own life.*

Bibliography

Lalor, Liz. *A Homeopathic Guide to Partnership and Compatibility.* Berkeley, California, North Atlantic Books, 2004, pp. 69-70. p. 184-185.

Schroyens, Frederik. M.D. *Synthesis.* London, Homeopathic Book Publishers, 1997.

Thuja

Abstract:

This is a case of a man who is not sure whether it is Jesus or the devil who is influencing him. *Thuja* is the only remedy listed in the *Delusion* rubric: *divided into two parts, which part he has possession on waking; and could not tell.*

Keywords:

Anxiety. Weakness. Fragility. 'Delusions of grandeur'. 'Delusions of original sin'.

Case Notes

First Consult: October 2008.

D.O.B. 1947.

Occupation: Christian Pastor.

Presenting Issue

- Physical weakness and exhaustion
- Pervasive sadness and crippling anxiety
- Frequent urination
- Food sensitivities

Mental and Emotional Symptoms of the Case

- He describes himself as having clinical depression.
- Pervasive sadness.
- Afraid of people. He will come into the church via the back door in order to avoid running into his parishioners.
- Fearful of parishioners finding out he is scared of people.
- Fearful of the legal responsibility he has as the parishioner of the church. He is terrified of a parishioner claiming against the church for injury. He has severe anxiety attacks, especially at night in regards to potential future public liability claims.
- Fearful of bureaucracy. He has dreams about being responsible for insurance claims.
- He is finishing his seminary thesis, and struggles with writing because he has learning difficulties.
- Has suffered with crippling depression and Chronic Fatigue Syndrome which contributed to him dropping out of society and moving to the hills to live in the 1970's.
- He was a vegetarian in the 1970's, but his wife insists on cooking meat which he doesn't like eating.
- He suffers with anxiety after he eats and is often in pain with gastritis.
- He hides his past life when he practiced vegetarianism, yoga, and meditation, from his parishioners because he is afraid of what they would think.
- He hides his psychic abilities from the church.
- He believes he is able to hear God's direction, and is following God's instructions by joining the church.
- He left society for twenty years and lived in isolation in the hills. He was subsequently rejected by his mother and father.
- He feels that he was being punished for having abandoned

his two young children when he left his first wife. He feels that God has forgiven him his sins because he has contact with his children. He feels that by taking care of his step-daughter he is making up for not having looked after his own children.

- He feels he is a failure because he is always depressed and overcome by crippling panic attacks. He thinks he will not be able to succeed at his role of pastor of a church because he is fearful of people.
- He feels that he is too weak to be able to deal with the stress and fear of running the business side of a parish church. He is terrified of dealing with public liability and the possibility of a parishioner suing him.

Physical Symptoms of the Case

- Frequent urination up to 6-8 times at night
- Frequency during the day, approximately hourly
- Thirsty (not diabetic)
- Extreme sensitivity to foods
- Anxiety after eating
- < Sugar, which causes bleeding gums
- < Fructose
- < Milk, lactose intolerant
- < Spices
- < Creamy sauces
- < Cheese
- < Mayonnaise
- Signs of Irritable Bowel Syndrome, (IBS)
- Belching
- Indigestion
- Bloating

- Difficulty swallowing
- Hot hands at night
- History of Chronic Fatigue Syndrome, (CFS)
- Adrenal gland exhaustion
- Feels weak and easily overcome with extreme tiredness
- Extreme sensitivity to chemicals

Notable Key Aspects of the Case

The patient was born into a wealthy well established family. He went to boarding school in Australia with Prince Charles. (He tells me this to highlight the fact that he was born into a socially prominent family.) His father was a barrister and his mother a well known socialite. Preceding his birth, his mother lost twin girls who died after birth in the hospital. His mother wanted a girl and was grief stricken that he was born a boy. She subsequently dressed him in girl's clothes until he was five years of age. His mother rejected him as a young child and made it clear she had never wanted a boy.

At six or seven years of age he was exposed to pictures of nuclear bombing on the television. He became crippled, and catatonic with fear of being annihilated, and has been classified as clinically depressed ever since. He has suffered suicidal feelings since his childhood, when he was overcome with guilt from seeing pictures of starving children on television, in a campaign called *Feed the Children*.

Before he saw the photos of starving children, he described himself as extremely fat. He told me that shortly after seeing the photos he gave up drinking milk and has been extremely thin ever since. He does not like it if he puts on any weight. His food sensitivities started after he gave up drinking milk, but he does not attribute his food sensitivities to experiencing the trauma of the pictures of starving children. He believes he always had food sensitivities, and this is what had made him fat as a child. He stopped eating after seeing the campaign *Feed the Children*. He still suffers with extreme fears of violence and, is extremely uncomfortable with stereotypical masculine men. His main reason for consulting me was his food sensitivities and his anxiety. He suffers from anxiety about being sued in his role as a parish priest and is struggling to embrace the role and responsibilities that the job entails. As a child he was intensely disgusted by his mother. He described her dress sense as being sexually inappropriate and *in the vein of Tina Turner style of dressing*. His mother would walk around the house naked and would go to the toilet in front of him as a child; he found this repugnant. He married a girl who he got pregnant at an early age, and had two children. His father was physically violent, and emotionally abusive towards his mother. He left his wife and children because she was schizophrenic and physically violent towards him. He escaped into living a hermit's life in the hills. He has been estranged from his family since he left his wife. He argued with his father about his lack of success. He has recurring dreams of being alone and terrified in a city, with no money. In the dream he eventually finds his way home and is not allowed into the family home. He wakes up in terror when he realizes that he is not able to enter the family home. He is on a disability pension from the government, and has suffered with clinical depression and Chronic Fatigue Syndrome. He is now finishing off his studies to become a Christian pastor. He has practiced yoga and meditation in the past, but joined the church because he wanted to gain spiritual recognition in a *more socially acceptable form of religion*. He is worried about whether it is *Jesus or the devil* who he can hear. He hopes that joining the Christian church will ensure that it is Jesus he can hear, and not the devil. He hides his past spiritual practices from his wife and his practitioners. His mother recently died, cutting him out of the family inheritance and denying that he was her child in the will. His brother and sister are the only children mentioned. He is contesting the will. Physically, he suffers from numerous food sensitivities.

He suffers from anxiety after eating. He is embarrassed by his urinary frequency; during the first consult he needed to go to the toilet three times. He describes himself as psychic and able to see images and auras. He suffers with learning difficulties which make his efforts to achieve his Master in theology extremely hard work.

Case Analysis

This case justifies the use of *Delusion* rubrics in the case-taking because the following four aspects have been noted in the patient's case-development.

1. Evidence of inner conflict and evidence of self-destruction and pathology. If a patient has intense food sensitivities there has to be inner turmoil fueling the reactivity. He has not been able to work because of crippling physical weakness, and sensitivity to his environment.

2. The psychological delusion is used in a disproportionate way. He over-reacted to his responsibilities towards solving the world's nuclear crisis, and starvation in the poor countries. He still over reacts to responsibility; this is evident in his fear of public liability responsibilities in regard to his parishioners. He is still crippled by the sin of having left his children.

3. The delusional stance is maintained because it is advantageous to feel too weak to be able to take responsibility. His anxiety about his role as a pastor is terrifying. It is advantageous to maintain the fragility because he is then able to avoid taking on responsibility. He also needs to maintain his feelings of fragility so that he can deny his past guilt for having fallen from grace.

4. The 'never-well-since-event' is the fear and subsequent depression he suffered when he learnt about the possibility of being annihilated by a nuclear bomb. He is still crippled

by suicidal depression and guilt, and pervaded by sadness, and extremely sensitive to suffering in himself and others. The campaign *Feed the Children* has filled him with guilt when he eats food.

The simillimum in this case must cover his exaggerated self-blame for his sins and the sins of the world.

Each remedy profile will present in one, or all, of the following five psychological stages.

If the constitutional remedy that the homoeopath has chosen has *Delusion* rubrics allocated into Denial, the patient *must* display psychological 'delusions of grandeur'. The simillimum in this case must pertain to the delusion that he is not sure whether it is Jesus or the devil who is influencing him.

- *Delusions*: *influence; one is under a powerful*: thuj.
- *Delusions*: *divided*: *two parts; into*: *which part he has possession on waking; and could not tell*: thuj. [1] 1.
- *Delusions*: *superhuman; is*: *control; is under superhuman*: Thuj.

These three rubrics can refer to illusions that one is under the control of Jesus (God) or the devil.

If the constitutional remedy that the homoeopath has chosen has *Delusion* rubrics allocated into Forsaken, the patient *must* display psychological 'delusions of abandonment' or 'delusions of persecution'. The simillimum must cover his feelings of being forsaken by his mother because she wanted a girl. The simillimum must cover the feelings of being an outcast, and his dreams about being abandoned and forsaken with no home to go.

- *Delusions*: *forsaken; is*: thuj.
- *Delusions*: *outcast; she were an*: thuj.
- *Delusions*: *friend*: *affection of; has lost the*: Thuj.

If the constitutional remedy that the homoeopath has chosen has *Delusion* rubrics allocated into Causation, the patient *must* display psychological 'delusions of original sin'. He is worried about whether it is *Jesus or the devil* who influences him. By joining the Christian church he is hoping that it is Jesus he can hear, and not the devil. He hides his past spiritual practices from his wife and his practitioners; this is the *Delusion* rubric: *he is dirty*. The simillimum must cover his feelings that he sinned by abandoning his children.

- *Delusions*: *dirty*: *he is*: thuj.
- *Delusions*: *criminal, he is a*: thuj.
- *Delusions*: *sinned; one has*: thuj.
- *Delusions*: *divided*: *two parts; into*: *which part he has possession on waking; and could not tell*: thuj. [1] 1.
- *Delusions*: *influence; one is under a powerful*: thuj.
- *Delusions*: *superhuman; is*: *control; is under superhuman*: Thuj.

These rubrics can refer to illusions that one is under the control of God or the devil.

If the constitutional remedy that the homoeopath has chosen has *Delusion* rubrics allocated into Depression, the patient *must* display psychological 'delusions of impending doom'. The simillimum must cover his feeling that he is not worthy enough to succeed as a Christian minister. Responsibility in *Thuja* confronts them with the terrifying fear of failure.

- *Delusions*: *worthless; he is*: thuj.

If the constitutional remedy that the homoeopath has chosen has *Delusion* rubrics allocated into Resignation, the patient *must* display psychological 'delusions of hypochondria'. The simillimum in this case must address his crippling feelings of being weak, emotionally, mentally, and physically.

Delusions: *body*: delicate, is: *Thuj*. [2] 1.

Delusions: *existence*: *longer; she cannot exist any*: thuj. [1] 1.

The advantage in identifying and understanding the psychological processing that your patient is moving through is that it allows you to narrow the remedies being considered to the remedies listed in those particular rubric-categories. I have no other information about this case other than what he has told above. By following these psychological stages, I have easily found the simillimum and understood the disturbance in this case.

Prescription: *Thuja* 30 C., dry pilule once a day, continuously.

Case Analysis: I used the following key points and headings in analyzing this case.

1. *Striking*, or *Peculiar* Signs and Symptoms; Organon 153
2. **Theme**
3. **Rubric-repertorisation**
4. **Materia Medica**
5. **Follow-up Consultations**
6. *How*, *Why*, and *When* Causations – the 'Never-well-since-event'.

1. *Striking*, or *Peculiar* Signs and Symptoms; Organon 153

Thuja are listed in the *Delusion* rubric: *under superhuman control*, but they have self-conflicting denial about who is influencing them. *Thuja* have the *Delusion* rubric: *being at war*. *Thuja* choose to abdicate personal responsibility for their power because they fear that the powerful influence is coming from 'the evil side', and not 'the good side'. This secret will be the underlying self-denial in every *Thuja* case. Another rubric to consider in a *Thuja* case would be the *Delusion* rubric: *someone calls*. The homoeopath needs to ask *who* is influencing them. All *Thuja* cases will have a divided self which they are trying to keep secret; this conflict will always cause eventual destruction of either the mind or body. *Thuja* are significantly the only remedy listed in the *Delusion* rubric: *divided into two parts, and which part he has possession of when he wakes he does not know*. *Thuja* have a strongly developed defense which manifest in their obsessive need for religion – *Mind* rubric: *fanaticism, too occupied with religious affections*. *Thuja* need to believe that they are being controlled by God or a 'good' higher being, otherwise they are overwhelmed by their own fears of immoral behavior. This *Thuja* (case) feared that the higher power with which he was in contact was the devil, and not Jesus. It was this fear which drove him to become a Christian pastor and give up his previous 'unconventional' spiritual life. If he had stayed in the alternative world of spirituality, the power influencing him could have been the devil. In the Christian ministry he felt he would be protected, and more assured that Jesus would influence him, and not the devil.

If a constitutional remedy has two opposing forces, they will be evident in the *Delusion* rubrics. *Thuja* have the *Delusion* rubric: *she is all powerful* in Stage one versus the *Delusion* rubric: *he is worthless* in Stage four. A person with such extreme conflicting polarities will move into a psychological process of self-denial; it is too painful to live with the self-realizations. The rubric-repertorisation, using the psychological model I am proposing is extremely worthwhile because it will always reveal the psychodynamic crisis within each remedy. The self-denial in *Thuja* is the precursor of their secrecy. *Thuja* have the *Mind* rubric: *secretive*. He hides his past spiritual practices from his wife and his practitioners.

2. Theme

- *Delusions: superhuman; is; control; is under superhuman*: He has religious fanaticism. He believes he is able to hears Jesus' direction and is following God's instructions by joining the church. He is in denial of how exhausted trying to be good and religiously acceptable has made him; he is crippled with tiredness. He believes that by being good and listening to God's instructions he will clear the slate of his sinful past. He hides his psychic spirituality from the church and his parishioners. He also hides his sadness and fear from his parishioners.

If the trauma inside of your patient starts with religious martyrdom and denial of the self, then immediately the simillimum is listed in the *Delusion* rubrics: *in communication with God*. Thuja believe they are *under a superhuman control*. This *Thuja* (case) is fearful of hell, damnation and the supernatural.

Thuja need to align themselves with God and religiosity with incredible fervor to overcome their fear of punishment.

- *Delusions: outcast; she were an*: He lived in isolation in the hills for twenty years. He was rejected by his mother and father.

- *Delusions: wrong; done wrong: he has*: He feels that he was punished for having abandoned his two young children. He feels that by taking care of his step-daughter he is making up for not having looked after his own children. He feels that God has forgiven him his sins now that he has contact with his children.

- *Delusions: worthless; he is*: He feels he is a failure because he is always depressed and overcome by crippling panic attacks. He thinks he will not be able to succeed at his role of pastor because he is fearful of people.

- *Delusions: body; continuity of body would be dissolved*: He feels that he is too weak to be able to deal with the stress and fear of running the business side of a parish. He is terrified of dealing with public liability and the possibility of a parishioner suing him.

Mostly, I have successfully used the homoeopathic remedy *Thuja* to treat very simple cases of the wart virus in patients.

Thuja have the *Mind* rubrics: *fear of others approaching them,* and *insanity will not be touched.* Both of these are internal dialogues and responses one would expect from someone who has warts all over their hands or face. Warts on the face or hands can make people feel like they do not want to be touched or feel like they need to hide from society.

The underlying disturbance within the *Thuja* profile is fragility. *Thuja* have the *Delusion* rubrics: *the body is lighter than air, the body is delicate, body is brittle,* and *body is thin.* The *Delusion* rubrics: *their body will be dissolved* and *she can no longer exist* indicate a core disturbance underpinning *Thuja*. Understanding the *Delusion* rubric: *body is dissolved* helped me understand the psychotherapeutic need in *Thuja* for the 'delusions of grandeur' which force them into believing they are *all powerful.*

In one *Thuja* patient who consulted me, his fear of being eliminated was formed deep within his psyche when he was brutally attacked in his first sexual encounter. His first sexual encounter formed the primary 'never-well-since-event'. His crippling fear of being killed [*no longer exist*] every time he had sex in the future resulted in pre-emptive, self-protective erectile dysfunction. The self-deluding need to avoid his underlying fear of extinction created huge psychological 'delusions of grandeur'. He consulted me but left without taking a remedy because he believed that nothing was physically or mentally wrong with him. He also refused to take the homoeopathic remedy in case it changed him in some way.

Thuja fear attack. *Thuja* have the *Delusion* rubric: *body is in danger of coming in pieces.* [1] 1. In this *Thuja* (case), the fear of no longer existing is the underlying psychological trauma underpinning the development of the patient's Chronic Fatigue Syndrome, and his mental and emotional breakdown later in life. His fear of being eliminated [*dissolved*] developed from the primary 'never-well-since-event' when he found out about nuclear extinction. His fear of nuclear extinction subsequently overwhelmed him with fear of his own extinction.

A little while after finding out about nuclear extinction,

he was confronted with world poverty and starvation. He subsequently went on to develop food allergies as a child. The food allergies justified his reduced intake of food so he could become very *thin*. *Thuja* frequently develop psychosomatic, empathic pathologies. *Thuja* have the *Delusion* rubric: *has lost the affection of a friend* – this rubric is reflective of a deep fear in *Thuja* of being *friendless* and isolated and *outcast*. As a result, *Thuja* often develop strong somatic, empathic responses to others' suffering, especially animals. *Thuja* have the *Mind* rubric: *love for animals, and cats*. The patient's Chronic Fatigue Syndrome developed from years of internal discord within himself.

Thuja have a profound contradiction between Stage one and Stage five in the five stage psychological model. On the one hand, *Thuja* manifest psychological 'delusions of grandeur' which allude to them being under God-like superhuman control, while on the other hand they have profoundly disabling psychological 'delusions of hypochondria' which cause them to feel that at any moment they will dissolve and die. The *Delusion* rubrics: *delicate, thin, about to die, diminished, disintegrating, emaciated*, are all examples of exaggerated predictions of physical decay. The inconsistencies and contradictions between Stage one and Stage five in *Thuja* are evidence of self-deluding psychosis. Psychosis is a severe mental derangement involving the whole personality. Psychosis is the precursor to the destruction of 'ego', and involves a complete loss of contact with reality. *Thuja* need to believe they are all powerful to avoid their fears of extinction. Religious fanaticism is common in *Thuja*. *Thuja* need a savior to save them from *diminishing*. *Thuja* have the *Mind* rubrics: *religious fanaticism, too occupied with religion, despair of religious salvation* and *reproaching oneself about one's own passion*. *Thuja* have the *Delusion* rubric: *is under superhuman control* and *she is all powerful*.

For the simillimum to be *Thuja* there has to evidence

that the patient is not aware of their own self-delusion. The psychological delusional stance of *Thuja* is locked in their unconscious mind. *Thuja* have the *Mind* rubric: *untruthful*. If *Thuja* are confronted in their conscious or sub-conscious mind with their underlying *disintegration* it will literally shatter a very *brittle* and fragile 'ego'. If *Thuja* are confronted by the homoeopath with their state of denial, it will overwhelm them. I have experienced a few *Thuja* patients who have walked away from my consultations without taking the remedy because they did not think there was anything wrong with them. *Thuja* have the *Mind* rubric: *secretive*. [2]. In psychosis, the mental derangement needs to remain hidden in the unconscious mind of the patient; to face the psychotic derangement would cause complete destruction. The simillimum will only be *Thuja* if the patient appears (to the homoeopath) mentally and emotionally fragile. *Thuja* will not believe *they* are fragile; they believe they are *powerful*. *Thuja* will acknowledge their physical fragility, but they will not acknowledge mental and emotional fragility.

1. Denial: *Delusion* rubric: *powerful: all powerful; she is*: thuj. *Delusion* rubric: *fancy, illusions of*: thuj. *Delusion* rubric: *superhuman; is*: *control; is under superhuman*: Thuj. [In relation to *Thuja* this rubric can be allocated to either God or the devil.]

2. Forsaken: *Delusion* rubric: *forsaken; is*: thuj. *Delusion* rubric: *appreciated, she is not*: Thuj. *Delusion* rubric: *friendless, he is*: Thuj. *Delusion* rubric: *outcast; she were an*: thuj.

3. Causation: *Delusion* rubric: *criminal; he is a*: thuj. *Delusion* rubric: *sinned; one has*: thuj.

4. Depression: *Delusion* rubric: *insane: he is insane*: Thuj. *Delusion* rubric: *worthless; he is*: thuj.

5. Resignation: *Delusion* rubric: *body: continuity of body would be dissolved*: thuj. [1] 1. *Delusion* rubric: *diminished: thin, he is too*: thuj. [1] 1. *Delusion* rubric: *body: pieces:*

coming in pieces; body is in danger of: thuj. [1] 1. *Delusion* rubric: *die: about to die; one was: Thuj. Delusion* rubric: *body: delicate, is: Thuj.* [2] 1. *Delusion* rubric: *dirty, he is:* thuj. *Delusion* rubric: *touched; he is: Thuj. Delusion* rubric: *flying: skin; out of his:* thuj. [1] 1.

Inconsistencies:

1. Denial: *Delusion* rubric: *powerful: all powerful; she is:* thuj. Versus

5. Resignation: *Delusion* rubric: *body: delicate, is: Thuj.* [2] 1.

Thuja is a homoeopathic remedy derived from the *Arbor vitae* tree. The wood is light, soft and brittle and vulnerable to splitting. *Thuja* have the theme of fragility and sensitivity in all spheres – emotional, mental, and physical. Because of the trees' tall growth, "longevity, incorruptible resin and ever-green leaves, cypress and thuja have been associated with immortality (Tree of Life)." [Vermeulen] *Thuja* have opposing sensitivities of weakness and strength (religious fervor).

Noted Theme Words used in the Consultation

- Weak
- Sensitive
- Fragile
- Anxious
- Suicidal
- Sad
- Depressed
- Fragile health
- Thin
- Afraid
- Fears of abandonment
- Guilty
- Fears of violence

- Fear of hell
- Fear of the supernatural
- Guilty of a crime
- Duty
- The right thing
- Spiritual
- Religious
- Morals
- God
- Sociably acceptable

3. Rubric-repertorisation

I have listed below an extensive list of rubrics which are reflective of 'ego' disintegration.

- *Delusions: bed: touch the bed when lying; as if she did not*: thuj.
- *Delusions: body: brittle, is: Thuj.*
- *Delusions: body: continuity of body would be dissolved*: thuj. [1] 1.
- *Delusions: body: delicate, is: Thuj. [2] 1.*
- *Delusions: body: immaterial, is*: thuj.
- *Delusions: body: lighter than air; body is*: thuj.
- *Delusions: body: pieces: coming in pieces; body is in danger of*: thuj.
- *Delusions: body: ugly; body looks: Thuj.*
- *Delusions: die: about to die; one was: Thuj.*
- *Delusions: die: time has come to*: thuj.
- *Delusions: diminished: thin, he is too*: thuj. [1] 1.
- *Delusions: dirty: he is*: thuj.
- *Delusions: divided: two parts; into*: thuj.

- *Delusions: divided: two parts; into: which part he has possession on waking; and could not tell of:* thuj. [1] 1.
- *Delusions: double: being:* thuj.
- *Delusions: emaciation; of:* thuj.
- *Delusions: existence: longer; she cannot exist any:* thuj. [1] 1.
- *Delusions: falling: height; from a: Thuj.*
- *Delusions: feet: touch scarcely the ground: walking; when:* thuj.
- *Delusions: floating: air, in:* thuj.
- *Delusions: flying: skin; out of his:* thuj. [1] 1.
- *Delusions: friendless, he is: Thuj.*
- *Delusions: glass: she is made of:* thuj.
- *Delusions: glass: wood, glass, etc.; being made of: Thuj.*
- *Delusions: ground: touch the ground; she would hardly:* thuj.
- *Delusions: head: belongs to another:* thuj.
- *Delusions: heavy; is:* thuj.
- *Delusions: identity: errors of personal identity:* thuj.
- *Delusions: influence; one is under a powerful:* thuj.
- *Delusions: insane: he is insane: Thuj.*
- *Delusions: intoxicated: is; he:* thuj.
- *Delusions: legs: glass; were made of: Thuj.* [2] 1.
- *Delusions: light: is light; he:* thuj.
- *Delusions: move: he moves: to and fro; he moves: sitting and lying; when:* thuj. [1] 1.
- *Delusions: outcast; she were an:* thuj.
- *Delusions: people: beside him; people are:* thuj.
- *Delusions: person: present; someone is:* thuj.
- *Delusions: poisoned: he: has been:* thuj.
- *Delusions: pursued; he was:* thuj.

- *Delusions: seat: moving; seat is: to and fro*: thuj. [1] 1.
- *Delusions: separated: body: mind are separated; body and*: thuj.
- *Delusions: separated: body: soul; body is separated from*: thuj.
- *Delusions: separated: world; from the: he is separated*: thuj.
- *Delusions: strange: familiar things seem strange*: thuj.
- *Delusions: strangers: seeing: Thuj.*
- *Delusions: thin: body is*: thuj.
- *Delusions: turn: she: had been turned: circle; in a*: thuj.
- *Delusions: worthless; he is*: thuj.
- *Delusions: wrong: something was wrong*: thuj.

Mind rubrics for *Thuja*

- *Mind: ailments from; neglected; being; mother; by one's*: thuj.
- *Mind: ailments from; quarrelling; father; with one's*: thuj.
- *Mind: anxiety: business; about*: thuj.
- *Mind: anxiety: conscience; anxiety of: Thuj.*
- *Mind: anxiety: eating ; after*: thuj.
- *Mind: anxiety: future, about*: thuj.
- *Mind: aversion; mother, to*: thuj. [1] 3. [positr. taosc.]
- *Mind: company: aversion to; sight of people; avoids the: Thuj.*
- *Mind: confidence: want of self-confidence; self-depreciation*: thuj.
- *Mind: eating; after; agg*: thuj.
- *Mind: fear: approaching; of; others; of; delirium, in: Thuj.*
- *Mind: fear: opinion of others, of*: thuj.
- *Mind: forsaken feeling; beloved by his parents, wife, friends; feeling of not being: Thuj.*

- *Mind*: *religious affections: too occupied with religion; fanaticism*: thuj.
- *Mind*: *reproaching oneself*: *Thuj.*
- *Mind*: *suicidal disposition*: thuj.
- *Mind*: *timidity: public; about appearing in*: thuj.
- *Urinary organs*: *complaints of urinary organs*: thuj.
- *Vision*: *colors before the eyes*: thuj.

This patient is a man who is physically weak and fragile. Emotionally, he is frightened of his parishioners, and terrified of taking responsibility. He has struggled with living in society. He has abandoned his two young children and his marriage. He is a psychic. He has lived his life believing the 'Age of Aquarius' was about to unfold. He is also starkly judgmental and moralistic in his portrayal of his 'Tina Turner' mother. He needs to discard his own psychic spirituality for the socially acceptable forms of religion found within the Christian church. He martyrs himself to his step-daughter to overcome his debt to his own children. He martyrs himself to his wife, who continues to feed him meat when he would prefer to be a vegetarian, because he needs to prove he will be conscientious and stay in the marriage.

Thuja struggle with opposing forces. On the one hand he is weak and frightened, and on the other hand he is fixed and rigid. On the one hand he has 'God on his side', and on the other he is terrified of *hell and judgment and the supernatural, and the devil. Thuja* have psychological 'delusions of grandeur' [religiosity] which leave them open and vulnerable, and needing to hide their psychological 'delusions of original sin'. *Thuja* develop psychoses because they need to hide from themselves, and others.

4. Materia Medica

"I have often found this feeling of fragility in *Thuja* expressed in the physical sphere, where the patient feels that any article of food or drink is surely bound to cause him problems, and that his system cannot take things such as drugs, allergens,

emotional stress or even a draught of air. He tries to avoid all these factors and attempts to keep himself covered from exposure to the same. These avoidances only reinforces the fear, and this vicious cycle goes on, making *Thuja* one of the main remedies for neurosis, with several obsessive-compulsive traits, fixed ideas and behavior patterns. In the emotional sphere, this feeling of fragility is manifest in the fear of losing face in society. The person believes that he has a certain image in society of being a religious, morally upright, clean, honest person, free from human failings such as dishonesty, sexual temptations (especially) when forbidden, etc. Thus he presents an elevated picture of himself and is afraid that any little slip on his part might reveal the real him or the bad part of him which he has tried so hard to cover up. In this "bad part" lies his dishonesty, sexual desires (which may even be for close relatives), his immoral or irreligious feelings. If this is discovered, he is going to fall down from his imagined elevated position and will be finished. Thus his survival depends on a complete cover up, and there is a tremendous anxiety of being exposed. Translated into expressions the Thuja person is secretive and talks to the physician as if sharing a secret; he is conscious of the presence of other persons, especially strangers. In rubrics, you have the feeling of floating in the air ("Delusion, body lighter than air") and dreams of falling from high places which represent his fear of falling from his elevated position. Thus Thuja seems to come from a situation of religious order in society or from any situation that demands rigidity in thinking, very fixed ideas. Theocracies, like those in the Middle East, would require this remedy. Also many of the strict religious leaders, with rigid ideas about sin, often have many skeletons in their cupboards, and many times require Thuja. In fact "Religious fanaticism" is one of the rubrics."
[Sankaran]

5. Follow-up Consultations

First Follow up Consult: November 2008.

I concentrate entirely on videotaping only the follow-up consultations. I usually commence videos after the patient has taken the remedy for some time and I am always vigilant of any new trauma which has sparked off their subconscious or unconscious memory because it is at that point that I find the meaning and relevance of every *Delusion* rubric. In this case, the transformation was so profound after just four weeks of taking *Thuja* 30 C., continuously, 1 dose a day, that I was compelled to ask the patient if I could record the first follow-up session. This is the first *Thuja* case which I have ever videotaped.

For the simillimum to be correct, the five stages of the psychological delusion of illness and loss must be noted to have changed.

- He realizes that he has been exhausted for years from pushing himself to be good.
- He reports that his spiritual confidence has grown.
- He reports he is *no longer sorry for the fact that he exists.*
- He is not as fearful of bureaucracy. He reports that he is dealing with stress much better. He has had only two anxiety attacks about bureaucracy and public liability responsibilities and was able to get out of the anxiety much better. He now thinks that the degree to which he feels responsible is an overreaction. He is not as afraid of his parishioners. He has started to be able to talk with people and organize to have coffee with his parishioners.
- His clinical depression is much improved.
- He no longer feels like he has an all pervasive sadness.
- His suicidal feelings have decreased substantially.
- He is finishing his seminary thesis. He doesn't feel like he is

struggling with writing as much, and feels confident about presenting his paper.

- He realized after the first consultation that he likes to be *slight and small* so people will not notice him. [*Delusions: body thin.*]

Follow-up Physical Symptoms of the Case

- Frequent urination is no longer an issue at night
- The frequency during the day is still present, but greatly reduced. In the first consult he went to the toilet three times, this consult he didn't go once
- The hot hands at night returned momentarily in two short-lasting panic attacks

Transcript from the Follow-up Consultation

Question: Can you tell me about the dream which you were talking about that was twenty years old?

It was a vivid dream. I was driving a car that was a white BMW. I was aware the car belonged to a blond lady who was into fashion. I was driving the car, and the car got out of control, and it crashed into the car in front of me. It was on the corner of Williams Road and High Street. I jumped out of the car and I was dressed in my 1970's clothes. I had on a moleskin top and shoulder bag. I reached into the car and on the consol of the car was a package of food like a rissole, and I took a handful of food and put it into my mouth, and there was a long hair attached to the food. Then my father arrived. He was a barrister in reality, and he actually used to do car accidents. He picked up the pieces of the accident and put them into a wall which was like a black filing cabinet, like the structures you see in mausoleums, and each compartment was the wreckage of the accident which he marked with a felt tipped pen. I had been aware that how I lived out the dream was that when I was just a young man in my early twenties. I had two daughters, but I didn't bring up my daughters. I left the family but for the last eight years I have a step-daughter. She lives with us and also for the last fifteen years I have actually been seeing my own daughters as well, we had reconnected. In the home where I live with my present wife often in the sink I find long hairs which belong to my step-daughter. I often feel, with my step-daughter that I am continually repaying the debt that I owe to my own daughters. The long hair, as I understand the dream, is a debt that I owe to life for not being there for my daughters. This is not part of the dream, but just recently I was in a café and a lady walked in and she began talking to me. Without me explaining my circumstances or how I was feeling, she told me that my debt had been repaid and it was time to move on and to not apologize. It is interesting that word the debt had been repaid, because there are various things like the family inheritance coming around at this time. If the debt has been repaid, then I feel like I want to connect to my spiritual life. I have spent my whole life repaying debts. The second dream that I have had has been quite instrumental in the way that I have lived, I met with a group of people on another plane, or in another place, and they were all dressed in long, white robes, and the reason why we were meeting is that we were preparing to leave the planet. We were surrounding a master, or a Christ like being, and we passed through the crowd. We had to go back, and the reason we had to go back was to retrieve a roll of plans that had been left in a rubbish tip. So the driver arrived in a Datsun station wagon, and his role was to drive us to where we were going to be dropped off on our mission. He had on the consol a can of Solo lemonade which had been spiked with alcohol. I said to him, 'You had better be careful drinking and driving.' His response was 'Look, if I am going to be doing this job then I am going to drink'. He let me off at the entrance to an underground cave and we were taken down in an escalator to this underground world. When I was in that underground world I was met by a man dressed in bishop's clothes. Everyone *in the chamber were acting out figurines or porcelains. I saw these two women on a cow or horse, and I said to her 'That figure you are acting out I have seen above,' and there was another lady laying on a grave. I thought I was clever knowing that, but it made the man showing me around very angry, very aggressive. Then what happened is that a red dome started to pulse and a bell started to ring. Then this shaft started to emit this gas and then this whole world was going to be set on fire. There was a real question at the end of the dream, 'Am I going to get out or not?'*

Do you remember that I asked you at what point do you think you became weak as a child, and you said it was from that point that you learnt about nuclear wars.

It wasn't weak, it was terrified, I mean terrified, suicidal with it. Also the idea of global starvation. We had that campaign Feed the Children. I remember those images and they really depressed me. It wasn't just for a few hours. I remained depressed and I have to this day.

So the difference that you feel in taking the remedy that I gave you is that you feel much stronger?

Yes, I do, and also much stronger in my physical presence. But I am not sure whether it is a physical or spiritual presence. I feel that my aura is strong enough to feel stronger with whatever environment that I am in. Like a confidence that wasn't there before. Also I don't know whether this is timing or the remedy, but I feel that it is time to move on. I am feeling a need to connect to my spiritual life. Why that is interesting is that at the time that I had those dreams, that was all I was interested in. I was immersed in meditation. I was a natural psychic but I have put all that aside, and I have done it quite intentionally. I want to be accepted by normal people. I want to be part of the human community, human people. That is why I have gone into the church. I can't tell them. Not many people think the way that I do. I wouldn't tell them some of the things that I have told you.

If I see someone's energy field it is not because I am trying to, but I would be lying if I said I didn't see it. The difference is that I have done years of hard core theology, and what I say now is: I see those things but I don't know what those things mean. That is where that loss of confidence is.

So, you said that since taking the remedy you felt less depressed and you said you felt that your eyes were much clearer?

Yes, definitely, and yes that was amazing. I have a mauve Shetland sweater, and after a few days of taking the remedy the sweater looked like it was covered in sequins. It was like a Monet seeing inner life in the colors. I have had times like that before, but not for a long, long time. When I went off to Daylesford, I went out running in the forest. There is this legend of St Patrick, that when St Patrick was fasting he had to tell the flowers to be quiet because they were so loud. Well, it reminded me of that. The colors of the greens were amazing. It still is, it hasn't left me. It is just that I am getting a bit more used to it. I am not sure if it is an optical thing or something else, but that is the first symptom that I noticed. It is seeing this incredible beauty in the world. It is not like it is something that is disturbing or anything.

Are you dealing with stress a lot better?

Yes I am, and it's crazy because at the moment I have far more reason to be stressed. Getting the thesis done, and the conflict that is happening in the church. Here I am sharing with you but I am often in your position, so you are talking to a lot of people and I find it very draining, particularly some people.

Have you felt as drained?

Now it is very interesting that you say that because I thought the draining was some sort of psychic thing that they were taking your energy in some way. But to have something which has been able to change that thing has made me think it has been part of me being weak or something, not robust. What I have been noticing is that so much of my lifestyle has been based around that weakness and the depression. One of the remedies you gave me was to overcome the sense of the body being fragile. I used to think, because I was vegetarian for so long, that I was undernourished. I don't know what it was in the remedies. I haven't been eating a whole lot more, but when I was in Daylesford I ran for five or six kilometers which I haven't been able to do for a long time. Much stronger at my age. I didn't think that could happen. That is part of me being in this negative state. What I have had a couple of times is panic attacks. We all went for a bike ride on the weekend, it was a recreational thing for the church. What happened is that a man who was part of the team jumped on someone else's bike. The bike fell over and he had an injury with his back; nothing serious but I had a huge panic attack late at night that he was going to sue me. What is different is that I recognized I am having a panic attack. So I could step back. I had another one since I have seen you. I bought a couple of computer monitors. I just gave the accountant the receipts, then about a week later I started to think the board might think, what do you think you are doing? I have had a panic attack about being arrested about these monitors. I talked to someone on the board and they didn't know what I was talking about. I can go and buy anything. My opinion is that it was because my father was a barrister, and I have a highly active super ego, guilt or something like that, or some sort of fear of authority. In this last month I have felt so much stronger and it has helped me even around the home. With my step-daughter and the rest of the extended family. It is improving the quality of my life because I am not avoiding people so much. Avoiding people in the position I am in is not a good thing to do. Because I have been feeling this wounded spirit, or rejection of some sort, like I told you I have been avoiding people. People would be surprised to hear that. They're not nasty people, that is the crazy thing. They're lovely people. But there is a robustness in the physicality of the people that I find hard to connect with. If they are physically robust, they might be guys and they do this bloke stuff, there is something of their energy which I find a bit distressing.

You know how you talked about your mother and father and the will. How do you feel about that now?

When I first read the will, it was like being left out of the Book of Life on the Day of Atonement. It was worse than money. I started to sweat, it had a chain reaction. I thought, well my wife is going to leave me as well. It was associated with a large rejection. It was a bit irrational as well because I knew what was going to be in the will. But when I read it, it was devastating. It was also doubly devastating because I got the news that my mother had died when I was in a hotel in Munich. Next, I was going to Israel. But because my mother had died I couldn't go to Israel, and I had quite a lot of torment over that because of the spiritual work I had to do in Israel. I knew my mother had dementia for eight years and I knew what the quality of our relationship was like. My wife said, 'You can't do that, it would bad', and when I thought about it, I couldn't do it either, so we came back to Melbourne. I had to do the eulogy, so reading the will was devastating, but it was the beginning of this turning around of paying back the debt. The solicitor asked me, 'Do you have any reason why you have been the victim of such a vindictive will?' I had to get the tissues out because I thought this situation is not normal. It made me realize that I have been the victim of a fairly negative attitude all my life. I am aware, Liz, that there is something really beautiful, and that life is really worth living. It is connected with what I have shared with you about my mother's death. What the solicitor said, and the ability to reflect on your experiences in that way makes you realize you are not crazy. Being with yourself, and being able to share things spiritually being psychic, is not encouraged. It is an area in which I am looking for some sort of reconciliation between Judeo-Christianity and 'New Age'. In my life it has both, so I am looking for some sort of balance or reconciliation.

Previously you used the word 'atonement'. Atonement means to me that something has been forgiven. That you have committed some sin, and that you have been forgiven and let back into paradise.

What does that look like? That idea of a crime having been committed comes to the surface quite a bit. A sense of guilt[30].

Where does that come from, what do you think you did?

I don't know where that starts from, but it is certainly an old one, right from the time I was little. I don't know, but I know how it has manifested. It has manifested as a fear of hell, and judgement, and things like that. It has been guilt to do with the supernatural and the devil.

6. *How*, *Why*, and *When* Causations – the 'Never-well-since-event'

To elicit the 'never-well-since-symptom', I ask leading and inquiring questions.

Do you think that guilt came from when you were a child?

It must have, because that is when it started to manifest. I have no idea of any incident other than what I told you my mother never wanted a boy, she wanted a girl. That was not just a little thing, it had a lot of energy in it. She had just lost two little girls. They didn't come out of the hospital. I think it is all tied in with needing to apologize for existing. This lady said don't apologize.

---

30 This case resonates with the patient's delusional expectation that if he is in communication with God he should be able to cure his present anxiety and physical weakness. If they can't cure his disease then he believes that his anxiety is a result of the sins he has committed, or that he is in communication with the devil, and not Jesus. He says, *I feel threatened they will find out about me. I can spend days in the presence of God. It is a blinding white light. The presence displaces me. It is ecstasy, nirvana. The problem is I don't know who it is. I don't know if it is God. I don't know if it is the devil which needs to be cast out of me. I don't know what it is. I can't tell my Christian friends and congregation because they will ask if it is Jesus who is in the white light and I don't know who it is, for all I know it could be the devil inside of me.*

When I first saw you, you were talking about your mother's grief and that she never wanted you as a boy. Do you think it is possible that a baby can pick up that sort of energy?

Absolutely. In fact, I have just had a lady in our church who has post-natal depression and she was holding the baby and she said one thing like, 'Maybe I won't be able to bring him up.' I had a reaction which really surprised me. It came out of left field I said 'Don't say that in front of him. He doesn't understand English but he can hear that you don't want him. But that was not out of my rational mind.

So, then you grow up, leave home, get married and leave your children, and then your life starts to really fall apart?

Can I tell you the story of the guitar? This is what happened: I married a young lady who was very troubled when I met her, psychiatrically. It was at a time when I was heavily into New Age. We thought the Age of Aquarius was coming. I had a more disciplined approach to it all, which is why I continued. For a lot of other people it was just like a fashion. One thing led to another, but because this lady was in the middle of a breakdown my mother told her she could come and stay at our place. Basically, to cut a long story short, the girl was very beautiful, and she got pregnant. (Please note he has not said he got her pregnant, which was what happened; he has distanced himself from his past sin.) *We began to live together, and the situation got worse; it got more explosive. I had a guitar which this grazer gave to me. I went to boarding school and because he knew I played guitar he rolled up one day with this guitar and the guitar was a very valuable guitar. The way the marriage ended was it was just another one of those explosive days, and she put her foot through the case. The broken guitar was like a metaphor of the marriage but more tragically what happened was it was like the end of the ideal.* [*Thuja* have the *Delusion* rubric: *illusions of fancy.*] *But I was very much in love with another woman at that time, but she didn't want to know about me because I was so dysfunctional. But one day the man who owned the guitar rang up one day, and wanted the guitar back. I had had it repaired and why he wanted this guitar was that he had married, and the person he married was the lady I was in love with. Years later, intentionally I started to make guitars and lived in the hills. All the time I was thinking of reconstructing my life because of this smashed up guitar. Years later, when I arrived in the church that I am in now, a lady that worshiped there had the same little guitar, and when I saw it I said, I have a case for you, and the case was the case that had the footprint on it. Maybe I have repaid the debt, but what happens next?*

If you go back to your religion when you repay the debt, then are you let back into paradise?

I think I am starting to know what that feels like. I think it is stopping the striving against those things like rejection.

The rejection from your mother?

Yes. After I read the will I took all the photos down. My present wife wanted me to have the photos up, in fact that is important to her; family. But what I think is that an idea that helped after the incident with the guitar, back when I was twenty-five years old, was: we do have a spiritual family. There are such wonderful goals in a spiritual life. People don't realize what the rewards are. I am not talking about God thinking you are a wonderful person, I am talking about a whole world of perception. Peace and a spiritual life which is really tangible.

The remedy I gave you is also for feeling abandoned and rejected and that you were not good enough. If there is a degree of being let back into paradise, you then asked, *What does that look like?* Paradise is when you start to feel like a worthy person. The remedy I gave you was for feeling unworthy for your assumption of sin. This is what you have felt all of your life since that event, rejected not only by your parents but by the whole of society, which is what you were talking about: wanting to be in the church, a conventional church, not a spiritual practice, because you wanted that acceptance.

Yes. Because it was part of getting back on the good side you see.

What the homoeopathic remedy is undoing is the issue of abandonment. Did you deal with the two panic attacks?

Yes. Basically, it didn't take long to deal with those, it was only five minutes of really intense. I feel like I have been intentionally trying to please people, but if you have lived your whole life like I have, then no-one trusts you. By the time I was forty, I had just lost so much credibility because I believed a spiritual life gave you permission. If I could make myself go back there I would tell myself I was going in the wrong direction. Why I am getting burnt out is that I am doing this just out of my own tank. I am intentionally forcing myself into right conduct and right attitudes, but I would like it to be spontaneous.

The secret revealed

Underlying the need for *Thuja* to maintain their secrecy is fear of being outcast from society.

I feel threatened they will find out about me. I can spend days in the presence of God. It is a blinding white light. The presence displaces me. It is ecstasy, nirvana. The problem is, I don't know who it is. I don't know if it is God. I don't know if it is the devil which needs to be cast out of me. I don't know what it is. I can't tell my Christian friends and congregation because they will ask if it is Jesus who is in the white light and I don't know who it is, for all I know it could be the devil inside of me. I had a dream. I was trying to go up some stairs and there were all these people on the stairs blocking the way. I knew that if I got in touch with the primitive beast inside of myself and just pushed these people out of the way I could get up the stairs. I have a lot of anger inside of me which I don't think I should have in my position as a pastor of a Christian ministry. If I was to do a mandala of my life there would be all these parts. My past life as a devotee, and my life as a Pastor. My life as a guitar maker, and then this anger which is inside and it shouldn't be there. If people get too close they are going to see that anger. I need to be in the presence of God, but I don't know what that is, it could be the devil. I don't know who it is. The presence displaces me. It is like the ecstasy you have in sex and you have an orgasm with your wife but this presence I can be in for days. How can I assure my parishioners that it is Jesus I am seeing?

I feel very threatened around people. I find it hard to be myself. I still feel that I am too broken, and damaged, and fragile, to be part of the human family. I think they will find out about me; that I don't really feel comfortable with people. Don't get me wrong, it is not that I don't like these people. I do, they are all good people. It is just that I have anger inside of me which, if I don't get away from people especially in the mornings, I am scared they will see. I am still very restless in the mornings. I can't stay at home. I need to leave the house and go and have a coffee. Even if I go to work, as soon as I get there I have to leave and go to the coffee shop. I am always looking for wide open spaces and anonymity. The anxiety is only there now in the mornings. By the afternoon and night I feel much better now, not so restless. I would like to change this. It is not that I am unusual in going to have a coffee in the mornings, lots of people do it. The thing is that if my wife was to disagree with it, would be something which would cause an argument. It is an obsession with me. I can't stay in the house. I am trapped and controlled by this need to get out of the house, and I would like that to change, it is an obsession.

Why do you have to leave the house?

There is something repugnant about people having breakfast in the morning, them having toast in their pajamas. I don't know if it just looks lazy, but I find it repugnant. (Here I am reminded of his feeling of repugnance that he had towards his mother when she would go to the toilet in front of him when he was a child.) *I get very angry with physical clumsiness and mess in the environment. Just seeing people eat toast in the morning in their pajamas is totally repugnant to me. I am totally threatened by my own organizational stress. I can go into my study and it is a mess. Don't get me wrong Liz, if you were to come to my house, everything is in order, but my desk is a mess. For example, if I did your job and had to have all the bottles you have in that cabinet in alphabetical order I would not be able to do it.* (My consulting room is extremely tidy. Patients are either confronted by it, or like it.) *I got a high distinction for my thesis and I can do my sermons, but I do them in the coffee shop in the morning. I am totally frozen with anxiety when I have to try to order my desk. My wife has put up a row of ugly files in the study. The reason I call them ugly is that I don't understand her system of filing and it overwhelms me. I feel very restless as soon as I wake up and I have to get out of the house. I can't deal with the laziness of what people look like in the morning eating toast in their pajamas. I need wide-open spaces, anonymity in the mornings.*

Case Analysis

Thuja have numerous *Mind* rubrics which reflect the same internal discord, for example: *disgust with his own body, aversion to being touched,* and *always washing her hands.* The psychotic patient can also develop delusional disorders, disorganized thinking, hallucinations, illusions, or paranoid delusional states. *Thuja* are extremely threatened by anything which reminds them of human decay. *Thuja* have the *Delusion* rubric: *he is dirty*[31]. *Thuja* need their religiosity to protect

31 I am currently treating another *Thuja* case, a woman whose reason for consulting me was to help her overcome her self-disgust and feelings of dirtiness after she has sex. Her disgust is so extreme that she has to shower for at least one hour after sex. Given the water restrictions that we have in place in Australia (after the longest drought in history), she was feeling racked with guilt, not only for having sex, but for also using so much water.

themselves from humanness. *Thuja* feel too delicate to be able to cope with any signs of gross human behaviors. *Thuja* are a victim of their own religiosity and conscientious sense of duty.

Treatment: continue with *Thuja* 30 C. dry pilule once a day, continuously.

Third Follow up Consult: January 2009.

- His stomach and digestion are greatly improved, no bloating or pain or indigestion.
- His frequency is greatly improved.
- He is also not as thirsty. He still came to the consultation with his drink bottle but he did not drink from it once. In the first consultation he drank obsessively, every twenty minutes. In the second consultation, he drank three times in a ninety minute consultation.
- He reports his confidence is greatly improved.
- He has less anxiety, and was able to deal with a legal issue at the church without it causing any panic attacks at all, which is the first time that has happened.
- The fact that he feels more stable he finds *remarkable*!
- He is dealing with more responsibility within the church, which he says he has never been able to cope with before.
- He reports his step-daughter has bought a house and is about to move out. He is far more open about the difficulties of living with a step-child. He no longer feels he is in karmic debt to her and is very happy she is moving out. He feels as if he has had to compensate for years. He feels that there has always been territorial tension over his *access rights to his wife* because the step-daughter has lived with them. He reports that it *feels remarkable to not feel so guilty*.
- He has started to reveal more about what he is keeping secret. His need to hide his past allegiances to the 'Aquarian Age' is less.

Conclusion

Follow-up: June, October, 2009.

He still contacts me from time to time, but they are mainly short phone consultations. He has continued on the remedy when *he* feels that he needs to repeat the remedy. He repeats the remedy for approximately a week at a time when he notices the anxiety returning. He rings to see what I think of his assessment of himself. He has finished his theological studies and has passed with distinction. He is seeking a permanent position in a church. After the will has been settled he wants to live in Germany and pursue more theological studies. He is much happier because he has started to teach his practitioners meditation. This indicates to me that his need to hide that part of himself is no longer an issue. He is extremely well physically, and no longer describes himself as having CFS or any other sort of physical weakness. He has allowed himself to gain a small amount of weight. He is still eating meat at home with his wife.

I have kept him on the same potency and daily dose: *Thuja* 30 C. 1/day, dry pilule, as needed.

Bibliography

Sankaran, Rajan. *The Soul of Remedies*. Santa Cruz, Bombay, Homoeopathic Medical Publishers, 1997. pp. 203-205.

Schroyens, Frederik. M.D. *Synthesis*. London, Homeopathic Book Publishers, 1997.

Vermeulen, Frans. *Prisma*. The Netherlands, Emryss bv Publishers, 2002. p.1337, pp.1375-1378.

Vermeulen, Frans. *Synoptic Materia Medica* 1. The Netherlands, Emryss Publishers, 1992. pp. 398-401.

Veratrum album

Abstract:

This is the case of a woman who did not seek treatment for her cancer because she saw the cancer as God's punishment, and she did not dare go against God's retribution. She believed if she sacrificed her life she would save the world from sin.

Keywords:

'Delusions of original sin'. 'Righteous Suicide'. God's judgment. 'New-Age' philosophy. Martyrdom. 'Delusions of grandeur'.

D.O.B. 1973.

- **First Consultation**: August 2005: Adenocarcinoma in left jaw; diagnosed 1992.She has had no medical treatment since diagnosis; at 22 years of age. She now has secondary tumors in both lungs. She is dying.

- **Appearance**: Pale, with dark rings under her eyes. Thin, and exhausted looking.

- **Presentation**: Weak voice, softly spoken, takes a long time to answer. Appears very depressed.

- **Father**: Lives in Italy. She tells me: *I am the result of an affair.*

- **Step-father**: Alcoholic.

- **Mother**: Diagnosed as Schizophrenic.

- **Brother**: *Committed suicide by putting his head under a moving train.*
- **Hobby**: Greek myths. [This becomes an important aspect of the case.]

Notes from the first consultation:

The woman informed me she did not want to pursue conventional radiotherapy treatment as advised by the medical doctors because she knew that she had the cancer as a result of the fact that I have never chosen to live. I sought medical advice following the first consultation. The general advice was that if she had had radiotherapy at the time of the first diagnosis in 1992, her success with this type of tumor would have been very favorable. Whether this advice was correct or not it is impossible to know; the essence of the case was she felt she did not *deserve* treatment. She found out she had cancer at the very young age of 22, when it can easily be said that most young adults don't know what direction they are taking in life. Her harsh judgment of herself immediately worried me. On finding out she had cancer, she was convinced she had caused it. *I asked what I have done to myself.* She was extremely sure that because she had *no passion to live,* and that she had never had any passion to live that she had *deserved the cancer. It is wrong to not know what to do with the gift of life, therefore I don't deserve it.*

I treat a lot of clients with cancer, and I had never seen such self-assuredness.

She was very sure that she *deserved* her condition. I mistook this for a *Carcinosin* depression and prescribed *Carcinosin*. As you read the transcript, the suppression of *Carcinosin* reverberates, but this is not the remedy as it clearly does not match the psychological delusion of God's wrath within the case.

She described her depression as: *I do not know if I want to live but I have no passion. I am used to having no passion, this has been my way to solve not wanting to live*: *I have no passion.* She is in a relationship, but she does not share with her partner how she feels. He did not go with her to any doctor's consultations. He is not aware of the seriousness of her cancer, or of how much pain she is in.

In all my years as a homoeopath I have never prescribed a remedy on the basis of the *physical* symptoms of a tumor but rather on the basis of the underlying psychodynamic crisis. The psychodynamic crisis is the 'never-well-since-event' in the case. I arrived at the correct prescription of *Veratrum album* by pure luck in the third consultation, when I gave her the remedy on the basis of the physical symptoms of the tumor itself. Until then, I had prescribed *Carcinosin* 200 C. x 2 doses.

Case Analysis: I used the following key points and headings in analyzing this case to arrive at the correct prescription of *Veratrum album*.

1. **Rubric-repertorisation**
2. **Follow-up Consultations**
3. *Striking*, or *Peculiar* **Signs and Symptoms; Organon 153**
4. **Theme**
5. *How*, *Why*, and *When* **Causations – the 'Never-well-since-event'**
6. **Materia Medica**

Third Consultation:

Presenting Symptoms

She had been complaining about the tumor and the level of discomfort at night.

- The area of the tumor she described as numb: *like waking up after a general or local anesthetic.*

- She described the bone pain as neuralgic shooting pains through her jaw, and running up the left side of her head. She described the pain as *like freezer burn*.

- She sleeps with her head bundled up to keep it warm. She sleeps in her lounge room each night as this is the only room where she is able to keep warm, *the only room that is not frigid*. She sleeps in two sleeping bags, covered with four blankets and a feather doona. She also wraps several woolen scarves around her face and jaw.

- She always has a thick woolen scarf wrapped around her jaw in the consultations (regardless of how warm the room is).

- In the consultations whenever she refers to how she feels she immediately pulls the woolen scarf up to cover her jaw and tumor.

- The pain at night was intense cold. Although she was sweating profusely, she was still cold.

- The tumor was growing and causing terrible pressure on her jaw bone. As a result of the tumor a large, cavernous ulcer in her gum had started to form.

- The ulcer was very infected and filled with pus.

- The infection was also causing nausea, vomiting and diarrhoea. [*Veratrum album*]

The Dreams: In the third consultation she relayed these dreams.

- Being outside and cold, and not asking to come inside.

- Her image in the mirror fading, and not being there anymore.

- Fighting to survive, but she knows she doesn't deserve to.

I had not used the dreams she had been having in the rubric selection, as I was focusing on relieving the infection in her jaw. She did not want to go to the doctor, and had refused antibiotics, so my intense focus was on finding the remedy to alleviate the pus in her jaw. In the follow-up consultations, the dream of fighting to survive but not feeling like she deserved to survive became pertinent to the explaining the delusion she had committed a crime by not knowing what she should do with her life.

1. Rubric-repertorisation

- *Chill*: *coldness*: *external parts*: **VERAT**.
- *Chill*: *coldness*: *single parts*: **VERAT**.
- *Chill*: *internal*: *night*: *cold air were streaming through the bones; as if*: verat. [1] 1.
- *Chill*: *icy coldness of the body*: *single; in*: *spots*: verat. [1] 4. [arg-met. par. petr.]
- *Chill*: *icy coldness of the body*: *skin; of*: *perspiration and also livid hands and feet; covered with a cold*: verat. [1] 2. [*Stram.*]
- *Chill*: *internal coldness*: *bones; as if in the*: verat.
- *Skin*: *coldness*: *icy*: *chill; during*: verat. [1] 1.
- *Skin*: *ulcers*: *painful*: *ulcerative*: *below surface of ulcer*: verat.
- *Generals*: *pain*: *cold parts, in*: *burning*: verat. [1] 2. [sec.]
- *Mouth*: *swelling*: *gums*: verat.

Prescription: I prescribed *Veratrum album* 200 C. 3 times a day for 3 days to help relieve the pain and the infected ulcer.

2. Follow-up Consultations

In that month, she had used the *Veratrum album* initially 3 times a day for 3 days and then one dose a day for 3 days. I repeated the remedy once a day for 3 days, via her phone consultations with me. She had been reporting in weekly that the remedy was giving her tremendous relief.

It was not until I consulted with her that I was completely overwhelmed by the transformation, and I realized that what I had thought was an acute prescription also covered the essence of the original delusion within her case.

At that consult, she told me *she wanted to live.*

3. *Striking*, or *Peculiar* Signs and Symptoms; Organon 153

Veratrum album is convinced that they have *committed a crime* or *done something wrong,* therefore they should be punished; this is exactly what she said to me in the first consult: *It is wrong to not know what to do with the gift of life, therefore I don't deserve it.*

4. Theme

Veratrum album use their belief that 'God is on their side' to protect themselves. Underlying their righteousness is fear of God's vengeance. *Veratrum album* have the opposing *Delusion* rubrics: *he is a messenger of God* versus *he has done wrong. Veratrum album* have the *Delusion* rubric: *hears the ringing of bells. Veratrum album* feel they are doomed to die. This *Veratrum album* (case) would not seek treatment for her cancer because she saw the cancer as God's punishment, and she did not dare go against God's retribution.

The simillimum will not be *Veratrum album* unless the patient believes that they are God-like or that they are in contact with divine, God-like energy. One of the hardest issue to tackle in *Veratrum album* is their belief in God's punishment. Another is their belief in their God-like status.

Veratrum album will not trust or work with the homoeopath unless they believe that the homoeopathic practitioner is in contact with 'divine energy' which is able to guide their prescription.

1. Denial: *Delusion* rubric: *God: communication with God; he is in*: verat. *Delusion* rubric: *God: messenger from God; he is a*: verat. [1] 1. *Delusion* rubric: *religious*: *Verat*. *Delusion* rubric: *Christ, himself to be*: **VERAT**. *Delusion* rubric: *Mary; Virgin: she is*: verat. *Delusion* rubric: *heaven: is in; talking with God*: verat. [1] 1. *Delusion* rubric: *distinguished; he is*: verat. *Delusion* rubric: *vow: keep it, must*: verat. [1] 1.

2. Forsaken: *Delusion* rubric: *home: away from home*; *he is*: verat. *Delusion* rubric: *enemy: surrounded by enemies*: verat. *Delusion* rubric: *murdered: will be murdered; he*: verat. *Delusion* rubric: *persecuted: he is persecuted*: verat. *Delusion* rubric: *pursued; he was*: verat.

3. Causation: *Delusion* rubric: *criminal, he is a*: verat. *Delusion* rubric: *wrong: done wrong; he has*: verat.

4. Depression: *Delusion* rubric: *doomed, being*: *Verat*. *Delusion* rubric: *misfortune: approaching; as if some misfortune were*: *Verat*. *Delusion* rubric: *misfortune: inconsolable over imagined misfortune*: *Verat*. [2] 2. [calc-s.] *Delusion* rubric: *unfortunate, he is*: verat. *Delusion* rubric: *ruined: is ruined; he*: verat.

5. Resignation: *Delusion* rubric: *disease: deaf, dumb and has cancer; he is*: verat. [1] 1. *Delusion* rubric: *die: about to die; one was*: verat. *Delusion* rubric: *cancer, has a*: verat. *Delusion* rubric: *sick: being*: verat. *Delusion* rubric: *bells; hears ringing of*: verat. [This rubric is reminiscent of the saying: 'The bell tolls for thee' or 'Do not ask for whom the bell tolls'.]

Identifying the psychological processes and the psychodynamic avoidances and self-delusions which come into play in each constitutional remedy not only explains the remedy and expands our knowledge – it is necessary for identifying the simillimum. When a patient is sick they are in conflict; when someone is in conflict they self-delude or avoid reality. When a patient is sick, they will move through the five psychological processes as they struggle to acknowledge or accept their illness. Identifying the prominence of one remedy in a particular psychological process will indicate the simillimum. *Veratrum album* are religiously and self-righteously consumed with their guilt.

This *Veratrum album* (case) highlights the consequences of being unable to accept one's illness. *Veratrum album* have the *Delusion* rubrics: *has a cancer,* and *will be murdered. Veratrum album* have the *Delusion* rubrics: *proud,* and *must keep a vow.* The hardest issue to tackle in a *Veratrum album* case is their belief in righteous self-punishment. Self-destructive behavior and self-blame is justified because it is God's punishment. If one is punished for sins committed, then one is worthy of being let into heaven. Punishment is redemption and purification. *Veratrum album* believe that they deserve to be *doomed* forever for the *crimes they have committed. Veratrum album* have the *Delusion* rubric: *compelled to suicide,* and the *Mind* rubric: *suicidal disposition from religious despair. Veratrum album* have religious convictions of martyrdom. *Veratrum album* have the *Mind* rubric: *religious psychotic preaching.* There is hubris in the way *Veratrum album* embrace punishment. All perceived faults cause them to flee into religious fanaticism so they can purify themselves; this is 'hubristic denial' and avoidance. *Veratrum album* have the *Delusion* rubric: *he is deaf and dumb, and has the disease cancer.* [1] 1. The simillimum will only be *Veratrum album* if the patient has a very low opinion of themselves when they are sick. *Veratrum album* believes illness is proof of having been evil. Underlying righteousness is fear of God's vengeance. The simillimum will only be *Veratrum album* if the patient believes that they deserve to be punished by being sick, and that the punishment (sickness) will purify their soul.

Follow-up Consultations

The following is transcribed from the consultation one month after I prescribed *Veratrum album*. It was a videotaped session.

Question: After you saw me, there were a lot of things that came up in relation to your brother?

No. I think it was more the fact that I was emotional about it. It was the first time in a long time I'd cried. I guess just that the grief came out and even now just thinking about it I'm feeling teary. I'm feeling teary about a lot of things, about the children's book, The Bear's Last Winter. *Well, you don't need to know what that is about. Oh my God, that is so sad. News articles, you know, just thoughts, what was the other? The feeling that came up was that I'd been trapped and I'd actually felt this all my life, and so I was finding that I was really trapped by my physical. Now I feel like I'm waking up a bit and coming out into my life at last, which I've never felt, except on two separate occasions for a week, if that. So now it's actually surfacing. It is understanding I've always felt trapped, but earlier in my life it was by circumstances that things were happening to me because so many things were happening outside of me and my family and to those I loved. I couldn't do anything about it, and it wasn't appropriate for me to think of myself, to run off somewhere, to hide to try and do things for myself or save myself because they came first. So I guess I tapped myself in that way.* [Here she is referring to her step-father who was an alcoholic; her mother, a Schizophrenic; and her brother, who committed suicide.] *That was the thing I had to do was to stay. And so I sort of disempowered. I became that victim. I disempowered[32] myself. I felt disempowered by the world because it didn't matter what I did. There was nothing I could do to help them; which I guess was just the realist coming out.*

The point being though that you now actually want to do

---

32 Depression: *Delusion* rubric: *doomed, being*: *Verat. Delusion* rubric: *misfortune: approaching; as if some misfortune were*: *Verat. Delusion* rubric: *misfortune: inconsolable over imagined misfortune*: *Verat.* [2] 2. [calc-s.] *Delusion* rubric: *unfortunate, he is*: verat. *Delusion* rubric: *ruined: is ruined; he*: verat.

something? As opposed to when you first came to see me you were very much like *I don't know what I wanted to do, I've never known what I want to do, and in fact don't know if I want to live.* [Here I am reading from my notes.]

Yes, well that's changed yeh! I've spoken to people and they've said you know, the first thing I thought after I was diagnosed that was an unusual thing because I didn't ask 'why me?' Because I knew, 'why me'. You know, it was to me, 'what have I done to myself?' And you know I have done[33] *this to myself, and you know I have created this and I will fix*[34] *it. That was the immediate thought. It was so clear, it was like a bell going off in my head. And for somebody who has suffered depression, who doesn't know their sort of thoughts and ideas because they've shut them out completely. Who has no opinion, because I have no ego, who doesn't feel emotion because, well it's just not appropriate to the condition you find yourself in. I mean, that was quite amazing. I had created myself, and even the dream that I had was illustrative of that, I think I told you about that a while ago.*[She had told me this dream in her first consultation. It is not until now that I finally understand the delusions in the dream.]

The dream was about a king who, in wanting to show his God that he had his level of devotion and love for him, took his son and killed his son. The God took notice and said he was surprised and honored by this, and so he gave not only the life of his son back, the son's life became immortal. So the boy grew up as an immortal being, and the king realized that the son had got out of control in some way, that he was waging

---

33 Causation: *Delusion* rubric: *criminal, he is a*: verat. *Delusion* rubric: *wrong: done wrong; he has*: verat.

34 Denial: *Delusion* rubric: *God: communication with God; he is in*: verat. *Delusion* rubric: *God: messenger from God; he is a*: verat. [1] 1. *Delusion* rubric: *religious*: Verat. *Delusion* rubric: *Christ, himself to be*: **VERAT**. *Delusion* rubric: *Mary; Virgin: she is*: verat. *Delusion* rubric: *heaven: is in; talking with God*: verat. [1] 1. *Delusion* rubric: *distinguished; he is*: verat. *Delusion* rubric: *vow: keep it, must*: verat. [1] 1.

wars and being a person out of his control. That he wasn't quite doing what the king had thought he wanted the boy to do. So he realized that he had to kill his son to stop this, and he also knew in the act that he might anger the God and he might die as well. But nevertheless he did it, and also he was about to do it, or he had done it, and the God turned around and said, 'What's this? Why would you do something like this after you had given your son's life to me and I have given him back?' So to me that was the consciousness who was the king.

I guess the consciousness who was the king, who thought he was doing the best thing for himself, who had created the life which is now, which is his son. And sub-consciousness is the God. And the God has realized that something is amiss here, that this is not exactly what should be going on, and obviously it was just a recognition of each other. It was a very powerful dream and it clarified exactly what was going on for me.

Analysis of Dream:

This dream is reflective of her feeling of having 'committed a crime' by not deciding what to do with her life. Her reason for not seeking treatment, and her resolve that this cancer was her 'due in life' is now self-explanatory. She has abused the gift of life, as did the son in her dream, hence she should die.

Veratrum album feature prominently in all the *Delusion* rubrics of grandeur to do with being one with God. The *Delusion* rubrics: *he is in heaven talking to God*, and *she is the Virgin Mary*, and *he is a prince*, indicate the elevated status that *Veratrum album* have for themselves. From such a lofty height, *Veratrum album* fall a long way when they acknowledge sin. *Veratrum album* have the *Delusion* rubric: *must keep a vow*.

This *Veratrum album* (case) highlights the intensity of the guilt they feel for having committed a sin. This patient did not feel she was worthy of treatment for her cancer because she had fallen so far in the eyes of God.

Veratrum album have numerous rubrics all of which indicate hubristic 'delusions of grandeur'. Their religious fanaticism is a 'hubristic denial' and arrogance which allows them to feel pure and purified in the eyes of God.

- *Delusion* rubric*: Christ, himself to be*: **VERAT**.
- *Delusion* rubric*: God: communication with God; he is in*: verat.
- *Delusion* rubric*: God: messenger from God; he is a:* verat. [1] 1.
- *Delusion* rubric*: great person, is a: Verat.*
- *Delusion* rubric*: heaven, is in: Verat.*
- *Delusion* rubric*: heaven, is in: talking with God: Verat.*[2] 1.
- *Delusion* rubric*: Mary; Virgin: she is*: verat.
- *Delusion* rubric*: prince; he is a: verat.* [1] 1.
- *Delusion* rubric*: power: all powerful; she is*: verat.
- *Delusion* rubric*: religious: Verat.*
- *Delusion* rubric*: rank; he is a person of*: verat.
- *Mind: egotism*[35]: *Verat.*

Fourth Consultation: Follow-Up Notes after the *Veratrum album*

- The tumor is smaller in size.
- The tumor is less painful at night. The pain is considerably less during the day.
- She is not so cold at night but she is still struggling with maintaining her body temperature.
- If she's too cold she becomes very exhausted.

---

35 I noted at the first consultation her self-assurance about refusing treatment. She appeared so arrogant about this that I should have seen that her arrogance was in fact an important indicator of the remedy picture.

- The numbness is less.

- The infection in her gum comes and goes, but it's not filled with pus anymore; the gums are red and inflamed, but not infected with pus.

She has decided that she wants to live. She wants to go on a trip to Italy to enjoy the sun and sea. She has decided that her family and father in Italy are important to her. She has decided that her relationship with her partner could be meaningful, and that he might be worthy of sharing more of her feelings with so he can know how she feels. He has responded positively to hearing how she feels. The outstanding change in her appearance is encouraging. She is no longer so pale and drawn. She responds quickly to questions. She is no longer depressed. *My family in Italy is very emotional, so I can see at this point that I have been a very emotional person but have been suppressed by my very logical other side, which is from my mother. Not that it's my mother's fault or anything like that, it's just something that I picked up from her, and it was a coping mechanism for the things that I wasn't able to cope with, I guess on an emotional level.* [Her mother was a Schizophrenic. She learnt early on, to associate all emotionalism with a potential onset of a Schizophrenic episode from her mother.] She now feels sad, or angry, or happy, in proportion to what would be the expected response to a particular situation; she can now allow herself to *feel*.

Dose: She is currently taking 3 doses of the *Veratrum album* 200 C. a day according to her need for pain relief. The same pattern of 3 days on and 3 days off seems to correspond to her need of the remedy. I am not concerned by the seemingly high dose. It is matching her physical need, and the intensity of the pain and physical exhaustion. She continues to improve emotionally, mentally, and physically.

Follow-up Consultation three months later, after her trip to Italy:

- The tumor is noticeably larger.
- The tumor is still cold.
- She is now in so much pain, she is on morphine patches.

Her belief in her father has been shattered. He did not look after her, and he was a huge disappointment. The healing and love she was imagining did not come to fruition. She is greatly distressed by her father's abandonment. She only slept in two hour blocks the whole time she was away. Her father did not help with providing food, or with cooking meals for her when she was unable to feed herself. When she first arrived, he gave her a healing. Her father is a religious healer who believes he has a connection to Jesus. As soon as he touched her he told her: *you do not have faith*. Soon after 'his healing' the tumor grew to three times its previous size. After one month of treatments, she asked her father to not touch her anymore; the tumor stopped growing after that. Most significantly, she did not take the *Veratrum album* whilst she was away.

She believes she is not worthy of homoeopathic treatment, nor is she worthy of life. God's vengeance has been absorbed into her psyche. She is frozen in her conviction that God is punishing her.

5. *How*, *Why*, and *When* Causations – the 'Never-well-since-event'

She told me her primary psychodynamic trauma in the very first consultation, when she described herself and her family of origin: *I am the result of an affair*. I am intensely reminded of her telling me she was conceived out of wedlock and, for a Italian girl who is very religious, I should have noted the terrible weight that sin has had in her life. She felt that her father was witness to the fact that she was not close to Jesus and she is convinced her father has the ability to see she is faithless. I am reminded of the *Delusion* rubric: *he has committed a crime.*

I have found in my practice that every patient who presents with any serious disease, whether it be emotional, mental, or physical, always presents with the *Delusion* rubrics of abandonment and the underlying guilt of being cast out of Paradise because they are evil. Each case presented also resonates with the patient's delusional expectation that if they are in communication with God or a 'higher being' or their 'inner spiritual spirit' they should be able to cure their disease. If they can't cure their disease then they believe that their disease is a result of God's judgment or karma for the sins they have committed. The assumption of the concept of 'original sin', and the attributing of personal blame will, in my experience, always present itself when a patient faces the loss of their health, regardless of whether it is fatal or non-fatal. If the trauma inside your patient starts with them feeling guilty and responsible for being sick, then the simillimum is listed in the *Delusion* rubrics: *he is sinful* and *he has committed a crime.*

The dose prescribed at this consultation was *Veratrum album* 200 C. x 1/dose a day.

She is exhausted, and she is dying. She promises to seek conventional treatment though her medical doctor.

Follow-up, 1 month later: She has not taken her homoeopathics for the last two weeks.

- The tumor has grown so large in the last two weeks that her cheek has developed an enormous abscess around the tumor.
- She has been on antibiotics and in incredible pain; she is now on morphine patches of 10 mg.
- The pus filled abscess has been aspirated. The infection is however, still present.

- Her weight loss is significant; she has not had enough energy to feed herself.
- She currently weighs 52 kilos.

She has once again retracted her promise to seek conventional treatment, even though her medical doctor is also insisting on this.

In this case, the self-destructive psychological delusion formed the first conscious thought of being in communication with God, or knowing more than anyone else that she deserved her cancer. The struggle to find her validation for existence continues.

Follow-up, 6 weeks later: She has once again decided to stop taking the remedy; again two weeks prior to the appointment.

Every time she stops the remedy, she goes back to the belief that she has done something wrong, and she has not yet learnt what the particular lesson is. In my experience of working with cancer patients, a common 'New-age' ideology is that they believe they deserve the cancer, or it has come as a result of needing a particular lesson. The essence of that feeling is of course mirroring the *Delusion* rubrics: *he is a criminal*, and *he has done wrong*.

The following is transcribed from the above consultation. It was a videotaped session.

Question: What do people want you to do?

Well, they want me to go to the hospital and they want me to try the chemotherapy. It was offensive being underestimated in that sense. So I guess it's that cross over between people caring, and where I have to justify what I am doing.

(In this statement, she is referring to her belief that she can cure herself, and to the continuing belief that when she has been punished enough by God, the tumor will stop growing.)

New Year's Eve I had one of those half-awake dreams again; possession-like ones. I was lying down mediating and a little girl came to me. She wanted to be held and I didn't know whether it was going to be a good thing. I asked the little girl, well if you are here as part of my healing and you are not here to harm me then that is okay. I didn't get an answer, but I feel as though she must have stepped in and I sort of felt calmness. That fear that has been so prevalent in everything that I have done has left. I have had a vision of a hanged girl and her mother. The girl is a great part of me that I had sacrificed myself.

Why are you suffering?

Because somehow I deserved it, or if I suffered then things would be okay for others. I needed to suffer for things to be okay.

(Here she refers to saving the world. The essence of what she is saying is reflective and reminiscent of the imagery of Jesus dying on the cross to save us from our sins. This is a psychological delusion of grandeur. *Delusion* rubric: *God: messenger from God; he is a:* verat. [1] 1.)

Physical Symptoms:

- She is no longer cold
- The tumor is no longer cold
- Her weight is down to 48 kilos
- The tumor has now grown to such a large size it is protruding at least four inches from her face. Her whole face is contorted
- She is suffering from congestive headaches, which is not surprising given the size of the tumor
- < Hot weather
- < Tumor hot to touch [*Veratrum viride*]
- < Headaches < hot weather
- Swelling
- Constrictive pain

- She is no longer able to chew and is now eating soft food
- Sleep is disrupted because of the increasing pain in her jaw
- Blood clots in the mouth from the tumor
- The tumor is hot to the touch and is reacting to the present hot weather
- The tumor is putting a lot of pressure on the jaw bone. Her temperature is not cold and she is no longer cold at night

Remedy Given: *Veratrum viride* 30 C., 3 times a day.

The simillimum *must* have *Delusion* rubrics which match the delusional state of mind of the patient.

The advantage in identifying and understanding the psychological processing that your patient is moving through is that it allows you to narrow the remedies being considered to the remedies listed in those particular rubric-categories. If the constitutional remedy that the homoeopath has chosen has *Delusion* rubrics allocated into Causation, the patient *must* display psychological 'delusions of original sin'. *Veratrum viride* was not the first simillimum because she clearly displayed numerous 'delusions of original sin'. *Veratrum viride* have no *Delusion* rubrics allocated in Causation. If the constitutional remedy that the homoeopath has chosen has *Delusion* rubrics allocated into Denial, the patient *must* display psychological 'delusions of grandeur'. *Veratrum viride* believe they understand everything and *possess infinite knowledge. Veratrum viride* have the *Mind* rubric: *insanity, megalomania*, and the *Delusion* rubric: *understands everything.* [1] 1. *Veratrum viride* believe that have infinite hubristic knowledge of the cause and cure of their illness.

Veratrum viride possess the infinite wisdom that Jesus possessed when he sacrificed his life to save humanity. She says: *that fear that has been so prevalent in everything that I have done has left. I have had a vision of a hanged girl and her mother. The girl is a great part of me that I had sacrificed myself.*

Question: Why are you suffering?

Because somehow I deserved it, or if I suffered then things would be okay for others. I needed to suffer for things to be okay.

She felt that her father was witness to the fact that she was not close to Jesus. Her father believes he has a connection to Jesus. As soon as he touched her, he told her: *you do not have faith.* Regardless of whether she eventually rejected his 'healing treatments', she left Italy having absorbed deep within her psyche that she was not close to Jesus, and that she did not deserve to live. There is no greater hubristic goal than sacrificing oneself to a higher being. Martyrdom is fueled by 'hubristic visions' of a grand persona. Being willing to become a martyr and suffer death for the advancement of a righteous cause can be analyzed as visionary or self-destructive.

All psychological delusions of martyrdom are a complex mixture of self-deceit fueled by paranoid fears of impotence. *Veratrum viride* righteously sacrifice themselves. There is hubris in their act of martyrdom. *Carcinosin* (which I gave her in the first consultation) in comparison use martyrdom self-righteously to excuse themselves for not taking personal power and control over their own lives.

If the constitutional remedy that the homoeopath has chosen has *Delusion* rubrics allocated into Forsaken, the patient *must* display psychological 'delusions of abandonment' or 'delusions of persecution'. *Veratrum viride* have numerous fears of doctors and medical treatment. They have the persecutory *Delusion* rubrics: *he is persecuted, pursued,* and *about to be poisoned.* Peculiar to *Veratrum viride* is the *Delusion* rubric: *clothes did not fit. Veratrum viride* believe that they are so great that nothing lowly can possibly apply to them.

1. Denial: *Delusion* rubric: *great person, is a*: verat-v. *Delusion* rubric: *knowledge; he possesses infinite*: verat-v. [1] 3. [cann-i. psil.] *Delusion* rubric: *understands: understands everything*: verat-v. [1] 1. *Delusion* rubric: *clothes: fit; did*

not: verat-v. [1] 1. [This rubric can pertain to perceptions of grandeur or persecution.]

2. Forsaken: *Delusion* rubric: *persecuted*: *he is persecuted*: verat v. *Delusion* rubric: *pursued; he was*: verat -v. *Delusion* rubric: *poisoned*: *he*: *about to be poisoned; he is*: verat-v. *Delusion* rubric: *clothes*: *fit; did not*: verat-v. [1] 1. [This rubric pertains to the *Veratrum viride* belief that they do not fit within society.]

3. Causation: NONE.

4. Depression*: Delusion* rubric: *confused; as if*: verat-v. [1] 2. [tub]

5. Resignation: *Delusion* rubric: *confused; as if*: verat-v. [1] 2. [tub] [This rubric can pertain to depression or resignation about illness.]

- *Mind*: *death*: *desires*: verat-v.
- *Mind*: *fear*: *doctors*: verat-v.
- *Mind*: *fear*: *poisoned*: *being poisoned; fear of*: verat-v.
- *Mind*: *insanity*: *megalomania*: *Verat-v.*

After taking the *Veratrum viride* she was able to seek medical treatment. *Veratrum album* moved her stance on whether she *deserved* to die. *Veratrum viride* subsequently moved her delusion of being able to cure her own cancer so she could forgive herself of her sins and die in peace.

6. Materia Medica

"Exalted opinion of her own ideas and powers." [Vermeulen]

Last Consultation, February 2007

The tumor has grown considerably. I stress very intensely that I am scared the tumor threatens her spinal cord and carotid artery[36]. For the first time, after the dose of *Veratrum viride* she

---

36 The tumor had in fact metastasized into her jaw, and was threatening her spinal cord and carotid artery.

acknowledges that she has been unable to cure the tumor. I do not believe that she would have admitted to not being able to cure her own cancer, if she had not taken the *Veratrum viride*. *Veratrum viride* have "Exalted opinion of her own ideas and powers."

She thanks me for my persistence with working with her, and admits that until taking the last remedy she has had an omnipotent belief in her ability to know what is best for her and her cure. Most importantly she acknowledges that she has in fact wished to die with this cancer.

She states that I have taken her from years of depression and of believing she deserved to die like her brother (he put his head under a train) to now wanting to live. She finally admits herself into the emergency section of the cancer ward and commences radiotherapy. For the first time, she starts to tell family and friends that she has failed in her attempts to cure herself, and that she is seeking medical intervention.

The essence of *Veratrum viride* was her "exalted opinion of her own ideas and powers". [Vermeulen] She has now 'moved' her hubristic stance on whether she can cure herself. She is now able to talk with me about the need to prepare herself for death. She tells me that for the first time in her life she is not depressed.

Conclusion: March 2007

I was still in contact with the patient, and helping her with palliative treatment through the conventional medical system. She tells me that for the first time in her life she is not depressed, and is co-operating with her doctors in their fight for her life.

This patient contracted the severe 2007 Influenza A virus in Australia that resulted in several deaths. She died seven hours after getting pneumonia. She weighed 46 kilos and was not able to resist the infection. Her last words to her partner were that she was sorry she was dying. This woman died of pneumonia, having moved her delusion of being evil. She died having lived life, and by receiving and feeling love for the first time in her life, she died wanting to live. This case resulted in death. I do not view this case as one in which I did not cure the delusion or original crisis; this was a true case of the spiritual healing of homoeopathy. This *Veratrum* case reverberates with a crisis of self-examination which reflects both the delusions of herself as God – *Delusion* rubric: *in communication with God*, and herself as the victim of God's judgment – *Delusion* rubric: *he has committed a crime*. In this case, the woman believed she deserved the Adenocarcinoma and she tragically sought no treatment. This was a suicide case. I believe her desire to resist treatment was reflective of her suicidal desire because she believed she did not deserve life. Her father's connection to Jesus, and his pronouncement as soon as he touched her, "You do not have faith", confirmed her own view that she deserved punishment from God. This acknowledgement of her sin resulted in her stopping the *Veratrum album*.

The hubristic delusion of being in communication with God will cause *Veratrum album* to stop the remedy. Patients with Schizophrenia have exactly the same behavior, mirroring the same delusions of exalted power. They profess hubristic communication with God and the devil. They often are directed by God to stop taking their medication.

In the first consultation she told me: *I am the result of an affair*. It is apt that this *Veratrum album* (case) is the last case analysis because it was the first case which emphasized for me the need to listen and truly understand the significance of what the patient tells me in the first consultation. It was also the first time I understood the need to ask leading questions of the patient. This patient came to see me at a point in her life when the cancer had already become fatal. She was already dying. However, what I have learnt from this case I have now crystallized into not only my practice with patients, but into writing *Homoeopathic Psychiatry*. In the cases, I emphasize repeatedly the need to understand the causation or the 'never-well-since-event'.

Bibliography

Schroyens, Frederik. M.D. *Synthesis*. London, Homeopathic Book Publishers, 1997.

Vermeulen, Frans. *Synoptic Materia Medica* 2. The Netherlands, Merlijin Publishers, 1992. p. 941.

Glossary

Conscious mind: knows and is aware of thoughts and feelings.

Delusion: a self-deluding and self-deceiving belief which avoids reality.

'Delusion of abandonment': an assumption or presumption that one will be abandoned or neglected.

'Delusion of deprivation': an over-exaggerated presumption of poverty.

'Delusion of grandeur': a delusion that one is greater or more powerful than is the case in reality.

'Delusion of hypochondria': a delusion that one could become ill or that one is already ill. Exaggerated fear of diseases and obsessive fear that one is going to die.

'Delusions of impending doom': assumptions and predictions of failure.

'Delusion of original sin': an assumption of presumed guilt for real or perceived wrongs committed in one's life.

'Delusion of persecution': also known as a **'persecution complex'**. A delusional belief that others are pursuing you in order to harm you. Incorrect perceptions and imaginings that someone is going to embarrass you or cause you embarrassment in society. Imagining rejection and abandonment. Pre-empting real or perceived rejection or abandonment and responding to this incorrect perception by either aggressive behavior or self-imposed exile.

'Delusion of superiority': a delusion that one is superior to others.

'Ego': Freud developed the concept of the 'id', 'ego', and 'super-ego'. The organized, realistic part of the psyche is the 'ego'. The use of the word 'ego' in *Homoeopathic Psychiatry* refers to the destruction of the 'ego' from the conflict between the psyche and the external world. If a remedy profile has a weakened 'ego' then their psyche is under threat. In modern-day society, ego is usually used to describe self-esteem or one's sense of self-worth. However, according to Freud, the 'ego' is used to describe the psyche.

Hallucination: illusory perceptions or imaginations not based in reality.

Hubris: an insolent pride or alignment with the Gods, leading to nemesis.

'Hubristic denial': the belief that God has bestowed upon one great powers of omnipotence. A patient suffering with 'hubristic denial' refuses to believe that they are sick, or could die. In relation to disease, and impending death, a patient suffering from 'hubristic denial' believes they will be cured by God. Often, they believe that they are so powerful they can cure themselves. 'Hubristic denial' is the denial of illness, or impending death, because one believes one is an omnipotent God.

'Hubristic visions': the *Delusion* rubric: *has visions* can indicate a need to create an illusion of oneself which is grander than reality. A 'hubristic vision' of oneself is the belief that one is aligned with God.

'Id': the unconscious, instinctual, unstructured inspiration in our somatic behavior is the 'id'. The 'id' is unconscious and is not restricted by social conventionality. The 'id' is unrestrained, selfish, self-gratification.

Illusion: a sense-perception which proves to be incorrect.

Illusions of fancy: the *Delusion* rubric: *illusions of fancy*, alludes to a psychological 'delusion of grandeur'. A patient who is suffering *illusions of fancy* has grand visions of persona: their expectations of what they can achieve, or what they *have* achieved, or who they are in the world, are exaggerated.

'Narcissism': the personality trait of excessive vanity or self-love. In psychology and psychiatry, narcissism is recognized as a severe personality disorder of excessive selfishness.

'Narcissistic neurosis': a pre-emptive cause of manic-depressive psychosis insofar as it is characterized by the withdrawal of energy from the realistic and rational 'ego'. Energy which is disproportionately redirected on to a narcissist persona causes 'delusions of grandeur'. Freud defined neurosis as a conflict between the 'ego' and the 'id'. 'Neuroses' relate to psychosomatic conditions, and 'psychoses' relate to mental conflict between the 'ego' and the external world.

Neurosis: a disproportionate adherence to unrealistic, deranged thoughts. An inability to take a rational, realistic approach to a particular subject.

'Nihilistic delusion': the delusion that everything, including the self, does not exist; a sense that reality and the somatic does not exist and that everything outside of the self is also unreal.

Paranoia: a fear of persecution which results in a disproportionate or abnormal tendency to suspect others; hence paranoiac or paranoid.

Primary Trauma: the first trauma in a patient's life. It usually occurs in childhood, and frequently forms the conscious, subconscious and unconscious responses which govern the assimilation and misinterpretation of the first pain in life.

Psychodynamic: the interplay between conscious, subconscious, and unconscious motivations in a patient's life, and the manifestation or evidence of those motivations in behavioral patterns. Psychodynamics is the study of the interrelationship between the conscious, subconscious, and unconscious mind, and the psyche, and how they process behavioral patterns at the conscious, subconscious and unconscious levels. The psychodynamic therapist aims to find evidence of the first maladaptive event or evidence of the first disproportionate response to an event or trauma in the patient's life. The assumption is that this primary event is the core basis of future delusional functioning which has influenced the patient's behavioral patterning within their conscious, subconscious, and unconscious mind. In homoeopathy, this event is called the 'never-well-since-event'.

Psychodynamic application of the *Delusion* rubrics in case-development: rubric evidence of the first 'never-well-since-event' and subsequent events in the patient's life. Rubric-repertorisation or evidence collected to explain the patient's behavioral patterning within their conscious, subconscious, and unconscious mind.

Psychotherapeutic: understanding the application, and need for, the psychological delusion in the patient's life. The understanding behind the practical reason why the patient has maintained the psychological delusional belief.

Psychotherapeutic meaning: the study of how each remedy profile listed under each rubric heading has used the delusional stance to its advantage.

Psychical: of the soul, phenomena outside of the emotional, mental or physical sphere.

Psyche: the personification of the soul, spirit and mind.

Psychology: the science that deals with emotional and mental processes and behaviors.

Psychological delusion: a perception or opinion which is exaggerated or disproportionate to reality.

Psychosis: according to Freud psychosis is a conflict between the 'ego' and the external world. A psychosis is a severe mental derangement. The *Delusion* rubrics which cover psychoses are the *Delusion* rubrics: forsaken, depression and resignation. These *Delusion* rubrics emphasize the threat that the world poses to the self or 'ego'. They contain the 'delusions of abandonment', 'delusions of persecution', 'delusions of impending doom', and the 'delusions of hypochondria', in that order. Psychosis results from a difficulty in the relationship between the 'ego' and the external world.

Psychosomatic: delusions of mind and body. Illusions which cause a physical manifestation of an imagined disease. A psychosomatic disease can be in response to the aggravations of stress.

'Somatic delusion': an incorrect delusion about physicality. A 'somatic delusion' is a delusion concerning the body image or parts of the body.

Subconscious mind: contains thoughts which are not fully conscious, and mental and emotional processes existing or operating in the mind beneath the easy reach of the conscious mind. Contains mental and emotional processes and motivations of which the person is not aware, but which are still able to influence, and offer explanations of behavior. The subconscious mind is easily accessed in any psychotherapeutic environment, including homoeopathic consultations, when the practitioner delves into the development of the primary trauma in a patient's life.

'Super-ego': the perfectionist critical function of all our moralistic and inspirational ideals, and spiritual goals, and conscience is the 'super-ego'.

'Transference': a psychological term which describes the projection process that can take place in all helping professions, including a homoeopathic consultation. In 'transference', the patient pressures the homoeopath into playing a role that mirrors their own delusional internal world.

'Transference neurosis': according to Freud, 'transference neurosis' is a conflict between the 'ego' and the 'id'. A neurosis is a disorder of the behavioral system in which one is unable to have a rational or realistic objective view of one's life. Transference is characterized by unconscious, self-deluding denial which allows for the redirection of feelings on to another person. A 'transference neurosis' can be found in the *Delusion* rubrics of 'hubristic denial' in which the patient transfers 'cause and effect' on to God or their own 'delusions of grandeur'. These are the *Delusion* rubrics: *in communication with God*. A 'transference neurosis' can also be found in the *Delusion* rubrics of sin in which the patient transfers 'cause and effect' on to the devil. These are the *Delusion* rubrics: *in communication with the devil*.

Unconscious mind: contains secrets, thought processes, emotional feelings, intuitions or perceptions, and behavioral patterns which are suppressed by the patient's conscious mind, even though they can still influence behavior and thoughts.

Zoanthropy: the delusion that you have assumed the form of an animal.

Bibliography

Allen, Timothy Field, M.D. LL.D. *Handbook of Materia Medica.* New Delhi, B. Jain Publishers, 1994. p.p. 450-456.

Bailey, Philip, M, M.D. *Homeopathic Psychology.* Berkeley, California, North Atlantic Books, 1995.

Boericke, William, M. D. *Pocket Manuel of Homoeopathic Materia Medica.* New Delhi, Motilal Banarsidass Publishers, 1996.

Clarke, John Henry, M.D. *A Dictionary of Practical Materia Medica.* Volume 11. New Delhi, B. Jain Publishers, 1994. p.p. 44-45.

Grieve, Mrs. M. *A Modern Herbal.* Middlesex, England, Penguin Books, 1980.

Hahnemann, Dr. Samuel, *The Chronic Diseases.* New Delhi, B. Jain Publishers, 1995.

Julian, O. A. *Dictionary of Homoeopathic Materia Medica.* New Delhi, B. Jain Publishers, 1984, p.p. 269-271.

Kent, J. T. *Lectures on Materia Medica.* New Delhi, B. Jain Publishers, 1994.

Kent, J. T. *Repertory of the Homoeopathic Materia Medica and a Word Index.* New Delhi, B. Jain Publishers, 1994.

Lalor, Liz. *A Homeopathic Guide to Partnership and Compatibility.* Berkeley, California, North Atlantic Books, 2004.

Morrison, Roger, M.D. *Desktop Guide*. Nevada City, CA, Hahnemann Clinic Publishing, 1993.

Phatak, Dr. S. R. *Materia Medica of Homeopathic Medicines*. New Delhi, Indian Books & Periodicals Publishers, p.p. 233-235.

Sankaran, Rajan. *The Soul of Remedies*. Santa Cruz, Bombay, Homoeopathic Medical Publishers, 1997. p.p. 47, 139, 59-60, 75-76, 141-143, 94-95, 109-110, 31, 49-50, 85.

Sankaran, Rajan. *An Insight Into Plants*. Santa Cruz, Bombay, Homeopathic Medical Publishers, 2002.

Shakespeare, William. *Shakespeare The Complete Works*, Volume III. England, Heron Books, 1995. pp.482-574.

Schroyens, Frederik, M.D. *Synthesis*. London, Homeopathic Book Publishers, 1997.

Tolkien, J.R.R. *The Lord of the Rings. The Fellowship of the Ring* London, HarperCollins Publishers, 1994.

(*The Lord of the Rings* is comprised of three books - *The Fellowship of the Ring, The Two Towers*, and the final book *The Return of the King*.)

Tumminello, Peter. *Twelve Jewels*. St. Leonards, NSW, The Medicine Way, 2005. p.p. 121, 125.

Vermeulen, Frans. *Synoptic Materia Medica*. The Netherlands, Emryss Publishers, Haarlem, 1992.

Vermeulen, Frans. *Synoptic Materia Medica 2*. The Netherlands, Merlijin Publishers, 1992. p.p. 149, 768-772, 722-723.

Vermeulen, Frans. *Prisma*. Emryss Publishers, Haarlem, 2002. p.p. 429-436, 646-649, 549, 1019.

Vithoulkas, George. The Science of Homeopathy. New Delhi, B. Jain Publishers, 1997.

Acknowledgements

I am indebted to the following people, without their support *Homoeopathic Psychiatry* would never have become a reality.

To Dale Emerson, the inspiration and creative force behind the development of Radar™. I am inspired by this innovative software because I found *Delusion* rubrics which I have never found before even though I have scrolled the repertory for years. I accessed all the *Delusion* rubrics used in *Homoeopathic Psychiatry* via Radar Schroyens F., Synthesis Treasure Edition, Millennium view (progressive). Dr. Frederik Schroyens's *Repertorium Homeopathicum Syntheticum* is the most reliable repertory which I refer to for all my rubric-repertorisation needs in case analyses.

To René Otter for his strong conviction in the need for homoeopaths to return to repertorising cases and his consistent personal support. I am forever indebted to him for his heartfelt generosity.

To the Australian representative for Radar™ Greg Cope, for all of his much needed technical support in developing *Homoeopathic Psychiatry* into an innovative case-taking tool for homoeopaths.

To my wonderful editor Vera Di Campli San Vito who has helped me with the finishing touches to the final editing of *Homoeopathic Psychiatry*.

To Thupten Lekshe who taught me about illness and death.

Finally, my deepest thanks go to my *Sulphur* partner for his inspiration and belief in me. I hope it has not been delusional!

Endnotes

1   The psychological terminology used in *Homoeopathic Psychiatry* are defined in the Glossary.

2   I accessed all the *Delusion* rubrics used in *Homoeopathic Psychiatry* via Radar© Schroyens F., *Synthesis Treasure Edition*, Millennium view (progressive).

3   "One of the great desires of *Sulphurs* is to discover a new thought or theory. *Sulphurs* have optimism and hopefulness in life. They either inspire or frustrate others, who might view their beliefs as impractical philosophizing about life and basically a lot of hot air. *Sulphurs* have an explosive anger and passionate temperament that others will view either as flashes of visionary insight or just a bad temper. *Sulphurs* have a self-obsession with their own processes in life that could be viewed as the eccentricity of a genius or the pure selfishness of an egomaniac. *Sulphurs* need the world to acknowledge their brilliance. If the world does not acknowledge them, it is the fault of everyone else in the world who lacks the insight into their quest for knowledge—it is never *Sulphurs'* fault. This drive for ego satisfaction can also be viewed as either inspirational genius or chauvinistic." Lalor, Liz, *A Homeopathic Guide to Partnership and Compatibility*, Berkeley, California, North Atlantic Books, 2004, p.227.

4   Conrad, Joseph, Great Short Works of Joseph Conrad. New York, Harper and Row Publishers, 1966,1967, p.353.

5   Dr. Constantine Hering, (1800-1880) formulated the law of the direction of symptoms pertaining to evidence of cure. This is known as 'Hering's Law of Cure'.

   1. From above downwards.

   2. From within outwards.

   3. From a more important organ to a less important one.

   4. In the reverse order of their coming.

6   In Anne Michaels's novel, *Fugitive Pieces*, one of the characters says of biography: "We're stuffed with famous men's lives; soft with the habits of our own. The quest to discover another's psyche, to absorb another's motives as deeply as your own, is a lover's quest. But the search for

facts, for places, names, influential events, important conversations and correspondences, political circumstances – all this amounts to nothing if you can't find the assumption your subject lives by." Anne Michaels, *Fugitive Pieces,* New York, Alfred A. Knopf, Inc., p.222

7   I am the originator of the Liz Lalor Fertility Program© based on the Vannier method. I teach this program to homoeopaths world-wide. To date my statistical success is significant, with 216 babies born out of a total of 247 women treated.

8   A maelstrom is a great whirlpool.

9   When I was studying homoeopathy, I was taught that if a remedy is graded as a *one* in a rubric heading, it meant the rubric heading was of little significance. My experience of the importance of the psychological delusions which are revealed in the *Delusion* rubrics has led me to disagree with that teaching. The *peculiar* rubrics which contain only one remedy are exquisite gems which I treasure because they are *the more striking, singular, uncommon and peculiar signs and symptoms* of that particular remedy only. [Aphorism 153 The Organon.] The *Delusion* rubrics which contain only one remedy are indicative of the conflicting psychological delusions in each constitutional remedy.

10 The *Delusion* rubric: *religious* reflects either disproportionate over-reactivity to the belief one is, or has been, 'bad' or the need to align oneself with God in order to absolve oneself of all wrong. Each remedy in the *Delusion* rubric: *religious* is listed below with their particular 'sin' or underlying Causation rubric also listed.

Alumina silicata: *Delusion* rubric: *crime: committed a crime; he had*: alum-sil.

Anacardium: *Delusion* rubric: *crime: committed a crime; he had*: anac.

Arsenicum album: *Delusion* rubric: *crime: committed a crime; he had*: ars.

Aurum metallicum: *Delusion* rubric: *sinned; one has: day of grace; sinned away his*: aur.

Belladonna: *Delusion* rubric: *devil*: Bell.

Crocus sativus: *Delusion* rubric: *business: unfit for, he is*: Croc. [2] 1.

Hyoscyamus: *Delusion* rubric: *wrong: done wrong; he has*: hyos.

Kali bromatum: *Delusion* rubric: *crime: committed a crime; he had*: kali-br.

Lachesis: *Delusion* rubric: *crime: committed a crime; he had*: lach.

Lycopodium: *Delusion* rubric: *wrong: done wrong; he has*: lyc.

Medorrhinum: *Delusion* rubric: *crime: committed a crime; he had*: med.

Mercurius: *Delusion* rubric: *crime: committed a crime; he had*: merc.

Nux vomica: *Delusion* rubric: *crime: committed a crime; he had*: nux-v.

Olibanum sacrum: *Delusion* rubric: *soul*: *exchanged; were*: olib-sac. [1] 1.

Platina: *Delusion* rubric: *devil*: *possessed of a devil*: *he is*: plat.

Pulsatilla: *Delusion* rubric: *crime*: *committed a crime; he had*: puls.

Stramonium: *Delusion* rubric: *sinned*; *one has*: *day of grace; sinned away his*: stram.

Sulphur: *Delusion* rubric: *sinned*; *one has*: *day of grace; sinned away his*: sulph.

Tarentula hispanica: *Delusion* rubric: *assaulted, is going to be*: tarent.

Veratrum album: *Delusion* rubric: *crime*: *committed a crime; he had*: Verat.

11 Frankincense is obtained from trees of the genus *Boswellia sacra*. Its aroma has traditionally been associated with religious rituals within the Jewish and Christian religions. Frankincense was one of four 'sweet scents' of the ceremonial incense in the Jewish religion. Frankincense is mentioned in the Pentateuch and formed part of the offering which was presented with the Shabbat bread on Sabbath. In the book of Exodus in the Old Testament it was an ingredient for incense. In the Gospel of Matthew, gold, frankincense and myrrh were among the gifts given to celebrate the birth of Jesus.

12 *Calcarea silicata* and *Asterias rubens* are the only two remedies listed in the *Delusion* rubric: *hearing voices and answers*. *Asterias rubens* is a sea remedy. Survival and protection, and constant awareness of predators is essential to survival. *Asterias rubens* are influenced psychically which is why they are able to hear voices. With *Asterias rubens* this rubric can undoubtedly be allocated to hubristic grandeur. With *Calcarea silicata*, because they have so many protection rubrics associated with seeing and talking to dead people, the rubric is more indicative of their need to look outside of themselves psychically for reassurance.

13 "The homeopathic remedy *Nux vomica* is derived from a dilution of tincture taken from the seeds of a poison nut *strychnos nux vomica*. It was commonly referred to as the poison strychnine because the nut itself contained a high percentage of the poison. Strychnine poisoning creates a fanatical degree of spasms and severe cramps. A poisoning overdose affects the gut and travels to the blood and spinal cord; the eyes bulge, the muscles contract, and the whole body goes into convulsions. Death comes as the convulsions get more violent, and the respiratory muscle spasms cause the respiratory system to shut down.

Nux vomicas carry in their psyche the inner threat of possible annihilation. Nux vomicas are always on guard, and only relax when safely at home away from the world. The inability for Nux vomicas to relax and let down their guard against possible attack is mirrored in the types of physical strain and tension they suffer. Nux vomicas are fanatically intense and driven to succeed; they need to secure their position in the world so they can ward off any possible annihilation or poisoning." Lalor, Liz, *A Homeopathic*

Guide to Partnership and Compatibility, Berkeley, California, North Atlantic Books, 2004, p.59.

14 Refugees and people escaping from invading armies frequently sew money into their clothes. Jews who were being deported to concentration camps sewed money into their clothes so they would have money to be able to bribe people for food, or shelter (protection). As a *Delusion* rubric: it can be used in a case analysis if the patient indicates that they often hide money in their wallet or bra in case they will be robbed. The *Delusion* rubric: *money sewed up in clothing*, indicates that the patient is suffering from fear of loss of security.

15 "Sallekhana (also Santhara, Samadhi-marana, Samnyasa-marana) is a Jain practice of voluntary death through fasting when the end of life is very near due to unavoidable circumstances, such as illness or old age. It is the act of calmly withdrawing from worldly preoccupations and attachments by a combination of meditation and abstaining from food and water. In accepting to do sallekhana, the person must take a special vow to ensure that the body and the soul will leave the world in harmony and complete peace of mind, without fear. The purpose is to purge old karmas and prevent the creation of new ones. Like most Dharmic religious traditions, Jainism considers suicide a wrong that only retains the karma from the current life and does not allow escape from the cycle of births and rebirths. Suicide involves an intentional act of harm against oneself with a known outcome that negatively affects those left behind. With Sallekhana, death is welcomed through a peaceful, tranquil process providing peace of mind for everyone involved." www.cuke.com/deathanddying/santhara.html

16 "The relevant homeopathic concept in choosing the right remedy to match your personality is 'like cures like'. Cancer arises from the abnormal and uncontrolled division, and overgrowth of undifferentiated, or poorly differentiated cells. The undifferentiated cells divide and duplicate quickly without controls. Initially, the malignant cells invade surrounding tissues; as the cancer grows it expands, and begins to compete with the surrounding tissues and organs for space. Eventually the tumor metastasizes and invades the surrounding body cavities, entering lymph or blood systems; this enables the cancer cells to travel unchecked and uncontrolled throughout the body. The reason I have outlined the above pathophysiology is that it is crucial to the understanding of the constitution Carcinosin. The image that comes to mind is one of an ungrounded or undifferentiated energy that is expanding and desperately pushing on all that surrounds it, in the attempt to find definition or containment. Carcinosins do not know their personal boundaries. The description of the pathology of cancerous growth mirrors and is 'like' the personality of the constitution Carcinosin. Carcinosins are on a journey of self-discovery. Carcinosins are not sure of themselves; they need to push very hard in life to be able to find definition. Consequently they are always expanding and pushing limits and boundaries to find out who they are. If you are content with yourself you are not Carcinosin, and if you know who you are you are not Carcinosin." Lalor, Liz, *A Homeopathic*

Guide to Partnership and Compatibility, Berkeley, California, North Atlantic Books, 2004, p.p. 23-24.

17 The *Mind* rubric: *desire to be magnetized*, refers to a somatic need to be influenced by a greater force outside of oneself. The need to be aligned with a greater force than oneself is fueled by 'hubristic visions' of persona.

18 The *Delusion* rubrics: *seeing people*, and *visions* and *fancy illusions* can be interpreted as the patient making alliances with good spirits or good ghosts of dead family members who are helping them, which is why I have allocated them to the section of rubrics: *in communication with God*. The *Delusion* rubrics: *horrible visions*, **CALC,** *sees ugly faces*, **CALC,** *sees frightful images and phantoms*, **CALC**, should be allocated to the section dealing with *Delusion* rubrics: *forsaken* or *Delusion* rubrics: *sin*. The *Delusion* rubrics: *seeing specters, ghosts, spirits*, should be assessed according to the individual remedy and how the visions are advantageous to each individual constitutional remedy. For example, *Agaricus* will use their visions of specters and ghosts to their advantage to protect them from feeling diminished. For *Calcarea carbonica*, visions of ghosts are a negative confirmation that they are all alone, away from home, and vulnerable to becoming the victim of ghosts and spirits. For *Kali bromatum* the alliance with ghosts and spirits strengthens their allegiance to the devil. *Cuprum* use their alliance with spirits to ward off potential attackers; conversely they can also feel persecuted by their ghosts and specters. Each constitutional remedy has to be assessed accordingly.

- *Delusions*: *specters, ghosts, spirits*; *seeing*: acon. agar. alum. am-c. ambr. ant-t. ars-met. *Ars*. atro. aur. **BELL.** bov. brom. *Calc. Camph.* carb-v. cocc. *Croc. Cupr-act. Cupr*. dig. dulc. hell. hep. hura. *Hyos.* hyper. ign. *Kali-br.* kali-c. kali-i. kali-sil. lach. lepi. lyc. merc. *Nat-c. Nat-m.* nit-ac. *Op.* phos. phys. plat. psor. puls. ran-b. sal-fr. sars. sep. sil. spig. *Stram. Sulph.* tarent. thuj. verb. visc. zinc.

19 Self-actualization is the ability to actualize and maximize one's capabilities and achievements. People that have reached self-actualization are characterized by certain behaviors: they must be able to face reality and problems, rather than deny the truth. They must be able to solve problems and actualize solutions in their life at the same time as having a realistic acceptance of themselves and others.

20 "The fact that this is a metal that cannot retain structure is reflected in the psyche of Mercurius. Mercurius constantly react and respond to every stimulus "like" a thermometer. People who are this constitutional type are unable to maintain order or predictability; their mercurial mind is changeable, and their emotional nature is unstructured. Reactivity is the theme of Mercurius. Exposure to high levels of mercury is toxic; it causes nervous system damage, neurological tremors, and alterations in personality and mood.

Mercurius will not always feel emotionally unstable; it is only when stressed or feeling undermined and threatened that Mercurius will feel emotive or reactive. The underlying changeability and sensitivity of Mercurius creates a constitutional picture that is hypersensitive and hyper vigilant to contradiction. Mercurius do not like to be contradicted, and will always interpret contradiction as a critical attack; Mercurius always react violently to being attacked. Mercurius fear exposure of emotional unpredictability, and the mercurial, impulsive reactivity continually undermines feelings of sanity. Depending on the strength of feeling, the reaction will be physical or verbal violence directed toward the person who is seen to have offended; violence toward oneself is also possible. The self-directed violence is a convoluted undermining of ego and self that results in Mercurius feeling confused and disintegrated. The Mercurius who is fatigued, confused, and unsure is the most common presentation of Mercurius in my practice. The most important emotional characteristic is how quickly Mercurius can feel overtaken or influenced by stronger personalities. The mercurial theme of thermometer reactivity is a good image to refer to in considering Mercurius as a constitution." Lalor, Liz, *A Homeopathic Guide to Partnership and Compatibility*, Berkeley, California, North Atlantic Books, 2004, p.p. 51-52.

21 "The homeopathic remedy *Pulsatilla* is derived from the *Pulsatilla nigricans* plant, commonly called a wind flower. The delicate flower sits so precariously at the end of a very fine stem that it is constantly vulnerable to the environmental force of the wind. Just as the flower constantly changes positions, so does the emotional state of Pulsatilla. Pulsatilla will not easily be confused with too many other constitutional pictures. Emotional sensitivity, emotive changeability, and mental unpredictability are the Pulsatilla themes that connect the delicate flower to the constitutional personality. Pulsatilla reacts sympathetically and emotively, whether the issue is happy or sad. The most important aspect of this constitutional persona is that Pulsatillas feel comfortable with their changeability. They compensate for emotional unpredictability by feeling comfortable with knowing they need continual reassurance. Pulsatillas are not willing to let go of anything that makes them feel needed or secure; if they feel deprived at all, or if one thing is not right, they are very likely to be peeved and burst into tears." Lalor, Liz, *A Homeopathic Guide to Partnership and Compatibility*, Berkeley, California, North Atlantic Books, 2004, p.65.

22 "Pulsatillas know they need to be looked after and the only dilemma for Pulsatillas is whether they are getting the love and affection they need. Pulsatillas will always endeavor to make sure they receive what they need in terms of assurance and security because if they feel alone or abandoned they truly despair. Pulsatillas delicately flirt, with the same quality of the flower allowing the wind to move it. Pulsatillas are extremely attractive and endearing in this process; they do not take without giving in return, but their desire for assurance and consolation is so strong they are constantly seeking attention. The exchange for Pulsatillas comes in their sweetness and nurturing. Pulsatillas are genuinely happy when they are devoted to their loved ones." Lalor, Liz, *A Homeopathic Guide to Partnership and Compatibility*, Berkeley, California, North Atlantic Books, 2004, p.133.

23 "The homeopathic remedy *Sepia* is derived from the ink that cuttlefish squirt out when they sense that danger is present. If cuttlefish feel hemmed in or threatened they need to quickly create a subterfuge so they can escape. The Sepia theme of escape and subterfuge runs through the presentation of the emotional, mental, and physical complaints." Lalor, Liz, *A Homeopathic Guide to Partnership and Compatibility*, Berkeley, California, North Atlantic Books, 2004, p.68.

24 "*Sepia* present with converse polarities. The healthy *Sepia* is self-actualized, and the unhealthy, ungrounded *Sepia* struggles to realize independence: the theme is dependence versus independence.

- Healthy Sepias are nonconformist.

- Need to find meaning and purpose in life—through career, occupation, or creative outlet.

- Freedom is crucial to feeling happy and secure.

- The Sepia love of space and freedom is often expressed in a love of dance, movement, or exercise.

- Often feel better if they are busy and active; even feel better if they rush around and clean the house.

- Healthy Sepias are creative and passionate.

- Need physical and emotional space to feel alive.

- All gender role expectations of wife and mother will threaten Sepia women.

- Unhealthy Sepias are irritable and defeated.

- When they feel distraught, can often present as typical nagging harridans.

- Unhealthy Sepias look and feel overburdened and exhausted.

- React to restrictions with anger.

- Feel emotionally disconnected if they feel overburdened.

- The cuttlefish need to create subterfuge has parallels in Sepias' feeling cut off and detached.

- Premenstrual tension, anger, and weepy depression are all worse if Sepias feel overburdened.

- Indifferent to everything when depressed and passionately creative when healthy.

- A Sepia woman who is able to walk away from family is healthy. Sepias often stay feeling overburdened out of a strong sense of duty; this is the type of self-suppression that will eventually lead the Sepia woman into crippling depression. It is, of course, far healthier for Sepia to know that some independence will prevent the need to walk away in the first place."

Lalor, Liz, *A Homeopathic Guide to Partnership and Compatibility*, Berkeley, California, North Atlantic Books, 2004, p.p. 69-70.

25 "The situation of Anacardium is that of a kind of child abuse. Over strict parents impose all their desires on the child and do not allow him to think or do anything on his own. He cannot take his own decisions, to the extent that he is not allowed even to decide what clothes he should wear. If he starts taking his own decisions or does not live up to the expectations placed upon him, he will be punished cruelly. So he tries to live up to these expectations by being obedient and angelic in his behavior, and by being excellent in his work. But he begins to develop a lack of self-confidence, and becomes nervous. He is irresolute, because the outcome of his decisiveness is usually a severe punishment. If the domination persists and he is compelled to put up with it, he starts reacting with cruelty, malice, want of moral feeling, and antisocial behavior. Here he may also develop a tremendous overconfidence with contempt for others. But Anacardium can be very hard and cruel, and at the same time have a lack of self-confidence. There are thus two sides to Anacardium. On the one hand he is good, angelic, obedient from fear of punishment. He is very orderly, fastidious, cannot rest till things are in their proper place. The other part of him is hard, malicious, violent, devilish, disgusted with himself. He becomes immoral, develops suicidal or homicidal tendencies, is abusive, stubborn and avoids the company of people. These two sides of Anacardium are constantly in opposition to each other: should he be an angel or a devil. Anacardium could be the wife of a selfish tyrant who rules with an iron fist, and does not allow her to take any decisions. She becomes irresolute, lacks in self-confidence, is confused - always has two wills. She becomes dull and very absent-minded (Anacardium has a marked absent-mindedness). She may be childish, idiotic and timid out of lack of self-confidence and fear. The fear can paralyze her thinking as can be seen when appearing for an examination." Sankaran, Rajan, *The Soul of Remedies*, Santa Cruz, Mumbai, Homoeopathic Medical Publishers, 1997, p. 7.

26 A bier is a movable frame with wheels on which the coffin or corpse is placed on so it can be taken to the grave site.

27 "The homeopathic remedy *Graphites* is derived from a dilution of the mineral graphite, a carbon containing a small amount of iron. The sphere of action *Graphites* affects is nutrition and circulation. Graphite the mineral is used in machinery to help resolve friction. Graphites' emotive sensitivity has the same theme, reflecting the sensitivity that allows graphite to resolve the friction of machinery parts. People who are the constitutional type Graphites are extremely sensitive and finely tuned to react to conflict and disharmony. When you spill the mineral graphite on the floor the small particles clump together. The same desire to clump together is part of the psyche of Graphites. People of this constitutional type are very happy when surrounded by family and friends." Lalor, Liz, *A Homeopathic Guide to Partnership and Compatibility*, Berkeley, California, North Atlantic Books, 2004, p.30.

28 "Dr. Samuel Hahnemann, the founder of homeopathy, listed some interesting dichotomies in the personality description of Lycopodium. The personality traits listed ranged from "great timidity" to "cannot bear the least contradiction ..." to "... breaking out in envy, pretensions and ordering others about." (Hahnemann, pp. 863–864). These personality contradictions run the whole way through the constitutional picture of Lycopodium. It is an interesting dilemma for Lycopodium to one minute feel a lack of confidence and, with the next breath, brim with enough bragging arrogance to be able to win over an entire roomful of people. The thread that ties the two sides of Lycopodium together is a desperate need to remain on top and survive. The only way Lycopodium can see to remain on top is to be very big and very important. The theme that ties the two parts together can be explained by the evolution of the plant from which Lycopodium the remedy is derived: *Lycopodium clavatum*. The underlying psychodynamic trauma of Lycopodium is that *Lycopodium clavatum* was, thousands of years ago, a large tree, and now it is a small club moss. Lycopodium carry this existential threat to their largeness in their psyche. The crisis of size is the theme of Lycopodium. Lycopodium are fearful of any threat to their potency and importance in this world." Lalor, Liz, *A Homeopathic Guide to Partnership and Compatibility*, Berkeley, California, North Atlantic Books, 2004, p.40.

29 "The main concern of, and theme for, Lycopodium in life is acquiring success and power in order to survive. Their main fear in life is the loss of power — the loss or failure of their business, the failure of their marriage, their loss of position in society. Lycopodium is a constitution that is acutely aware of needing to succeed and perform. Lycopodium do not outwardly acknowledge feeling vulnerable. When you meet a Lycopodium this is not the personality picture that is presented. The need to be successful and to win favor in society is so paramount, they overcompensate, and present as bragging and arrogant. The anxiety of failure is so threatening, they literally bust their gut to prove to themselves and the world that they are not a failure. Their hard work usually pays off; Lycopodium are good and they know it. They are also good because they have had to work harder than others to achieve their success. Lycopodium are under continual stress and strain. Every new situation is a potential threat to their existence, and every new encounter could potentially undermine their authority and position. It is not easy for Lycopodium to continually struggle with the feeling that one mistake could undermine their very existence. It is possible, then, to understand why they present with over inflated opinions of themselves. If Lycopodium convince the world that they are good, they also convince themselves." Lalor, Liz, *A Homeopathic Guide to Partnership and Compatibility*, Berkeley, California, North Atlantic Books, 2004, p.p. 109-110.

30 Howard Hughes was one of the wealthiest people in the world, and one of the most well known sufferers of Obsessive Compulsive Disorder (OCD). Howard Hughes' megalomania alternated between self-exalted passion for grandiose perfection and self-deprecating insanity.

31 "The homeopathic remedy *Sulphur* is derived from the element sulfur. Sulfur is a yellow crystalline solid that is found underground and is only able to be mined and forced to the surface in molten form at extremely high temperatures of 115°Celsius. The degree of intense heat that is needed to extract sulfur can be seen as the motivational theme in the psyche of the constitution Sulphur. The explosive, expansive heat needed to extract sulfur is matched by Sulphur constitutionally and mirrored by their reactive genius and creative self-absorption.

It is important to understand and know the core motivations behind each constitution. If you only look on the surface, it is possible to confuse Nux vomica with Lycopodium, or Lycopodium with Sulphur. All three constitutions are essentially egoistical, but the egotistical motivation of each is different. Nux vomica needs ego to eliminate possible threats, and builds ego to win. Lycopodium needs ego for survival and security, and builds ego for greatness. Sulphur's relationship with ego is distinctive. Sulphurs are altruistically inspired by a sense of greatness and a need to inspire the rest of the world to see the beauty they see. Sulphur uses ego as fuel for an unfaltering, inspirational desire to light the fire of knowledge and creativity in humanity.

The psychodynamic force behind Sulphur's passion and intensity is the heat and power of the element sulfur. Sulphur has conjured up so much force behind the exploding volcano that to not be recognized is crippling. If the world is not inspired and Sulphur is ignored, Sulphur sinks into intensely acrid, cynical depression." Lalor, Liz, *A Homeopathic Guide to Partnership and Compatibility*, Berkeley, California, North Atlantic Books, 2004, p.p. 79-80.

32 "Introduced into homoeopathy by Drysdale in 1880, pyrogenium was obtained by the following mode of preparation: Half a pound of chopped lean beef is put into a pint of tap water and macerated on the sunny side of a wall for two or three weeks, so that a pellicle may form and the maceration fluid assume a reddish, thick, and fetid appearance. Then: strain through muslin and filter; evaporate the filtered liquid to dryness in a water bath at boiling heat. The dry residue, which forms a brown, caky mass, rub up in a glass mortar with 2 ounces of rectified spirit, and allow to digest for two hours; boil for five minutes this spirituous maceration, filter, and thoroughly dry in the warm chamber the residue that is on the filter, which forms a hard, brownish mass, weighing 54 grains. Rub this with 540 minims of distilled water; allow to stand an hour an a half, and then filter. This clear amber-coloured liquor which passes through is the watery extract or solution of sepsin." Vermeulen, Frans. *Prisma*. The Netherlands, Emryss bv Publishers, 2002. p. 1112.

33 "Phosphorus is a mineral that plays a conductive role in every chemical reaction in the body. Physiologically, phosphorus enables cells to utilize carbohydrates, fats and proteins; phosphorus is also used for the maintenance and repair of cells, and for production of cellular energy. Phosphorus is a non-metallic element that is luminous in the dark and is

unique because of its ability to produce light. Within the persona of the constitution Phosphorus is the essence of phosphoric conductivity and light. The phosphoric nature of the element phosphorus is reflected in the luminescent, sparkling ability to stimulate others and be stimulated by them. The conductive nature of phosphorus, the mineral, is reflected in phosphoric, enthusiastic involvement and ability to bubble and bob enthusiastically from one thing in life to another.

The theme of Phosphorus is conductive; Phosphorus needs to stimulate, enthuse, and receive. They need continual acknowledgment, excitement, and stimulation to be able to be healthy and shine. Phosphorus is a mineral that is essential for the production of cellular energy. A deficiency of phosphorus can cause rapid weight loss, mental and emotional fatigue, nervous disorders, and irregularities in breathing. The dark side or unhealthy side of Phosphorus is emotional anxiousness, overexcited nervousness, and mental indifference to everything in life. Phosphorous is affectionate, loving of self and others, joyful, carefree, and childlike — but only when receiving necessary affection and attention. In partnerships, Phosphorus needs to gravitate toward people who are going to give the most amount of attention." Lalor, Liz, *A Homeopathic Guide to Partnership and Compatibility*, Berkeley, California, North Atlantic Books, 2004, p.p. 62-63.

34 Samsāra in Buddhism refers to the continual suffering associated with the cycle of birth and death. This continual 'wheel of life' can only be escaped through achieving enlightenment.

35 "*Spigelia Anthelmia*, Linné (*Anthelmia quadriphylla*), Demerara pinkroot. An annual of the West Indies and South America. The root has been used by the natives of those countries for centuries as an anthelmintic. It is the form of spigelia official in the *Homoeopathic Pharmacopoeia* (1890), and possesses decidedly narcotic qualities. It was introduced into Europe by Dr. Browne, in 1751. The French gave it the name *Brinvilliers*, after the Marchioness de Brinvillière, the celebrated poisoner, executed in 1676, and who is said to have used this drug upon her victims. The fresh plant is very poisonous, and contains the volatile alkaloid, *spigeliin* (Boorsma, in Dragendorff's *Heilpflanzen*, 1899). This drug is said to act specifically upon the heart, and particularly the endocardium. It is valued by some practitioners in *cardiac palpitation* and *endocarditis*, especially the rheumatic form, and to guard against relapses of *cardiac rheumatism*. *Painful conditions of the heart*, the pain extending along the arm, *angina pectoris*, and *cardiac neuralgia*, with palpitation, are conditions in which it is employed with asserted success. Large doses debilitate the heart. Browne (1751) compared its narcotic power to that of opium."

From the internet page: www.henriettesherbal.com/eclectic/kings/spigelia.html

36 I have treated one *Aurum metallicum* patient. Her 'never-well-since-event' came from an experience she had when her mother abandoned her and her siblings when she was five years of age. She became the sole carer

of all her siblings as well as her father. She never forgave herself for not being able to protect her brother from sexual abuse from her father. She was also sexually abused by her father, but this was not the source of her anguish; it was that she was not able to protect her little brother who was only four years old. Her brother later committed suicide by hanging himself when he was seven years old. *Aurum metallicum* assume responsibility for 'delusions of original sin'. *Aurum metallicum* have the *Mind* rubric: *too occupied with religion from melancholia remorse*. When the patient came to me she was heavily medicated on anti-depressants and anti-psychotics and under the psychological management of a psychiatrist and psychologist. The psychologist understood homoeopathy and recommended her to me. Periodically, she would climb on to the roof of an office building in the city and ring her psychologist who after some time worked out that what had stopped her from jumping was six repeated doses of *Aurum metallicum* 200 C. She would only take the *Aurum metallicum* 200 C if she was literally about to jump. She would not take the remedy at any other time because she did not believe it worked. *Aurum metallicum* have the *Delusion* rubric: *obstacles in his way*. [1] 1. *Aurum metallicum* also have the *Mind* rubric: *desires death during convalescence* and the *Mind* rubrics: *doubtful of recovery* and *doubtful of salvation*. The patient was an alcoholic. She consumed four bottles of Vodka per day. Three months after consulting me, she haemorrhaged to death from a ruptured stomach ulcer after a particularly bad bout of excessive drinking.

- *Mind*: *anguish*: *self-destruction; leading to*: aur. [1] 1.
- *Mind*: *anxiety*: *suicidal disposition, with*: *Aur.*
- *Mind*: *cheerful*: *death, while thinking of*: aur.
- *Mind*: *death*: *desires*: **AUR.**
- *Mind*: *death*: *desires*: *evening*: **AUR.**
- *Mind*: *death*: *desires*: *convalescence, during*: *Aur.*
- *Mind*: *death*: *thoughts of*: *Aur.*
- *Mind*: *insanity*: *suicidal disposition, with*: aur.
- *Mind*: *jumping*: *impulse to jump*: *Aur.*
- *Mind*: *jumping*: *impulse to jump*: *pregnancy, during*: **AUR.** [3] 1.
- *Mind*: *jumping*: *Aur.*
- *Mind*: *laughing*: *alternating with*: *death; desire for*: aur. [1] 1.
- *Mind*: *mania*: *suicidal*: *sexual symptoms; with*: aur. [1] 1.
- *Mind*: *sadness*: *suicidal disposition with*: **AUR.**
- *Mind*: *suicidal disposition*: **AUR.**
- *Mind*: *suicidal disposition*: *evening*: aur.
- *Mind*: *suicidal disposition*: *anxiety, from*: aur.

- *Mind: suicidal disposition: car; throwing himself under a: Aur.*
- *Mind: suicidal disposition: drowning, by: Aur.*
- *Mind: suicidal disposition: hanging, by: aur.*
- *Mind: suicidal disposition: hypochondriasis, by: aur.*
- *Mind: suicidal disposition: knife: with a knife: aur.*
- *Mind: suicidal disposition: love; from disappointed: Aur.*
- *Mind: suicidal disposition: pains, from:* **AUR.**
- *Mind: suicidal disposition: perspiration, during:* **AUR.**
- *Mind: suicidal disposition: pregnancy, during: aur.* [1] 1.
- *Mind: suicidal disposition: sadness, from:* **AUR.**
- *Mind: suicidal disposition: shooting, by: aur.*
- *Mind: suicidal disposition: thinking about suicide amel.:* **AUR.**
- *Mind: suicidal disposition: thoughts:* AUR.
- *Mind: suicidal disposition: throwing: height; himself from a:* **AUR.**
- *Mind: suicidal disposition: throwing: windows, from:* **AUR.**
- *Mind: suicidal disposition: throwing: windows, from: delivery; during:* aur. [1] 1.
- *Mind: suicidal disposition: throwing: windows, from: pain; from: Aur.* [2] 1.

37 "The homeopathic remedy *Mag-carb* is often the first remedy I would think of using for the anxieties of an orphaned or abandoned child. The same remedy can also be applicable for adults who feel like they were abandoned as a child. A child does not need to have physically lost its parents to experience abandonment. Children are spending long days in childcare or are being left at home with nannies, while their parents spend long days at work. Not every child will feel abandoned if left with a nanny or at childcare, but the child who does absorb this experience as an abandonment trauma will often grow up to become the constitution Mag-carb. Mag-carbs experience a sense of underlying dread and apprehension of potential rejection and abandonment. This anxiety is reflected in the need that Mag-carbs have to protect themselves from conflict or disharmony". Lalor, Liz, *A Homeopathic Guide to Partnership and Compatibility*, Berkeley, California, North Atlantic Books, 2004, p.238.

38 "The homeopathic remedy *Magnesium carbonica* (shortened to *Mag-carb* for both remedy and constitutional type) is derived from a dilution of carbonate of magnesia, which contains the mineral magnesium. A tissue salt deficiency of magnesium results in loss of nervous system function. A person suffering from a physical magnesium deficiency will experience muscle cramping and tremors, as well as emotional apprehensiveness, confusion, and disorientation. The theme of a person who is suffering from

nerve fiber contraction is reflected in the emotional and physical action and nature of Mag-carb. Mag-carbs literally shut down feelings to avoid feeling anxious. Mag-carbs experience a sense of underlying apprehension and anxiety that they then experience as fear of rejection and abandonment. This is reflected in the need that Mag-carbs have to protect themselves from conflict or disharmony. Often the effort of dealing with anxiety and the effort of holding down feelings of apprehensiveness result in Mag-carbs suffering from depression. The anxiety that Mag-carbs suffer is so intense that they end up suppressing it just to be able to function. When Mag-carbs suppress their emotional feelings they often then experience the effects of the suppression physically, in muscular cramps and neuralgic pains that reflect magnesium deficiency". Lalor, Liz, *A Homeopathic Guide to Partnership and Compatibility*, Berkeley, California, North Atlantic Books, 2004, p.44.

39 One of my *Spongia* patients described this feeling of being crowded as: *there is interference in my space. I feel that the only way I can survive is to become a 'snow queen'. This allows me to remain detached from afar. I am not taking part. I am judging from afar. I am sad and depressed. I feel exposed. I am not comfortable in my place of living. My mother had dementia, I am afraid of getting dementia. I have enormous sadness. I am awkward in society and fearful of people. I do not function well in a group environment. I feel detached and feel like I do not belong anywhere. Not grounded. I have a feeling of despair periodically in the evening which is accompanied by a desire to weep and hopelessness. Everything is a burden, I drag myself through life. I feel different to everyone and do not belong anywhere. I was much happier living in overseas rather than in Australia because I need a strong sense of community and strong spiritual connection and direction from God otherwise I feel afloat with no direction. I also think I can be rude and harsh and oblivious and judgmental and dictatorial. I am judging from afar. I feel that all my complaints have a psychosomatic origin which comes from too much negative thinking. I have a fear of doing something wrong because of the punishment.* Mentally, she suffers from periods of dullness, no thoughts and finds it hard to concentrate. Physically, she has no energy and is tired. *Spongia* have a psychodynamic need to separate from themselves and from the world in order to protect themselves from being enveloped by and encroached upon by their own inner fears and negativities. A major cause of her current depression is that she does not feel comfortable living in Australia. In the Australian community she feels *suffocated and stifled* and *not able to be myself*. Her biggest fear is that she will lose her mental freedom and be trapped like her mother who had dementia. I asked her how she felt as a child. Her reply was: *I never belonged there either. I felt like I couldn't breathe.*

40 The second *Spongia* case I had was a patient who came to see me for *all consuming* waves of hot flushes and heart palpitations associated with the onset of menopause. Her health history included high blood pressure and heart palpitations which are consistent with the homoeopathic

remedy profile of *Spongia*. The 'never-well-since-event' or psychodynamic causation in this case was *being set free* by her mother who sent her overseas when she was fifteen. *I felt trapped in France, I couldn't go home I had no choice.* She felt like she had *been swimming against the tide ever since. Spongia* psychologically need to feel attached (anchored to the sea bed) to their home. Sea creatures only feel safe when they are alone and hiding in a safe place [*home*]. *Spongia* have the *Mind* rubric: *desires to go home* and the *Mind* rubric: *ailments from fright*. Since she was fifteen this woman had been experiencing crippling panic attacks. The panic attacks left her *feeling immobilized*. Her biggest anxiety was at work, her boss would ask her a question and she felt so scared that she was unable to speak. She *felt insecure, without a voice, trapped and with no choice*. She hated working in offices because of the fact that everyone would be able to look at her all day. *Spongia* have the *Mind* rubric: *cannot bear to be looked at*. She felt paranoid about what others would be thinking about her. All of her life since she was fifteen she thought she was a *dumb twit* and a *stupid girl* because she couldn't talk. *Spongia* have the *Larynx* and *Trachea* rubric: *nervous aphonia, lost voice*. She also felt awkward in all social communication. *I blush terribly. I feel like people are on a different wave length, there are things that I just don't understand. I can't talk about myself socially. I also struggle to understand things socially; I get confused a lot. Spongia* somaticize all of their anxieties, which is why *Spongia* as a homoeopathic remedy is used for heart palpitations and difficulties in breathing as a result of anxiety and fear. The only time this *Spongia* patient felt like she could *escape* her anxiety was when she was singing. *Spongia* have the *Mind* rubric: *loathing of work alternating with singing.* [1] 1.

41 *Spongia* make very good therapists, especially if they are working with individuals or groups who have suffered persecution. Their capacity to *see something as though he saw through someone else's eyes,* gives them an inbuilt capacity to understand how it feels to be persecuted.

42 'Dissociation' is a normal response to the trauma of illness. If the patient dissociates, it allows themselves space to distance themselves from the feelings which are overwhelming them. 'Dissociative disorder' on the other hand is a far more complex disorder in which the patient creates multiple personalities which allow their psyche protection from what they perceive to be potentially traumatic situations, within and outside of themselves.

43 "Staphisagrias suppress feelings by not allowing any expression of anger or rage; they are proud of the fact that they are able to remain nice and sweet. Staphisagrias have developed justifiable reasons for why they need to suppress their feelings; they are protecting a very painful history of some form of abuse. The theme of suppression and composure has healthy and unhealthy advantages, as well as disadvantages and consequences for Staphisagria. Staphisagrias eventually always lose control because their suppression is challenged by the equally powerful force of their anger and rage at being continually abused and repressed. When Staphisagria lose control they are abusive because the build-up of emotion is overwhelming.

Staphisagrias then sink into remorseful self-abuse that mirrors their history of abuse. Within Staphisagria is the theme of abuse, out-of-control abuser, and the remorseful self abuser." Lalor, Liz, *A Homeopathic Guide to Partnership and Compatibility*, Berkeley, California, North Atlantic Books, 2004, p.76.

44 See www.hominf.org/posi/posifr.htm. The proving of *Positronium* is written by Misha Norland.

45 "Positronium is an "exotic" atom made of matter and antimatter: an electron and a positron (anti-electron) bound together without a nucleus. Since researchers have already made positronium atoms and ions, the next step would be to coax the atoms to interact through collisions, and ultimately to form molecules. While there are always occasional collisions in positronium gas, researchers haven't succeeded in making it dense enough for frequent collisions--enough to affect the gas's properties.

But a team of physicists led by Allen Mills of the University of California at Riverside may have done just that. They collected and compressed positrons in a magnetic trap and then fired super-intense positron pulses at a thin film of "nano-porous" silica, a material riddled with myriad microscopic pores. Positrons hitting the film liberate electrons and can bind with them to make positronium atoms. These atoms live for a brief time as tiny gas clouds, trapped within the material's pores, until the electrons and positrons inevitably annihilate with one another in a burst of gamma-rays. Mills and his colleagues detected these gamma rays to measure the rate of annihilation, or "decay," and probe the underlying physics."

Written by Mark Buchanan, a freelance science writer from Cambridge, England. From the internet site: focus.aps.org/story/v16/st16

46 "Compression and oppression" are the two opposing themes Misha Norland identifies in the proving of *Positronium*.

47 **Oedipus Complex** is a son's largely unconscious sexual attraction toward his mother accompanied by jealousy toward his father. Austrian psychiatrist Sigmund Freud first used the term. Oedipus is the hero of the ancient Greek play *Oedipus Tyrannus* by Sophocles, which tells the story of how Oedipus was abandoned at birth by his parents and returned as an adult to kill his father and marry his mother. Freud suggested that if this complex is not resolved in the young child, it contributes to neurosis in later life. Swiss psychologist Carl Jung suggested that such feelings were not restricted to boys but that girls could also experience a similar complex.

48 Allen, in *Handbook of Materia medica,* notes the tendency of *Asterias rubens* to abandon themselves to stronger influences: "melancholy to give herself up to mental or bodily work, to walk or engage in violent exercise, species of moral intoxication. Anguish from noon till 3 p.m. as if a misfortune were impending or he were going to hear bad news, and he then feels as if he should give way to tears." Allen, Timothy Field, M.D. LL.D. *Handbook of Materia Medica*. New Delhi, B. Jain Publishers, p. 146. 1994.

49 Boericke notes that the homoeopathic remedy "has an unquestionable influence over cancer disease." It is easy to see the psychosomatic themes in all spheres — emotionally, mentally, and physically. Cancer patients often relay that the cancer has consumed them and that they have abandoned themselves to the cancer. Their body has surrendered to the cancer and the smell of death itself has invaded their body. They often report that they smell dirty, and that death is consuming them. *Asterias rubens* are the only remedy listed in the *Mind* rubric: *fear of Mammae cancer*. Boericke, William, M. D. *Pocket Manual of Homoeopathic Materia Medica*. New Delhi, Motilal Banarsidass Publishers. p. 94. 1996.

50 The other remedy in the *Delusion* rubric: *conscious of the suffering of women through the ages* is *Lac-Lupinum*. From the proving of this remedy a strong personality characteristic which merged was the need to protect and take responsibility for the group (pack) and the children within the group. Wolves are very family (pack) orientated. Within all the Lac remedies there is a struggle between the group versus the individual.

51 The 'never-well-since-event' in *Sepia* will occur in childhood, specifically pre-verbal. *Sepia* experiences abandonment quite often as a baby.

52 *Borax* is one of the homoeopathic remedies I use in my Liz Lalor Fertility Program. *Borax* is the *Drainage* remedy that I prescribe most commonly. It is the remedy which addresses disturbance within the *function* of the organ – *Borax* improves mucus quality because it increases low levels of Estradiol. The *Mind* rubric: *starting during menses* is reflective of the fear of failing which is predominant in the psyche of women faced with infertility.

- *Female genitalia/sex* rubric: *menses: return: ceased; after the regular menstrual cycle has: Borx.*

- *Female genitalia/sex* rubric: *menses: short, too: one day: borx.*

53 Allen notes in his *Encyclopedia of Pure Materia Medica* that *Carboneum hydrogenisatum*, the homoeopathic remedy is derived from Carburetted Hydrogen, Ethene, and Olefiant gas. Allen does not make a distinction whether it is all three or just Carburetted Hydrogen. It is also debatable given the research done by William Henry whether Allen assumed that all three were the same substance. Boericke states *Carboneum hydrogenisatum* is derived from Carburetted Hydrogen.

"William Henry was very interested in the gases produced by the destructive distillation of coal and oil. He analyzed their constituents and studied their suitability for lighting. He showed that such gases were a mixture of carbonic oxide (carbon monoxide), carburetted hydrogen (methane), hydrogen, olefiant gas (ethene) with some carbonic acid gas (carbon dioxide) and sulphuretted hydrogen (hydrogen sulphide). As a result he found himself at variance with some other authors who maintained that olefiant gas was the sole compound of carbon and hydrogen and that coal gas contained only a mixture of olefiant gas and hydrogen. In 1821 William Henry published in the *Philosophical Transactions* a proof of his original views. John Dalton, Humphrey Davy, Dr. Thomson and himself had all examined the gases bubbling to the surface in marshes and from coal mines and found them to be the same substance which they called carburetted hydrogen.

William Henry then proceeded to show that carburetted hydrogen was different from olefiant gas by examining their reactions with chlorine." www.thornber.net/cheshire/ideasmen/henry.html

54 Willow wood (amongst wand collectors) is the most desired of the Celtic woods. Willow wood is supposedly aligned to conducting magical energy. Willow wood reacts to the energy and will of the one using the wand. It is for this reason that there are numerous internet webpages which are dedicated to the sale of magical wands made from willow wood. It is questionable if one can use Harry Potter in a text on homoeopathy, however, the owner of the willow wand in the Harry Potter books was Ron Weasley. Ron Weasley's wand broke because he could not force the wand to yield to his power. "Wands are capable of changing masters. When a wand's master is disarmed, stunned, or killed, but not had their wand snatched from their hand, the wand will accept the old master's attacker as its new master. This will occur even if the wand in question is not in the possession of either of the two people involved."

From the internet webpage: harrypotter.wikia.com/wiki/Wand

55 From Stirling's notes listed on Radar: "Jilted Lovers: Virtually all the provers experienced some tensions in their primary relationship. Maybe this is common in a proving. The general feeling was one of "drawing the line". Situations that previously had been unresolved but tolerated either became intolerable or spontaneously moved towards a solution. Out of the members of the group who actually took a remedy, one prover's partner started seeing a counselor to resolve his problems, another couple split up temporarily during the proving, one couple came together and moved in together really quickly, one couple split up shortly after the proving, one prover nearly started an affair, and another got her partner to discuss the issue of having children, which they had been avoiding for years. My own seven year marriage, which had appeared very stable, split dramatically and my husband left, a few weeks before the proving group finished meeting, to start a relationship with someone he met the week after the proving started."

56 From Stirling's notes listed on Radar: "The tree is also associated with fertility and easing childbirth, and in herbal lore is used for the ailments of the newborn and the aged."

57 Exanthema: feverish diseases with notable eruptions on the skin.

58 According to Genesis, the first five books of Moses, Adam was the first man created by God and is acknowledged in Jewish, Christian and Islamic Religions. Adam and Eve appear in many books besides Genesis, such as the Quran, The Life of Adam and Eve, The Talmud and Gnostic texts.

59 In Genesis it is the serpent which tempts Eve to eat from the tree of knowledge of good and evil. In Christianity the serpent was interpreted as Satan. Early Christian interpretations also held Eve responsible for the fall of Adam because she tempted him to eat the forbidden fruit. In Gnostic tradition the fall meant man was delivered up to evil. In Islam, Adam is considered the first prophet of God and the expulsion of Adam and Eve from Eden was the first act of revenge from Satan for disobeying God. In the Islamic religion resisting 'original sin' is rewarded by being allowed into Paradise. In Judaism, Islamic, and Christian doctrine, man was born pure but was then corrupted and cast out from Paradise. The belief in Buddhism is that man is born impure or unenlightened and that a human reincarnation is viewed very favorably as it allows man to seek enlightenment. In Hindu religions good actions and thoughts are aimed at improving your chances of a fortuitous human rebirth.

60 A 'persecution complex' is psychological terminology applied to an array of complex behaviors that specifically deal with the feeling of being persecuted for various possible reasons, imagined or real. A self-imposed persecution complex is applied to the patient who deliberately instigates predetermined 'delusions of persecution'. 'Delusions of persecution' is applied to the patient who believes that the whole world is against them. 'Delusions of persecution' can justify retaliation acts excused by the presumed hostility of the world. The acts of hostility become a self-fulfilling prophecy: the person is rejected by the world for their acts of hostility.

61 I have previously written an essay in *Links* (Winter 2005) analyzing Frodo as *Anacardium* in the Tolkien story, *The Lord of the Rings*. Below in an extract from that essay.

The Lord of the Rings is a story of man's irresistible desire for control and power. Tolkien is concerned with telling a tale of great bravery, and with recounting a tale of how evil and the desire for hubristic power affects a simple person. The moralistic message that comes across in *The Lord of the Rings* is that all dark power will eventually destroy and neither good will, nor purpose, will be able to resist the dark power of hubristic evil. Frodo is in an *Anacardium* state because the Ring has matched his desire for acknowledgement and acceptance and thrown him into a 'like' *Anacardium* energy. The most interesting aspect of Frodo is that the 'like' *Anacardium* state of good versus evil means that only an *Anacardium* Frodo can resist the power of the One Ring and be chosen for the Quest to save Middle-earth. Frodo already displays a need to have the world acknowledge his importance by proving himself a notable person within the shire. Frodo is an orphan and as a result of his Uncle Bilbo choosing to adopt and favor him, Frodo is acknowledged within the shire as an important person. Frodo is chosen for the Quest because he has a powerful need to prove himself and all the council can see that if the Quest is to succeed it will require all the strength and power behind Frodo's need. Within Frodo is an *Anacardium* desire to prove himself and be important. Whether Frodo was in an *Anacardium* state before he came into possession of the Ring is not possible to ascertain from the story as told by Tolkien. The mere fact of Frodo's orphaned state, his adoption by Bilbo, and the fact that he has stayed in his position within the shire with Sam as his servant, sets the scene for Frodo's emotional propensity to move into *Anacardium* or to be vulnerable to an *Anacardium* 'layer'.

Frodo's struggle with the possession of the Ring is the struggle of good over evil; it is an integral struggle that goes on within the nature of *Anacardium* all the time. *These two sides of Anacardium are constantly in opposition to each other: should he be an angel or a devil.* [Sankaran] *Anacardium* has an *angel* on one side, and a *devil* on the other side. As *Anacardium*, Frodo has a good side which is able to give strength and purpose to the Quest to destroy the Ring; he also has a dark side which causes him not to choose at the end of the journey to throw the Ring into the Fires of Mount Doom. Frodo displays the two sides of *Anacardium* when he becomes aware of the two powers of good and evil pulling him apart and tempting him: *he heard himself crying out: Never, never! Or was it: Verily I come, I come to you?... The two powers strove in him.* p.527. *The Fellowship of the Ring.* It is also his desire to prove himself that makes Frodo vulnerable to the power of the Ring. The *fear and enmity* eventually come to the fore in Frodo; the evil in the Ring eventually overcomes the struggle for *good* and Frodo cannot stop moving into the *evil* [Kent] side of *Anacardium*. Frodo needs the power of the Ring to bring importance and self-confidence to a self that is devoid of the 'I'. *Anacardium* need recognition and fear being ignored, even more than they fear their cruel side. *Anacardium* suffer intense fears of being 'left out in the cold' and shunned by the world. *Anacardium* have no 'I' within the self. A delusion *peculiar* to *Anacardium* is that they see everyone's face in the mirror except their own. *Anacardium* suffers from loss of identity. The disintegration of 'I' or 'self' drives *Anacardium* to do the 'right' thing. *Anacardium* only know who they are when they receive praise from the world for their actions. Frodo, before he came into possession of the Ring, saw himself as insignificant. After the adventure and Quest is over he once again sinks into insignificance in the shire, and Pippin and Merry and Sam become the heroes of the Quest. Frodo's need to be the Ring-bearer, and offer himself to the council, is reflective of an *Anacardium* need to be praised. *Anacardium* suffer from a fear that there is something wrong with them, and they continually need to strive to prove it is not correct.

- *He is at odds with the world, and has little confidence in himself being able to accomplish what is demanded of him.* p.279. [Hahnemann].

Anacardium suffer from anxiety about being judged or found out to be flawed.

- *Internal anguish, which did not allow him to rest, he troubled himself about every trifle, as if it would cause great injury, with solicitude about the future.* p.279. [Hahnemann].

Frodo is the first to admit to Sam at the end of the journey, at the chasm of the Fires of Mordor, that he has failed in his Quest. Gandalf had been right in predicting the role of Gollum and the power of the Ring over Frodo. If had not been for the obsessive Gollum grabbing the Ring off Frodo at the last minute, and accidentally falling into the Fires of Mordor he would have failed in the Quest because he could not choose to relinquish the power and fame the Ring offered him. Throughout the journey as they draw nearer to the Fires of Mount Doom, Frodo looses his ability to resist the power of the Ring. Frodo on the chasm of Mount Doom declares, *I will not do this deed. The Ring is mine!* p.265 *The Return of the King.*

Anacardium can be sweeter and nicer than most people, but it is important to note that they are driven by the desire to prove they are worthy people and by their anxiety about being judged. *Anacardium literally has two wills, one bad, one good.* [Vermeulen] It is literally the good will within Frodo that can resist the Ring and is able to push him always onwards towards the Fires of Mordor. In deciding if Frodo is *Anacardium* you have to see his struggle in resisting the 'bad' in the Ring i.e. *the two powers strove in him,* and you also have to see within Frodo his decision to claim the evil for himself. *I am almost in its power now. I could not give it up, and if you tried to take it I should go mad,* is reflective of the struggle near the end of the Quest, but then Frodo declares, *The Ring is mine!* and this is the choice Frodo makes. The fact that it takes Frodo until the chasm of Mount Doom to give in to the power within the Ring is significant especially when taking into consideration that Elrond, Gandalf and Galadriel have all acknowledged they could not be Ring-bearers. The quality of the 'good' within *Anacardium* is the quality that Sankaran refers to as "a compensated *Anacardium*".

Whereas Anacardium is known for its hard-heartedness, cruelty, want of moral feeling, a compensated Anacardium cannot be cruel even when the situation demands. He will, perhaps, be unable to kill even an irritating mosquito. p.7. [Sankaran].

Bibliography

Bailey, Philip, M, M.D. *Homeopathic Psychology.* Berkeley, California, North Atlantic Books, 1995.

Boericke, William, M. D. *Pocket Manual of Homoeopathic Materia Medica.* New Delhi, Motilal Banarsidass, Publishers, 1996.

Grieve, Mrs. M. *A Modern Herbal.* Middlesex, England, Penguin Books, 1980.

Hahnemann, Dr. Samuel. *The Chronic Diseases.* New Delhi, B. Jain Publishers, 1995.

Kent, J. T. *Lectures on Materia Medica.* New Delhi, B. Jain Publishers, 1994.

Kent, J. T. *Repertory of the Homoeopathic Materia Medica and a Word Index.* New Delhi, B. Jain Publishers, 1994.

Morrison, Roger, M.D. *Desktop Guide.* Nevada City, CA, Hahnemann Clinic Publishing. 1993.

Sankaran, Rajan. *The Soul of Remedies*. Santa Cruz, Bombay, Homoeopathic Medical Publishers, 1997.

Schroyens, Frederik, M.D. *Synthesis*. London, Homeopathic Book Publishers, 1997.

Tolkien, J.R.R. *The Lord of the Rings*. London, HarperCollins Publishers, 1994.

(*The Lord of the Rings* is comprised of three books: *The Fellowship of the Ring, The Two Towers, The Return of the King*.)

Vermeulen, Frans. *Synoptic Materia Medica*.The Netherlands, Merlijn Publishers, 1992.

Vermeulen, Frans. *Prisma*. The Netherlands, Emryss bv Publishers, 2002.

62 I have written an essay in *Links* (Winter 2005) analyzing Gollum as *Mancinella* in Tolkien's story of *The Lord of the Rings*. Below is an extract from that essay.

Mancinella fear the world. *Mancinella* develop convoluted, obsessive compulsive habits and belief systems as a way of having superstitious power over the world. The thought of being alone in the world without anything to protect them can send them into a very real intense fear of losing their sanity. *Mancinella* obsess over how many times they turned the key in a lock, or how many cracks they stand on in the street, or the favorable position of the planets in astrology. All are merely devices of external power to protect their weakness of will and mind. *Mancinella* fear the world controlling their mind, and they fear losing control over their own mind in the world. The key sensation and theme of *Mancinella* is obsession with fear of possession by the devil.

The hold the One Ring has on Gollum is integrally tied to how he came to acquire it. When Gollum first sees the Ring in Déagol's hand, he is insane with his desire to possess it. Déagol refuses to hand the Ring over and Gollum kills him in a moment of "insanity" [Kent]. Gandalf, in the telling of the history of the One Ring, emphasizes to Frodo that the Ring had given Gollum power only according to his existing stature. Gollum only used the invisibility powers of the Ring to find out secrets and deceits, and use them to his advantage over others. The Ring gives Gollum the power and protection he as *Mancinella* needs. The Ring also fuels his mania and madness. The fear of having to face the world without his "precious" drives Gollum to the brink of insanity. Gollum takes the Ring and moves deep underground away from all contact with his family, who he fears might take his present or discover the murder and how he came into possession of the Ring.

Mancinella suffer from a weakness of will. They fear being possessed precisely because they are too weak to be able to defend their own mind from attack. Gollum was so obsessed with the Ring it became a sadistic love and hate relationship. Gollum agreed to become the servant of Frodo and call him "master"; granted Frodo was the master of his "precious" and Gollum wanted to stay near his "precious", but Gollum, when tamed by the power of the Ring, is timid and cowering in its presence. This is the vulnerability of the unstable mind of *Mancinella* when confronted with what they see as their protector from the Devil. It is not until Gollum is aware of Frodo's intent, and sure of Frodo's vulnerability, that he wholeheartedly makes an attack to retrieve his "precious" on the chasm of Mount Doom.

Everyone who comes into contact with Gollum is overcome with his torment and pain. Frodo comments that upon seeing Gollum he is overcome with pity for him. Gollum is a pathetic creature tortured by his own lack of will to defend himself against his own *Mancinella* madness and mania. *Mancinella* are victims of their own obsessions, they have no will or strength to resist their temptations, or their own thoughts. When Gollum first spies the Ring he has no strength of will not to follow his own mania and kill his friend. *Mancinella* cannot let a thought or obsession go, which is why I earlier drew a parallel between Gollum and *Mancinella*, and a person suffering from dissociative identity disorder, or an obsessive compulsive disorder.

The closer that Frodo comes to the Fires of Mount Doom, the greater the mania and dissociative split grows within Gollum's mind; his fear is an overwhelming mania of not being able to survive without his "precious" to protect him. He becomes tortured by his desire to once again possess his "precious". "We wants it, we wants it, we wants it!" p.296. [Tolkien] *The Two Towers*. Morrison says of *Mancinella*, "There is an obsession with evil forces, with the devil, or with ideas of demoniac possession. Also sexual ideas may be mingled with obsessions." When Gollum on the chasm of Mount Doom manages to take the Ring from Frodo, "Gollum cried. 'My Precious! O my precious!' And with that, even as his eyes were lifted up to gloat on his prize, he stepped too far." Even as Gollum falls into the depths of Mount Doom his last words were "precious". In the film *The Lord of The Rings*, directed by Peter Jackson, the ecstatic pleasure in Gollum's face and eyes as he finally holds his desired love, and exclaims "O my precious!" reveals the sexual crossover between the "demoniac possession", "mingled with obsessions" that Morrison refers to. Gollum is in love with his "precious", and he also hated it; it was a *Mancinella* relationship of obsession and possession.

Bibliography

Bailey, Philip, M, M.D. *Homeopathic Psychology*. Berkeley, California, North Atlantic Books, 1995.

Boericke, William, M. D. *Pocket Manual of Homoeopathic Materia Medica*. New Delhi, Motilal Banarsidass, Publishers, 1996.

Grieve, Mrs. M. *A Modern Herbal*. Middlesex, England, Penguin Books, 1980.

Hahnemann, Dr. Samuel. *The Chronic Diseases*. New Delhi, B. Jain Publishers, 1995.

Kent, J. T. *Lectures on Materia Medica*. New Delhi, B. Jain Publishers, 1994.

Kent, J. T. *Repertory of the Homoeopathic Materia Medica and a Word Index*. New Delhi, B. Jain Publishers, 1994.

Morrison, Roger, M.D. *Desktop Guide*. Nevada City, CA, Hahnemann Clinic Publishing. 1993.

Sankaran, Rajan. *The Soul of Remedies*. Santa Cruz, Bombay, Homoeopathic Medical Publishers, 1997.

Schroyens, Frederik, M.D. *Synthesis*. London, Homeopathic Book Publishers, 1997.

Tolkien, J.R.R. *The Lord of the Rings*. London, HarperCollins Publishers. 1994.

(*The Lord of the Rings* is comprised of three books: *The Fellowship of the Ring, The Two Towers, The Return of the King.*)

Vermeulen, Frans. *Synoptic Materia Medica.*The Netherlands, Merlijin Publishers, 1992.

Vermeulen, Frans. *Prisma*. The Netherlands, Emryss bv Publishers, 2002.

63 "Causticum is excitable, stimulating, and restless. Causticum is also, conversely, stuck, paralyzed, and anxious. Causticums are an interesting mix of emotional sensitivity, empathic reactivity, and mental and emotional stagnation. The more over stimulated Causticums are, the more likely they are to shut down emotionally. In my practice I have used *Causticum,* the remedy, when patients' response to a deep loss or grief has been so totally overwhelming or paralyzing that they literally cannot get on with their own life, even after what would be seen as an acceptable mourning period. Causticums have such a strong mindset that they are completely obsessed. The most extreme picture of this type of person is a religious fundamentalist terrorist, while the not-so-extreme picture might be a vegetarian activist. Obviously, the manifestation of the passionate views of Causticum can be varied. Most commonly, the picture I see of Causticums in my practice are those who are so committed to a particular cause that they cannot 'loosen up' emotionally. This is the unhealthy, contracted picture of Causticum." Lalor, Liz. *A Homeopathic Guide to Partnership and Compatibility*. Berkeley, California, North Atlantic Books, 2004. p.27-28

64 I recently had an anorexia case. The woman had had extensive psychotherapy and had attended a clinic for eating disorders. She told me she felt that she would never be able to rid herself of the anorexia, nothing had ever worked: *It feels like a problem which comes over me and I can't change it, I think I will always have it. I am crippled by it.*

The initial rubrics used in the rubric-repertorisation are listed below:

• *Mind* rubric: *anorexia nervosa.*

- *Delusion* rubric: *doomed, being.*
- *Delusion* rubric: *troubles: great troubles had just come over him:* cycl. [1] 1.
- *Delusion* rubric: *paralyzed; he is.*

I asked her why she thought she was still suffering with her anorexia and bulimia. This question was aimed at finding the cause of her self-destruction. If a patient's case reveals self-destruction, there is self-punishment. If there is self-punishment there are psychological delusions of real or perceived sins which she has committed. I already know from what she has told me that she believes she is doomed to have this complaint all of her life and that she is crippled by it. *Cyclamen* have the *Delusion* rubric: *doomed* and the *Delusion* rubric: *is paralyzed.* This is the *Delusion* rubric layer pertaining to Depression. Preceding the Depression layer is the layer of Causation or sin. In this layer is her 'never-well-since-event'. I know this because inherent within the illness anorexia is self-dislike. Self-dislike is maintained to cover up and reinforce psychological 'delusions of original sin'. I add the *Delusion* rubric: *has done wrong*, even though I am not sure yet what it is she has done wrong, or even if she is going to tell me. Conclusion: the remedy is *Cyclamen.*

This is a very simple case in which following the five psychological steps allowed me to uncover the simillimum in just fifteen minutes.

This was her reply:

Liz, don't try to psychoanalyze me because it does not work and I don't like it. Everyone has tried and it hasn't worked. I don't like to talk about myself. I don't want to reveal anything more about myself to you.

- *Mind* rubric: *taciturn.*

My next question was simply phrased as an intellectual query; this bypassed her refusal to reveal anything about herself but also sensitively respected that she was feeling emotionally distraught. I asked: why didn't you like the clinic?

Because they criticized me and threatened me and told me I had to do this and that otherwise I would be in trouble.

What did you feel like when they threatened you?

Like I do with my mother.

What happened with your mother?

It is not fair. I made one mistake and I have been on a path of self-destruction ever since. [cries]

What did you do?

I got drunk when I was sixteen and she came to the hospital. I was so drunk I ended up in hospital, and she screamed at me that I was disgusting. When I got home she had thrown all my things out of the house.

Do you think you are disgusting?

Yes.

I repertorised this case using the following rubric-repertorisation:

- *Mind* rubric: *anorexia nervosa*: *Cycl.*
- *Delusion* rubric: *doomed, being*: cycl.
- *Delusion* rubric: *troubles: great troubles had just come over him*: cycl. [1] 1.
- *Delusion* rubric: *paralyzed; he is*: cycl.
- *Mind* rubric: *taciturn. Cycl.*
- *Delusion* rubric: *crime: committed a crime; he had*: cycl.
- *Delusion* rubric: *criminal, he is a*: cycl.
- *Delusion* rubric: *neglected: duty; he has neglected his*: cycl.
- *Delusion* rubric: *wrong: done wrong; he has*: cycl.
- *Mind* rubric: *reproaching, oneself*: cycl.

65 "The homeopathic remedy *Ignatia* is derived from a dilution of the seeds of the St. Ignatius bean. The seeds contain a high level of the poisons strychnine and brucine. Strychnine is also an ingredient in the homeopathic remedy *Nux vomica.* As with *Nux vomica, Ignatia* produces a characteristic excessive sensibility of the senses and a tendency to produce convulsive spasms. The levels of strychnine are far stronger in *Ignatia* and the result is a far more destructive picture than with *Nux vomica.* The destructiveness is manifested in the more extreme, unstable emotionalism of Ignatia in comparison to the emotional control of Nux vomica. The constitution Ignatia mirrors the nature of strychnine in the sense that mental, emotional, and physical sensations are cramped inside and struggle for expression. Because the emotions are more aggravated in Ignatia, pressure often builds to the point of being hysterical." Lalor, Liz. *A Homeopathic Guide to Partnership and Compatibility.* Berkeley, California, North Atlantic Books, 2004. p. 33.

66 "The homeopathic remedy *Lachesis* is derived from a dilution of the poison of the Surukuku snake of South America, commonly known as the bushmaster. As the name implies, this snake is the master of its territory and has a reputation when disturbed of chasing its victim and attacking. It is known as one of the most poisonous and vicious snakes purely because the majority of snakes will choose to run rather than fight. The dilution of bushmaster snake venom was first made by the famous homeopath Hering, whose first experiments with the remedy were made when working in the Amazon as a zoologist. The poison was so toxic that just in the process of physically preparing the homeopathic remedy it was potent enough to throw Hering into a coma-like state with delirium and fever. Because homeopathy is based on the principle of "like cures like", the personality of a Lachesis constitution has to match the personality of the

bushmaster snake. Lachesis has the ability to disarm, charm, entice, and seduce victims. Lachesis is a personality state that has the same stunning and disabling qualities of the bushmaster poison and a theme that is reflective of the hyper-vigilance of the bushmaster snake. Across all levels Lachesis do not like restriction or control. Lachesis does not relax; even when charming and enticing, Lachesis is continually aware of any sort of perceived competition or threat to autonomy or territory." Lalor, Liz. *A Homeopathic Guide to Partnership and Compatibility.* Berkeley, California, North Atlantic Books, 2004. p. 36.

67 "Silicea as a constitution presents with the same theme of the vulnerability of shattered glass, but with a seemingly converse dichotomy of being strong enough to hold up the stem of a plant. The same theme of searching for connective structure is also visible in the psyche of Silicea. Siliceas suffer from shyness and lack of self-confidence, yet they overcome these by forming strong moral codes and by holding onto strong ideas and beliefs that help them find structure and inner strength. Siliceas are conscious of their assimilation faults, and are very conscientious about trying to eradicate them. Siliceas spend a lot of time creating a perfect outer image to try to reinforce their internal shakiness. This process creates a personality that is very refined and delicate, yet very exacting. This dichotomy of strong inner convictions juxtaposed with a seemingly delicate fragile outer presentation is the theme of Silicea. Siliceas are shy and appear outwardly as if they acquiesce because they do not argue or disagree; however, internally Siliceas never acquiesce and they never change their beliefs and morals." Lalor, Liz. *A Homeopathic Guide to Partnership and Compatibility.* Berkeley, California, North Atlantic Books, 2004. p.72-73.

68 "The drive to cover up inner weakness and conflict brings about anxiety that is unique to Medorrhinums. If you do not have a point of reference, there are always unlimited horizons you can travel to. Medorrhinums can appear to others to lack self-control. If someone else tries to enforce controls or their concepts of conventions in the form of taking responsibility, Medorrhinums are likely to want to escape.

If inside of themselves, Medorrhinums know they do not have a solid grip on reality, they will push in the opposite direction to make sure all possible weaknesses are covered up. At the time Medorrhinums are feeling most unsure and vulnerable, they will often act as if nothing scares or affects them. Medorrhinums are extreme in everything. It is possible to either catch them on the flight out of themselves when they present as the extrovert or on the flight into themselves when they present as the introvert. The essence is the same; they have to always be exceeding all limits. If you do not have an orientation point or boundary that contains you, then you will always alternate between extremes." Lalor, Liz. *A Homeopathic Guide to Partnership and Compatibility.* Berkeley, California, North Atlantic Books, 2004. p.194.

69 "The homeopathic remedy *Calcarea carbonica* (shortened to *Calc-carb*)

is derived from a dilution of carbonate of calcium, prepared from the inner layer of an oyster shell. The most obvious function of the oyster shell is to provide protection for the soft oyster inside. Calc-carbs carry the same theme of needing protection of a soft, inner emotional being. The problem is Calc-carbs do not have the protection of the oyster shell; consequently, they seek outward protection in the world. Because Calc-carbs struggle with issues of security and protection in the world, they will obviously change a lot depending on how secure they feel. Calc-carbs will be a lot more fearful in a relationship with a constitution that does not take into consideration how potentially threatened they feel being in the world without a shell to protect them.

The most important thing to ask yourself, if you think you are Calc-carb, is how do you feel about being in the world by yourself? Do you think you would cope if you did not have the support of family? If you feel that financial stability, a secure home, and a supportive partnership, are absolutely crucial to your health, then it is more than likely that you are Calc-carb. The oyster is the slowest creature in the ocean. This same tentativeness and lack of surety is a theme within Calc-carb. Calc-carbs know that the partner they choose in life must be able to protect and look after them." Lalor, Liz, *A Homeopathic Guide to Partnership and Compatibility*, Berkeley, California, North Atlantic Books, 2004.p. 19.

70 Psychological 'delusions of deprivation' are illusions and delusions of poverty. Generally speaking, survivors of war, refugees or displaced persons, are noted for their desire to work exceedingly hard if they have been fortunate enough to immigrate to a stable country. Australia is a country built on its waves of refugees from China, Italy, Greece, and Vietnam, to list just a few. After the Second World War, Melbourne, where I live, became home to the largest community of Holocaust survivors per capita outside Israel. Each new group has a strong need to reestablish themselves in a new country and to make themselves feel as secure as possible by accumulating great wealth. They usually like to have large families to reinforce a sense of the survival of their family, especially if they have lost a lot of their family in wars. They also like to accumulate numerous real estate properties to give themselves a solid sense of belonging. Psychologically, they never lose their somatic memories of deprivation and loss. It is not unusual for a survivor of war to always have a refrigerator full of food and panic if they leave any uneaten food on their plate, regardless of how much food they have access to, or regardless of how much they have already eaten. It is also not unusual for a refugee in a new country to still continue to feel anxious about not having accumulated enough money, regardless of how much wealth or property they own. Within the Jewish community for example, numerous psychological studies have looked at the effects of the decimation of families and the Jewish race on the survivors themselves as well as the second and third generations of Holocaust survivors. It has been noted that psychological 'delusions of deprivation' continue in the following generations regardless of existing wealth or regeneration. It is also common for abandoned children to grow up with a burning desire to

accumulate wealth and property, and they often marry into large families. It has also been noted that each new wave of refugees, Greek, Italian, and Vietnamese refugees have followed similar patterns of accumulating wealth, property and having large extended families.

71 This *Delusion* rubric is a recent addition to *Natrum sulphuricum* from Rajan Sankaran. I accessed this *Delusion* rubric via Radar© Schroyens F., *Synthesis Treasure Edition*, Millennium view (progressive).

72 The *Delusion* rubric: *one will become insane* is a recent addition to *Natrum sulphuricum*. I accessed this *Delusion* rubric via Radar© Schroyens F., *Synthesis Treasure Edition*, Millennium view (progressive). When Frans Vermeulen discussed *Natrum sulphuricum* in *Prisma* he noted: "Nat-s. is in NONE of the delusion rubrics." In Kent's *Repertory of the Homoeopathic Materia Medica* the *Delusion* rubric: *she will become insane*, does not include *Natrum sulphuricum,* nor is the remedy listed in the primary *Delusions* rubric. I do not view this addition to *Synthesis* as contentious because I believe the *Delusion* rubrics: *one will become insane* and *she is disgraced* both reflect and confirm the self-effacing passive-aggressive behavior I have observed in *Natrum sulphuricum.* If a patient shows signs of self-destructive behavior there has to be a *Delusion* rubric attached to the constitutional remedy profile. Out of immense respect to Frans Vermeulen I have discussed *Natrum sulphuricum* and the addition of the *Delusion* rubrics with Frans.

73 Freud developed the concept of the 'id', 'ego', and 'super-ego'. The instinctual inspirations in our somatic behavior is the 'id'. The organized realistic part of the psyche is the 'ego'. The perfectionist critical function of all our moralistic and inspirational ideals and spiritual goals and conscience is the 'super-ego'. The reference and use of the word 'ego' in the *Rubric-categories* refers the destruction of the 'ego' from the conflict between the psyche and the external world. The psyche is the personification of the soul, spirit, and mind. If a remedy profile has a weakened 'ego' then their psyche is under treat. Freud outlined that psychoses are a conflict between the 'ego' and the external world. A psychosis is a severe mental derangement. The *Delusion* rubrics which cover psychoses are the *Delusion* rubrics: forsaken, depression and resignation. All these *Delusion* rubrics emphasize the threat that the world poses to the self or 'ego'. All these *Delusion* rubrics contain the 'delusions of abandonment', 'delusions of persecution', 'delusions of impending doom' and the 'delusions of hypochondria', in that order.

74 For *Gelsemium* the *Delusion* rubric: *enlarged*, confirms their exaggerated tendency to anxiety and fears and forebodings. That is not the case for all the other remedies listed in the *Delusion* rubric: *enlarged*. For example, *Aranea*, a homoeopathic remedy derived from a Cross spider, use the delusion of being *enlarged* to increase the sense of their size and therefore their sense of power. Increased size in turn increases their social standing and their disregard for social conventionality. *Platina* use the *Delusion* rubric: *enlarged*, to vilify their righteous belief in their own

grandeur. In *Hyoscyamus* the *Delusion* rubric: *enlarged*, is reflective of their imaginations of desirability. Each remedy can be listed in a rubric but each constitutional remedy will psychologically process the same rubric in different ways depending on the delusional need within their psyche.

- *Delusion* rubric: *enlarged*: acon. alum. apis. *Aran.* arg-met. *Arg-n. Bapt.* bell. berb. *Bov.* caj. **CANN-I.** coc-c. con. euph. ferr. *Gels.* glon. hydrog. *Hyos.* irid-met. kali-ar. kali-bi. kali-br. kola. lach. laur. limest-b. loxo-recl. mang. nat-c. nux-m. nux-v. *Op.* ox-ac. *Par.* phos. pic-ac. pip-m. *Plat.* puls. rhus-t. sabad. spig. stram. zinc.

75 *Tarentula hispanica* are noted for their plotting and cunning revenge. The motivation behind that revenge is the causation or 'never-well-since-event' relevant to the case analysis. The core causation of *Tarentula hispanica* is unrequited love. *Tarentula hispanica* is the only remedy listed in the *Mind* rubric: *insanity from disappointed love*. The character of Iago in the William Shakespeare play *Othello*, a tale of love, jealousy and vengeful hate, is a wonderful portrayal of that *insanity from unrequited love*. When Othello, The Moor, overlooks Iago for the role of Lieutenant, instead giving the position to Cassio, the enraged Iago sets out on a calculated course of murderous revenge. Fueled by "hate" at his perceived insult, "I know my price", Iago sets out to right his insult by destroying the Moor and his love, Desdemona. Iago, through cunning and opportunistic means, convinces Othello that his sweet wife Desdemona is deceiving him with Cassio, hence entrapping Cassio and causing the deepest of injury to Othello who is passionately in love with Desdemona. Desdemona's own father provides the fuel and the wick for his plan when he venomously warns "look to her, Moor, if thou hast eyes to see: she has deceived her father, and may thee". Iago plants the seeds of Desdemona's unfaithfulness, and "poisons" the Moor's passionate sulfuric nature so that he "burn like the mines of sulphur" with sexual jealousy. The nature of the Moor "is of a free and open nature", but his "black" blood is of the most sulfuric inflammable kind, and once poisoned by "jealousy...the green-eyed monster", he is blinded with his need to "loathe her". Tragically, Othello kills Desdemona before he finds out that he was beguiled by the cunning Iago. *Tarentula hispanica* have the slow and calculative resolve of Iago to cunningly and methodically carry out revenge and destruction because of their perceived insult and hurt at being overlooked for a promotion. The revenge of Iago is impressive in its unrelenting resolve to cause pain to Othello; he sets his plan of action and he never falters in his attack.

Iago Act I, Scene I

I know my price, I am worth no worse a place: But he; as loving his own pride and purposes, Evades them, with a bombast circumstance

- *Delusion* rubric: *insulted, he is*: tarent.

Iago Act I, Scene iii

I hate the Moor.

- *Mind* rubric: *cynical:* tarent.
- *Mind* rubric: *hatred: revengeful; hatred and*: tarent.

Tarantula (Lycosa tarantula) does not spin its web as a snare but as a subterfuge to hide behind as it waits for prey to walk past its burrow. The Tarantula is renowned for its wolf-like hunting ability to suddenly pounce undetected on its prey from behind the hidden entrance of its burrow. It digs a deep burrow and covers the entrance with a layer of silk web. The first symptom reported after being bitten is a state of depression and lethargy which the sufferer will usually only come out of if they are roused by music and dance. Through a series of the most cunning methods of deception, Iago plots his plan of action. Iago waits at the entrance of his burrow, waiting patiently to strike when his victims present themselves.

Iago

The Moor is of a free and open nature,
That thinks men honest that but seem to be so,
And will as tenderly be led by the nose

Iago Act II, Scene I

[Aside] *He takes her by the palm: ay, well said,*
whisper: with as little a web as this will I
ensnare as great a fly as Cassio.

The Moor already changes with my poison:
Dangerous conceits are, in their natures, poisons
Which at the first are scarce found to distaste,
But with a little act upon the blood.

Iago cleverly manipulates each member of the play as an animal would its prey. The language he uses reflects the remedy sitting in the animal kingdom. The themes of entrapment "led by the nose", "ensnare", "fools are caught", and "changes with my poison", are themes of attack, and aggressor; 'him versus me'. Iago's presiding stimulus of being overlooked, "I know my price, I am worth no worse a place", contains the main theme of the animal kingdom. Animals need to maintain hierarchy and supremacy within the group in order to survive.

Spider Themes:

- Cunning, plotting, revengeful
- Manipulation
- Persecution
- Jealousy
- Hate
- Hysteria, complaining
- Identity – asocial individuals, <u>feel on outer</u>
- Activity, restlessness and a need to hurry

- Short sexual life

Iago Act IV, Scene I

My medicine, work! Thus credulous fools are caught.

- *Mind* rubric: *cunning*: tarent.
- *Mind* rubric: *deceitful*: *Tarent.*
- *Mind* rubric: *delirium, raging* : tarent.
- *Mind* rubric: *exhilaration*: **TARENT**.
- *Mind* rubric: *industrious, mania for work*: **TARENT**.
- *Mind* rubric: *laughing*: *Tarent.*
- *Mind* rubric: *malicious*: tarent.
- *Mind* rubric: *mischievous*: *Tarent.*

Iago Act III, Scene iii.

O, beware, my lord, of jealousy;
It is the green-eyed monster which doth mock
The meat it feeds on; that cuckold lives in bliss

Iago presents the concept of jealousy to Othello, adding fuel to the fires of sulphur, even before Othello has conceived of the emotion within his own heart. Vermeulen quotes Tyler in *Prisma*: "Sudden violent, or sly destructive movements are absolutely characteristic, and unique to the drug". "Threatening, destructive, unexpected behavior, but cunning". [Vermeulen]

Iago has no time for his wife Emilia. He constantly attacks and belittles her, except for when she has a part to play in his plot by stealing Desdemona's scarf so Iago can use it to incriminate Cassio. In my experience of *Tarentula hispanica* patients, this is a true reflection of their relationship patterning. They want a relationship but it must be at arm's length, so they can stay alone. Love and relationships appear to irritate and annoy, and interfere with their routine. ("Annoying, intruding, interfering". [Vermeulen]) I was not surprised when I read the courting habits of Tarantula in Vermeulen's *Prisma*. The fact that the male needs to leave immediately after mating, and that the courtship is potentially life threatening for him, reflects the relationship history of my *Tarentula hispanica* patients. *Tarentula hispanica* will attack in response to all sexual or emotional advances; it is part of their emotional foreplay. In the case below, the patient could only be released from her depression by first attacking me, her counselor; then she would go into an almost hysterical explosion of emotion that would end in exhilaration and release from the depression. The key aspect of *Tarentula hispanica* is that they do not like to be unnoticed in love.

Iago cunningly feeds Othello the concept of jealousy and slowly manipulates the Moor's insecurities to his own personal advantage. No one more than Iago, the *Tarentula hispanica,* has the Achilles heel of feeling overlooked. It is always interesting to sit back in a consultation when a patient is 'venting their spleen', and just make a note of all 'key words'. It is a gross generalization of 'New-Age psycho-babble' to assume that everything hated in someone else is a reflection of the patient themselves. However, there is an interesting element of truth in that assumption in a homeopathic consultation. Rajan Sankaran reported in a conference I attended that he had made a similar observation of wives complaining about their mother-in-laws in India. Often, he commented that what they accused the mother-in-laws of was a reflection of a 'key word' within the case. Iago knows how to fuel the fire of jealousy in the burning, sulfuric Othello because he identifies with the jealousy he has towards Cassio for receiving what was his due. Iago's hate is only matched by the intensity of the love he had for Othello. Iago's jealousy of Desdemona does not come from his own love of Desdemona or jealousy of the "black" Moor with a fair Desdemona, as has been suggested by literature critics, but from his own spurned, unreciprocated love of Othello.

- *Mind* rubric: *insanity: love; from disappointed*: tarent.

- *Mind* rubric: *hatred: revengeful; hatred and*: tarent.

Rajan Sankaran in *The Soul of Remedies* says: "characteristic of *Tarentula* is the feeling of unreciprocated love or affection. The person has the feeling they are not attractive enough and therefore does not get the attention he craves for. So in *Tarantula* you have many features that have to do with attractiveness. Also mischievousness, cunning, hysterical behavior, lasciviousness, shamelessness, exposing himself and even threatening – all with the intention to attract attention." *Tarentula hispanica* want *all* the love and attention within *all* relationships. Iago hated Desdemona because it was she who took his master Othello away from noticing *him*. Iago also hated Cassio because it was he who took his master Othello away from noticing *him*. This is why *Tarentula hispanica* is the only remedy listed in the *Mind* rubric: insanity from disappointed love – this is the causation of *Tarentula hispanica* – and it is something that is often missed when we just concentrate on the nature of that revenge. Iago loved Othello before he hated him. The 'never-well-since-event' of *Tarentula hispanica* is unrequited love.

Sankaran, Rajan, *The Soul of Remedies*. Santa Cruz, Bombay, Homoeopathic Medical Publishers, 1997. p. 199.

Schroyens, Frederik, M.D. *Synthesis*, London, Homeopathic Book Publishers, 1997.

Shakespeare, William. *Shakespeare The Complete Works*, Volume IV, England, Heron Books, 1995.p.p. 82-162.

Vermeulen, Frans, *Prisma*. The Netherlands, Emryss bv Publishers, 2002. p.p.1337-1348.

76 This *Tarentula hispanica* patient came to me predominantly for counselling. I did not tell her until the second consultation that the remedy given was *Tarentula hispanica*. She suffers from a horrendous fear of spiders, Tarantulas in particular.

Presenting issue: She had suffered from depression her whole life. She had previously tried several counselors but they had not worked out; *they did not understand her, or the nature of her depression.* She had always stopped going. She was extremely *lonely,* and she desperately wanted a relationship. She had only experienced a relationship once, and that was short-lived. *I have been depressed ever since he left me.* She couldn't take any form of anti-depressants as they made her *anxious* and *restless,* more depressed than she is already, and *paranoid.* Both of her parents suffer from depression. Her father is Bi-polar, but her mother also suffers from clinical depression. She feels *that the world and everyone has been unfair to her. There must be something wrong with me as I have never had anyone want to be in a relationship with me; this is what depresses me and what can you do about that?* The last statement was said forcefully as a provocation.

Key words noted:

- Lonely
- Anxious
- Restless
- Paranoid
- Unwanted / rejected

Notes from the first Consultation:

Question: I asked – what do you mean by paranoid?

I am different from other people, they are not honest. They do not like me at work; my new boss does not like me. For example, other people at work use their work mobile for private use; I do not do that. I notice people in the morning getting on the tram they don't buy a ticket. I would never do that. I like to be left alone at work; that way I get things done. I am much more efficient that way. I do not want to be noticed. The new boss does not like me and wants to get rid of my position. No one notices me when I go to work parties; no one comes and talks to me, no one wants to have a relationship with me.

Question: You have had one relationship? What happened in that relationship?

He didn't want me after a short amount of time. I would not have a relationship with me; I would not have a relationship with someone who was fat. After twenty years of no one having a relationship with me there must be something wrong with me. I do not like therapy, you are not very nice, it is not easy talking about things that upset me; you are very cruel. It is hard to come here and cry like this. I do not belong; I am not the same as everyone else; no one wants me, I am alone and no one is ever going to want to have a relationship with me. My first and only relationship has left me with the viral infection of genital herpes. I feel this will always make me sick and that no-one will ever want to have a relationship with me ever again. I belong to a herpes support group. I will not have a relationship with anyone for fear of passing it on to someone else. I am crippled by this infection. I do not think I should have a relationship with anyone ever again, I am infectious.

[The patient is now crying.]

Question: Do you have a memory of not belonging like this before?

When I was five my mother took me to the library. She wanted to leave. I said I didn't want to go – I had just started to read. She did not talk to me for one week. I didn't know what I had done wrong.

[The patient is still crying.]

Question: One week! How did this make you feel? Did she often do that?

All the time she would often not speak to me for up to five days. [This is the 'never-well-since' causation.]

I didn't know what I had done wrong but I knew that she didn't love me.

- *Mind* rubric: *insanity: love; from disappointed:* tarent. [1] 1.

She was very somber, dressed in black, very emotionally intense. She had a very 'heavy feeling'. She was provocatively challenging me to reject her. She whole heartedly accepted her depression and felt intensely alone and she thought she will always be like this. In the consultation she remembers several events in her life which prove she is not liked, and will never be liked. One of the strongest memories is of a nativity play at kindergarten when she was not chosen and was rejected by the teacher. Other memories are of having to wear a skirt and top that was knitted with wool by her mother to school, and having to face rejection and ridicule. I asked why she wears black as I was certain the remedy picture was a spider. She doesn't like being exposed or noticed, and if she is in black then she won't draw attention to herself. *Tarentula hispanica* is listed under the rubric: colors: *aversion black.* In this case the black color of her clothing enhanced her ability, given her large size, to be able to hide. This is an example of the need to always ask the reason behind something that strikes you as unusual.

Key words extended:

- Persecuted
- Attacked
- Alone
- Noticed
- Efficient
- Sexual life-short.

Physicals: No appetite! *I do not eat anything.* This shocked me considering her size. It was immediately obvious that I was shocked. She explains she only like to eat one particular brand of potato chips. I asked what she likes about potato chips.

She replied, *I feel very relaxed and calm when I hear the* <u>*crunch in my mouth*</u>.

Menstrual periodicity: Head aches / menstrual pain / severe depression post ovulation until her menses.

Severe daily hang-over: She also drinks an excessive amount of alcohol every night, which would explain the weight issue. I asked her about why she thinks she drinks so much. She doesn't want to stop the drinking, she needs it to deal with the pain and hurt from work; when people upset her. She told *I think a lot about what to do the next day and how I am going to get them back, so they notice me.*

Muscular pains: knees / neck / back.

Daily headaches.

Weekly migraines.

Constipation.

Remedy: 1st consult: *Tarantula hispanica* 30 1/day x 1 month.

2nd consult 1 month later increased to 200 potency x 1 dose only

3rd consult 1 month later increased to 1m. potency x 1 dose only.

She has since stayed on a dose of 30 1/day. Treatment so far has lasted six years.

She is now far less depressed. She no longer cries with the same disturbing sadness. Her crying is shorter-lasting, cathartic hysterical releases from her depression. People who have been bitten by a Tarantula spider report going into a maniacal spasm of hysterical weeping. She is still coming for consultations with me, which is the longest time she has ever trusted anyone. She is not as depressed with rejection at work, imagined or real. Her constipation is gone. Migraines are less frequent now monthly, as opposed to 3 a week. She is drinking less, but can still go through periods of drinking daily; *Tarentula hispanica* love the effects of alcohol. She still has headaches, especially after drinking a lot on a weekend. The reason for coming to see me: ill effects from unreciprocated love, is still the dominant cause of her depression, but it is not the overwhelming cause of daily depression that it used to be. She has just started a new work position, which is also a big move because *Tarentula hispanica* in my experience do not come out of their burrows; i.e. what they know to be safe, whether it be a physical work place or an emotional state of depression. Six years into treatment and she recently wore a light pink top under her black jacket. She has recently decided to lose weight to make *herself more attractive so she can wear brighter clothes*. She is now able to stop drinking for three month periods. This case continues.

77 This *Delusion* rubric can be allocated into Denial or Resignation. In Denial the remedy profile would use the perception that they are light to avoid 'heavy' or probing feelings. In Resignation the remedy profile would use this perception to reinforce physical weakness.

78 This *Delusion* rubric can be allocated into Depression or Resignation. In Depression it pertains to mental and emotional feelings of emptiness. In Resignation it pertains to the feeling that one's body (health) has deserted one.

79 This *Delusion* rubric can be allocated into Denial or Resignation. In Denial the remedy profile would use the perception that their body is light so they can escape. In Resignation the remedy profile would use this perception to reinforce physical weakness.

80 Psychosis refers to an abnormal or incorrect perceptions of the mind. Psychosis involves the patient 'losing contact with reality'. Patients experiencing psychosis may report hallucinations, religious visions, or delusional beliefs, and hear or see visions. Many people experience visions and they do not have abnormal behavior or perverted perceptions of reality. Psychosis is an incorrect judgement of reality which manifests and causes abnormal behavior.

81 "The **glass delusion** was an external manifestation of a psychiatric disorder recorded in Europe in the late middle ages (15th to 17th centuries). People feared that they were made of glass "and therefore likely to shatter into pieces". One famous early sufferer was King Charles VI of France who refused to allow people to touch him, and wore reinforced clothing to protect himself from accidental 'shattering'." http://en.wikipedia.org/wiki/Glass_delusion

82 *Conversations with God* is a sequence of nine books written by Neale Donald Walsch, written as a dialogue in which Walsch asks questions and God (speaking through Walsch) answers.